AF380667

Management of Bladder Cancer

Badrinath R. Konety • Sam S. Chang

Editors

Management of Bladder Cancer

A Comprehensive Text With Clinical Scenarios

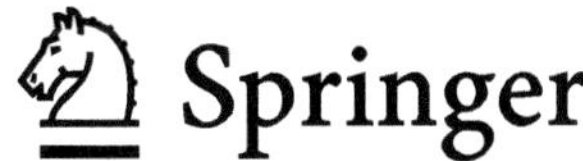

Springer

Editors
Badrinath R. Konety
Department of Urology
University of Minnesota
Minneapolis, MN, USA

Sam S. Chang
Department of Urologic Surgery
Vanderbilt University Medical Center
Nashville, TN, USA

ISBN 978-1-4939-1880-5   ISBN 978-1-4939-1881-2 (eBook)
DOI 10.1007/978-1-4939-1881-2
Springer New York Heidelberg Dordrecht London

Library of Congress Control Number: 2014954231

Springer is part of Springer Science+Business Media (www.springer.com)

For my parents, my wife, and my children none of whom I can ever thank enough.

Badrinath R. Konety

For my parents and family who provide unbelievable understanding, never-ending support, and most importantly, undying love.

Sam S. Chang

Preface

The clinical scope of bladder cancer is well known. As the second most frequent genitourinary malignancy, it is the most expensive cancer to care for from diagnosis to death. Significant improvements in diagnosis and management of this disease provide hope but need to permeate the clinical practice. This textbook provides a single, comprehensive reference source that incorporates all the latest information regarding bladder cancer and will serve as an easy and complete guide for researchers, clinicians, individuals in training, allied health professionals, and medical students. It includes a thorough discussion of all aspects and of all types of bladder cancer. The text covers topics ranging from epidemiology, natural history, diagnosis, risk-stratified management to the latest findings regarding genetics and molecular biology of bladder cancer. Diagnostic and staging evaluation of both non-muscle invasive and invasive bladder cancer are discussed. Guideline-based approaches are analyzed and summarized. Controversies in management of high-grade minimally invasive bladder cancer as well as muscle invasive disease are identified and explained. The application of chemotherapy and multimodality therapy for muscle invasive and advanced disease is outlined and highlighted. Finally gaps in current knowledge and areas for future research are discussed.

The unique feature of this book is the incorporation of clinical scenario-based examples which are discussed by experts in the field who outline their management approach. This would be particularly helpful to practicing physician seeking help in managing controversial aspects of bladder cancer which are fairly commonplace. Several key educational concepts have been incorporated in the framework of patient situations and these chapters are interspersed amidst chapters that provide more complete discussion of subject areas. It is our sincere hope that this book will become a "go to" reference source for all individuals with an interest in the management of bladder cancer.

Minneapolis, MN, USA
Nashville, TN, USA
Badrinath R. Konety
Sam S. Chang

Acknowledgments

We would like to thank Amy Nelson and Mariah Gumpert for their administrative and editorial assistance in putting this book together.

Contents

Contributors

Zeeshan Ahmad, M.D. Division of Hematology, Oncology and Transplantation, Department of Medicine, University of Minnesota, Minneapolis, MN, USA

Department of Internal Medicine, Unity Hospital, Fridley, MN, USA

Division of Hematology, Oncology and Transplantation, Department of Medicine, University of Minnesota, Minneapolis, MN, USA

Jennifer J. Ahn, M.D. Department of Urology, New York-Presbyterian Hospital, Columbia University, New York, NY, USA

Department of Urology, Columbia University Medical Center, Herbert Irving Pavilion, New York, NY, USA

Christopher B. Anderson, M.D. Department of Surgery, Urology Service, Memorial Sloan Kettering Cancer Center, New York, NY, USA

Richard M. Bambury, M.B., M.R.C.P.I. Department of Genitourinary Medical Oncology, Sidney Kimmel Center for Prostate and Urologic Cancers, Memorial Sloan Kettering Cancer Center/Weill Cornell Medical College, New York, NY, USA

Daniel A. Barocas, M.D., M.P.H. Department of Urologic Surgery, Center for Surgical Quality and Outcomes Research, Vanderbilt University Medical Center, Nashville, TN, USA

Jeffrey C. Bassett, M.D., M.P.H. Department of Urology, Kaiser Permanente Southern California, , Anaheim, CA, USA

Stephen W. Bickler, M.D., D.T.M. &. H., F.A.C.S. Rady Children's Hospital, University of California San Diego, San Diego, CA, USA

Bernard H. Bochner, M.D., F.A.C.S. Department of Urology, Memorial Sloan-Kettering Cancer Center, Kimmel Center for Prostate and Urologic Tumors, New York, NY, USA

Stephen A. Boorjian, M.D. Mayo Clinic, Rochester, MN, USA

Maurizio Brausi Department of Urology Ausl Modena, B. Ramazzini Hospital, Carpi-Modena, Italy

Amanda N. Calhoun, M.S. Department of Urology, Ohio State University Wexner Medical Center, Columbus, OH, USA

Daniel J. Canter, M.D. Urologic Institute of Southeastern Pennsylvania, Einstein Healthcare Network, Philadelpia, PA, USA

Jorge Raul Caso, M.D., M.P.H. Department of Urology, University of Miami, Bar Harbour, FL, USA

Erik P. Castle, M.D., F.A.C.S. Department of Urology, Mayo Clinic Arizona, Phoenix, AZ, USA

Albert J. Chang, M.D., Ph.D. Department of Radiation Oncology, Helen Diller Family Comprehensive Cancer Center, University of California, San Francisco, CA, USA

Peter E. Clark, M.D. Vanderbilt University Medical Center, Nashville, TN, USA

Michael S. Cookson, M.D., M.M.H.C. University of Oklahoma Medical Center, Oklahoma City, TN, USA

Colin P. Dinney, M.D. Department of Urology, MD Anderson Cancer Center, The University of Texas, Houston, TX, USA

Jose L. Dominguez-Escrig, L.M.S., M.D., F.R.C.S. (Urol) Servicio de Urología, Fundacion Instituto Valenciano de Oncologia, C. Profesor Beltrán Báguena, Valencia, Spain

Tracy M. Downs, M.D. Department of Urology, University of Wisconsin School of Medicine and Public Health, Madison, WI, USA

Nilay M. Gandhi, M.D. James Buchanan Brady Urological Institute, Johns Hopkins Medical Institutions, Baltimore, MD, USA

Maurice Marcel Garcia, M.D., M.A.S. Department of Urology, (Moffit-Long, Mount Zion), San Francisco General Hospital and The San Francisco Veteran's Adminstration Hospital, University of California San Francisco, San Francisco, CA, USA

Joseph A. Gillespie, M.D. Department of Urology, University of Iowa, Iowa City, IA, USA

Alvin C. Goh, M.D. Department of Urology, Houston Methodist Hospital, Houston, TX, USA

Christopher S. Gomez, M.D. Department of Urology, University of Miami Miller School of Medicine, Miami, FL, USA

Mark L. Gonzalgo, M.D., Ph.D. Department of Urology, University of Miami Miller School of Medicine, Miami, FL, USA

John L. Gore, M.D., M.S., F.A.C.S Department of Urology, University of Washington, Seattle, WA, USA

Fred Hutchinson Cancer Research Center, Seattle, WA, USA

Joshua G. Griffin, M.D. Department of Urology, University of Kansas Medical Center, Kansas City, KS, USA

Donna E. Hansel, M.D., M.S.H.S. Department of Pathology, University of California at San Diego, La Jolla, CA, USA

Farnaz Hasteh, M.D. Department of Pathology, University of California at San Diego, La Jolla, CA, USA

Richard E. Hautmann, M.D., M.D. hon. University of Ulm, Neu-Ulm, Germany

Jeffrey M. Holzbeierlein, M.D. University of Kansas Hospital, Kansas City, KS, USA

Gautam Jha, M.B.B.S., M.S. Division of Hematology, Oncology and Transplantation, Department of Medicine, University of Minnesota, Minneapolis, MN, USA

Merce Jorda, M.D., Ph.D., M.B.A. Department of Pathology, University of Miami Miller School of Medicine, Miami, FL, USA

Samuel D. Kaffenberger, M.D. Department of Urologic Surgery, Vanderbilt University, Medical Center North, Nashville, TN, USA

Thomas E. Keane, M.B., Ch.B., F.R.C.S.I., F.A.C.S. Department of Urology, Medical University of South Carolina, Charleston, SC, USA

Adam S. Kibel, M.D. Division of Urology, Department of Surgery, Brigham and Women's Hospital, Harvard Medical School, Boston, MA, USA

Timothy Kim, M.D. Department of Genitourinary Oncology, Moffitt Cancer Center, Tampa, FL, USA

Luis A. Kluth, M.D. Department of Urology, New York Presbyterian Hospital, Weill Cornell Medical College, New York, Germany

Department of Urology, University Medical-Center Hamburg-Eppendorf, Hamburg, Germany

Ramdev Konijeti, M.D. Division of Urology, Department of Surgery, Brigham and Women's Hospital, Harvard Medical School, Boston, MA, USA

Laura-Maria Krabbe, M.D. Department of Urology, University of Texas Southwestern Medical Center, Dallas, TX, USA

Department of Urology, University of Muenster Medical Center, Muenster, NRW, Germany

Donald L. Lamm, M.D. BCG Oncology, University of Arizona, Phoenix, AZ, USA

Cheryl T. Lee, M.D. Department of Urology, University of Michigan, Ann Arbor, MI, USA

Daniel J. Lee, M.D. James Buchanan Brady Department of Urology, Weill Cornell Medical College, New York Presbyterian Hospital, New York, NY, USA

J. Joy Lee, M.D. Department of Urology, Stanford University School of Medicine, Stanford, CA, USA

Seth P. Lerner, M.D. Scott Department of Urology, Beth and Dave Swalm chair in Urologic Oncology, Multidisciplinary Bladder Cancer Program, Baylor College of Medicine, Houston, TX, USA

Yair Lotan, M.D. Department of Urology, University of Texas Southwestern Medical Center, Dallas, TX, USA

Amber Mackey, D.O. Department of Pathology, University of California at San Diego, La Jolla, CA, USA

Sean McAdams, M.D. Department of Urology, University of Minnesota, Minneapolis, MN, USA

James M. McKiernan, M.D. Department of Urology, Columbia University Medical Center, Herbert Irving Pavilion, New York, NY, USA

Edward Messing, M.D. Department of Urology, University of Rochester Medical Center, Rochester, NY, USA

Todd M. Morgan, M.D. Department of Urology, University of Michigan, Ann Arbor, MI, USA

Eduardo Solsona Narbón Servicio de Urología, Fundacion Instituto Valenciano de Oncologia, C. Profesor Beltrán Báguena, Valencia, Spain

Michael A. O'Donnell, M.D. Department of Urology, University of Iowa, Iowa City, IA, USA

Dipen J. Parekh, M.D. Department of Urology, University of Miami Miller School of Medicine, Miami, FL, USA

Manish I. Patel, M.B.B.S., Ph.D., F.R.A.C.S. Westmead Hospital, University of Sydney, Westmead, NSW, Australia

David F. Penson, M.D., M.P.H. Department of Urologic Surgery, Center for Surgical Quality and Outcomes Research, Vanderbilt University Medical Center, Nashville, TN, USA

Kamal S. Pohar, M.D., F.R.C.S.C. Department of Urology, Ohio State University Wexner Medical Center, Columbus, OH, USA

Sima P. Porten, M.D., M.P.H. Department of Urology, MD Anderson Cancer Center, The University of Texas, Houston, TX, USA

Raj S. Pruthi, M.D. Department of Urology, Chapel Hill, NC, USA
UNC School of Medicine at Chapel Hill, Chapel Hill, NC, USA

Adam C. Reese, M.D. Assistant Professor, Department of Urology, Temple University School of Medicine, Philadelphia, PA, USA

Michael C. Risk, M.D., Ph.D. Department of Urology, University of Minnesota, Minneapolis, MN, USA
Department of Urology, Minneapolis VA Medical Center, Minneapolis, MN, USA

Chad R. Ritch, M.D., M.B.A. University of Miami, Miller School of Medicine, Miami, FL, USA

Mack Roach III, M.D. Department of Radiation Oncology, Helen Diller Family Comprehensive Cancer Center, University of California, San Francisco, CA, USA

Claus Rödel, M.D. Department of Radiotherapy and Oncology, University Hospital, Goethe University, Frankfurt am Main, Germany

Claudia P. Rojas, M.D. Department of Pathology, University of Miami Miller School of Medicine, Miami, FL, USA

Jonathan E. Rosenberg, M.D. Department of Genitourinary Medical Oncology, Sidney Kimmel Center for Prostate and Urologic Cancers, Memorial Sloan Kettering Cancer Center/Weill Cornell Medical College, New York, NY, USA

James S. Rosoff, M.D. Department of Urology, Yale School of Medicine, New Haven, CT, USA

Douglas S. Scherr, M.D. James Buchanan Brady Department of Urology, Weill Cornell Medical College, New York Presbyterian Hospita, New York, NY, USA

Florine W.M. Schlatmann, M.D. Department of Urology, Radboud University Nijmegen Medical Center, Nijmegen, The Netherlands

Mark Schoenberg, M.D. The Department of Urology, Albert Einstein College of Medicine and The Montefiore Medical Center, Bronx, NY, USA

Anne K. Schuckman, M.D. USC Institute of Urology, Keck Medical Center of the University of Southern California, Los Angeles, CA, USA

Emil Scosyrev, Ph.D. Department of Urology, University of Rochester Medical Center, Rochester, NY, USA

John D. Seigne, M.B. Division of Urology, Dartmouth-Hitchcock Medical Center, Lebanon, NH, USA

Wade J. Sexton, M.D. Department of Genitourinary Oncology, Moffitt Cancer Center, Tampa, FL, USA

Shahrokh F. Shariat, M.D. Department of Urology, New York Presbyterian Hospital, Weill Medical College of Cornell University, New York, NY, USA

Division of Medical Oncology, New York Presbyterian Hospital, Weill Cornell Medical College, New York, NY, USA

Professor of Urology, Department of Urology, Medical University of Vienna, New York, NY, USA

Robert B. Sims, M.D. Department of Genitourinary Medical Oncology, Sidney Kimmel Center for Prostate and Urologic Cancers, Memorial Sloan Kettering Cancer Center/Weill Cornell Medical College, New York, NY, USA

Eila C. Skinner, M.D. Department of Urology, Thomas A. Stamey Research Chair of Urology, Stanford, CA, USA0

Norm D. Smith, M.D. Surgery/Urology, University of Chicago, Chicago, IL, USA

Mark S. Soloway, M.D. Department of Urology, University of Miami Miller School of Medicine, Miami, FL, USA

Guru Sonpavde, M.D. Department of Hematology/Oncology, University of Birmingham Alabama, Birmingham, AL, USA

Division of Hematology and Oncology, University of Alabama, Birmingham, AL, USA

Gary D. Steinberg, M.D., F.A.C.S. Section of Urology, Department of Surgery, The University of Chicago Medicine, Chicago, IL, USA

Robert S. Svatek, M.D., M.S.C.I. Department of Urology, University of Texas Health Science Center San Antonio, San Antonio, TX, USA

Paul D. Sved, M.B.B.S., M.S., F.R.A.C.S. Royal Prince Alfred Hospital, University of Sydney, Newtown, NSW, Australia

Christian Thomas Department of Urology, University Medical Center, Johannes Gutenberg University Mainz, Mainz, Germany

Joachim W. Thüroff, M.D. Department of Urology, University Medical Center, Johannes Gutenberg University Mainz, Mainz, Germany

Christopher J. Weight, M.D., M.S. Department of Urology, University of Minnesota, Minneapolis, MN, USA

Christian Weiss, M.D. Department of Radiotherapy and Oncology, University Hospital, Goethe University, Frankfurt, Germany

J. Alfred Witjes, M.D., Ph.D. Department of Urology, Radboud University Nijmegen Medical Center, Nijmegen, The Netherlands

Michael Woods, M.D. Department of Urology, The University of North Carolina Chapel Hill, Chapel Hill, NC, USA

Joseph Zabell, M.D. Department of Urology, University of Minnesota, Minneapolis, MN, USA

Part I

General Concepts

Edward Messing and Emil Scosyrev

1.1 Bladder Cancer Incidence and Mortality

The incidence of bladder cancer in different populations worldwide varies considerably according to geographic region, demographic characteristics such as age, sex, and race, smoking history, history of certain environmental exposures, and likely poorly understood genetic susceptibilities. Some of these factors also influence disease-specific mortality in patients diagnosed with bladder cancer. The roles of these factors are reviewed in the following sections.

1.1.1 Geographic Distribution

According to estimates available from the most recent World Health Organization's GLOBOCAN project, in the year 2008, when all regions of the World were considered together, bladder cancer was the 7th most frequently diagnosed malignancy in men, with approximately 297,000 new cases and 112,000 deaths, while in women it was the 18th most commonly diagnosed malignancy, with approximately 89,000 new cases and 37,000 deaths [1, 2]. The incidence of bladder cancer shows considerable regional variation, which can likely be attributed to regional differences in exposures, although differences in reporting may also play a role. In general, the incidence tends to be higher in the developed countries compared with less developed regions (Fig. 1.1). One explanation for variation in incidence in countries with similar demographics and exposures is a reporting issue where some countries do not record stage Ta low-grade (LG) papillary urothelial cancers and urologic tumors of low malignant potential (LMP) and others do. In the US, according to the most recent estimates available for the year 2013, bladder cancer will be diagnosed in approximately 54,600 men and 18,000 women and will be reported as the cause of death in 10,800 men and 4,400 women [3]. The US incidence counts do include LG and LMP stage Ta tumors as urothelial cancers. The average lifetime risk of bladder cancer in the US is currently estimated at 3.8 % for men and 1.2 % for women [3]. It is also estimated that more than 500,000 people in the US are now living with histories of bladder cancer diagnosis [4]. Many of these patients experience frequent recurrences of non-muscle-invasive cancers and require continuous cystoscopic surveillance and therapy.

E. Messing, M.D. • E. Scosyrev, Ph.D. (✉)
Department of Urology, University of Rochester
Medical Center, 01 Elmwood Ave, Box 656,
Rochester, NY 14642, USA
e-mail: Edward.messing@urmc.rochester.edu;
emelian_scosyrev@urmc.rochester.edu

B.R. Konety and S.S. Chang (eds.), *Management of Bladder Cancer:*
A Comprehensive Text With Clinical Scenarios, DOI 10.1007/978-1-4939-1881-2_1,
© Springer Science+Business Media New York 2015

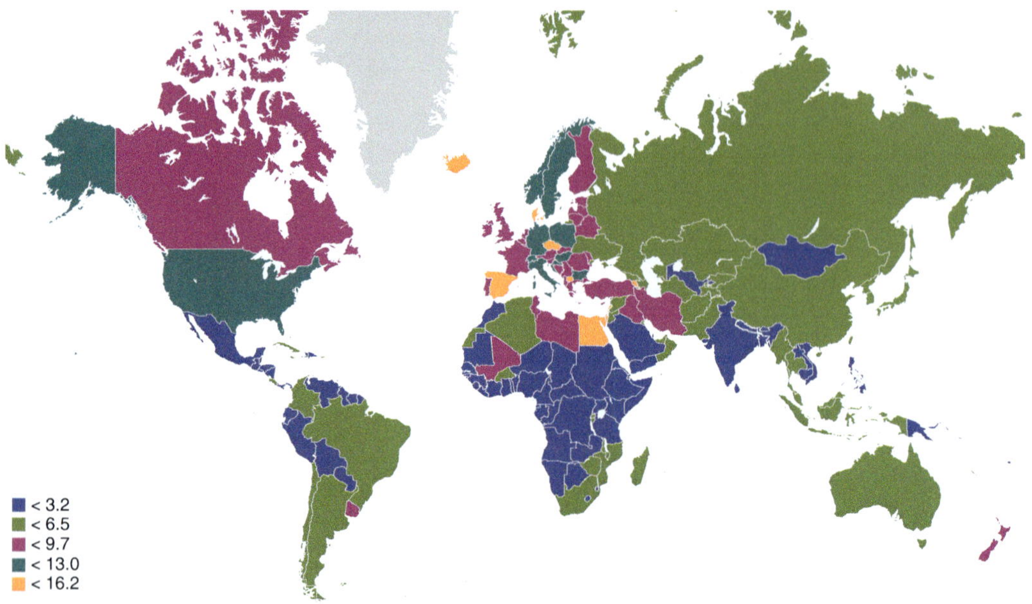

Fig. 1.1 Age-standardized annual incidence rates for bladder cancer (per 100,000 persons) according to geographic region (both sexes, all ages). Adapted from Ferlay J, Shin HR, Bray F, Forman D, Mathers C and Parkin DM. GLOBOCAN 2008 v2.0, Cancer Incidence and Mortality Worldwide: IARC CancerBase No. 10 [Internet]. Lyon, France: International Agency for Research on Cancer; 2010. Available from: http://globocan.iarc.fr

1.1.2 Smoking

Cigarette smoking appears to be one of the most important modifiable risk factors for bladder cancer. The risk of bladder cancer among current smokers is two to five times greater than the risk among never smokers (Table 1.1) [5–11]. Smoking cessation substantially reduces the risk, but the former smoker's risk remains higher than the risk of a person who never smoked [11]. For example, in a recently published study conducted by the National Institutes of Health (NIH), smoking status at baseline was assessed for 281,394 men and 186,134 women, who were then followed for a 10-year period from 1996 to 2006 [11]. During the follow-up, bladder cancer was diagnosed in 3,896 men (1.38 %) and 627 women (0.34 %). Among men, compared with the never smokers, the risk of bladder cancer was 3.89 times higher in the current smokers (95 % CI: 3.46–4.37) and 2.14 times higher in the former smokers (95 % CI: 1.92–2.37). Among women, compared with the never smokers, the risk of

bladder cancer was 4.65 times higher in the current smokers (95 % CI: 3.73–5.79) and 2.52 times higher in the former smokers (95 % CI: 2.05–3.10) [11]. In both sexes, there was clear evidence of a dose–response relationship between the quantity and duration of smoking and the risk of bladder cancer; however, even in those individuals who smoked <10 cigarettes per day and stopped smoking more than 10 years before the baseline assessment, the risk of bladder cancer was significantly higher than in those who never smoked. Population attributable risk for ever smoking in this study was 0.50 for men and 0.52 for women (i.e., smoking was responsible for about one-half of all bladder cancer cases documented in the study cohort) [11]. Among various chemical compounds present in cigarette smoke, polycyclic aromatic hydrocarbons, 4-aminobiphenyl (4-ABF), and unsaturated aldehydes have been identified as bladder carcinogens [12, 13]. Inter-personal variability in the structure and function of certain enzymes such as N-acetyltransferase 2 (NAT2) and glutathione

Table 1.1 Relative risk of bladder cancer in the current smokers versus the never smokers according to prospective cohort studies completed in the US

Study	Sex	Years	No. never smokers	No. current smokers	Relative risk	Lower 95 % CL	Upper 95 % CL
Alberg 2007 [5]	Both	1963–1978	11,722	20,037	2.70	1.60	4.70
Chyou 1993 [6]	Men	1965–1991	2,410	3,495	2.86	1.67	4.91
Mills 1991 [7]	Both	1976–1982	26,059	1,129	5.67	1.73	18.61
Alberg 2007 [5]	Both	1975–1994	15,249	17,006	2.60	1.70	3.90
Tripathi 2002 [8]	Women	1986–1998	24,723	5,619	4.23	2.76	6.70
Michaud 2001 [9]	Men	1986–1998	24,035	4,648	2.81	1.85	4.27
Cantwell 2006 [10]	Women	1987–2000	27,691	7,826	2.44	1.56	3.80
Freedman 2011 [11]	Both	1995–2006	166,154	67,853	4.06	3.66	4.50

CL confidence limit

S-transferase-M1 (GTSM1) which are involved in metabolism of bladder carcinogens seems to modify the risk of smoking-induced bladder cancer [14–17]. Exposure to second-hand smoke was not definitively associated with increased risk of bladder cancer in a meta-analysis of seven observational studies (risk ratio = 0.99, 95 % CI: 0.86–1.14) [18].

1.1.3 Occupational Risk Factors

Among occupational risk factors, exposure to beta-naphthylamine, benzidine, and 4-ABF has been shown to be strongly associated with development of bladder cancer [19]. Occupational exposure to these chemicals occurred most frequently in the textile dye and rubber manufacturing industries. In the 1970s, the Occupational Safety and Health Administration (OSHA) recognized beta-naphthylamine as a human carcinogen and imposed strict regulations on the use of this compound. Similar regulations were applied to benzidine and 4-ABF [19]. Although occupational exposure to these chemicals has been nearly completely eliminated in the US, exposure to other potential bladder carcinogens (e.g., *o*-toluidine) may still occur among workers involved in the manufacturing of dyes, rubber, pharmaceuticals, and pesticides (Markowitz [20]). According to recent estimates, about 7 % of bladder cancer cases in men and 2 % in women may be attributed to occupational exposures in the developed countries [21].

1.1.4 Age

The incidence of bladder cancer increases with age and most patients are over age 65 at diagnosis. This is typical of most other cancers and is likely due to accumulation of mutations as a consequence of increasing cumulative exposure to carcinogens and reduced DNA repair mechanisms, although anti-neoplastic capabilities of the immune system may also decrease with age. In the US, median age at bladder cancer diagnosis is 70 years for men and 72 years for women [22]. Older age is also associated with increased disease-specific mortality in patients diagnosed with bladder cancer [23–25]. Some of this may be explained by decreased ability of the older patients to tolerate and/or accept aggressive treatments, although the disease itself may also be more aggressive in the elderly [23–25].

1.1.5 Sex

In all geographic regions, the risk of bladder cancer diagnosis is higher in men than in women (Fig. 1.2, Table 1.2). The reasons for this difference are not well understood. Two main factors have been investigated in this context: different patterns of smoking and industrial carcinogen exposure in men and women, and differences in hormonal and other biologic factors between the sexes. Historically, the prevalence of smoking among men was higher than in women. Additionally, men were more likely to be

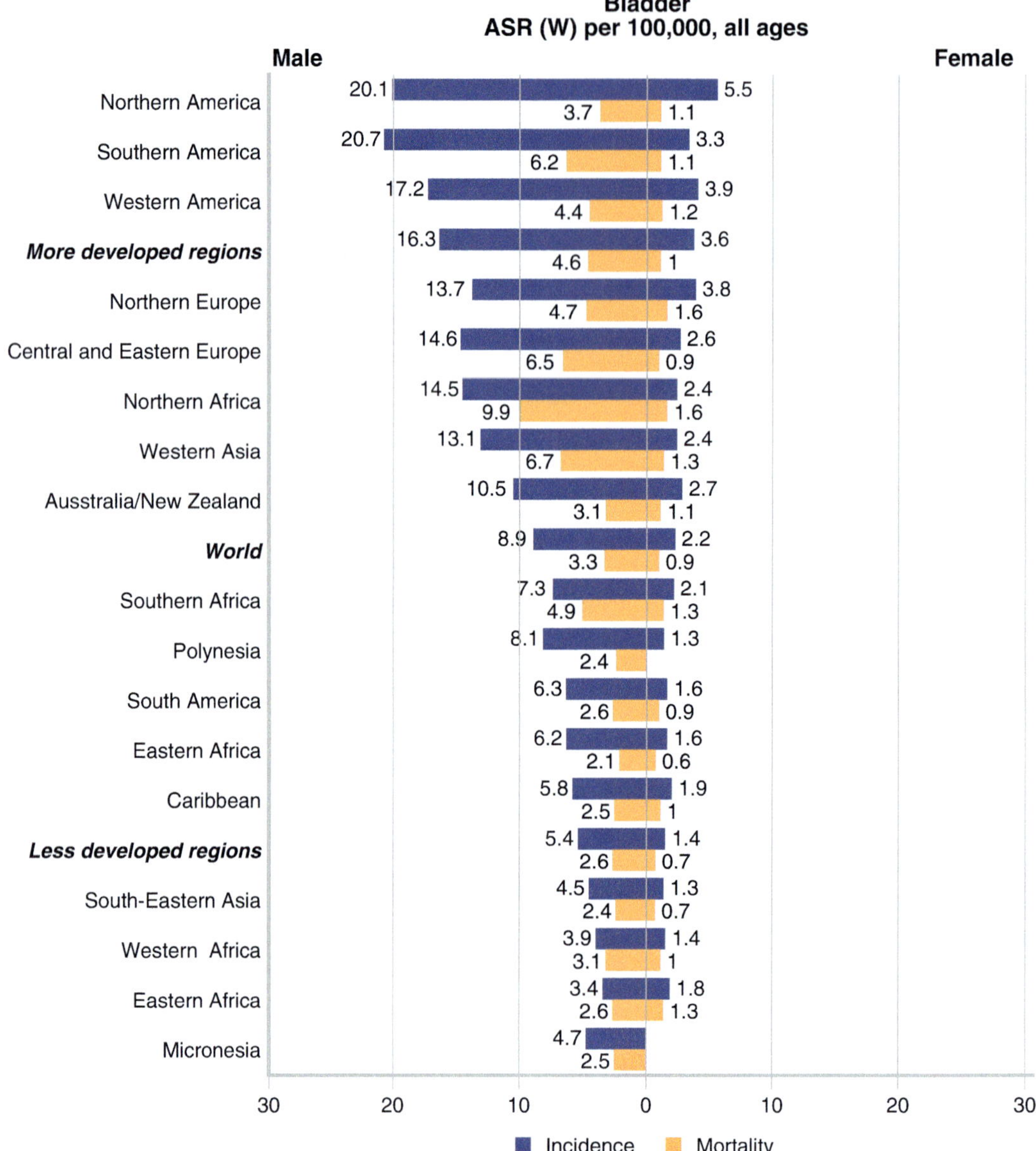

Fig. 1.2 Bladder cancer incidence and mortality according to sex and geographic region, age-standardized rates (ASR). Adapted from Ferlay J, Shin HR, Bray F, Forman D, Mathers C and Parkin DM. GLOBOCAN 2008 v2.0, Cancer Incidence and Mortality Worldwide: IARC CancerBase No. 10 [Internet]. Lyon, France: International Agency for Research on Cancer; 2010. Available from: http://globocan.iarc.fr

exposed to industrial carcinogens. This was believed to explain much of the sex differences in bladder cancer incidence. However, during the second half of the twentieth century, the proportion of smoking women steadily increased and approached the proportion of smoking men in developed countries [26]. Furthermore, women increasingly entered the traditionally male workplace. Despite these changes, the sex difference in the incidence of bladder cancer has continued to remain large in magnitude [27]. In the early 1990s, it was recognized that although smoking and occupational exposures accounted for some of the sex difference in the incidence of bladder cancer, even in the absence of

Table 1.2 Male-to-female incidence ratios for bladder cancer: data from the GLOBOCAN 2008 database [1]

Country	Incidence ratio (M/F)	Lower 95 % CL	Upper 95 % CL	Country	Incidence ratio (M/F)	Lower 95 % CL	Upper 95 % CL
Spain	6.30	6.00	6.63	Australia	3.03	2.77	3.31
France	5.16	4.90	5.43	Peru	3.02	2.50	3.65
Belarus	4.78	4.09	5.58	Uzbekistan	3.02	2.42	3.76
Greece	4.77	4.28	5.33	Canada	2.97	2.78	3.18
Israel	4.38	3.85	4.97	Venezuela	2.93	2.44	3.52
Ukraine	4.36	4.06	4.67	Mexico	2.93	2.67	3.22
Argentina	4.33	3.95	4.74	Brazil	2.91	2.76	3.07
Belgium	4.23	3.79	4.72	USA	2.91	2.86	2.96
Italy	4.22	4.05	4.39	Slovakia	2.90	2.47	3.40
Kazakhstan	4.14	3.48	4.91	Norway	2.89	2.53	3.30
Romania	4.10	3.75	4.48	Germany	2.85	2.77	2.94
S Korea	4.08	3.74	4.45	Sweden	2.84	2.58	3.12
Bulgaria	3.91	3.45	4.43	Denmark	2.76	2.48	3.08
Lithuania	3.90	3.14	4.85	UK	2.69	2.57	2.81
Russia	3.69	3.54	3.85	Austria	2.68	2.41	2.99
China	3.49	3.42	3.56	Czech R	2.65	2.44	2.89
Switzerland	3.33	2.98	3.73	Serbia	2.62	2.33	2.95
Poland	3.28	3.10	3.46	Philippines	2.39	2.04	2.80
Portugal	3.24	2.92	3.60	C Taipei	2.33	2.12	2.55
Japan	3.20	3.09	3.31	Hungary	2.30	2.10	2.53
Cuba	3.19	2.75	3.70	Colombia	2.11	1.88	2.38
Finland	3.18	2.71	3.72	Chile	2.09	1.82	2.40
Netherlands	3.16	2.90	3.45	Ireland	2.00	1.70	2.35
N Zealand	3.13	2.57	3.81	Viet Nam	1.31	1.13	1.53
Croatia	3.05	2.63	3.54				

CL confidence limit

exposure to cigarettes or occupational hazards, men were about 2.7 times more likely to develop bladder cancer when compared with women of the same age [28]. It was hypothesized that the unexplained excess risk of bladder cancer among men could be related to biologic differences between the sexes, particularly those involving sex hormones and hormone receptors. Data from basic research suggest that androgen and androgen receptors as well as estrogens and estrogen receptors may be involved in bladder carcinogenesis and progression [29, 30], although their exact roles remain unclear.

In recent years, numerous observational studies suggested that the risk of bladder cancer in women may be influenced by certain reproductive factors. For example, compared with nulliparous women, parous women may have a 25–35 % lower risk of bladder cancer according to two meta-analyses, with reported hazard ratios of 0.73 (95 % CI: 0.63–0.85) [31] and 0.66 (95 % CI: 0.55–0.79) [32]. In another recent meta-analysis of observational studies, use of estrogen plus progestin was associated with substantially lower risk of bladder cancer compared with no hormonal therapy (HR=0.61, 95 % CI: 0.47–0.78); however, use of estrogen alone was not associated with increased or decreased risk compared with no hormonal therapy (HR=1.03, 95 % CI: 0.87–1.24) [33]. Early age at menopause was also associated with increased risk of bladder cancer in a meta-analysis [32].

Although women have a lower life-time risk of bladder cancer than men, among patients diagnosed with bladder cancer, women tend to have less favorable outcomes in terms of disease-specific mortality, relative survival, and years of potential life lost [22, 27, 33, 34]. For example, according to data from the US SEER program, men diagnosed with BC on average lose approximately one-third (33 %) of their expected remaining years of life to BC, while for women, the respective estimate is close to one-half (47 %) [34]. These patterns could not be completely explained by differences in stage or other tumor characteristics at presentation, or variation in treatment modalities [33, 34]. Among patients diagnosed with BC in Europe, women also seem to have increased disease-specific mortality compared with men, at least according to data reported from some cohorts [35–37]. In a recent analysis of the GLOBOCAN 2008 data contributed by 49 countries representing all major geographic regions except Africa, in patients diagnosed with bladder cancer, disease-specific mortality was significantly higher in women than in men in 26 countries (53 %), significantly lower in women than in men in two countries (4 %), and not significantly different between the two sexes in 21 countries (43 %) [27]. The median relative risk was 1.21 (inter-quartile range: 1.04–1.41) [27]. Hence, excess mortality in women compared with men appears to be a common, although not a universal phenomenon. The origins of this phenomenon are not entirely clear, although delay in diagnosis in women and as a consequence more advanced stage at presentation may play a role.

1.1.6 Race

In the US, the incidence of bladder cancer is approximately two times lower in African Americans compared with Caucasians of the same sex; however, among patients diagnosed with bladder cancer, African Americans tend to present at more advanced stage and experience higher disease-specific mortality. In one SEER study of 96,540 white and 4,709 black patients newly diagnosed with bladder cancer, muscle-invasive or more advanced disease at presentation was found in 22 % of white men, 30 % of black men, 25 % of white women, and 43 % of black women [22]. African Americans of both genders also had a higher incidence of non-urothelial histologies than Caucasians, although

non-urothelial cancers still represented a small minority of newly diagnosed bladder cancers (5.9 % in African American men and 10.5 % in African American women) [22]. Compared with white patients, black patients of the same sex had increased disease-specific mortality, particularly within the first 2 years from diagnosis, when most patients presenting with micro-metastases die (black men vs. white men HR = 1.73, 95 % CI: 1.58–1.90; black women vs. white women HR = 2.04, 95 % CI: 1.85–2.25) [22]. These differences are likely explained by delay in diagnosis and more limited access to/utilization of medical care among African Americans.

1.1.7 Other Risk Factors

Other factors associated with increased risk of bladder cancer include therapeutic radiation to the pelvis, certain types of chronic bladder inflammation, exposure to cyclophosphomide, heavy use of phenacetin (banned by the FDA in 1983), and use of Chinese herb *Aristolochia fangchi*, which contains a nephrotoxin and a urothelial carcinogen known as aristolochic acid [38, 39]. Recently, use of anti-diabetic drug pioglitazone was also found to be associated with increased risk of bladder cancer [40].

Therapeutic radiation to the pelvis is often administered for prostate cancer in men and for uterine or cervical cancer in women, increasing the risk of bladder cancer by approximately 70 % in men and by about twofold in women, at least according to observational data [41–45]. In the Middle East (particularly in Egypt) many cases of bladder cancer are attributed to bladder inflammation due to chronic infection with a urinary parasite, *Schistosoma haematobium*. In the US, chronic inflammation of the bladder often occurs in patients with indwelling catheters, such as those suffering from a spinal cord injury. Unlike urothelial carcinoma, which is the most common histologic type of bladder cancer seen almost everywhere in the World, bladder cancer arising in the setting of chronic inflammation is often of squamous cell histology. Compared with urothelial carcinoma, squamous cell carcinoma of the bladder usually presents at much more advanced stage and is associated with poor prognosis [46].

Recently, some observational studies also reported an association between use of a common anti-diabetic drug pioglitazone (Actos) and increased risk of bladder cancer [40, 47]. In a meta-analysis of six observational studies with a total of 215,142 pioglitazone users and a median follow-up of 44 months, use of pioglitazone was associated with a 23 % relative increase in the risk of bladder cancer (HR = 1.23, 95 % CI: 1.09–1.39) [40].

1.2 Natural History of Bladder Cancer

Urothelial carcinoma of the bladder, which is by far the most common histologic type of bladder cancer in most parts of the world, is a very heterogeneous disease with a highly variable natural history. On the one side of the spectrum are the small solitary low-grade cancers (or LMPs) confined to the urothelium which rarely progress and typically do not pose a threat to patient's life, while on the other side are the high-grade muscle-invasive lesions that produce early metastases and cause death despite aggressive treatment. It should be recognized that the true natural history of untreated bladder cancer in the modern era remains largely unknown. Because bladder cancer is rarely found incidentally at autopsy, it is highly likely that its preclinical duration (the interval between when it could be detected if looked for and the onset of signs and symptoms leading to diagnosis) is very brief and that clinical statistics from tumor registries report something very close to its real incidence in the covered populations. However, since almost all bladder cancers cause signs and symptoms and become diagnosed, and virtually all bladder cancers are treated at least by transurethral resection, we only know the "treated history" (at least partially treated) of bladder cancer. However, we will not focus on the details of therapy, leaving this up to other chapters in this book. In the section which follows, we will describe the expected clinical course of bladder cancer, focusing mainly on cancers which are predominantly or purely urothelial carcinomas. Other bladder cancers which are primarily non-urothelial (e.g., squamous, small cell, or adenocarcinomas) or unusual variants of urothelial histology (e.g., micropapillary or nested variant) are not discussed as extensively. However, in general, non-urothelial cancers and unusual variants of urothelial cancers have prognoses similar to or worse than that of the most aggressive forms of urothelial cancer with standard therapies.

1.2.1 Low-Grade Non-muscle-Invasive Bladder Cancer

These tumors represent between 50 and 60 % of all newly diagnosed bladder cancer cases in the US [22]; the majority are confined to the urothelium (stage Ta) and rarely pose a threat to a patient's life. However, even low-grade Ta tumors have several significant features necessitating medical intervention. First, these tumors tend to produce microscopic and gross hematuria, which is the most common finding leading to the initial diagnosis of bladder cancer. Hematuria resulting from bladder cancer often leads to the bladder outlet obstruction, requiring clot evacuation. Hence, unlike low-grade prostate cancer, low-grade bladder cancer is almost always clinically significant eventually, and is rarely if ever found incidentally at autopsy. The second significant feature of these lesions is that they tend to recur, necessitating cystoscopic surveillance and repeated transurethral resections of bladder tumors (TURBTs). Large (e.g., >3 cm) and multifocal tumors are more likely to recur than smaller solitary tumors [48]. Furthermore, tumors that were initially diagnosed as low grade, stage Ta may undergo grade and/or stage progression on recurrence. For example, in one study of 82 recurring tumors, all originally of low grade, 9 (11 %) recurred as high-grade tumors [49]. Low-grade Ta tumors may also progress to stage T1 without a grade progression, although further progression of low-grade tumors to stage T2 without grade progression is very uncommon. Almost all muscle-invasive bladder tumors are high grade.

Table 1.3 The EORTC nomogram predicting the risk of recurrence and progression of Ta/T1 bladder tumors: prediction scores

Factor	Recurrence	Progression
No. of tumors		
Single	0	0
2 to 7	3	3
≥7	6	3
Tumor size		
<3 cm	0	0
≥3 cm	3	3
Prior recurrence rate		
Primary	0	0
1 rec/year	2	2
>1 rec/year	4	2
T category		
Ta	0	0
T1	1	4
CIS		
No	0	0
Yes	1	6
Grade		
G1	0	0
G2	1	0
G3	2	5
Total score	0–17	0–23

From: Sylvester RJ, van der Meijden AP, Oosterlinck W, et al. Predicting recurrence and progression in individual patients with stage TaT1 bladder cancer using EORTC risk tables: a combined analysis of 2596 patients from seven EORTC trials. Eur Urol 2006; 49(3):466-5., reproduced with permission from Elsevier

Table 1.4 The EORTC nomogram predicting the risk of recurrence and progression of Ta/T1 bladder tumors: estimated probabilities

Recurrence score	Prob recurrence 1 year (95 % CI)	Prob recurrence 5 years (95 % CI)
0	15 % (10 %, 19 %)	31 % (24 %, 37 %)
1–4	24 % (21 %, 26 %)	46 % (42 %, 49 %)
5–9	38 % (35 %, 41 %)	62 % (58 %, 65 %)
10–17	61 % (55 %, 67 %)	78 % (73 %, 84 %)
Progression score	Prob progression 1 year (95 % CI)	Prob progression 5 years (95 % CI)
0	0.2 % (0 %, 0.7 %)	0.8 % (0 %, 1.7 %)
2–6	1.0 % (0.4 %, 1.6 %)	6 % (5 %, 8 %)
7–13	5 % (4 %, 7 %)	17 % (14 %, 20 %)
14–23	17 % (10 %, 24 %)	45 % (35 %, 55 %)

From: Sylvester RJ, van der Meijden AP, Oosterlinck W, et al. Predicting recurrence and progression in individual patients with stage TaT1 bladder cancer using EORTC risk tables: a combined analysis of 2596 patients from seven EORTC trials. Eur Urol 2006; 49(3):466-5., reproduced with permission from Elsevier

The European Organization for Research and Treatment of Cancer (EORTC) used a database of 2,596 patients to create a nomogram predicting recurrence and progression to muscle-invasive disease of non-muscle-invasive Ta and T1 bladder cancer (Tables 1.3 and 1.4) [48]. For example, for a newly diagnosed solitary low-grade Ta bladder tumor <3 cm in diameter, the estimated probability of recurrence would be 15 % in the first year and 31 % in the first 5 years of follow-up, while the estimated risk of progression would be 0.2 % in the first year and 0.8 % in the first 5 years. If this tumor was >3 cm in diameter and invaded the lamina propria (stage T1) the 1- and 5-year risk of recurrence would increase to 24 % and 46 %, respectively, while the 1- and 5-year risk of progression would increase to 5 % and 17 %, respectively. It should be noted however that the risk of progression was estimated in the population of patients who were under regular surveillance after initial diagnosis and were treated at recurrence. In the absence of surveillance and treatment, the progression rates would likely be much higher. The EORTC trials also used chemotherapy as the primary adjuvant intravesical therapy. Given that intravesical BCG may achieve lower recurrence and progression rates compared to chemotherapy, the predicted rates of recurrence and progression using the EORTC tables may be higher than that observed in patient treated with adjuvant intravesical BCG therapy. Also, it is now recognized that recurrence status at 3 months from TURBT is a strong predictor of subsequent recurrence, with much lower risk in those with a negative cystoscopy at 3 months [50, 51].

1.2.2 High-Grade Non-muscle-Invasive Bladder Cancer

These tumors account for 20–25 % of all newly diagnosed bladder cancer cases in the US [22]. High-grade lesions in the bladder can be flat (so-called carcinoma in situ, CIS) or elevated. Pure CIS is uncommon, but it is frequently found along with the elevated sessile or papillary lesions. Presentation of high-grade non-muscle-invasive bladder cancer is similar to that of low-grade tumors, with initial diagnosis usually triggered by microscopic or gross hematuria, although irritative bladder symptoms may also be present, particularly in the presence of CIS. These are much less common with low-grade bladder cancer. All or nearly all high-grade lesions in the bladder if left untreated have a tendency to invade deep into the bladder wall, eventually producing metastases, although the latter usually does not occur until the tumor extends at least to detrusor muscle (stage T2). In particular, despite presence of vascular and lymphatic spaces in the lamina propria, patients treated with cystectomy for high-grade lamina-propria invasive bladder cancer (i.e., stage T1 as the highest clinical or pathologic stage) usually have a favorable prognosis, particularly if no lymphovascular invasion (LVI) or CIS is identified microscopically. For example, in one recent study of 101 cystectomy patients with stage T1 as the highest clinical or pathologic stage, only six patients (6 %) had LVI, but with median follow-up of 38 months, four of these (67 %) experienced disease recurrence and three (50 %) died from bladder cancer [52]. In patients without LVI, recurrence and mortality rates were 8 % and 3 % respectively. In this study, all recurrences occurred in the patients who had either LVI or CIS [52].

Because high-grade bladder cancer usually does not produce metastases until the detrusor muscle is invaded, the initial management of high-grade, clinical stage Ta/T1 tumors is often conservative, consisting of TURBTs and intravesical therapy. Nevertheless this approach has been a subject of controversy, because the risk of progression to muscle-invasive disease is high, particularly in the presence of concurrent CIS (Tables 1.3 and 1.4). Isolated CIS when found in the absence of other lesions is also associated with a significant risk of progression if left untreated or if treatment fails to completely eradicate it [53, 54]. Another issue with conservative management of high-grade non-muscle invasive

bladder cancer is the problem of understaging. Some of these tumors, particularly those invading the lamina propria based on the TURBT pathology, are under-staged T2 if not more advanced lesions. For example, in patients diagnosed with high-grade T1 bladder cancer on initial TURBT which involved sampling of the detrusor muscle, repeated TURBT revealed presence of T2 disease in 14 % of the cases [55], while cystectomy, when performed resulted in upstaging to stage T2 or greater in 23 % of the cases [56]. If initial TURBT specimen did not contain the detrusor muscle, but lamina propria invasion was present, upstaging to stage T2 may occur in up to 50 % of all high-grade T1 cases on repeated TURBT [55]. Because high-grade T1 lesions are associated with high risk of progression and some of these cancers in fact represent under-staged T2 if not more advanced disease, radical cystectomy is considered an option for some patients presenting with high-grade T1 bladder cancer, particularly those with large tumors and concurrent CIS [51].

1.2.3 Muscle-Invasive Bladder Cancer

These tumors account for 20–25 % of all bladder cancer cases diagnosed in the US. Almost all are of high grade, with highly aggressive natural histories. Invasion of detrusor muscle is a critical event in disease progression because at that point, the risk of lymphatic and hematogenous spread becomes very high. Lymphatic spread usually occurs to the internal and external iliac chains, and obturator nodes, and less commonly to sacral, presacral and presciatic nodes. The common iliac chain and the retroperitoneal nodes can be involved later in the course of disease. Distant metastases usually develop in the lungs, liver, and bone [57, 58]. Presentation of muscle-invasive bladder cancer may involve microscopic and gross hematuria, as well as symptoms resulting from direct tumor extension or metastases.

In the US, the first-line therapy for muscle-invasive bladder cancer in the absence of known metastases is radical cystectomy with pelvic lymphadenectomy [59]. Systemic platinum-based combination chemotherapy can be given before or after surgery for treatment of micro-metastases which are unfortunately very common. Multimodality bladder-sparing protocols consisting of aggressive TURBTs, systemic multidrug chemotherapy and pelvic radiation also exist, but these have not been directly compared to radical cystectomy in randomized trials. Partial cystectomy may be an option in some patients [59]. Overt metastatic disease is treated with systemic chemotherapy [59].

Unfortunately, extravesical involvement by direct extension and discontinuous spread usually occurs early in the natural history of muscle-invasive bladder cancer but often cannot be detected at initial diagnosis by currently available methods of clinical staging. In particular, patients with biopsy-confirmed muscle-invasive bladder cancer are evaluated for evidence of extravesical disease by physical examination, liver function tests, computed tomography (CT) of the abdomen and pelvis, a chest x-ray (or CT of the chest), and a bone scan. It is possible that magnetic resonance imaging (MRI) and 18F-fluorodeoxyglucose positron emission (PET) CTs may improve local and regional staging to some degree, but this has to be shown in large prospective studies in which all subjects are surgically staged. Currently, imaging results in substantial under-staging of the true extent of muscle-invasive disease. For example, in one recent study, among 135 patients with biopsy-confirmed muscle-invasive bladder cancer treated with radical cystectomy without neo-adjuvant chemotherapy, only 29 patients (21 %) had evidence of direct extravesical extension (stage T3/T4) based on clinical staging, but pathologic stage T3/T4 was found in 85 of the patients (63 %) [60]. Similarly, any regional adenopathy was present by imaging in only 15 of 135 patients (11 %), but pathologically positive nodes were found in 58 patients (43 %) [60]. During a median follow-up of 32 months, 44 of 135 patients (33 %) died from bladder cancer, and this percentage would undoubtedly increase with longer follow-up [60]. Similar or more extreme under-staging and treatment failure rates have been reported from other recent series [61–63]. Such high failure rates of definitive local treatment are primarily explained by presence of occult micro-metastatic disease in many patients with muscle-invasive bladder cancer. According to SEER data, overall case-fatality for muscle-invasive bladder cancer in the US (all stages combined) is approximately 45 % for men and 55 % for women [34].

Although all muscle-invasive bladder tumors should be considered of high risk in terms of disease-specific mortality, there are several tumor characteristics that clearly modify this risk. As would be expected, patients presenting with visceral metastases generally have very poor prognosis, with median survival of approximately 10 months despite systemic multi-agent chemotherapy [58], although even in this high-risk group, average survival varies to some extent according to the number of metastatic sites, the baseline performance status, and presence of leukocytosis [64]. In the M0/MX patients, the presence and the extent of nodal metastases, the T stage, and the presence of LVI are important predictors of the clinical course of the disease.

Node-positive M0/MX bladder cancer is a very aggressive disease generally associated with poor prognosis (even with cystectomy), although outcomes vary to some extent according to the degree of nodal involvement [65], the extent of lymphadenectomy [66], the T-stage [67], and the use of systemic chemotherapy [68]. The average 5-year survival of patients with node-positive bladder cancer is between 20 and 40 %, depending on the above-mentioned factors [62, 67]. The prognosis may be relatively more favorable for those with only one or two positive nodes out of 20 or more nodes examined and no direct extra-vesical extension of the tumor. Administration of adjuvant chemotherapy may also improve outcomes, although the quality of level 1 evidence on this has been debated [68]. Lymphadenectomy in itself is believed to be potentially curative in some patients with nodal involvement [66, 69]. For example, in one study, 84 patients all with grossly (palpable) and pathologically node-positive bladder cancer were treated with radical cystectomy with extended pelvic lymph node dissection and followed for at least 10 years [69]. Systemic chemotherapy was given at recurrence but none of the patients received it adjuvantly. Despite this, at 10 years of follow-up, 20 (24 %) of the patients had no history of recurrence, of which 16 were alive and 4 died from causes other than bladder cancer. The remaining 64 (76 %) patients died from bladder cancer [69]. These findings strongly suggest that nodal metastases of bladder cancer may occur in the absence of distant spread and can be resected at least in some patients. Indeed, in many observational studies the extent of pelvic lymphadenectomy was positively correlated with overall survival [66, 70]. A clinical trial of standard versus extended pelvic lymphadenectomy during cystectomy for muscle-invasive bladder cancer (NCT01224665) is underway.

The depth of the bladder wall invasion is also a strong predictor of clinical behavior of muscle-invasive bladder cancer, predicting the risk of nodal metastases as well as that of disease-specific mortality in patients with a given nodal status. For example, in one SEER study of 2,388 patients with pT2b-pT3b bladder cancer treated with radical cystectomy, the risk of nodal metastases increased with increasing T sub-stage in a dose–response fashion (pT2b = 20 %, pT3a = 36 %, pT3b = 48 %, trend $P < 0.001$) [67]. In this study, penetration of the bladder wall by direct extension of the tumor (even if microscopic) was also a strong predictor of disease-specific and overall survival in patients with a given nodal status. For example, compared with stage pT2b, stage pT3a was associated with a twofold increase in disease-specific mortality in node-negative patients (HR = 2.00, 95 % CI: 1.89–2.53) and a more than 50 % increase in disease-specific mortality in node-positive patients (HR = 1.57, 95 % CI: 1.16, 2.13), after adjusting for the number of nodes examined and the number of positive nodes [67].

Association of the T stage with disease-specific and overall survival independent of the nodal status and other prognostic factors has also been reported in many other studies [62, 65, 66]. This is probably because more advanced T stage increases the risk of distant hematogenous spread as well as the risk of local recurrence in addition to its effect on the risk of nodal metastases. Interestingly, some patients with biopsy-confirmed muscle-invasive disease treated with radical cystectomy have no residual tumor in the cystectomy specimen (stage pT0). In the absence of systemic neo-adjuvant chemotherapy, this occurs in about 5–15 % of all patients, while with platinum-based neo-adjuvant chemotherapy, the frequency of stage pT0 has been reported at 20–38 % [60, 71, 72]. Despite invasion of detrusor muscle in the TURBT specimen, patients with stage pT0 at the time of cystectomy have very favorable prognosis, with overall 5-year survival of approximately 85 % [71].

Another factor that may help predict the behavior of muscle-invasive bladder cancer is the presence of lymphovascular invasion (LVI). For example, in one study, in 374 patients with pathologically organ-confined bladder cancer (stage <T3 with negative nodes), 5-year survival was 75 % in those without LVI and 52 % in those with LVI [73]. In patients with direct extravesical extension with negative nodes, and in patients with positive nodes, presence of LVI was also associated with decreased survival [73]. Similar results were reported from many other studies, with LVI as an independent predictor of survival in patients with a given T stage and a given nodal status [60, 74–76].

In summary, muscle-invasive bladder cancer is usually a life-threatening illness with highly aggressive natural history. Prognosis is particularly poor for those presenting with distant metastases, but even among patients with a negative metastatic workup at presentation, positive nodes are frequently found at the time of cystectomy, and distant recurrences involving the lungs, liver, or bone are common. Patients with direct extravesical extension of the tumor and with evidence of lymphovascular invasion are at particularly high risk for metastatic disease. On the other hand, those with no residual disease in the cystectomy specimen generally have favorable prognosis.

References

1. Ferlay J, Shin HR, Bray F, Forman D, Mathers C, Parkin DM. GLOBOCAN 2008 v2.0, Cancer incidence and mortality worldwide: IARC CancerBase No. 10 [Internet]. Lyon, France: International Agency for Research on Cancer; 2010. http://globocan.iarc.fr.
2. Ferlay J, Shin H, Bray F, Forman D, Mathers C, Parkin DM. Estimates of worldwide burden of cancer in 2008: GLOBOCAN 2008. Int J Cancer. 2010;127: 2893–917.

3. Siegel R, Naishadham D, Jemal A. Cancer statistics, 2013. CA Cancer J Clin. 2013;63(1):11–30.
4. American Cancer Society. Bladder cancer. http://www.cancer.org/acs/groups/cid/documents/webcontent/003085-pdf.pdf. Accessed 3 June 2013.
5. Alberg AJ, Kouzis A, Genkinger JM, et al. A prospective cohort study of bladder cancer risk in relation to active cigarette smoking and household exposure to secondhand cigarette smoke. Am J Epidemiol. 2007;165(6):660–6.
6. Chyou PH, Nomura AM, Stemmermann GN. A prospective study of diet, smoking, and lower urinary tract cancer. Ann Epidemiol. 1993;3(3):211–21.
7. Mills PK, Beeson WL, Phillips RL, Fraser GE. Bladder cancer in a low risk population: results from the Adventist Health Study. Am J Epidemiol. 1991;133(3):230–9.
8. Tripathi A, Folsom AR, Anderson AE, Iowa Women's Health Study. Risk factors for urinary bladder carcinoma in postmenopausal women. Cancer. 2002;95(11):2316–23.
9. Michaud DS, Clinton SK, Rimm EB, Willett WC, Giovannucci E. Risk of bladder cancer by geographic region in a U.S. cohort of male health professionals. Epidemiology. 2001;12(6):719–26.
10. Cantwell MM, Lacey Jr JV, Schairer C, Schatzkin A, Michaud DS. Reproductive factors, exogenous hormone use and bladder cancer risk in a prospective study. Int J Cancer. 2006;119(10):2398–401.
11. Freedman ND, Silverman DT, Hollenbeck AR, et al. Association between smoking and risk of bladder cancer among men and women. JAMA. 2011;306(7):737–45.
12. Bartsch H, et al. Black (air cured) and blond (flue-cured) tobacco cancer risk. IV. Molecular dosimetry studies implicate aromatic amines as bladder carcinogens. Eur J Cancer. 1993;29:1199–208.
13. Bernardini S, et al. Influence of cigarette smoking on p53 gene mutations in bladder carcinomas. Anticancer Res. 2001;21:3001–4.
14. Risch A, Wallace DM, Bathers S, et al. Slow N-acetylation genotype is a susceptibility factor in occupational and smoking related bladder cancer. Hum Mol Genet. 1995;4(2):231–6.
15. Cui X, Lu X, Hiura M, Omori H, Miyazaki W, Katoh T. Association of genotypes of carcinogen-metabolizing enzymes and smoking status with bladder cancer in a Japanese population. Environ Health Prev Med. 2013;18(2):136–42.
16. Bell DA, Taylor JA, Paulson DF, et al. Genetic risk and carcinogen exposure: a common inherited defect of the carcinogen-metabolism gene glutathione S-transferase M1 (GSTM1) that increases susceptibility to bladder cancer. J Natl Cancer Inst. 1993;85(14):1159–64.
17. García-Closas M, Malats N, Silverman D, Dosemeci M, Kogevinas M, Hein DW, Tardón A, Serra C, Carrato A, García-Closas R, Lloreta J, Castaño-Vinyals G, Yeager M, Welch R, Chanock S, Chatterjee N, Wacholder S, Samanic C, Torà M, Fernández F, Real FX, Rothman N. NAT2 slow acetylation, GSTM1 null genotype, and risk of bladder cancer: results from the Spanish Bladder Cancer Study and meta-analyses. Lancet. 2005;366(9486):649–59.
18. Van Hemelrijck MJ, Michaud DS, Connolly GN, Kabir Z. Secondhand smoking, 4-aminobiphenyl, and bladder cancer: two meta-analyses. Cancer Epidemiol Biomarkers Prev. 2009;18(4):1312–20.
19. Verma DK, Purdham JT, Roels HA. Translating evidence about occupational conditions into strategies for prevention. Occup Environ Med. 2002;59:205–14.
20. Markowitz SB, Levin K. Continued epidemic of bladder cancer in workers exposed to ortho-toluidine in a chemical factory. J Occup Environ Med. 2004;46:154–60.
21. Rushton L, Hutchings SJ, Fortunato L, Young C, Evans GS, Brown T, Bevan R, Slack R, Holmes P, Bagga S, Cherrie JW, Van Tongeren M. Occupational cancer burden in Great Britain. Br J Cancer. 2012;107 Suppl 1:S3–7.
22. Scosyrev E, Noyes K, Feng C, Messing E. Sex and racial differences in bladder cancer presentation and mortality in the US. Cancer. 2009;115(1):68–74.
23. Nielsen ME, Shariat SF, Karakiewicz PI, Lotan Y, Rogers CG, Amiel GE, Bastian PJ, Vazina A, Gupta A, Lerner SP, Sagalowsky AI, Schoenberg MP, Palapattu GS, Bladder Cancer Research Consortium (BCRC). Advanced age is associated with poorer bladder cancer-specific survival in patients treated with radical cystectomy. Eur Urol. 2007;51(3):699–706.
24. Resorlu B, Beduk Y, Baltaci S, Ergun G, Talas H. The prognostic significance of advanced age in patients with bladder cancer treated with radical cystectomy. BJU Int. 2009;103(4):480–3.
25. Fairey AS, Kassouf W, Aprikian AG, Chin JL, Izawa JI, Fradet Y, Lacombe L, Rendon RA, Bell D, Cagiannos I, Drachenberg DE, Lattouf JB, Estey EP. Age ≥ 80 years is independently associated with survival outcomes after radical cystectomy: results from the Canadian Bladder Cancer Network Database. Urol Oncol. 2012;30(6):825–32.
26. Fiore MC, Novotny TE, Pierce JP, et al. Trends in cigarette smoking in the US: the changing influence of gender and race. JAMA. 1989;261:49–55.
27. Donsky H, Coyle S, Scosyrev E, Messing EM. Sex differences in incidence and mortality of bladder and kidney cancers: national estimates from 49 countries. Urol Oncol. 2014;32:40.e23–31.
28. Hartge P, Harvey EB, Linehan WB, et al. Unexplained excess risk of bladder cancer in men. J Natl Cancer Inst. 1990;82:1636–40.
29. Miyamoto H, Yang Z, Chen YT, et al. Promotion of bladder cancer development and progression by androgen receptor signals. J Natl Cancer Inst. 2007;99(7):558–68.
30. Miyamoto H, Yao JL, Chaux A, Zheng Y, Hsu I, Izumi K, Chang C, Messing EM, Netto GJ, Yeh S. Expression of androgen and oestrogen receptors and its prognostic significance in urothelial neoplasm of the urinary bladder. BJU Int. 2012;109(11):1716–26.

31. Davis-Dao CA, Henderson KD, Sullivan-Halley J, Ma H, West D, Xiang YB, Gago-Dominguez M, Stern MC, Castelao JE, Conti DV, Pike MC, Bernstein L, Cortessis VK. Lower risk in parous women suggests that hormonal factors are important in bladder cancer etiology. Cancer Epidemiol Biomarkers Prev. 2011; 20(6):1156–70.

32. Dietrich K, Demidenko E, Schned A, Zens MS, Heaney J, Karagas MR. Parity, early menopause and the incidence of bladder cancer in women: a case-control study and meta-analysis. Eur J Cancer. 2011;47(4):592–9.

33. Scosyrev E, Trivedi D, Messing E. Female bladder cancer: incidence, treatment, and outcome. Curr Opin Urol. 2010;20:404–8.

34. Scosyrev E, Golijanin D, Wu G, Messing EM. The burden of bladder cancer in men and women: analysis of the years of life lost. BJU Int. 2012;109(1):57–62.

35. Horstmann M, Witthuhn R, Falk M, et al. Gender-specific differences in bladder cancer: a retrospective analysis. Gend Med. 2008;5:385–94.

36. Tilki D, Svatek RS, Karakiewicz PL, et al. Characteristics and outcomes of patients with pT4 urothelial carcinoma at radical cystectomy: a retrospective international study of 583 patients. J Urol. 2010;187:87–93.

37. Palou J, Sylvester RJ, Faba OR, Parada R, Peña JA, Algaba F, Villavicencio H. Female gender and carcinoma in situ in the prostatic urethra are prognostic factors for recurrence, progression, and disease-specific mortality in T1G3 bladder cancer patients treated with bacillus Calmette-Guérin. Eur Urol. 2012;62(1):118–25.

38. Kirkali Z, et al. Bladder cancer: epidemiology, staging and grading, and diagnosis. Urology. 2005;66(6 Suppl 1):4–34.

39. Stiborová M, Martínek V, Frei E, Arlt VM, Schmeiser HH. Enzymes metabolizing aristolochic acid and their contribution to the development of aristolochic acid nephropathy and urothelial cancer. Curr Drug Metab. 2013;14:695–705.

40. Ferwana M, Firwana B, Hasan R, Al-Mallah MH, Kim S, Montori VM, Murad MH. Pioglitazone and risk of bladder cancer: a meta-analysis of controlled studies. Diabet Med. 2013;30:1026–32. doi:10.1111/dme.12144.

41. Kumar S, Shah JP, Bryant CS, et al. Second neoplasms in survivors of endometrial cancer: impact of radiation therapy. Gynecol Oncol. 2009;113:233–9.

42. Brown AP, Neeley ES, Werner T, Soisson AP, Burt RW, Gaffney DK. A population-based study of subsequent primary malignancies after endometrial cancer: genetic, environmental, and treatment-related associations. Int J Radiat Oncol Biol Phys. 2010;78:127–35.

43. Lonn S, Gilbert ES, Ron E, Smith SA, Stovall M, Curtis RE. Comparison of second cancer risks from brachytherapy and external beam radiation therapy after uterine corpus cancer. Cancer Epidemiol Biomarkers Prev. 2010;19:464–74.

44. Abern MR, Dude AM, Tsivian M, Coogan CL. The characteristics of bladder cancer after radiotherapy for prostate cancer. Urol Oncol. 2012;31:1628–34.

45. Kukreja B, Scosyrev E, Brasacchio R, Toy E, Messing E, Wu G. Bladder cancer incidence and mortality in patients treated with radiation for uterine cancer. Abstract presented at AUA 2013.

46. Scosyrev E, Yao J, Messing E. Urothelial carcinoma versus squamous cell carcinoma of bladder: is survival different with stage adjustment? Urology. 2009;73(4):822–7.

47. Lewis JD, Ferrara A, Peng T, Hedderson M, Bilker WB, Quesenberry Jr CP, Vaughn DJ, Nessel L, Selby J, Strom BL. Risk of bladder cancer among diabetic patients treated with pioglitazone: interim report of a longitudinal cohort study. Diabetes Care. 2011;34(4): 916–22.

48. Sylvester RJ, van der Meijden AP, Oosterlinck W, et al. Predicting recurrence and progression in individual patients with stage TaT1 bladder cancer using EORTC risk tables: a combined analysis of 2596 patients from seven EORTC trials. Eur Urol. 2006;49(3):466–5.

49. Borhan A, Reeder JE, O''onnell MJ, Wright KO, Wheeless LL, di Sant'Agnese PA, McNally ML, Messing EM. Grade progression and regression in recurrent urothelial cancer. J Urol. 2003;169(6):2106–9.

50. Aldousari S, Kassouf W. Update on the management of non-muscle-invasive bladder cancer. Can Urol Assoc J. 2010;4(1):56–64.

51. Babjuk M, Oosterlinck W, Sylvester R, et al. Guidelines on non-muscle-invasive bladder cancer. European Association of Urology 2012. http://www.uroweb.org/gls/pdf/05_TaT1_Bladder_Cancer.pdf. Accessed 3 May 2013.

52. Tilki D, Shariat SF, Lotan Y, Rink M, Karakiewicz PI, Schoenberg MP, Lerner SP, Sonpavde G, Sagalowsky AI, Gupta A. Lymphovascular invasion is independently associated with bladder cancer recurrence and survival in patients with final stage T1 disease and negative lymph nodes after radical cystectomy. BJU Int. 2013;111:1215–21. doi:10.1111/j.1464-410X.2012.11455.x.

53. Compérat E, Jacquet SF, Varinot J, Conort P, Roupret M, Chartier-Kastler E, Bitker MO, Witjes JA, Cussenot O. Different subtypes of carcinoma in situ of the bladder do not have a different prognosis. Virchows Arch. 2013;462(3):343–8.

54. Lamm DL. Carcinoma in situ. Urol Clin North Am. 1992;19(3):499–508.

55. Herr HW. The value of a second transurethral resection in evaluating patients with bladder tumors. J Urol. 1999;162(1):74–6.

56. Dutta SC, Smith JA, Shappell SB, et al. Clinical understaging of high risk nonmuscle invasive urothelial carcinoma treated with radical cystectomy. J Urol. 2001;166(2):490–3.

57. Shinagare AB, Ramaiya NH, Jagannathan JP, Fennessy FM, Taplin ME, Van den Abbeele AD. Metastatic pattern of bladder cancer: correlation with the characteristics of the primary tumor. AJR Am J Roentgenol. 2011;196(1):117–22.

58. Von Der Maase H, Sengelov L, Roberts JT, Ricci S, Dogliotti L, Oliver T, Moore MJ, Zimmermann A, Arning M. Long-term survival results of a randomized

trial comparing gemcitabine plus cisplatin, with methotrexate, vinblastine, doxorubicin, plus cisplatin in patients with bladder cancer. J Clin Oncol. 2005; 23(21):4602–8.

59. Clark PE, Agarwal N, Biagioli MC, et al. NCCN clinical practice guideline in oncology: bladder cancer. Version I. 2013. http://www.nccn.org/professionals/physician_gls/pdf/bladder.pdf. Accessed 3 June 2013

60. Scosyrev E, Messing EM, van Wijngaarden E, Peterson DR, Sahasrabudhe D, Golijanin D, Fisher SG. Neo-adjuvant gemcitabine-cisplatin chemotherapy for locally advanced urothelial cancer of the bladder. Cancer. 2012;118(1):72–81.

61. Green DA, Rink M, Hansen J, Cha EK, Robinson B, Tian Z, Chun FK, Tagawa S, Karakiewicz PI, Fisch M, Scherr DS, Shariat SF. Accurate preoperative prediction of non-organ-confined bladder urothelial carcinoma at cystectomy. BJU Int. 2013;111(3):404–11. doi:10.1111/j.1464-410X.2012.11370.x. Epub 2012 Jul 13.

62. Power NE, Kassouf W, Bell D, et al. Natural history of pT3-4 or node positive bladder cancer treated with radical cystectomy and no neoadjuvant chemotherapy in a contemporary North-american multi-institutional cohort. Can Urol Assoc J. 2012;6(6):E217–23.

63. Turker P, Bostrom PJ, Wroclawski ML, van Rhijn B, Kortekangas H, Kuk C, Mirtti T, Fleshner NE, Jewett MA, Finelli A, Kwast TV, Evans A, Sweet J, Laato M, Zlotta AR. Upstaging of urothelial cancer at the time of radical cystectomy: factors associated with upstaging and its effect on outcome. BJU Int. 2012;110(6):804–11.

64. Galsky MD, Moshier E, Krege S, Lin CC, Hahn N, Ecke T, Sonpavde G, Godbold J, Oh WK, Bamias A. Nomogram for predicting survival in patients with unresectable and/or metastatic urothelial cancer who are treated with cisplatin-based chemotherapy. Cancer. 2013;119:3012–9. doi: 10.1002/cncr.28146. [Epub ahead of print].

65. Tarin TV, Power NE, Ehdaie B, Sfakianos JP, Silberstein JL, Savage CJ, Sjoberg D, Dalbagni G, Bochner BH. Lymph node-positive bladder cancer treated with radical cystectomy and lymphadenectomy: effect of the level of node positivity. Eur Urol. 2012;61(5):1025–30.

66. Herr HW, Faulkner JR, Grossman HB, Natale RB, deVere WR, Sarosdy MF, Crawford ED. Surgical factors influence bladder cancer outcomes: a cooperative group report. J Clin Oncol. 2004;22(14):2781–9.

67. Scosyrev E, Yao J, Messing E. Microscopic invasion of perivesical fat by urothelial carcinoma: implications for prognosis and pathology practice. Urology. 2010; 76(4):908–13.

68. Advanced Bladder Cancer (ABC) Meta-analysis Collaboration. Adjuvant chemotherapy in invasive bladder cancer: a systematic review and meta-analysis of individual patient data. Eur Urol. 2005;48: 189–201. Discussion 199–201.

69. Herr HW, Donat SM. Outcome of patients with grossly node positive bladder cancer after pelvic lymph node dissection and radical cystectomy. J Urol. 2001;165(1):62–4. Discussion 64.

70. Tilki D, Brausi M, Colombo R, Evans CP, Fradet Y, Fritsche HM, Lerner SP, Sagalowsky A, Shariat SF, Bochner BH. Lymphadenectomy for bladder cancer at the time of radical cystectomy. Eur Urol. 2013;pii: S0302-2838(13): 0042–1. doi: 10.1016/j.eururo.2013.04.036. [Epub ahead of print]

71. Grossman HB, Natale RB, Tangen CM, Speights VO, Vogelzang NJ, Trump DL, deVere White RW, Sarosdy MF, Wood Jr DP, Raghavan D, Crawford ED. Neoadjuvant chemotherapy plus cystectomy compared with cystectomy alone for locally advanced bladder cancer. N Engl J Med. 2003;349(9): 859–66.

72. Yuh BE, Ruel N, Wilson TG, et al. Pooled analysis of clinical outcomes with neoadjuvant cisplatin and gemcitabine chemotherapy for muscle invasive bladder cancer. J Urol. 2013;189:1682–6.

73. Quek ML, Stein JP, Nichols PW, Cai J, Miranda G, Groshen S, Daneshmand S, Skinner EC, Skinner DG. Prognostic significance of lymphovascular invasion of bladder cancer treated with radical cystectomy. J Urol. 2005;174(1):103–6.

74. D'Souza AM, Pohar KS, Arif T, Geyer S, Zynger DL. Retrospective analysis of survival in muscle-invasive bladder cancer: impact of pT classification, node status, lymphovascular invasion, and neoadjuvant chemotherapy. Virchows Arch. 2012;461(4): 467–74.

75. Gondo T, Nakashima J, Ozu C, Ohno Y, Horiguchi Y, Namiki K, Yoshioka K, Ohori M, Hatano T, Tachibana M. Risk stratification of survival by lymphovascular invasion, pathological stage, and surgical margin in patients with bladder cancer treated with radical cystectomy. Int J Clin Oncol. 2012;17(5):456–61.

76. Palmieri F, Brunocilla E, Bertaccini A, Guidi M, Pernetti R, Morselli-Labate AM, Martorana G. Prognostic value of lymphovascular invasion in bladder cancer in patients treated with radical cystectomy. Anticancer Res. 2010;30(7):2973–6.

Laura-Maria Krabbe, Robert S. Svatek,
and Yair Lotan

2.1   Introduction

Bladder cancer is the 4th most common cancer in males (6 % of all cancers diagnosed) and the 11th most common cancer in females in the US in 2013 [1]. Overall, bladder cancer is the sixth most common cancer in the US with 72,570 estimated new cancer cases (54,610 in males and 17,960 in females) and 15,210 estimated deaths (10,820 in males and 4,390 in females) in 2013 [1]. Non-muscle-invasive bladder cancers account for approximately three-fourth of all new diagnosed bladder cancers, and can be subdivided into low-grade and high-grade disease. Low-grade disease

L.-M. Krabbe, M.D.
Department of Urology, University of Texas
Southwestern Medical Center,
5323 Harry Hines Blvd., Dallas, TX
75390-9110, USA

Department of Urology, University of Muenster
Medical Center, Albert-Schweitzer-Campus 1,
Gebaeude A1, Muenster, NRW 48149, Germany
e-mail: lauramaria.krabbe@ukmuenster.de

R.S. Svatek, M.D., M.S.C.I.
Department of Urology, University of Texas Health
Science Center San Antonio, 7703 Floyd Curl Dr.,
San Antonio, TX 78229, USA
e-mail: svatek@uthscsa.edu

Y. Lotan, M.D. (✉)
Department of Urology, University of Texas
Southwestern Medical Center, 5323 Harry Hines
Blvd., Dallas, TX 75390-9110, USA
e-mail: yair.lotan@utsouthwestern.edu

usually lacks the tendency to progress into muscle-invasive disease and remains rather indolent and not threatening to survival despite its tendency for frequent recurrence. In contrast, high-grade disease can progress to muscle invasion, which carries a significantly worse prognosis and can lead to severe morbidity due to the need for aggressive therapy to eradicate the disease from the bladder. The lifetime probability (from birth to death) of developing bladder cancer is 3.81 % in males and 1.15 % in females [1]. Depending on the stage of cancer at time of diagnosis the survival rates vary. Unfortunately, approximately one-fourth of all patients present with muscle-invasive or metastatic disease at diagnosis which leads to a poor prognosis for these patients. Patients with organ confined muscle-invasive bladder cancer at diagnosis have an estimated 70 % 5-year survival rate, while the patients with presence of regional or distal metastasis have approximately 33 % and 6 % 5-year survival, respectively [1]. Outcomes for patients with bladder cancer have not significantly improved in the last 25 years, so better methods for detection of bladder cancers before invasion or metastasis as well as better treatment options are needed to improve survival [2].

2.1.1   Basic Rationale for Screening

The concept underlying screening is to diagnose diseases in an asymptomatic population before

B.R. Konety and S.S. Chang (eds.), *Management of Bladder Cancer:*
A Comprehensive Text With Clinical Scenarios, DOI 10.1007/978-1-4939-1881-2_2,
© Springer Science+Business Media New York 2015

symptoms of the disease develop and to improve outcomes compared to the natural history of the disease. One test or a combination of different tests can be used, which should be cost-effective and accurate. Since screening focuses on an asymptomatic population at variable risk for the disease, the invasiveness of the diagnostic tests should be as low as possible so benefits will outweigh risks of screening. The National Cancer Institute published a statement in which three requirements were determined to be fulfilled to have efficacy of screening [3]:

1. Screening leads to earlier disease detection than if the cancer would have been detected because of symptoms.
2. Earlier detection and therefore earlier treatment can improve the overall outcome of the disease.
3. Prospectively collected screening results show a decrease in disease-specific mortality and an improvement in overall survival.

There are potential issues with screening that need to be considered. There is a risk for overdiagnosis of indolent disease which may lead to overtreatment. This is particularly problematic in prostate cancer as diagnosis often results in treatment with either radical prostatectomy or radiation therapy. Therapy for prostate cancer results in significant morbidity and decreased quality of life for many patients due to issues such as erectile dysfunction, urinary incontinence, urinary voiding dysfunction, or anxiety. One potential advantage of screening in bladder cancer is the relative minimal morbidity associated with removing bladder tumors. Second, the accuracy of the screening test is also important since false-positive results can lead to patient anxiety and unnecessary testing with attendant complications and cost. Furthermore, false-negative findings in a cohort at risk may lead to a false sense of security. Finally, benefits of population-based screening should outweigh the risks and show cost-efficacy before widespread utilization.

Interpretation of the benefit of screening based on provided data is subject to important biases termed lead- and length-time bias. Lead-time bias is a statistical distortion of results which can occur because a disease is diagnosed earlier than it would have if it was diagnosed following the onset of symptoms. The additional "lead time" could be falsely interpreted as an increase in survival. Length-time bias occurs because screening studies are more likely to detect patients with slower growing, less aggressive tumors simply because these patients have a longer period of time in the asymptomatic phase than faster growing tumors. Since these slower growing tumors are less likely to result in cancer-related death than the faster-growing tumors, persons with cancer detected through screening will seem to do better than persons with tumor detected without a screening test.

2.1.2 Basic Rationale for Screening for Bladder Cancer

Demographic facts have to be taken into account when discussing screening for bladder cancer. A screening test is most effective when the targeted disease either displays a high incidence or a high mortality [4]. Bladder cancer has a lower incidence and mortality than breast and colon cancer, but higher incidence rates than cervical cancer [1]. However, the incidence rates include all grades (low and high grade) and stages (invasive as well as non-invasive). Since the low-grade cancers are in most cases not life-threatening, their early detection will have minimal impact on survival and the impact of screening on the detection of high-grade or invasive cancers is most critical [2]. Based on the current incidence and the fact that low-grade non-invasive tumors constitute approximately 40–50 % of all bladder cancers, screening the whole population is unlikely to be effective. In order for bladder cancer screening to be considered, a high-risk cohort needs to be identified. There are several well-known risk factors for bladder cancer including increasing age and male gender [1]. The risk to develop bladder cancer increases significantly with rising age (probability of developing bladder cancer: 0.37 % in men under 60 years old and 3.69 % in men over 70 years old). Also the incidence of bladder cancer is significantly higher in men (37.5/100,000 men vs. 9.3/100,000 women).

Most bladder cancers result from smoking or less frequently environmental exposures. Risk factors for bladder cancer can be acquired through exposure to a carcinogen such as cigarette smoke, aromatic amines, or polycyclic aromatic hydrocarbons [5, 6]. These carcinogens can be subdivided in occupational (aromatic amines, polycyclic aromatic hydrocarbons) and non-occupational risk factors (smoking). Smokers have a four- to fivefold higher risk of developing bladder cancer compared to non-smokers [5]. Other risk factors can be determined genetically, like a positive family history or known predisposing syndromes like the Lynch Syndrome [7–9]. The probability of overdiagnosis of bladder cancer with screening seems negligible since invasive bladder cancers found at autopsies are extremely rare, suggesting that most invasive cancers become symptomatic in a rather short timeframe [10].

2.2 Urine Markers: What Possible Tools Do We Have And How Good Are They?

At this time bladder cancer is diagnosed in patients who are found to have blood in the urine. As such, the most commonly used tool to screen for bladder cancer has been to look for microscopic blood in the urine. Several urine-based tumor markers have also been investigated for their potential role in screening for bladder cancer, detection of bladder cancer in patients with micro-hematuria as well as for surveillance of recurrent bladder cancer. To date, none of them could demonstrate sufficient performance (sensitivity, specificity, and positive predictive value) to be recommended for screening. In this chapter, we will review the data available for tests that have been previously utilized for bladder cancer screening.

2.2.1 Dipstick Hematuria Testing

Dipstick testing of freshly voided urine is used commonly to evaluate the presence or absence of micro-hematuria, is inexpensive and gives immediate results. It can be done in the office or at home by the patients themselves after only little training. The test does not require intact red blood cells and can detect micro-hematuria with a sensitivity of 0.91 and a specificity of 0.99 [11, 12].

Unfortunately, there is a high prevalence of microscopic hematuria in the adult population (as high at 10–14 %) and most do not have bladder cancer with rates of 2–5 % in referred populations [13]. As such, the low positive predictive value (PPV) results in many unnecessary work-ups with resultant cost and anxiety. Unfortunately, dipstick performance in detection of bladder cancer is even less effective and results in a sensitivity of 0.52 and a specificity of 0.82 over all stages and grades [14]. Sensitivity is better for higher grade and higher stages of disease.

2.2.2 Cytology

Cytology is used high frequently to assess malignant, suspicious, or atypical cells in voided urine samples. It is a subjective procedure with high intra-observer variability and the results are not available immediately. Overall sensitivity of cytology is very low (approximately 34 %) but can be as high as 80–90 % for high-grade disease. It benefits form a very high specificity of 95–99 % which exceeds all available markers [14]. Cytology has not been studied sufficiently in the screening setting to determine its performance, especially when considering that many screened tumors may be smaller than those detected symptomatically. Furthermore, the test is relatively expensive since requires preparation and a pathologist to interpret results.

2.2.3 Nuclear Matrix Protein 22 (NMP-22)

The BladderChek NMP-22 test (Alere Inc., Waltham, MA, USA) is a point-of-care assay in which freshly voided urine is tested for presence or absence of nuclear matrix proteins, which are preferentially released into the urine during cell destruction as commonly present in malignancies.

Because of its superior sensitivity compared to cytology, the US food and drug administration (FDA) approved NMP-22 for detection of bladder cancer in patients with hematuria and surveillance of patients with a positive history of bladder cancer [15, 16]. Overall sensitivity is 0.73 and specificity is 0.80, also with better performance in higher grades and higher stages [14]. As other markers, the performance of NMP-22 has been primarily assessed in patients with bladder cancer or at risk for bladder cancer and needs to be better defined in a screened population.

2.2.4 Fluorescence In Situ Hybridization Assay (FISH)

The UroVysion FISH assay (Abbott Inc., Abbott Park, IL, USA) is a laboratory multi-target essay that detects aneuploidy of chromosomes 3, 7, and 17 as well as loss of 9p21 and in cells in voided urine with an overall sensitivity of 0.71 in patients with a history of bladder cancer and a specificity of 0.95 in healthy volunteers without a history of bladder cancer [17]. The specificity is generally lower in patients undergoing evaluation for bladder cancer (between 0.84 and 0.94) [18]. Furthermore, the lab-based assays have a considerably higher cost then point-of-care tests and this has a detrimental impact on their cost-effectiveness in the setting of screening large populations.

2.2.5 ImmunoCyt Test

Bladder cancer markers present on exfoliated cells in voided urine are detected by various fluorescent antibodies (19A211, M344, and LDQ10) of the ImmunoCyt test (DiagnocureInc, Québec, QB, Canada/Scimedx, Denville, NJ, USA) and evaluated in conjunction with cytology. This test is FDA-approved for surveillance of bladder cancer and not for detection at this time. Unfortunately this test is a laboratory test only, but reaches a sensitivity of 0.86 and a specificity of 0.79. Noteworthy is its overall good performance regardless of grade or stage of the tumors [19].

2.2.6 Bladder Tumor Antigen (BTA)

BTA-Stat and BTA-Trak are semi-quantitative and quantitative immunoassays detecting complement factor H (CFH) and related proteins (CFH-rp) in voided urine as a point-of-care test [20, 21]. BTA-Stat has a sensitivity of 0.71 and a specificity of 0.73 whereas BTA-Trak has a sensitivity of 0.69 and a specificity of 0.90 overall [14]. Best performance of both tests is in detection of tumors with higher grades and higher stages [14].

2.3 Screening for Bladder Cancer: What Data Is Out There?

2.3.1 Screening of the General Population

There have been only few studies investigating screening for bladder cancer in the general population (Table 2.1). Messing et al. tested 1,575 men (45 % of men solicited), older than 50 years for hematuria via repetitive home screening with urine dipstick testing [22]. The patients were advised to carry out daily urine testing for 14 days and if results were all negative, to repeat testing 9 months later for another 14 days. Patients with one or more positive tests were recommended to have a complete workup including intravenous urogram, cystoscopy, and cytology. A control group ($n=509$) was formed with data from the Wisconsin Cancer Reporting System (WCRS) which is a population-based tumor registry. Screening and control population had a similar mean age of 64.8 and 64.0 years and a comparable amount of smokers 15.9 and 22.0 % for current smokers at the time of study and 44.0 and 47.0 % former smokers. In the screening group 258 (16.4 %) men had positive dipstick testing and underwent evaluation as mentioned above. A total of 21 bladder cancers (1.33 %) were found on these evaluations and were treated according to tumor stage and grade. There was no significant difference found in the detected bladder cancers in proportion of low-grade and

Table 2.1 Screening for bladder cancer in the general population and heavy smokers

Study author	Country	Study time	Population targeted	No. of total patients in study	Primary test	No. of positive tests (%)	Further tests	No. of positive further tests (%)	Diagnostic procedure	No. of diagnostic procedures	No. of bladder cancer found	% of bladder cancer found in total population
General population												
Messing et al. [22]	USA	1989–1992	Men >50 years	1,575	Dipstick	258 (16.4)	–	–	Cystoscopy	258	21	1.33
Britton et al. [24]	UK	1989–1992	Men >60 years	2,356	Dipstick	474 (20.1)	–	–	Cystoscopy	317	17	0.72
Hedelin et al. [26]	Sweden	Before 2006	Men 60–70 years	1,096	Dipstick	174 (15.9)	–	–	Cystoscopy (white-light + fluorescent)	174	7	0.64
Bangma et al. [31]	The Netherlands	2008–2009	Men 50–75 years	1,747	Dipstick/UBC	409 (23.4)	NMP-22, MA, FGFR3, CH3	75 (18.3)	Cystoscopy	71	4	0.23
Total	–	–	Men >50 years	6.774	Dipstick	1.315 (19.4)	–	–	Cystoscopy	820	49	0.72
Heavy smokers												
Steiner et al. [35]	Austria	2007	Smokers ≥40 PY	183	Dipstick, NMP-22, Cytology, FISH	75 (40, 9)	–	–	Cystoscopy	75	3	1.64
Lotan et al. [36]	USA	2006–2007	>50 years, smoking >10 years, occupational exposure >15 years	1,502	NMP-22	85 (5.7)	–	–	Cystoscopy	69	3[a]	0.13
Total	–	–	Heavy smokers	1,685	Various	160 (9.4)	–	–	Cystoscopy	144	6	0.36

[a] 1 marked atypia

high-grade cancers between the screening (52.4 % vs. 47.7 %) and control group (60.3 % vs. 39.7 %), but the proportion of invasive high-grade cancers was significantly lower in the screening group (10 % vs. 60 % of all high-grade tumors detected and 4.8 % vs. 23.5 % of all cancers detected, $p=0.02$) [23]. The long-term outcomes showed that none of the men who had a cancer detected through screening died of bladder cancer, while 20.4 % of the patients with bladder cancer in the control group died of disease ($p=0.02$) and suggested a significant reduction in mortality from bladder cancer.

In a similar effort Britton et al. screened 2,356 men, older than 60 years, with weekly urine dipstick testing for a total of 10 weeks, without any repeat testing when results were negative [24]. Similar to Messing et al. [22], 474 (20 %) had a positive urine dipstick for hematuria and 319 underwent evaluation of hematuria. There were 17 (0.7 % of total study population and 3.5 % of men with hematuria) patients diagnosed with bladder cancer (out of which ten men had a positive cytology). As in the Messing cohort, approximately 53 % (9 of 17) of patients had high-grade disease but screening resulted in a significant reduction in the detection of muscle-invasive disease with no patients found by Britton to have muscle-invasive disease. Outcome results did not match the results of the Messing study however, since five of nine (56 %) patients with high-grade bladder cancer progressed to muscle-invasive bladder cancer, and three (33.3 %) died of disease as well as three died from unrelated causes [25]. No control group was available in this study, so understaging at the time of diagnosis or undertreatment of disease for high-grade tumors is a possibility.

In 2006, Hedelin et al. reported about a cohort of asymptomatic men (age 60–70 years) from Scandinavia [26]. They included 1,096 (55 % of invited men) and used urine dipstick, urinary bladder cancer test (UBC), and international prostate symptom score (IPSS) as screening tools. Patients with a positive urine test or IPSS >10 were evaluated with white-light and fluorescence cystoscopy. Seven tumors were detected with white-light cystoscopy, all in patients that had a history of smoking (two in patients without hematuria, but positive UBC test). No additional tumors were detected with fluorescence cystoscopy. The authors concluded that UBC and fluorescence cystoscopy were not useful in screening, and the high rate of micro-hematuria (25 %), without corresponding malignant disease, made screening of the general population ineffective.

The most recent study comes out of the Netherlands. With the aim to see if general population screening is feasible and to find a way to reduce cystoscopies, Roobol et al. initiated a prospective trial in which Dutch men aged 50–75 could participate [27]. A total of 6,500 men were invited to participate and were trained to conduct 14 consecutive, daily home urine dipstick testing. If one or more results were positive, participants were recommended to undergo further evaluation consisting of more urine tests using molecular markers in the first instance. Further urine tests consisted of NMP-22, microsatellite analysis (MA), fibroblast growth factor receptor (FGFR3), and multiplex ligation-dependent probe amplifications (MLPA) [28–30]. Recently, the final results were reported [31] with 1,747 men undergoing hematuria testing of which 409 men (23.4 %) tested positive with urine dipstick. Of these, 385 (94.1 %) men underwent subsequent testing for the other urine markers mentioned and 75 (18.3 %) had one or more positive test results and were referred for cystoscopy. Cystoscopy was performed on 71 (94.7 %) subjects and four bladder cancers (0.2 % of total population tested and 1 % of men with positive dipstick) and one kidney tumor were detected. Patients with positive markers, but negative cystoscopy were asked to undergo rescreening 6 months later. From linkage with the Dutch Cancer Registry one bladder cancer and one kidney cancer were missed by the screening protocol. Interestingly, three of four detected bladder cancers by protocol were in non-smokers, whereas the cohort had 58 % former smokers and 17.1 % current smokers. Also 36 % of the cohort stated a history of occupational exposures, but there was no significant difference between positive dipstick or positive molecular markers and smoking or occupational exposure. While use of a second-step combination of molecular urine markers resulted in a significant reduction of cystoscopies with very few missed cancers, the low number of cancers detected and high cost demonstrated minimal benefit of screening an asymptomatic unselected population.

2.3.2 Screening of Non-occupational High-Risk Populations

Targeted screening of high-risk patients increases the cancer yield and reduces the number of unnecessary evaluations. Identification of risk is an important component of screening for all cancers. Age is the primary risk factor in deciding when to screen for colon, breast and prostate cancer since cancer is typically a disease of the elderly. Similarly, any strategy to screen for bladder cancer will require a determination of risk and will be limited to the highest risk cohort, which will allow screening to be practical and cost-effective.

2.3.2.1 Definition of High-Risk Populations

As mentioned above (Sect. 2.2) various risk factors increase the chance for developing bladder cancer. A positive family history generates a two- to sixfold increased relative risk (RR) to develop bladder cancer, but this only accounts for around 2 % of total bladder cancer diagnoses [7]. Also tumor predisposing syndromes like the Lynch syndrome (see section "Screening in Patients with Lynch syndrome") increase the RR for developing bladder cancer up to 5.42 depending on genetic mutation present [3]. Non-genetic, acquired risk factors include smoking, occupational exposure and others like certain medications (thiazolidinediones, cyclophosphamide, and phenacetin), radiation exposure, exposure to herbs containing aristolochic acids, infections and chronic irritation due to indwelling catheters. Smoking is the leading cause of bladder cancer with an increased RR for former and current smokers (defined as >10 cigarettes/day). RR for current smokers is 4–5 times higher than for non-smokers and even former smokers kept an

increased RR of 1.3–2.7 for men and 1.8–3.8 for women, depending on intensity of former smoking, with the tendency to persist through time after quitting [5, 32]. Occupational exposure to aromatic amines or polycyclic aromatic hydrocarbons has an elevated RR between 1.16 and 1.23. The attributable risk is the amount of disease incidence that can be attributed to a specific exposure. Attributable risk is calculated by taking the difference in incidence of disease between exposed and non-exposed individuals. The attributable risk of bladder cancer from occupational exposures is 4.2–7.4 % [33]. There is also a gender and age-associated risk with men and older subjects exhibiting higher rates of bladder cancer as noted previously.

There have been attempts to quantify the degree of risk by establishing predictive models. A study by Wu et al. including 678 white bladder cancer patients and 678 controls found that significant risk factors for bladder cancer included pack-years smoked and exposures to diesel, aromatic amines, dry cleaning fluids, radioactive materials, and arsenic [34]. This model yielded good discriminatory ability (AUC=0.70; 95 % CI, 0.67–0.73) but improved to 0.80 (95 % CI, 0.72–0.82) when mutagen sensitivity data were incorporated. Mutagen analysis is expensive at this time and may not be practical for broad-based screening. Furthermore, this will need to be validated in prospective studies. Decision-analysis techniques were applied by Vickers et al. based on the occurrence of high-grade or invasive bladder cancer in the Prostate, Lung, Colorectal and Ovarian Cancer Screening Trial (PLCO) [7]. The PLCO included 149,619 individuals of 55–75 years of age and a risk score for bladder cancer was defined that consisted of four variables that could sum up to reach 0–11 points total (2 points for age >65; 2 points for smoking history >10–19 pack-years, 4 points for smoking history >20 pack-years, 4 points for male sex and 1 point for positive family history). If people with >6 points (around 25 % of the population) were screened for bladder cancer, 57 cases of high-grade or invasive bladder cancer per 100,000 people could be detected. Screening the total population would detect only 38 further cases at much higher costs. The assumption is that earlier detection would also reduce mortality if the cases can be identified before the cancer became invasive.

2.3.2.2 Evidence of Screening on high-risk populations

Few studies have been published concerning high-risk populations for bladder cancer. Two groups have presented results of screening in a high-risk smoking population (Table 2.1) and very diverse studies have shown conflicting results in screening people with occupational exposure (Table 2.2).

2.3.2.2.1 Heavy Smokers and Occupational Exposed People

The rationale for screening heavy smokers is that the majority of patients with bladder cancer are previous or current smokers and tobacco exposure is the most significant risk factor for the disease. Steiner et al. screened 183 heavy smokers (>40 pack years) using urine dipstick test, NMP-22, cytology, and FISH [35]. Participants with one or more positive test results were further evaluated including cystoscopy and imaging. Seventy-five men (40.9 %) had one or more positive test results and in further evaluation, 18 men (24 % of men with positive test results and 9.8 % of total cohort) were detected as having an abnormal histologic condition. Of those lesions 15 were in the urinary bladder (1 pT1 low-grade, 2 carcinoma in situ (CIS), 11 dysplastic lesions, and 1 inverted papilloma) and 2 upper tract urothelial tumors and 1 renal cell carcinoma. Thus a total of 6 men (3.3 %) had urinary tract malignancy and 12 (6.6 %) displayed a possible precancerous lesion of the urinary tract. The authors considered screening of this population efficient and the most efficient screening tool was the combination of FISH, cytology and urine dipstick testing. However, there are questions regarding cost implications of using multiple tests and their incidence of disease far exceeded that of any other screening study to date.

A larger study by Lotan et al. screened a high-risk population, defined as ≥ 10 years history of smoking ($n = 1,298$) or ≥ 15 years of occupational status ($n = 513$) using the NMP-22 BladderChek test [36]. In case of a positive NMP-22 result, the participants were advised to undergo evaluation with cystoscopy and cytology. NMP-22 was positive in 85 participants (5.7 %) and 69 underwent further evaluation, the other 16 declined. Of those that underwent further testing, three (3.5 %) participants were found to have lesions, including one pTa high grade, one pTa low grade, and one marked atypia. This represented 0.16 % of the total cohort. In the 12 months of follow-up period (range 0.9–25.5 months), 2 of 1,309 (0.15 %) participants developed low-grade non-invasive bladder cancer. The low incidence of cancer suggests that the selection criteria for bladder cancer risk were too low. Furthermore, women were included in the screening ($n = 327$) and all the cancers were confined to men.

Occupational exposure is known to increase the risk for development of bladder cancer. Still, various studies on screening of workers have shown that bladder cancer incidence is low and those studies lack information regarding time of exposure and smoking histories. Furthermore, they frequently were underpowered due partly to low acceptance rates of workers for screening (Table 2.2) [37–44]. While regulations have reduced exposure to potential carcinogens in the Western world, there is still concern for potential exposures in developing societies.

2.3.2.2.2 Aristolochic Acid

Zlotta et al. reported about screening a cohort of persons that had been exposed to aristolochic acid (present in certain Chinese herbs) and were diagnosed with aristolochic acid nephropathy (AAN) [45]. Patients exposed to aristolochic acid show a rapidly progressive renal interstitial fibrosis alongside with renal failure as well as a high incidence of upper tract urothelial cancers and bladder cancers. In their study, a total of 43 patients were screened for bladder cancer biannually for 10 years via cystoscopy and mapping biopsies. Bladder cancer was diagnosed in 25 patients (52 %). The vast majority (22 patients) were diagnosed with non-muscle-invasive cancer and none

Table 2.2 Screening for bladder cancer in workers

Study author	Country	Study time	Population targeted	No. of total patients in study	Primary test	No. of positive tests (%)	Diagnostic procedure	No. of diagnostic procedures	No. of Bladder cancer found	% of Bladder cancer found in total population
Davies et al. [37]	UK	1970	Workers	4,636	Urine microscopy	84 (1.8)	Repeat urine-test and Cystoscopy	–	3	0.06
Pesch et al. [38]	Germany	2003–2010	Workers exposed to AA	1,323[a]	Dipstick, Urine-sediment, Cytology, NMP-22, FISH	493 (37.2)	Cystoscopy	–	14[b]	1.06
Crosby et al. [39]	USA	Before 1991	Workers exposed to AA	541	Cytology	64 (11.8)	Cystoscopy	24	7	1.29
Marsh and Cassidy [40]	USA	1986–2001	Workers exposed to AA	277	Urinalysis, Cytology, Quantitative Fluorescence	51 (18.4)	Cystoscopy	40	3	1.08
Hemstreet et al. [41]	China	1991–1997	Workers exposed to B	1,788	Dipstick, Cytology, DNA ploidy, p300	153 (8.6 %)	Cystoscopy	116	28	1.57
Ward et al. [42]	USA	1969–1979	Workers exposed to BD	385	Dipstick, Cytology	60 (15.6)	Cystoscopy	200	3	0.78
Chen et al. [43]	Taiwan	Before 2005	Workers exposed to BD	70	Dipstick, Cytology, NMP-22	15 (21.4)	Cystoscopy	15	0	0.00
Giberti et al. [44]	Italy	2006–2008	Workers exposed to PAH	152	Dipstick, Cytology, ImmunoCyt	18 (11.8)	Cystoscopy	18	0	0.00
Total	–	–	Workers exposed to AA, B, BD, PAH	9,172	Dipstick, Cytology and others	938 (29, 37)	Cystoscopy	413	58	0.63

AA aromatic amines, *B* benzidine, *BD* benzidine derivates, *PAH* polycyclic aromatic hydrocarbons

[a]21 patients with history of BC included

[b]3 patients with history of BC

died of bladder cancer. However, three patients declined further screening and subsequently developed muscle-invasive and metastatic disease and died from bladder cancer. These results suggest that aggressive screening (consisting of urine markers alongside cystoscopy) in a population with these high incidences of bladder cancer and urothelial carcinoma in general seems obligate and effective.

2.3.2.2.3 Screening in Patients with Lynch Syndrome

Patients with Lynch syndrome express mutations in MLH1 and MSH2 (90 %) as well as MSH6 (10 %) and are at high risk of developing various cancers, which differ by mutation present [46]. These patients have the highest risk of developing colorectal cancer and endometrial cancer alongside with ovarian cancer, with age and mutation-dependent cumulative risks up to 49 % for colorectal cancer, 57 % for endometrial cancer and 38 % for ovarian cancer. But also other cancer entities are found more frequently in patients with Lynch syndrome like gastric cancer, small bowel cancer, biliary tract cancer, and urothelial cancer. Cumulative risk for urothelial cancer at the age of 70 years is estimated to a total of 1.9 % over all mutations, but up to 8 % for MSH2 mutations. In a recent publication by Skeldon et al., cancer incidences of patients with Lynch syndrome were compared to the general Canadian population and bladder cancer as well as upper tract urothelial cancer (UTUC) incidences were significantly higher in patients with MSH2 mutation (6.21 % for bladder cancer and 3.95 % for UTUC, both $p < 0.001$), but without statistical significance for MLH1 mutations [47]. Since patients and families with Lynch syndrome are under close observation for different cancers, patients with MSH2 mutations should be offered screening for bladder cancer and UTUC. Which testing and at what intervals has yet to be defined. Because of the considerably lower incidence of bladder cancer in the other mutations (MLH1 and MSH6), it will be important to consider the cost-benefit of screening these patients.

2.4 Cost and Cost-Effectiveness of Screening for Bladder Cancer

Cost and cost-effectiveness research is an important consideration when evaluating the feasibility and practicality of screening for bladder cancer. Currently, bladder cancer is estimated to cost approximately $3.98 billion and estimates have been projected at nearly $5 billion by 2020 (in 2010 dollars) [48].

Screening for other cancers such as breast and prostate cancer is widely practiced and from a cost perspective is considered reasonable but can result in costs up to US$50,000 per life year saved [49, 50]. Prevalence of disease, benefit of screening, performance of the test used and costs of the test play into the calculation, because a more expensive test has to perform significantly better than a cheaper test in order to maintain cost-effectiveness [51]. Cost for urine marker tests vary significantly with point of care tests such as NMP-22 BladderChek test or BTA stat costing approximately US$20–24 in comparison with laboratory tests such as FISH or ImmunoCyt that account for over US$200 per test. With lack of prospective studies up until now looking at cost-effectiveness of screening for bladder cancer, decision-analytic models are used to determine benefit of screening, which has the advantage of being able to vary certain factors such as marker cost, incidence of disease, and marker performance [51]. A Markov model, used to estimate cumulative cancer-related costs and efficacy of screening vs. no screening of a high-risk population for bladder cancer using a urine-based marker over a 5-year period, found that screening in a population with a bladder cancer incidence of >1.6 % would improve overall survival as well as result in potential cost savings [52]. This is unique and is bound to the fact that detecting high-grade tumors before muscle invasion results in survival advantage and also a cost-benefit due to lower costs for treatment of non-muscle-invasive tumors (transurethral resection of bladder tumors (TUR-BT) and intravesical therapy including follow up) compared to muscle-invasive tumors (cystectomy in combination with chemotherapy). Still, these results depend highly on cancer incidence. The relatively low incidence of bladder cancer, even in high-risk populations, remains the biggest challenge for a screening paradigm. Also performance of the markers used weigh heavily into the equation. While a higher sensitivity improves cost-effectiveness by improving survival due to earlier detection of cancer, a higher specificity increases cost-effectiveness by decreasing the number of unnecessary work-ups [51]. Also, cost of the test used has a major influence on cost-effectiveness for screening, since the cost of every test used will be transferred to each person screened.

2.5 Conclusions and Perspectives

Though screening for bladder cancer may be feasible in high-risk populations, there is currently no significant evidence to recommend such, because of lack of sufficient data to define screening protocols as well as lack of availability of high-performance urine markers reaching cost-effectiveness. There are few exceptions in which screening should be considered, consisting of patients with AAN due to their extremely elevated risk of urothelial disease. Furthermore, patients with Lynch syndrome and verified mutation of MSH2 likely have sufficient risk to justify screening for bladder cancer but the best screening practice is yet to be determined.

Demonstration of a survival benefit or at a minimum downstaging from muscle invasion to non-muscle-invasive disease is necessary before bladder cancer screening can be recommended. To demonstrate this would require a large prospective study targeting a population at sufficient risk and would ideally incorporate a cost-effective endpoint. One advantage of screening in bladder cancer however, unlike prostate cancer, is that the risks associated with unnecessary work-ups may be costly but have minimal risks. In prostate cancer the damage of unnecessary screening includes all the negative consequences associated with

prostate cancer diagnosis and treatment such as erectile dysfunction, urinary incontinence, and anxiety.

References

1. Siegel R, Naishadham D, Jemal A. Cancer statistics, 2013. CA Cancer J Clin. 2013;63(1):11–30. Epub 2013/01/22.
2. Larre S, Catto JW, Cookson MS, Messing EM, Shariat SF, Soloway MS, et al. Screening for bladder cancer: rationale, limitations, whom to target, and perspectives. Eur Urol. 2013;63(6):1049–58. Epub 2013/01/15.
3. NCI. NCI cancer screening overview. 2007. http://www.cancer.gov/cancerinfo/pdq/screening/overview. Accessed 26 Aug 2007.
4. Wilson J, Jungers GE. Principles and practice of screening for disease. Geneva, Switzerland: World Health Organization; 1968. p. 163.
5. Freedman ND, Silverman DT, Hollenbeck AR, Schatzkin A, Abnet CC. Association between smoking and risk of bladder cancer among men and women. JAMA. 2011;306(7):737–45. Epub 2011/08/19.
6. Silverman DT, Hartge P, Morrison AS, Devesa SS. Epidemiology of bladder cancer. Hematol Oncol Clin North Am. 1992;6(1):1–30. Epub 1992/02/01.
7. Vickers AJ, Bennette C, Kibel AS, Black A, Izmirlian G, Stephenson AJ, et al. Who should be included in a clinical trial of screening for bladder cancer? A decision analysis of data from the Prostate, Lung, Colorectal and Ovarian Cancer Screening Trial. Cancer. 2013;119(1):143–9. Epub 2012/06/28.
8. Garcia-Closas M, Malats N, Silverman D, Dosemeci M, Kogevinas M, Hein DW, et al. NAT2 slow acetylation, GSTM1 null genotype, and risk of bladder cancer: results from the Spanish Bladder Cancer Study and meta-analyses. Lancet. 2005;366(9486):649–59. Epub 2005/08/23.
9. Engel C, Loeffler M, Steinke V, Rahner N, Holinski-Feder E, Dietmaier W, et al. Risks of less common cancers in proven mutation carriers with lynch syndrome. J Clin Oncol. 2012;30(35):4409–15. Epub 2012/10/24.
10. Kishi K, Hirota T, Matsumoto K, Kakizoe T, Murase T, Fujita J. Carcinoma of the bladder: a clinical and pathological analysis of 87 autopsy cases. J Urol. 1981;125(1):36–9. Epub 1981/01/01.
11. Messing EM, Young TB, Hunt VB, Wehbie JM, Rust P. Urinary tract cancers found by homescreening with hematuria dipsticks in healthy men over 50 years of age. Cancer. 1989;64(11):2361–7. Epub 1989/12/01.
12. Rodgers M, Nixon J, Hempel S, Aho T, Kelly J, Neal D, et al. Diagnostic tests and algorithms used in the investigation of haematuria: systematic reviews and economic evaluation. Health Technol Assess. 2006;10(18):iii–iv, xi–259. Epub 2006/05/30.

13. Buteau A, Seideman CA, Svatek RS, Youssef RF, Chakrabarti G, Reed G, et al. What is evaluation of hematuria by primary care physicians: use of electronic medical records to assess practice patterns with intermediate follow-up. Urol Oncol. 2014;32:128–34. Epub 2012/11/17.

14. Lotan Y, Roehrborn CG. Sensitivity and specificity of commonly available bladder tumor markers versus cytology: results of a comprehensive literature review and meta-analyses. Urology. 2003;61(1):109–18. Discussion 18. Epub 2003/02/01.

15. Grossman HB, Messing E, Soloway M, Tomera K, Katz G, Berger Y, et al. Detection of bladder cancer using a point-of-care proteomic assay. JAMA. 2005;293(7):810–6. Epub 2005/02/17.

16. Grossman HB, Soloway M, Messing E, Katz G, Stein B, Kassabian V, et al. Surveillance for recurrent bladder cancer using a point-of-care proteomic assay. JAMA. 2006;295(3):299–305. Epub 2006/01/19.

17. Sarosdy MF, Schellhammer P, Bokinsky G, Kahn P, Chao R, Yore L, et al. Clinical evaluation of a multitarget fluorescent in situ hybridization assay for detection of bladder cancer. J Urol. 2002;168(5):1950–4. Epub 2002/10/24.

18. Lotan Y, Bensalah K, Ruddell T, Shariat SF, Sagalowsky AI, Ashfaq R. Prospective evaluation of the clinical usefulness of reflex fluorescence in situ hybridization assay in patients with atypical cytology for the detection of urothelial carcinoma of the bladder. J Urol. 2008;179(6):2164–9. Epub 2008/04/22.

19. Messing EM, Teot L, Korman H, Underhill E, Barker E, Stork B, et al. Performance of urine test in patients monitored for recurrence of bladder cancer: a multicenter study in the United States. J Urol. 2005;174(4 Pt 1):1238–41. Epub 2005/09/08.

20. Sarosdy MF, Hudson MA, Ellis WJ, Soloway MS, deVere WR, Sheinfeld J, et al. Improved detection of recurrent bladder cancer using the Bard BTA stat Test. Urology. 1997;50(3):349–53. Epub 1997/09/25.

21. Thomas L, Leyh H, Marberger M, Bombardieri E, Bassi P, Pagano F, et al. Multicenter trial of the quantitative BTA TRAK assay in the detection of bladder cancer. Clin Chem. 1999;45(4):472–7. Epub 1999/04/02.

22. Messing EM, Young TB, Hunt VB, Gilchrist KW, Newton MA, Bram LL, et al. Comparison of bladder cancer outcome in men undergoing hematuria home screening versus those with standard clinical presentations. Urology. 1995;45(3):387–96. Discussion 96–7. Epub 1995/03/01.

23. Messing EM, Madeb R, Young T, Gilchrist KW, Bram L, Greenberg EB, et al. Long-term outcome of hematuria home screening for bladder cancer in men. Cancer. 2006;107(9):2173–9. Epub 2006/10/10.

24. Britton JP, Dowell AC, Whelan P, Harris CM. A community study of bladder cancer screening by the detection of occult urinary bleeding. J Urol. 1992;148(3):788–90. Epub 1992/09/01.

25. Mayfield MP, Whelan P. Bladder tumours detected on screening: results at 7 years. Br J Urol. 1998;82(6):825–8. Epub 1999/01/12.

26. Hedelin H, Jonsson K, Salomonsson K, Boman H. Screening for bladder tumours in men aged 60-70 years with a bladder tumour marker (UBC) and dipstick-detected haematuria using both white-light and fluorescence cystoscopy. Scand J Urol Nephrol. 2006;40(1):26–30. Epub 2006/02/03.

27. Roobol MJ, Bangma CH, el Bouazzaoui S, Franken-Raab CG, Zwarthoff EC. Feasibility study of screening for bladder cancer with urinary molecular markers (the BLU-P project). Urol Oncol. 2010;28(6):686–90. Epub 2010/11/11.

28. van Oers JM, Lurkin I, van Exsel AJ, Nijsen Y, van Rhijn BW, van der Aa MN, et al. A simple and fast method for the simultaneous detection of nine fibroblast growth factor receptor 3 mutations in bladder cancer and voided urine. Clin Can Res. 2005;11(21):7743–8. Epub 2005/11/10.

29. van Rhijn BW, Lurkin I, Kirkels WJ, van der Kwast TH, Zwarthoff EC. Microsatellite analysis–DNA test in urine competes with cystoscopy in follow-up of superficial bladder carcinoma: a phase II trial. Cancer. 2001;92(4):768–75. Epub 2001/09/11.

30. Zuiverloon TC, Beukers W, van der Keur KA, Munoz JR, Bangma CH, Lingsma HF, et al. A methylation assay for the detection of non-muscle-invasive bladder cancer (NMIBC) recurrences in voided urine. BJU Int. 2012;109(6):941–8. Epub 2011/07/16.

31. Bangma CH, Loeb S, Busstra M, Zhu X, Bouazzaoui SE, Refos J, et al. Outcomes of a bladder cancer screening program using home hematuria testing and molecular markers. Eur Urol. 2013;64:41–7. Epub 2013/03/13.

32. Welty CJ, Wright JL, Hotaling JM, Bhatti P, Porter MP, White E. Persistence of urothelial carcinoma of the bladder risk among former smokers: Results from a contemporary, prospective cohort study. Urol Oncol. 2014;32:25.e21–5. Epub 2013/03/20.

33. Kogevinas M, 'tMannetje A, Cordier S, Ranft U, Gonzalez CA, Vineis P, et al. Occupation and bladder cancer among men in Western Europe. Cancer Causes Control CCC. 2003;14(10):907–14. Epub 2004/01/31.

34. Wu X, Lin J, Grossman HB, Huang M, Gu J, Etzel CJ, et al. Projecting individualized probabilities of developing bladder cancer in white individuals. J Clin Oncol. 2007;25(31):4974–81. Epub 2007/11/01.

35. Steiner H, Bergmeister M, Verdorfer I, Granig T, Mikuz G, Bartsch G, et al. Early results of bladder-cancer screening in a high-risk population of heavy smokers. BJU Int. 2008;102(3):291–6. Epub 2008/03/14.

36. Lotan Y, Elias K, Svatek RS, Bagrodia A, Nuss G, Moran B, et al. Bladder cancer screening in a high risk asymptomatic population using a point of care urine based protein tumor marker. J Urol. 2009;182(1):52–7. Discussion 8. Epub 2009/05/20.

37. Davies M. Final diagnoses after urinary screening of apparently normal workmen. Proc R Soc Med. 1970;63(3):242. Epub 1970/03/01.

38. Pesch B, Nasterlack M, Eberle F, Bonberg N, Taeger D, Leng G, et al. The role of haematuria in bladder cancer screening among men with former occupational exposure to aromatic amines. BJU Int. 2011;108(4):546–52. Epub 2011/01/13.

39. Crosby JH, Allsbrook Jr WC, Koss LG, Bales CE, Witherington R, Schulte PA, et al. Cytologic detection of urothelial cancer and other abnormalities in a cohort of workers exposed to aromatic amines. Acta Cytol. 1991;35(3):263–8. Epub 1991/05/01.

40. Marsh GM, Cassidy LD. The Drake Health Registry Study: findings from fifteen years of continuous bladder cancer screening. Am J Ind Med. 2003;43(2):142–8. Epub 2003/01/24.

41. Hemstreet 3rd GP, Yin S, Ma Z, Bonner RB, Bi W, Rao JY, et al. Biomarker risk assessment and bladder cancer detection in a cohort exposed to benzidine. J Natl Cancer Inst. 2001;93(6):427–36. Epub 2001/03/22.

42. Ward E, Halperin W, Thun M, Grossman HB, Fink B, Koss L, et al. Screening workers exposed to 4,4'-methylenebis(2-chloroaniline) for bladder cancer by cystoscopy. J Occup Med. 1990;32(9):865–8. Epub 1990/09/01.

43. Chen HI, Liou SH, Loh CH, Uang SN, Yu YC, Shih TS. Bladder cancer screening and monitoring of 4,4'-methylenebis(2-chloroaniline) exposure among workers in Taiwan. Urology. 2005;66(2):305–10. Epub 2005/08/16.

44. Giberti C, Gallo F, Schenone M, Genova A. Early results of urothelial carcinoma screening in a risk population of coke workers: urothelial carcinoma among coke workers. Biomed Environ Sci BES. 2010;23(4):300–4. Epub 2010/10/12.

45. Zlotta AR, Roumeguere T, Kuk C, Alkhateeb S, Rorive S, Lemy A, et al. Select screening in a specific high-risk population of patients suggests a stage migration toward detection of non-muscle-invasive bladder cancer. Eur Urol. 2011;59(6):1026–31. Epub 2011/04/05.

46. Bonadona V, Bonaiti B, Olschwang S, Grandjouan S, Huiart L, Longy M, et al. Cancer risks associated with germline mutations in MLH1, MSH2, and MSH6 genes in Lynch syndrome. JAMA. 2011;305(22):2304–10. Epub 2011/06/07.

47. Skeldon SC, Semotiuk K, Aronson M, Holter S, Gallinger S, Pollett A, et al. Patients with Lynch syndrome mismatch repair gene mutations are at higher risk for not only upper tract urothelial cancer but also bladder cancer. Eur Urol. 2013;63(2):379–85. Epub 2012/08/14.

48. Mariotto AB, Yabroff KR, Shao Y, Feuer EJ, Brown ML. Projections of the cost of cancer care in the United States: 2010-2020. J Natl Cancer Inst. 2011;103(2):117–28. Epub 2011/01/14.

49. Redaelli A, Cranor CW, Okano GJ, Reese PR. Screening, prevention and socioeconomic costs associated with the treatment of colorectal cancer. Pharmacoeconomics. 2003;21(17):1213–38. Epub 2004/02/28.

50. Krahn MD, Coombs A, Levy IG. Current and projected annual direct costs of screening asymptomatic men for prostate cancer using prostate-specific antigen. CMAJ Can Med Assoc J. 1999;160(1):49–57. Epub 1999/02/06.

51. Lotan Y, Svatek RS, Malats N. Screening for bladder cancer: a perspective. World J Urol. 2008;26(1):13–8. Epub 2007/11/22.

52. Lotan Y, Svatek RS, Sagalowsky AI. Should we screen for bladder cancer in a high-risk population? A cost per life-year saved analysis. Cancer. 2006;107(5):982–90. Epub 2006/07/25.

Amber Mackey, Farnaz Hasteh, and Donna E. Hansel

3.1 Introduction

Bladder cancer represents a broad diagnostic category that includes classic urothelial carcinoma and a spectrum of morphologic variants. In addition to urothelial carcinoma, less common primary tumors include pure squamous cell carcinoma, adenocarcinoma, and small cell carcinoma [1]. Challenges arise in surgical pathology diagnosis due to subtleties in recognizing uncommon variants, artifacts associated with tissue sampling and processing, and limitations in available ancillary techniques to aid in the diagnosis.

Tissue-based diagnosis of bladder cancer includes evaluation of biopsy, transurethral resection (TUR), and cystectomy/cystoprostatectomy specimens. Cytology is a useful adjunct in patient diagnosis in many instances, especially in patients with high-grade disease. Cytology specimens include both voided urine and bladder washes [2]. Each specimen type has limitations, risks, and benefits to be considered by the clinician. Diagnostic features and criteria differ between specimen types and often require an accurate clinical history and cystoscopy report for accurate diagnosis. Specifically, patient risk factors, prior treatment, cystoscopy findings, and the location of the lesion should be communicated clearly to the pathologist to provide the most accurate diagnosis [3, 4].

3.2 Non-neoplastic Urothelium

The urothelium is formed by 2–3 (distended) to 6–7 (contracted) layers of cells, which include umbrella cells (superficial layer), intermediate cells (mid portion of the urothelium), and basal cells (abutting the basement membrane; Fig. 3.1). Umbrella cells are elliptical with abundant eosinophilic cytoplasm and align in a single row to make up superficial most layer of the urothelium. These cells may distend or contract and are coined "umbrella" because when distended they stretch over several cells in the layer below. The presence of these cells is often reassuring that the lesion is either non-neoplastic or low-grade, as they are absent in most high-grade neoplasms. Intermediate cells may be cuboidal to low-columnar in shape with distinct cell borders, smooth nuclear contours, and stippled fine chromatin. Basal cells are cuboidal and form a single row of cells [5, 6].

Variation within the normal urothelium is common and may include a spectrum of benign proliferative and metaplastic processes that may

A. Mackey, D.O. • F. Hasteh, M.D.
Department of Pathology, University of California at San Diego, La Jolla, CA, USA
e-mail: anmackey@ucsd.edu; fhasteh@ucsd.edu

D.E. Hansel, M.D., Ph.D. (✉)
Department of Pathology, University of California at San Diego, 9500 Gilman Drive, MC 0612, La Jolla, CA 92093, USA
e-mail: dhansel@ucsd.edu

B.R. Konety and S.S. Chang (eds.), *Management of Bladder Cancer:*
A Comprehensive Text With Clinical Scenarios, DOI 10.1007/978-1-4939-1881-2_3,
© Springer Science+Business Media New York 2015

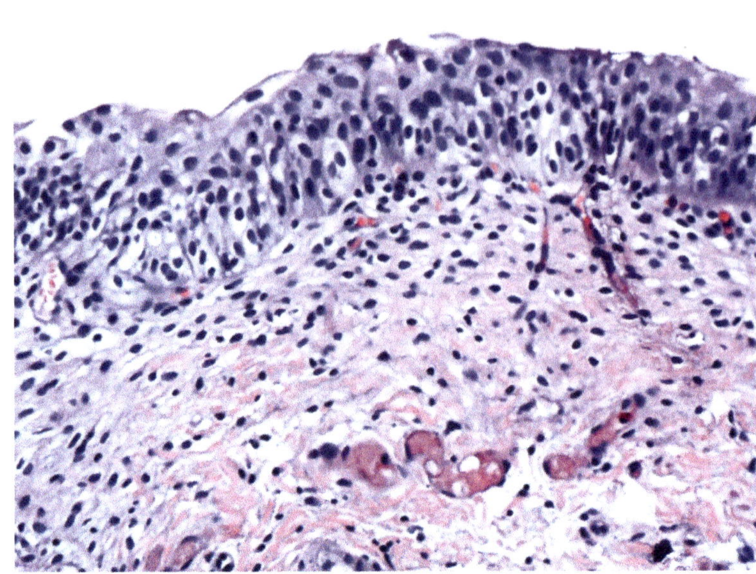

Fig. 3.1 Hematoxylin and eosin stain (H&E) of normal urothelium. Superficial umbrella cells (U) overlie layers of intermediate urothelial cells (UC). A single layer of basal cells (B) abuts the basement membrane. The underlying lamina propria (LP) is comprised of loose connective tissue filled with lymphatics and blood vessels

be diagnostically challenging [4–7]. Urothelial invaginations into the lamina propria, or von Brunn nests, are common in adult patients (Fig. 3.2a). These nests may become hyperplastic (von Brunn nest hyperplasia) or may dilate into cysts (cystitis cystica et glandularis) [8]. When florid, these conditions may mimic an early invasive carcinoma with or without glandular differentiation; however, the lack of involvement of deeper layers of the lamina propria and/or muscularis propria favors a benign process [6, 7]. Squamous metaplasia occurs frequently in the trigone of females and is often considered a benign alteration in the absence of keratinization (Fig. 3.2b) [9, 10]. In some instances, squamous metaplasia associated with reparative changes may lead to the development of squamoid "tongues" that extend into the lamina propria, a benign morphologic finding termed pseudocarcinomatous hyperplasia due to its ability to mimic invasive cancer (Fig. 3.2c) [11].

Cytologic variation also occurs under inflammatory or irritative conditions and is termed "reactive atypia." Reactive urothelial cells may have enlarged nuclei but typically have smooth nuclear contours, fine chromatin, and occasional small nucleoli (Fig. 3.2d). Polarity is maintained and mitotic figures may be present but not atypical and confined to the basal layers [6]. Umbrella cells are typically retained in the absence of denudation. Radiation therapy is a common cause of reactive atypia and also a risk factor for bladder neoplasia, thus making the differential diagnosis more challenging. The presence of smudgy, degenerative nuclear features, lack of mitotic figures, and an association with inflammation and vascular changes in the lamina propria aid in the correct diagnosis. Chemotherapy and Bacillus Calmette-Guerin (BCG) have been associated with atypia of the urothelium, with the latter showing characteristic granulomatous inflammation in the lamina propria. Finally, catheterization or other chronic injury can lead to squamous or glandular metaplasia or denudation of the epithelium, all of which may mimic neoplastic lesions [4].

3.3 Cystitis

Cystitis is inflammation of the urothelium and can be due to infectious or noninfectious causes. Infections may be bacterial, viral, fungal, or parasitic. Bacterial cystitis is comprised of mixed

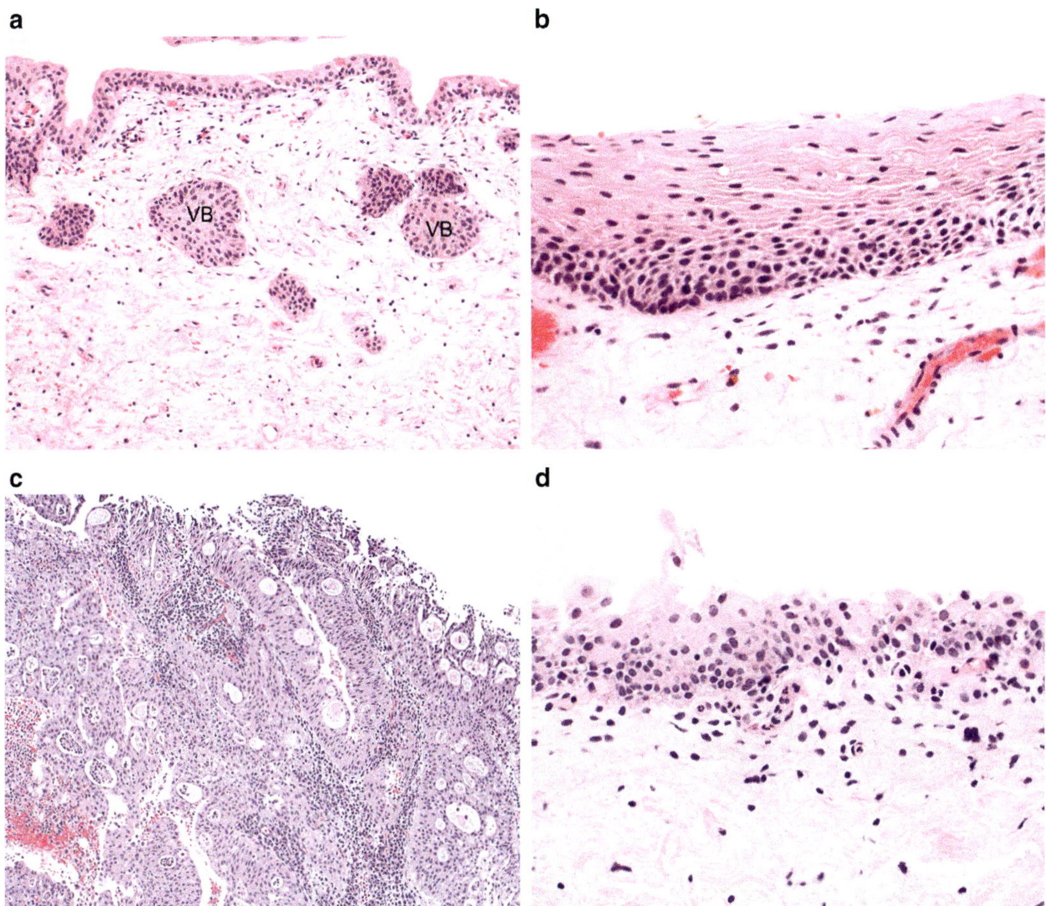

Fig. 3.2 Non-neoplastic features of the urothelium include (**a**) von Brunn nests (VB) are common in the adult bladder and represent invaginations of the urothelium; (**b**) non-keratinizing squamous metaplasia is considered a normal finding in the trigone of women; (**c**) pseudocarcinomatous hyperplasia is a reactive epithelial change that can mimic carcinoma; (**d**) reactive nuclear atypia is defined by enlarged nuclei with smooth nuclear contours, inconspicuous nucleoli and fine chromatin

inflammatory infiltrate. Viral cystitis has a background of inflammation with viral cytopathic features characteristic of the pathogen, including cystitis caused by herpes (large, multinucleated, glassy nuclei) and BK virus (enlarged, dark smudgy nuclei). Immunohistochemical staining targeted at viral antigens may be utilized to confirm the diagnosis [6].

Noninfectious cystitis encompasses a variety of unrelated entities that have distinct morphologic features and clinical associations. Interstitial cystitis often affects younger women and is associated with mucosal ulceration (Hunner's ulcers) and underlying focal hemorrhage; the etiology is unknown and likely autoimmune. Polypoid cystitis is associated with various inflammatory processes and catherization and is associated with bulbous, edematous protrusions of the urothelium that may grossly mimic a papillary neoplasm (Fig. 3.3a) [7]. Malakoplakia is associated with bacterial infection of the bladder and may represent a defect in the host histiocytic response to these organisms (Fig. 3.3b). This lesion is associated with nodular thickening of the mucosa and is defined by the presence of histiocytes with granular abundant cytoplasm (von Hansemann cells) and Michaelis-Gutmann bodies (concentric hydroxyapatite intracytoplasmic inclusions that

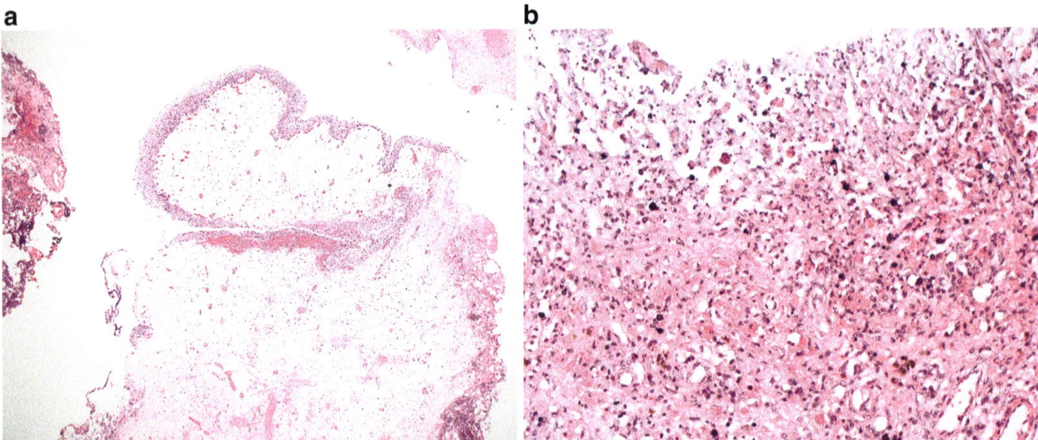

Fig. 3.3 (**a**) Polypoid cystitis shows broad-based, bulbous projections of urothelium with underlying edematous stroma; (**b**) Malakoplakia contains diffuse inflammation including histiocytes containing abundant granular cytoplasm and small round Michaelis-Gutman bodies

stain positively for calcium and iron) [6]. In general, these lesions are often distinct from carcinoma, but correct diagnosis is required for appropriate patient management.

3.4 Non-invasive Urothelial Neoplasms

3.4.1 Papillary Lesions

Papillary lesions are categorized in the US according to the 2004 WHO/ISUP classification scheme, which includes papilloma, papillary urothelial neoplasm of low malignant potential (PUNLMP), low-grade papillary urothelial carcinoma (LGTCC), and high-grade papillary urothelial carcinoma (HGTCC) [12]. Risk of recurrence and progression increase proportionately with grade using this schema. The lowest end of the spectrum is urothelial papilloma, which is morphologically defined as exophytic discrete (non-fused) papillary excrescences with thin fibrovascular cores (Fig. 3.4a). These fibrovascular cores are covered by essentially normal urothelium that lacks cellular atypia and shows limited to no mitotic figures. Umbrella cells are common and may be frequently vacuolated. These lesions have very low risk of recurrence or progression. PUNLMP is the next category of papillary lesions and is defined by urothelium with markedly increased thickness (often greater than ten layers) but no cellular atypia (Fig. 3.4b). LGTCC is defined as urothelium of any thickness that retains overall architecture and polarity but with scattered hyperchromatic nuclei and occasional mitotic figures that are normal and restricted to the lower layers of the urothelium (Fig. 3.4c). Finally, HGTCC is defined by moderate to marked architectural disturbance that includes frequent branching and fusion of papillary fronds. Loss of polarity, nuclear pleomorphism, irregular chromatin distribution, and prominent nucleoli are frequently present. In addition, denudation may be marked, resulting in naked fibrovascular cores without any adherent urothelium (Fig. 3.4d) [12, 13].

3.4.2 Flat Lesions

Urothelial dysplasia covers a spectrum of morphologies and its diagnosis is often challenging and subjective. By definition, dysplasia shows mild cellular and architectural changes that may include loss of polarity, nuclear crowding, and hyperchromasia. Mitoses are rare and mostly confined to the basal layer. Whereas dysplasia

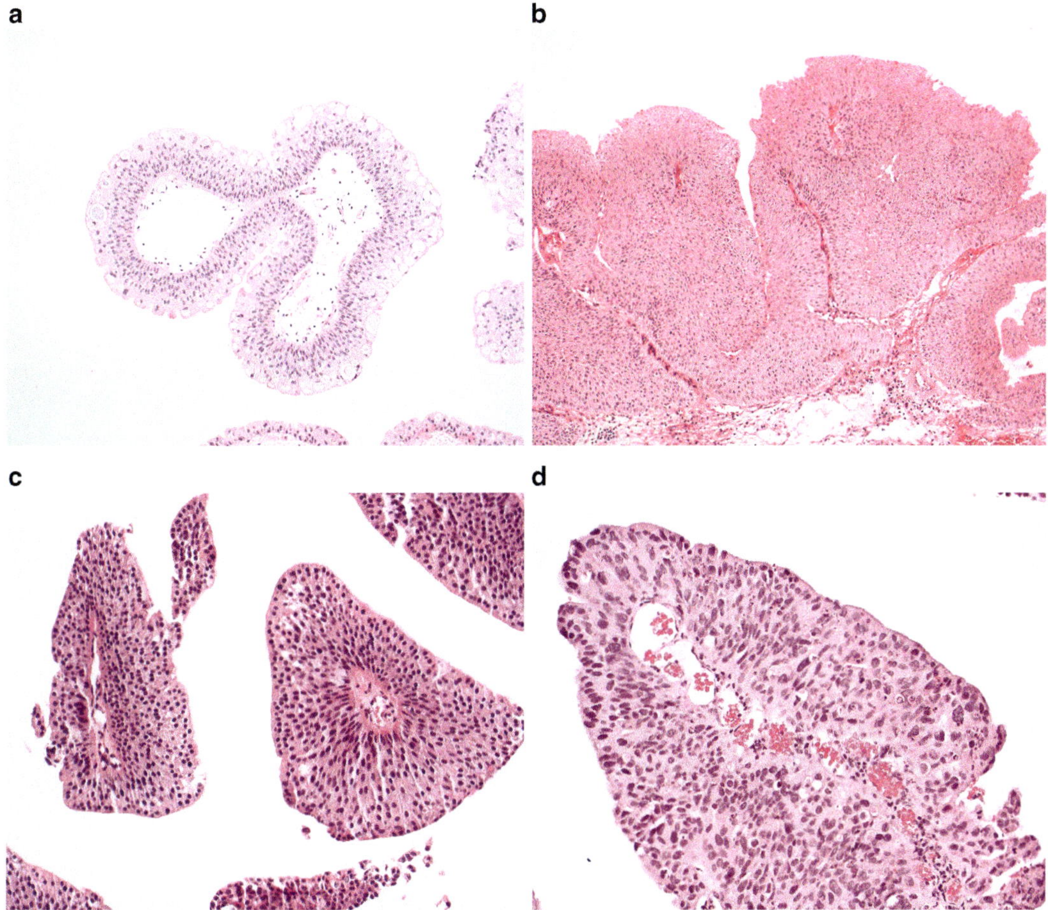

Fig. 3.4 Papillary lesions include (**a**) Urothelial papilloma with normal cytology and vacuolization of the umbrella cell layer; (**b**) PUNLUMP with marked thickness of the urothelium; (**c**) LGTCC showing scattered hyperchromatic nuclei but no disorganization; (**d**) HGTCC with marked nuclear atypia and loss of polarity

represents a precursor to the development of cancer in up to 20 % of cases, the remaining cases do not show progression; the atypical features seen in such instances likely represent a spectrum of reactive changes to early, limited neoplasia [14, 15].

Flat urothelial carcinoma in situ (CIS) represents a pre-invasive lesion in many instances and shares histologic features with HGTCC. In the classic form, disrupted polarity, nuclear pleomorphism and enlargement, prominent nucleoli and frequent mitotic figures high in the urothelium are often present (Fig. 3.5a). Numerous variants of CIS have been described and include micropapillary CIS (complex branching pattern),

clinging CIS (single layer of CIS cells attached to the surface), and pagetoid CIS to describe a few (Fig. 3.5b). Although most cases of CIS may be readily identified by light microscopy, immunohistochemical stains may be helpful in challenging cases (Table 3.1). Specifically, full thickness cytokeratin 20 expression, loss of basal CD44, and strong nuclear p53 expression in the majority of cells can help support the diagnosis [14, 16, 17]. These immunostains may also be applied to cases of dysplasia; however, the results are often variable and mixed and generally do not readily define a pre-neoplastic phenotype. CK20 is a low-molecular weight cytokeratin, representing intermediate filaments providing structural support

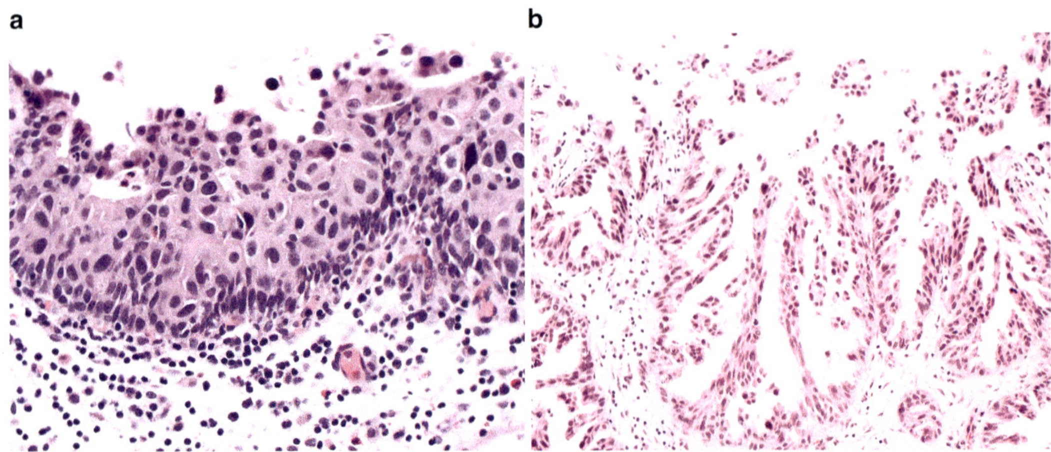

Fig. 3.5 CIS has numerous variants including (**a**) conventional CIS with enlarged hyperchromatic nuclei and architectural distortion and (**b**) micropapillary CIS showing complex branching papillary fronds that lack fibrovascular cores

Table 3.1 Immunohistochemical stains in the diagnosis of CIS [17]

Stain	Function	Pattern in normal urothelium	Pattern in CIS
p53	Tumor suppressor	Patchy cytoplasmic stain in urothelial cells	Intense nuclear expression in a large proportion of cells
CK20	Cytokeratin	Umbrella cell layer	Full thickness of urothelium
CD44	Cell surface receptor for hyaluronate	Basal cell layer	Absent
E-cadherin	Cell adhesion molecule	Cell membrane of urothelial cells	Absent or decreased
Ki67	Proliferation marker	Occasional patchy staining in urothelial cells	Increased throughout full thickness

to superficial umbrella cells. In neoplastic process it is expressed throughout the entire thickness of the urothelium and is not restricted to the superficial layer. Additional markers that have been described in CIS include loss of E-cadherin and increased Ki67, although these markers may not be as specific as the panel described above [18].

3.5 Invasive Urothelial Carcinoma

Conventional urothelial carcinoma (>90 % of bladder cancers) may demonstrate a range of morphologies and may be associated with flat CIS or HGTCC. In general, the presence of invasion associated with LGTCC is low; a recent study has identified focal high-grade features in the in situ component associated with these lesions, suggesting invasion occurs only in the presence of background high-grade disease [19]. Conventional urothelial carcinoma shows invasive nests of nondescript urothelial cells that may show minimal to marked nuclear atypia. In up to a third of cases, however, urothelial carcinoma variants may be present that can mimic virtually any other tumor type in the body (Table 3.2). Up to one-third of urothelial carcinomas may show divergent differentiation, with squamous differentiation present in two-thirds of these cases [12, 13]. Although beyond the scope of this discussion, several variants have been suggested to harbor a more aggressive disease course (e.g., micropapillary, nested) or limited response to therapy (e.g., squamous differentiation).

Table 3.2 Variants of urothelial carcinoma [12]

Urothelial carcinoma with squamous differentiation	Intercellular bridging and keratinization
Urothelial carcinoma with glandular differentiation	True glandular spaces; may appear colonic, tubular, mucinous or signet ring in appearance
Nested	Bland appearance; often missed at diagnosis
Large nested	Large bland nests
Microcystic	Microcysts admixed with macrocysts >1–2 mm
Urothelial carcinoma with small tubules	Bland, irregular small tubules
Lymphoepithelioma-like	Syncytial growth of tumor cells with vesicular nuclei; may be obscured by prominent associated inflammation
Lipoid-rich	Multiple large cytoplasmic vacuoles containing lipid
Glycogen rich/clear cell	Large tumor cells with clear cytoplasm
Urothelial carcinoma with rhabdoid features	Individual cells with perinuclear inclusion, eccentric nuclei, prominent nucleoli
Plasmacytoid	Individual cells with pink cytoplasm and eccentric nuclei
Sarcomatoid	Spindled cells and occasional osteoid production
Undifferentiated forms	May contain trophoblastic giant cells, osteoclastic giant cells, or giant cells NOS

3.6 Non-urothelial Bladder Cancer Forms

When conventional urothelial carcinoma occurs as an admixture with a variant, the carcinoma is considered to be urothelial in nature. However, when other bladder cancer subtypes are present in pure form (i.e., squamous cell carcinoma, adenocarcinoma, and small cell carcinoma) they are classified separately. It is likely that the pathogenesis of these entities are closely related and, in fact, pure forms of non-urothelial bladder cancer likely represent an outgrowth of a more conventional form [20]. For the purposes of this discussion, these entities are listed individually below with defining features and significant associations.

Squamous cell carcinoma is diagnosed when the invasive component of the lesion is associated with pure squamous differentiation (Fig. 3.6a). Lesions are graded based on the extent of differentiation, with well and moderately differentiated lesions showing the presence of intercellular bridges and keratin formation. In poorly differentiated lesions, keratinization may be scant and the diagnosis may be based primarily on the presence of desmosomes and dense pink cytoplasm. The in situ components associated with these carcinomas may vary and range from true in situ squamous cell carcinoma to high-grade urothelial carcinoma. Whereas pure squamous cell carcinoma occurs in only 5 % of the US population, squamous differentiation in the background of urothelial carcinoma is common. Recent gene expression profiling has shown that squamous and urothelial carcinomas share a significant proportion of dysregulated genes, suggesting a common origin to these two lesions [20].

Pure adenocarcinoma of the bladder comprises only 2 % of bladder cancers in the US and may originate from either the urachus or from glandular changes of the urothelium proper [12, 21]. In many instances, these tumors are large when discovered and the site of origin may be difficult to ascertain. The morphology of glandular differentiation in these carcinomas varies and may include adenocarcinoma NOS, signet ring cell, mucinous, clear cell, hepatoid, and mixed forms (Fig. 3.6b). The major differential diagnosis in this subset of bladder cancer includes spread of adenocarcinoma from the colon into the bladder. Although many groups have studied the utility of immunohistochemical stains in differentiating these two primary sites, application of these stains to individual patients remains challenging. In addition, a reduction in immunoreactivity may be evident in some variants, such as signet ring cell carcinoma [22]. A variety of in situ components, including urothelial CIS, may be present in association with invasive adenocarcinoma. Commonly, in situ glandular lesions including villous adenomas may be identified.

Small cell carcinoma occurs in <1 % of bladder cancers and consists of high-grade neuroendocrine carcinoma cells. Cells are small and

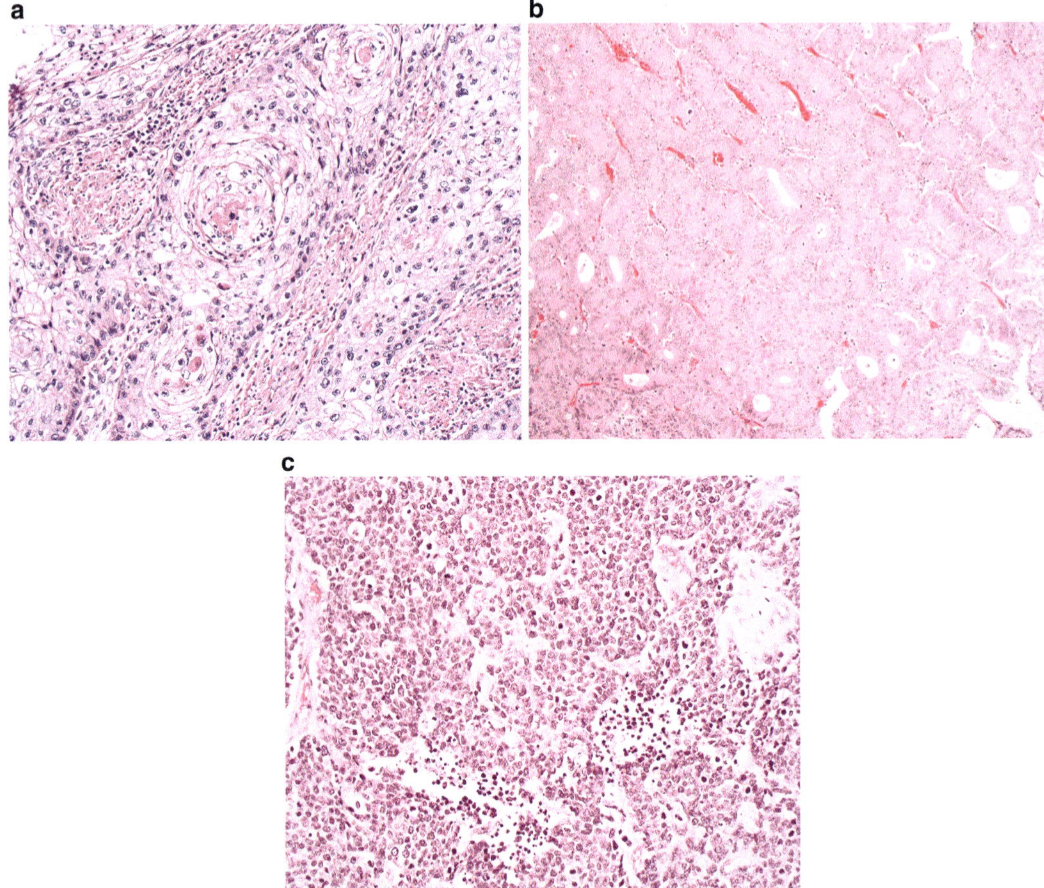

Fig. 3.6 Other primary carcinomas of the bladder include (**a**) squamous cell carcinoma showing intercellular bridges, keratinization and squamous pearls; (**b**) adenocarcinoma with colonic-type gland formation; and (**c**) small cell carcinoma defined by cells with increased nuclear/cytoplasmic ratio, "salt-and-pepper" chromatin and frequent mitotic figures

uniform with stippled chromatin, inconspicuous nucleoli, show nuclear molding and scant cytoplasm (Fig. 3.6c). Mitoses are frequent and necrosis may be present [12]. These lesions are often quite aggressive and may derive from a background urothelial carcinoma [13].

3.7 Staging of Bladder Cancer

The bladder consists of the urothelium and the underlying layers of lamina propria, muscularis propria (detrusor muscle) and perivesical fat, surrounded in parts by the adventitia. Bladder cancer staging follows these layers with increasing depth of invasion associated with increasing pathologic stage (Table 3.3) [13, 15, 23].

pT1 disease is defined by invasion into the lamina propria, which consists of loose connective tissue containing blood vessels, lymphatics and thin, wispy muscle called muscularis mucosae. This smooth muscle layer is generally thin and discontinuous; however, under some circumstances such as bladder stress or inflammation, these muscle bundles may undergo hypertrophy. This is clinically relevant, as the distinction between this hypertrophic muscularis mucosae layer and the detrusor muscle layer on biopsy or transurethral resection may be difficult to distinguish. pT2 disease involves cancer invasion into

Table 3.3 Bladder cancer staging [23]

pTx	Assessment of invasion cannot be performed due to limited specimen or cautery artifact
pT0	No residual in situ or invasive disease; often employed after neoadjuvant therapy or precedent BCG/TUR
pTa	Non-invasive high-grade papillary urothelial carcinoma
pTis	Flat CIS
pT1	Invasion into the lamina propria; includes invasion into the fibrovascular core of a papillary lesion
pT2	Invasion into the muscularis propria (detrusor muscle)
pT2a	Invasion of inner half of muscularis propria
pT2b	Invasion extends beyond inner half of muscularis propria
pT3	Invasion into the perivesical fat; performed on cystectomy only
pT3a	Invasion detected microscopically
pT3b	Macroscopically visible extravesicular mass
pT4	Invasion into adjacent organs
pT4a	Invasion into prostatic stroma or uterus or vagina
pT4b	Invasion into pelvic or abdominal walls

the large smooth muscle bundles of the muscularis propria (detrusor muscle). Identification of pT2 disease is critical in most patients for the decision to perform cystectomy versus conservative therapy. Whereas several studies have attempted to identify immunohistochemical markers specific for this muscle layer of the bladder (e.g., smoothelin), the utility of these stains has proven challenging due to a number of technical issues in various labs [24, 25]. Staging beyond pT2 can only be performed on cystectomy specimens, as fat may be present in all layers of the bladder wall; thus identification of pT3 disease is only possible when full thickness sections of the bladder wall are available for review.

Correct bladder cancer staging may be challenging for a number of reasons [26]. Limitations may occur at the time of sample collection, if only limited material is obtained (scant specimen) or if extensive cautery is used when obtaining the specimen. In such cases, the specimen may be staged as a pTx lesion, as inadequate evaluation of the lamina propria can be undertaken. Poor orientation of the specimen during embedding may lead to tangential sections and challenges in assessing the base of any in situ lesion for invasive cells. Finally, prior therapy may lead to morphologic variations that cause challenges in interpretation; this category includes prior chemotherapy, radiation therapy, or inflammation that leads to pseudocarcinomatous hyperplasia.

3.8 Utility of Cytology in Bladder Cancer Diagnosis

Cytology is commonly utilized for the screening and monitoring of bladder cancer. It is an inexpensive and minimally invasive procedure that provides ample information. It is most commonly utilized in screening high-risk patients (occupational exposure), monitoring recurrence, or for the workup of hematuria. Cytology is not frequently used for screening asymptomatic patients or intermediate risk patients. Cytology is most useful to provide basic information, such as the presence of atypical or malignant cells, and some characterization of the neoplasm, such as low or high grade. Accuracy of diagnosis in bladder neoplasia increases with higher grade disease or a greater extent of bladder involvement. In lower-grade neoplasia (LGTCC), false negatives are a potential error, and reactive or degenerative changes can lead to false positives.

3.9 Types of Cytology Specimens

Specimen types include voided urine, catheter-collected urine, and washing or brush samples. Voided specimens are easiest to obtain, need to be clean catch, obtained preferably 3–4 h after the last urine, and should not include the first urine in the morning [27]. While non-invasive and simple to obtain, the voided sample often provides few cells and these cells are poorly preserved and can be contaminated by the squamous cells from the genital tract. Cellularity is increased in many conditions like urolithiasis, urothelial neoplasia, and reparative processes after treatment and instrumentation [2, 27, 28].

Catheter specimens collect urine into a pooled container. They are more difficult to obtain, requiring a minimally invasive procedure and carry a risk of infection. Instrumentation artifact, bacteria, inflammatory cells, and pooling of urine with degenerated cells can lead to poor quality specimens. However, they provide more cells than voided urine and with less contamination from the genital tract. Bladder washings utilize a catheter in which saline is pulsed into the bladder and then collected. This method provides a superior specimen to voided or catheter specimens in that it provides higher numbers of well-preserved cells with little-to-no contamination but with known artifact [27]. It also carries the same risks of catheterization (minimally invasive procedure with risk of infection and instrumentation artifact) and is more expensive. Directed washing (upper tract) and brush procedures provide a similar sample to bladder washings but with direct selective sampling of the suspicious area. However, these are more difficult and expensive procedures, carrying inherent risks associated with an invasive procedure.

In patients who have undergone cystectomy, an ileal loop/conduit may be utilized for urine screening after cystectomy. This can be useful for monitoring recurrence in the ureter or renal pelvis [27, 28]. However, these specimens are often difficult to interpret and usually show contamination from the intestinal lining cells and bacteria that can obscure background cancer cells.

3.10 Nomenclature/Reporting of Cytology Specimens

In order to provide useful information to the clinician, nomenclature and reporting has to be clear and applied using standardized terminology (Table 3.4). Specimen adequacy has not been well defined; however, unsatisfactory specimens are defined as those with severe cellular degeneration or the presence of marked obscuring inflammatory cells or lubricants.

If no malignant cells or atypical cells are identified, the specimen is termed "negative for malignancy" on the diagnostic line. When mild

Table 3.4 Nomenclature of urine cytology specimens [27, 28]

Term	Definition
Non-diagnostic or unsatisfactory specimen	Cellularity too limited or obscuring inflammation
Negative for malignancy	No malignant cells identified
Atypical cells present	Clusters of urothelial cells in voided urine or mildly atypical urothelial cells. May indicate reparative process, instrumentation, stone or low-grade (papilloma, PUNLMP) papillary neoplasm
Suspicious for urothelial carcinoma	Highly atypical urothelial cells concerning for malignancy but lacking enough nuclei or adequate preservation for definitive diagnosis
Positive for malignancy	Clear cut atypical features that support a diagnosis of urothelial carcinoma

cellular atypia is present, the diagnosis of "atypical cells present" is rendered. Atypical cells could represent a low-grade lesion or reactive changes. When moderate atypia is present, but the cells are lacking criteria for a diagnosis of malignancy, they are termed "suspicious." Finally, when the features are conclusive for malignancy the diagnostic line reads "positive." [28] Whereas the diagnostic extremes are easy to interpret, the utility of atypia in predicting the presence of subsequent neoplasia varies somewhat between pathologists.

3.11 Cytologic Diagnostic Criteria

Low-grade lesions including hyperplasia, papilloma, or PUNLUMP are nearly impossible to differentiate from each other on cytology because they, by definition, lack cytologic atypia and rarely are associated with the denudation common in high-grade lesions. Certain features may give clues to low-grade lesions, such as clustering of urothelial cells with crowding and loss of honeycombing, especially when present in voided urine [27]. In addition, umbrella cells are often retained in these low-grade lesions. Rarely papillary fronds with delicate fibrovascular cores may provide a clue to the diagnosis of a papillary neoplasm. Overall, these lesions are rarely diagnosed on cytology.

In LGTCC, the specimen may show increased cellularity with cells forming loose-to-crowded clusters in a haphazard growth pattern (Fig. 3.7). Cells show atypia with mild variation including cellular enlargement, eccentric nuclei, increased nuclear/cytoplasmic ratio, and irregular and thickened nuclear membranes. The chromatin is uniform, dark and granular with small, inconspicuous nucleoli. Infrequent mitotic figures are seen. The cytoplasm is typically homogenous without vacuoles. These findings are often diagnosed as suspicious [2, 27, 28]. Clues to a diagnosis of urothelial neoplasia include coy cells (small single cells with high N/C ratio), bird's eyes (entosis, or cells wrapped around another cell), pyknotic cells, and eccentric nuclei.

High-grade urothelial lesions are diagnosed more frequently as CIS rather than HGTCC. High-grade cells show obvious malignant features and are present as individual cells or in small clusters (Fig. 3.8a, b). The frequent denudation in high-grade lesions makes detection of this category more common on cytology. The cells appear overlapped, with crowded large nuclei showing a high nuclear/cytoplasmic ratio (Fig. 3.9a, b). The chromatin is coarse and dark with large nucleoli and frequent indentation of the nuclear membrane. Mitosis or atypical mitotic figures may occur. The cytoplasm is often very small and sometimes vacuolated. Umbrella cells are absent in these lesions and there is often a background tumor diathesis [27, 28].

Variants are common in urothelial neoplasia and are generally associated with high-grade lesions. As described previously, squamous and glandular differentiation occur most commonly. The presence of such divergent differentiation is common in high-grade urothelial tumors and cannot be used to distinguish a pure adenocarcinoma or squamous cell carcinoma from urothelial carcinoma with

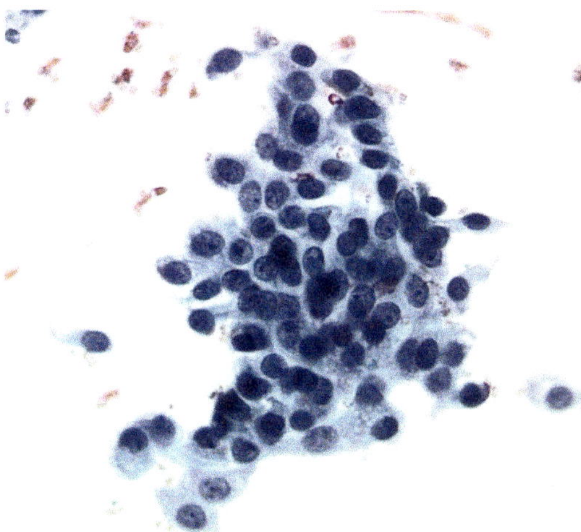

Fig. 3.7 Low-grade papillary urothelial carcinoma shows clusters of cells with loss of honeycombing, with enlarged and variable nuclei on cytology

a　　　　　　　　　　　　　　　　　b

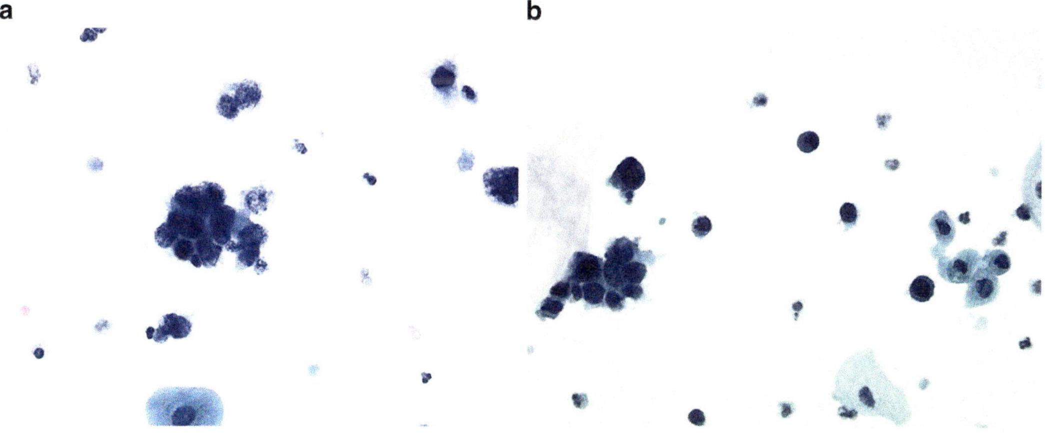

Fig. 3.8 High-grade urothelial carcinoma at cytology shows hyperchromatic, pleomorphic, irregularly shaped nuclei and coarse chromatin. (**a**) Clusters or (**b**) individual cells may be present

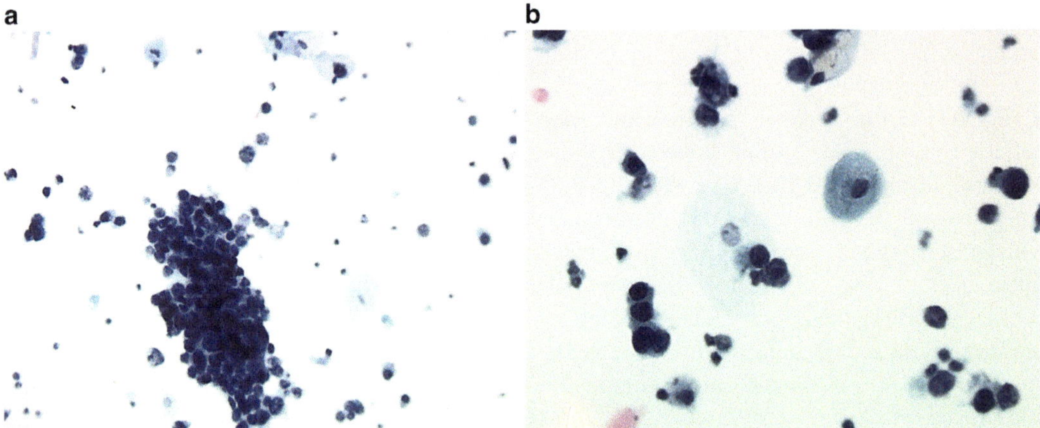

Fig. 3.9 High-grade urothelial carcinoma at cytology show (**a**) clusters of overlapped and crowded nuclei and (**b**) individual cells with hyperchromatic, pleomorphic, irregularly shaped nuclei and coarse chromatin

divergent differentiation on cytology. Finally, invasion cannot be accurately determined on cytology due to the lack of tissue-based orientation inherent in these specimen types.

3.12 Benign Urinary Tract Diseases on Cytology

Benign urinary tract diseases and conditions include infectious and noninfectious causes and may mimic malignancy in cytology or histology specimens. In many of these cases, the features that appear most obvious in cytology specimens may be more difficult to ascertain in biopsy or TUR specimens.

Infections may be bacterial (malakoplakia), fungi, parasitic (*Trichomonas vaginalis*), or viral such as herpes simplex virus (HSV), cytomegalovirus (CMV), polyomavirus, or human papilloma virus (HPV). Viral infections have characteristic cellular changes that can mimic malignancy. For example, the "decoy cell" found in polyomavirus has increased nuclear size, hyperchromasia and high N/C ratio and are named due to its ability to mimic malignant features (Fig. 3.10). The presence of ground glass chromatin, round and smooth nuclear membranes assists in a benign diagnosis.

Noninfectious findings include crystals, casts, nonspecific reactive changes, and therapeutic

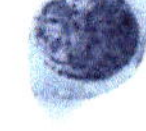

Fig. 3.10 Polyomavirus (decoy cell) cells have increased cellular size but with round, smooth nuclear contours. Note the glassy homogenous nuclear appearance due to intranuclear viral inclusions

effects [2, 27, 28]. Nonspecific reactive changes are similar to those identified in tissue specimens and include enlarged nuclei, prominent nucleoli, coarsely vacuolated cytoplasm but an absence of nuclear atypia such as dense chromatin, irregular nuclear contours, and high N/C ratio. Calculi may cause damage creating cellular changes including increased cellularity, variable N/C ratio, frayed cytoplasm, dark coarse chromatin, and irregular nuclear contours.

Therapeutic changes occur secondary to chemotherapy, radiation, and BCG changes. Changes due to radiation or chemotherapy typically include cellular and nuclear enlargement, but without change in N/C ratio, nuclear vacuolization, and smudged chromatin, with retention of smooth nuclear contours. BCG effects can leave multinucleated giant cells in a granulomatous background.

3.12.1 UroVysion

The UroVysion (®) assay is a commercially available kit that utilizes fluorescence in situ hybridization (FISH) using multiple probes to detect aneuploidy in chromosomes 3, 7 and 17, and loss of 9p21. It is utilized in urine cytology cases of urothelial atypia to help differentiate reactive from malignant processes. A negative result supports the diagnosis of a benign reactive process. A positive test result in cytology specimens that lack morphologic high-grade features may indicate the presence of urothelial carcinoma but is not always specific and does not identify the location within the urinary tract [29, 30].

References

1. Siegel R, Naishadham D, Jemal A. Cancer statistics, 2013. CA Cancer J Clin. 2013;63:11–30.
2. Renshaw A. Urine and bladder washings. In: Cibas E, Ducatman BS, editors. Cytology diagnostic principles and clinical correlates. 3rd ed. Philadelphia: Saunders Elsevier; 2009. p. 105–27.
3. Hansel DE, Miller JS, Cookson MS, Chang SS. Challenges in the pathology of non-muscle-invasive bladder cancer: a dialogue between the urologic surgeon and the pathologist. Urology. 2013;81(6):1123–30.
4. Lopez-Beltran A, Luque RJ, Mazzucchelli R, Scarpelli M, Montironi R. Changes produced in the urothelium by traditional and newer therapeutic procedures for bladder cancer. J Clin Pathol. 2002;55:641–7.
5. Rosai J. Rosai and Ackerman's surgical pathology. 10th ed. Philadelphia: Elsevier; 2011.
6. Harik LR, O'Toole KM. Nonneoplastic lesions of the prostate and bladder. Arch Pathol Lab Med. 2012;136(7):721–34.
7. Young RH. Tumor-like lesions of the urinary bladder. Mod Pathol. 2009;22:S37–52.
8. Smith AK, Hansel DE, Jones JS. Role of cystitis cystica et glandularis and intestinal metaplasia in development of bladder carcinoma. Urology. 2008;71(5):915–8.
9. Lagwinski N, Thomas A, Stephenson AJ, Campbell S, Hoschar AP, El-Gabry E, Dreicer R, Hansel DE. Squamous cell carcinoma of the bladder: a clinico-pathologic analysis of 45 cases. Am J Surg Pathol. 2007;31:1777–87.
10. Ozbey I, Aksoy Y, Polat O, Bicgi O, Demirel A. Squamous metaplasia of the bladder: findings in 14 patients and review of the literature. Int Urol Nephrol. 1999;31:457–61.
11. Lara HR, Merino C, Coindre JM, Amin M, Pedeutour F, Weiss SW. Pseudosarcomatous myofibroblastic proliferations of the bladder: a clinicopathologic study of 42 cases. Am J Surg Pathol. 2006;30:787–94.
12. Eble JN, Sauter G, Epstein JI, Sesterhenn IAE. World Health Organization classification of tumours: pathology and genetics of tumours of the urinary system and male genital organs. Lyon: IARC Press; 2004.
13. Amin MB, McKenney JK, Paner GP, Hansel DE, Grignon DJ, Montironi R, Lin O, Jorda M, Jenkins LC, Soloway M, Epstein JI, Reuter VE. ICUD-EAU International Consultation of Bladder Cancer 2012: pathology. Eur Urol. 2013;63:16–35.
14. Hodges KB, Lopez-Beltran A, Davidson D, Monitroni R, Cheng L. Urothelial dysplasia and other flat lesions of the urinary bladder: clinicopathologic and molecular features. Hum Pathol. 2010;41(2):155–62.
15. Babjuk M, Burger M, Zigeuner R, Shariat SF, van Rhijn BWG, Comperat E, Slvester RJ, Kaasinen E, Bohle A, Redorta JP, Roupret M. EAU Guidelines on non-muscle-invasive urothelial carcinoma of the bladder: update 2013. Eur Urol. 2013;64(4):639–53. doi:10.1016/j.eururo.2013.06.003. Epub 2013 Jun 12.
16. Nikiforova MN, Nikiforov YE. Molecular anatomic pathology: principles, techniques and application to immunohistologic diagnosis. In: Dabbs D, editor. Diagnostic immunohistochemistry. Philadelphia: Saunders Elsevier; 2010. p. 49–50.
17. Coleman JF, Hansel DE. Utility of diagnostic and prognostic markers in urothelial carcinoma of the bladder. Adv Anat Pathol. 2009;16(2):68–78.
18. Kamat AM, Hegarty PK, Gee JR, Clark PE, Svatek RS, Hegarty N, Shariat SF, Xylinas E, Scmitz-Drager BJ, Lotan Y, Jenkins LC, Droller M, van Rhijn BW, Karakiewicz PI. ICUD-EAU International Consultation on Bladder Cancer 2012: screening, diagnosis, and molecular markers. Eur Urol. 2013;63:4–15.
19. Watts KE, Montironi R, Mazzucchelli R, van der Kwast T, Osunkoya AO, Stephenson AJ, Hansel DE. Clinicopathologic characteristics of 23 cases of invasive low-grade papillary urothelial carcinoma. Urology. 2012;80:361–6.
20. Hansel DE, Zhang Z, Petillo D, Teh BT. Gene profiling suggests a common evolution of bladder cancer subtypes. BMC Med Genomics. 2013;6:42.
21. Zhong M, Gersbach E, Rohan SM, Yang XJ. Primary adenocarcinoma of the urinary bladder: differential diagnosis and clinical relevance. Arch Pathol Lab Med. 2013;137(3):371–81.
22. Thomas AA, Stephenson AJ, Campbell SC, Jones JS, Hansel DE. Clinicopathologic features and utility of immunohistochemical markers in signet-ring cell adenocarcinoma of the bladder. Hum Pathol. 2009;40:108–16.

23. Edge SB, Byrd DR, Compton CC, Fritz AG, Greene FL, Trotti A. AJCC cancer staging manual. 7th ed. New York: Springer; 2010.

24. Paner GP, Brown JG, Lapetino S, Nese N, Gupta R, Shen SS, Hansel DE, Amin MB. Diagnostic use of antibody to smoothelin in the recognition of muscularis propria in transurethral resection of urinary bladder tumor (TURBT) specimens. Am J Surg Pathol. 2010;34:792–9.

25. Hansel DE, Paner GP, Nese N, Amin MB. Limited smoothelin expression within the muscularis mucosae: validation in bladder diverticula. Hum Pathol. 2011;42:1770–6.

26. Hansel DE, Amin MB, Comperat E, Cote RJ, Knuchel R, Montironi R, Reuter VE, Soloway MS, Umar SA, Van der Kwast TH. A contemporary update on pathology standards for bladder cancer: transurethral resection and radical cystectomy specimens. Eur Urol. 2013;63:31–2.

27. Demay RM. Urine. In: Demay RM, editor. The art & science of cytopathology. 2nd ed. ASCP: Chicago, IL; 2012. p. 436–89.

28. Rosenthal DL, Raab SS. Cytologic detection of urothelial lesions, essentials in cytopathology series, vol II. New York: Springer; 2006.

29. Dimashkeih H, Wolff DJ, Smith TM, Houser PM, Nietert PJ, Yang J. Evaluation of UroVysion and cytology for bladder cancer detection: a study of 1835 paired urine samples with clinical and histologic correlation. Cancer Cytopathol. 2013;121(10):591–7. doi:10.1002/cncy.21327. Epub 2013 Jun 25.

30. Smith GD, Wilson A, Gopez EV, Tripp SR, Pasi A. A retrospective review of UroVysion FISH interpretations over 8.6 years: a major shift in the patient test population. Diagn Cytopathol. 2012;41(5):437–47.

Sean McAdams and Michael C. Risk

4.1 Introduction

Bladder cancer is the fourth most common cancer in men and tenth most common in women in the US, with an estimated 72,570 new cases diagnosed in 2013 (about 54,610 in men) and an estimated 15,210 deaths (about 10,820 in men) [1]. Bladder cancer is 3–4 times more likely in men than women, and is diagnosed twice as often in whites compared to African-Americans [2] for reasons that are not understood.

Histologically, 95–97 % of bladder cancer in the US and European countries is urothelial cell cancer (UCC) [3], which will be the focus of this chapter. Clinically, bladder cancer can be broadly divided into non-muscle invasive (NMIBC) or muscle invasive (MIBC), and NMIBC accounts for about 75 % of disease at initial diagnosis. NMIBC is further classified based on the tumor, node and metastases (TNM) system as Ta (confined to epithelium), carcinoma in situ (Tis or CIS), or T1 (invasion of the lamina propria). Additionally, tumors are often divided into low- and high-grade disease based on cellular differentiation. Low-grade disease is almost universally non-invasive, and accounts for about 60 % of NMIBC. The remainder of NMIBC (high-grade Ta, T1 and CIS) is high-grade, as is all MIBC. These categories (high-grade vs. low-grade) correspond to distinct histologic phenotypes that present different risks for recurrence and progression and thus direct management of those with NMIBC. Low-grade disease (including papillary urothelial neoplasm of low malignant potential (PUNLMP) and low-grade Ta) demonstrates a high rate of recurrence but a low risk of progression to MIBC and is often amenable to transurethral resection alone. In contrast, high-grade NMIBC (including CIS and high-grade Ta-T1) carries a high rate of recurrence and a high risk of progression, and therefore requires more aggressive management with intravesical therapy and close surveillance. MIBC has a high risk of metastatic progression and mandates radical treatments such as cystectomy and chemotherapy. MIBC carries a poor prognosis, with overall survival at 5 years of approximately 50 %.

UCC has an established association with increasing age and a variety of environmental exposures, including cigarette smoke. Cigarette smoking is the strongest and most common risk factor for bladder cancer conferring a twofold

S. McAdams, M.D.
Department of Urology, University of Minnesota,
420 Delaware St. SE, MMC 394, C512 Mayo
Building, Minneapolis, MN 55455, USA
e-mail: mcad0022@umn.edu

M.C. Risk, M.D., Ph.D. (✉)
Department of Urology, University of Minnesota,
420 Delaware St. SE, MMC 394, C512 Mayo
Building, Minneapolis, MN 55455, USA

Department of Urology, Minneapolis VA Medical
Center, One Veterans Drive (112D), Minneapolis,
MN 55417, USA
e-mail: mcrisk@umn.edu; mchlrisk@yahoo.com

B.R. Konety and S.S. Chang (eds.), *Management of Bladder Cancer:
A Comprehensive Text With Clinical Scenarios*, DOI 10.1007/978-1-4939-1881-2_4,
© Springer Science+Business Media New York 2015

increased risk for former smokers and a fourfold increased risk for current smokers. Smoking is associated with up to 50 % of new cancer cases in both US males and females [4]. Yet only a small percentage of those with environmental exposures develop bladder cancer, suggesting there may be a genetic predisposition. Some investigations into genetic contributions to bladder cancer give insight into the mechanisms of bladder carcinogenesis.

4.2 Familial and Genetic Risk

Epidemiologic studies have demonstrated that the risk of bladder cancer is approximately doubled in the case for first-degree relatives [5], yet familial aggregation has been reported in only 5 % of bladder cancer cases [6]. One common mechanism to identify genes involved in carcinogenesis is to analyze familial cases, yet to date familial studies have failed to identify a mode of inheritance, genetic site specificity, or an ethnic predilection [7]. Despite negative results from familial studies, high-penetrance genes associated with bladder cancer have been identified. Hereditary retinoblastoma (RB1) gene carriers may have the greatest genetic risk for bladder cancer. Fletcher et al. [8] studied 144 survivors of hereditary retinoblastoma and found a 26-fold increased rate of bladder cancer mortality in these patients compared to the general population. A germline translocation of the oncogene CDC91L1 (20q11) has been identified in 30 % of bladder cancers, though the protein it encodes for and its role in the biologic behavior of bladder cancer is not understood [9]. Lynch syndrome, or hereditary non-polyposis colorectal cancer (HNPCC) is an autosomal dominant genetic disorder that carries a relative risk of 14–22 times the general population and cumulative 2.6 % lifetime risk of urothelial cell cancer of the renal pelvis and ureter, with occurrence 10–15 years earlier than the typical age for upper tract UCC [10, 11]. While the risk of upper tract urothelial cancer with HNPCC is well established, data are inconsistent regarding the risk for bladder tumors. Two recent studies have suggested that patients with HNPCC carrying a germline mutation in MSH2, a mismatch repair gene, are at increased risk for bladder UC [12, 13] though a third study failed to find this association [14].

Despite a lack of explanation of familial bladder cancer cases aside from genetic syndromes, several low-penetrance genes have been identified as possible factors in developing bladder cancer through genome-wide association studies (GWAS). Three large GWAS studies [15–17] of European and American Caucasian subjects have resulted in the identification of eight novel single-nucleotide polymorphisms (SNPs) that convey a significant risk for developing bladder cancer, as well as confirmation of GSTM1 and NAT2, two genetic loci previously identified by candidate gene studies (Table 4.1). GSTM1 and NAT2 are the most studied loci, and lie at the crossroads between environmental exposure and genetic susceptibility.

N-acetyltransferases (NATs) are involved in bio-activation, detoxification, and enhanced secretion of aromatic amines, which are considered the most potent bladder carcinogens in tobacco smoke. NAT2 is normally expressed in the liver, and known genetic polymorphisms affect the acetylation function of NAT2. Depending on the alleles, individuals may have a rapid, intermediate or slow acetylation phenotype, which results in differing ability to clear aromatic amines. Various studies have found that individuals with the slow-acetylation phenotype carry a higher risk of developing bladder cancer from smoking than the rapid or intermediate acetylation phenotypes. Risk of bladder cancer in the slow-acetylator phenotype is limited to smokers (OR 1.2), with those who never smoked having no increased risk [15].

GSTM1 is an enzyme involved in detoxification of electrophiles by glutathione conjugation for a wide variety of substances. Numerous candidate gene studies have confirmed that deletion of GSTM1 (null) leads to a 50 % increased risk for developing bladder cancer [15–17]. Data pooled in the largest GWAS study to date demonstrate that the risk varies based on categories of smoking history. The odds ratio for GSTM1-null individuals for developing bladder cancer was

Table 4.1 Established urothelial cell cancer susceptibility loci

Gene	Chromosome	SNP location	Risk allele (frequency)	Allelic OR (95 % CI)	p-value	Reference
MYC	8q24.21	rs96428890	0.45	1.22 (1.15–1.29)	7.8×10^{-12}	[16]
TP63	3q28	rs710521	0.73	1.18 (1.12–1.24)	1.8×10^{-10}	[16]
PSCA	8q24.3	rs2294008	0.46	1.15 (1.10–1.20)	2.0×10^{-10}	[17]
CLPTM1L, TERT	5p15.33	rs2736098	0.54	1.11 (1.07–1.16)	5.0×10^{-7}	[48]
FGFR3, TACC3	4p16.3	rs2294008	0.19	1.24 (1.17–1.32)	9.5×10^{-12}	[16]
APOBEC3A, CBX6	22q13.1	rs1014971	0.38	0.88 (0.85–0.91)	8.4×10^{-12}	[15]
CCNE1	19q12	rs8102137	0.33	1.13 (1.09–1.17)	1.7×10^{-11}	[15]
UGT1A	2q37.1	rs11892031	0.08	0.84 (0.79–0.89)	1.0×10^{-7}	[15]
NAT2 (slow acetylator)	8p22	rs1495741	0.20	1.40 (1.30–1.50)	8.0×10^{-12}	[15]
GSTM1 (null)	1p13.3	Deletion assay	0.53	1.47 (1.38–1.57)	5.0×10^{-31}	[15]

1.7 in never smokers, 1.6 in former smokers, and 1.2 in current smokers [15]. Thus certain GSTM1 and NAT2 phenotypes may lead to individual susceptibility to the damaging effects of aromatic amines through formation of DNA adducts, and increased likelihood of entering the path to bladder carcinogenesis.

Larger studies are expected to uncover additional bladder cancer susceptibility SNPs, likely of similar significance to currently known SNPs [15]. The clinical value of SNPs identified by GWAS is yet to be demonstrated, as attempts to incorporate SNP analysis with traditional epidemiologic factors to predict the risk of developing bladder cancer have been unsuccessful. [18]. Future studies may provide not only the ability to predict bladder cancer risk, but also further insight into the mechanisms involved in the initial steps of bladder carcinogenesis.

4.3 Genetic Instability

Genetic instability is an important contributor to bladder carcinogenesis, and in fact appears to be one of the earliest events in this process. Additionally, increasing genetic instability is associated with higher grade and advanced stage in bladder tumors. Comparative genomic hybridization (CGH) studies evaluating the relative number of chromosomal gains and losses across the genome have revealed marked differences between Ta and T1 carcinomas, while the differences between T1 and MIBC were much smaller [19]. In general low-grade tumors have a lesser degree of genetic instability, permitting recurrence but rarely progression to high-grade disease. High-grade papillary cancer and CIS have more unstable genomes, leading to greater capacity for development of invasion and metastatic spread.

A variety of investigators have found frequent losses of 9p and 9q in PUNLMP and low-grade Ta tumors. This loss of heterozygosity (LOH) of chromosome 9 is thought one of the earliest events in bladder carcinogenesis, as chromosome 9 alterations can be found in papillary hyperplasia, considered a precursor to low-grade bladder cancer [20]. There are a number of candidate genes on 9p and 9q that may have a significant role in bladder carcinogenesis, which are discussed later.

T1 features LOH at chromosome 9 at a similar rate, but also has frequent losses of 8p, 11p, 11q and 13q, as well as gains of 1q, 8q, 17q and 20q. The total number of genetic alterations in stage T2-4 tumors is not significantly more than that of T1, suggesting T1 carcinomas are more closely related to T2-4 than to Ta at the genetic level [21]. Also, because the relative similarity in the amount of genetic changes in T1 and MIBC, genes associated with the progression to muscle invasiveness have been difficult to isolate [22]. Though the chromosomal aberrations are frequent, particularly in high-grade bladder cancer, a number of investigators have been able to identify key genes and/or signaling pathways associated with particular subsets of UCC, and allowed for the molecular characterization of bladder cancer.

4.4 Pathways to Carcinogenesis

The differences in clinical outcomes seen between low-grade, non-invasive urothelial carcinoma and high-grade, invasive urothelial carcinoma are manifested at a molecular level. Two distinct molecular pathways to the development of bladder cancer have been described [23] based on specific genetic changes that occur between each type of urothelial tumor development. The "Ta pathway" is the development of papillary, non-invasive low-grade disease from normal urothelium whereas the "CIS pathway" includes the development of high-grade tumors, not necessarily papillary, that often progress to MIBC. The origin of high-grade Ta tumors is currently not understood, and they may arise de-novo from flat dysplasia or from an increase in grade from low-grade Ta tumors. Figure 4.1 depicts the current model of pathogenesis for the major groups of bladder tumors. This model of two general molecular pathways provides a framework for discussion of the pathogenesis of bladder cancer, though progress in genetic and epigenetic studies suggests that with further discovery this model will become more complex.

The above molecular pathways are classified either by genetic alterations or pathologically in terms of grade and progression to invasiveness. Somatic mutations in fibroblast growth factor receptor-3 (FGFR3) and RAS have been strongly correlated with development of low-grade and low-stage bladder cancer, whereas TP53 and Rb mutations are associated with CIS, high-grade, and muscle invasive bladder cancer [24]. FGFR3 and TP53 mutations are almost mutually exclusive [25] and help to define the two pathways to formation of bladder cancer. Table 4.2 shows the frequency of notable genes that have a demonstrated involvement in the pathogenesis of Ta and MIBC.

4.4.1 The Ta Pathway

The Ta pathway is the development of papillary, non-invasive low-grade disease from normal urothelium. Genetic changes in the Ta pathway are associated with hyperplasia and growth. Normal urothelium transforms into low-grade papillary cancer through activation of proto-oncogenes, resulting in phenotypic changes that are histologically named papilloma, papillary urothelial neoplasia of low malignant potential (PUNLMP), hyperplasia, and low-grade urothelial cancer. Characteristic changes of the Ta pathway include LOH of chromosome 9, and mutations in FGFR3, RAS, and PI3K.

4.4.2 Chromosome 9

The deletion of parts or all of chromosome 9 is likely the earliest mutation seen in low-malignant potential (PUNLMP) and non-invasive bladder cancer, and is associated with hyperplasia. Deletions in 9p and 9q are also seen frequently in CIS and other high-grade tumors including MIBC. A variety of known tumor suppressor genes can be found at 9p and 9q. Deletion of 9p leads to loss of CDKN2A (9p21), which codes for TP16 (INK4a) and TP14 (ARF). INK4a is a negative regulator of RB, and ARF is an inhibitor of TP53, both pathways normally associated with the high-grade disease. Deletions in 9q involve the tumor suppressor genes TSC1 (tuberous sclerosis 1), PTCH (patched homologue 1), and DBC1 (deleted in bladder cancer gene 1). TSC1 (9q34) deletions activate oncogenic potential through signaling pathways such as the PI3K pathway (discussed below), and are seen in approximately 15 % of UCC [26], but studies to date show no apparent association with tumor grade or stage. Both PTCH (9q22) and DBC1 (9q33) are affiliated with increased cellular proliferation and these deletions are seen in up to

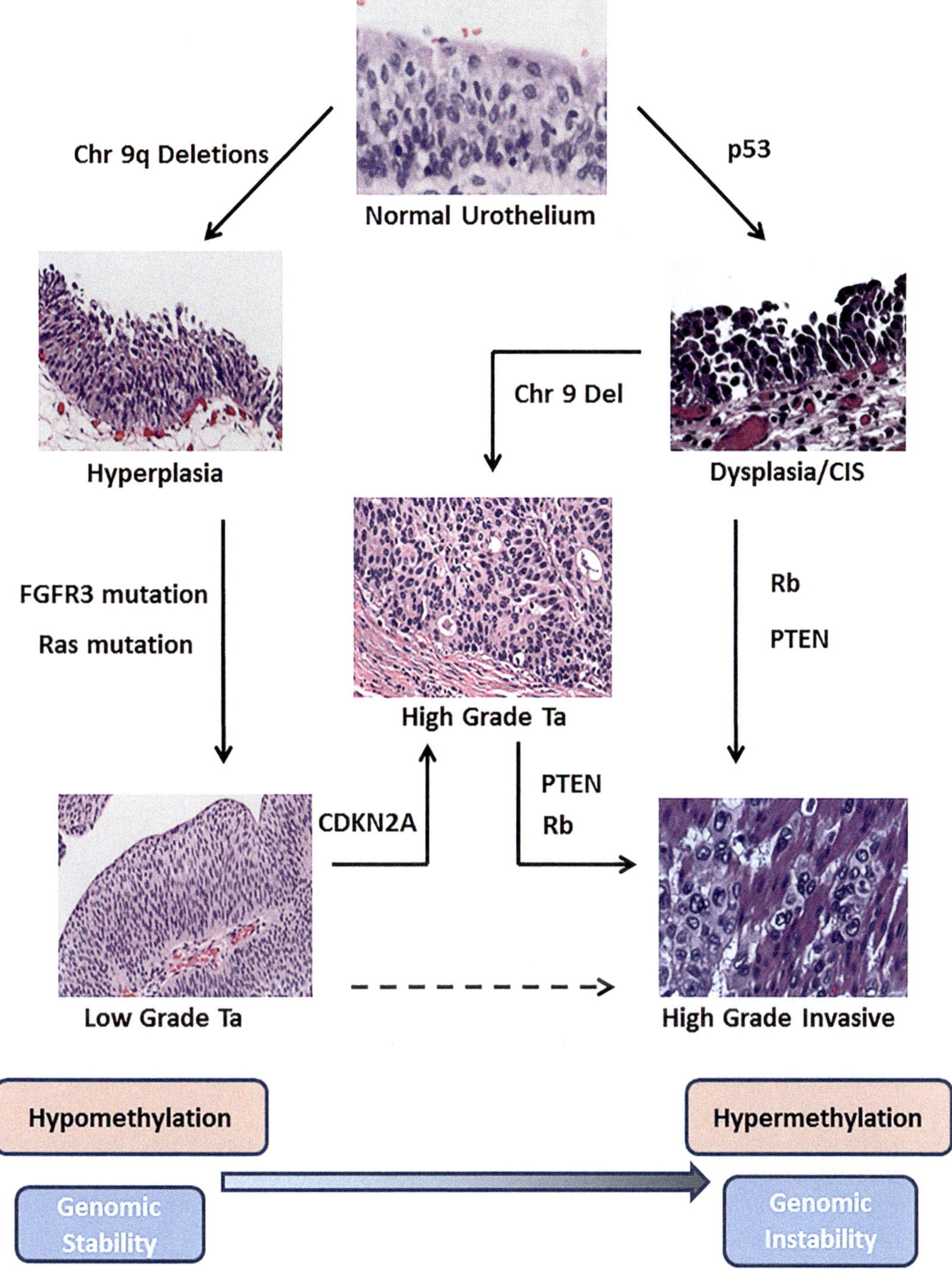

Fig. 4.1 Pathways of urothelial cell tumorigenesis. High-grade invasive disease is associated with greater genetic instability and hypermethylation compared to low-grade non-invasive disease

Table 4.2 Frequency of genetic alterations in select genes for Ta and MIBC tumors

Gene	Cytogenic location	Alteration	Frequency in Ta tumors	Frequency in MIBC tumors
Chromosome				
	9p	Deletion	36–47 %	21–30 %
	9q	Deletion	44–66 %	17 %
Oncogenes				
HRAS	11p15	Activating mutation	15 %	10–15 %
FGFR3	4p16	Activating mutation	60–80 %	~50 % Overexpression 15 % Mutation
PIK3CA	3q26	Activating mutation	35–65 %	25 %
MDM2	12q13	Overexpression	30 %	4 % Overexpression
Tumor suppressor genes				
TP53	17p13	Deletion or mutation	~0 % Ta, 20 % of T1	70 %
RB1	13q14	Deletion or mutation	~0 %	37 %
PTEN	10q23	Homozygous deletion or mutation	Infrequent	LOH 30–35 % Mutation 17 %
CDKN2A	9p21	Homozygous deletion or methylation or mutation	HD 20–30 % LOH ~60 %	HD 20–30 % LOH ~60 %
PTCH	9q22	Deletion or mutation	LOH ~60 % Mutation rare	LOH ~60 % Mutation rare
DBC1	9q32-33	Deletion or methylation	LOH ~60 %	LOH ~60 %
TSC1	9q34	Deletion or mutation	LOH ~60 % Mutation ~15 %	LOH ~60 % Mutation ~15 %

60 % of UCC due to LOH of 9q. Interestingly, PTCH1 is the gene in Gorlin Syndrome, a rare congenital syndrome associated with pediatric bladder cancer.

4.4.3 FGFR3

Somatic mutations in fibroblast growth factor receptor-3 (FGFR-3) are strongly correlated with development of low-grade and low-stage bladder cancer and are the hallmark mutation of the Ta pathway. FGFR-3 (4p16) is a tyrosine kinase receptor involved with regulation of several cellular processes including cell growth, differentiation, migration, wound healing, and angiogenesis, depending on the target cell type and the developmental stage. The receptor is one of the four FGFR members, and the structure is common to many receptor types. FGFR3 has an extracellular portion containing three immunoglobulin (Ig)-like domains, a hydrophobic transmembrane domain, and an intracellular domain containing a tyrosine kinase involved in signal transduction.

A variety of mutations have been described, with the majority found in exons 7, 10 and 15, and include alterations in the extracellular, transmembrane, and intracellular domains [27]. Many of these mutations lead to ligand-independent dimerization or autophosphorylation and activation of downstream signaling pathways, including the Ras-MAPK pathway and PI3K pathway. The most common of these, accounting for over 70 % of FGFR3 mutations, is S249C. This mutation results in cross-linking of adjacent receptors via disulfide bonds and ligand-independent dimerization [28].

Somatic mutations in FGFR-3 are found in 70–75 % of low-grade Ta urothelial cell cancer [29] and at a similar frequency in papilloma and PUNLMP. Papilloma is a benign exophytic growth covered with phenotypically normal appearing urothelium. In one study of 12 patients with urothelial papilloma, 9 were found to harbor the FGFR3 mutation (75 %) [30]. This has not been confirmed by additional studies, and further understanding is needed to explain why this lesion harbors the FGFR3 mutation but remains benign.

In bladders with both PUNLMP and low-grade Ta tumors, biopsies of these lesions have the same genetic alterations in most cases [31]. In fact, there are no genetic markers that consistently distinguish these entities, supporting the common belief that PUNLMP is a likely precursor to low-grade bladder cancer. Despite the high rate of recurrence for low-grade cancer, no study to date has definitely developed a relationship between mutant FGFR3 and tumor recurrence [32].

FGFR3 mutations are found in only 21–38 % of T1 disease, 0 % of primary CIS, and in about 10–15 % of T2-4 tumors [27, 33]. Despite a lower rate of FGFR3 mutations in higher-stage disease, overexpression of FGFR3 protein is more common in higher stage disease when compared to Ta disease and normal controls. In a study of micro-dissected tumor cells from 172 patients, overexpression of FGFR3 was found in 39 % of muscle invasive tumors despite most samples lacking the FGFR3 mutation, suggesting FGFR3 signaling may contribute to this phenotype, and that both wild-type and mutant FGFR3 may provide valid therapeutic targets in both NIMBC and MIBC [27].

A number of FGFR-targeted therapeutic agents have been tested in bladder cancer cell lines in vitro and in vivo [34–36]. Studies using siRNA or shRNA knockdown or specific antibodies to block FGFRs activity have shown that some UC cell lines are FGFR3-dependent. Overall, the in vivo and in vitro studies confirm that FGFR inhibitors may be of clinical relevance in the treatment of bladder cancer but also raise some crucial issues, particularly the requirement for biomarkers of FGFR dependence to predict response to treatment and the need for combination therapy with other agents due to the likely recurrence and/or resistance after treatment withdrawal.

4.4.4 RAS

RAS is the most common oncogene in human cancer, and is mutated in 10–20 % of bladder cancers. There are three activating mutations in the RAS family with KRAS and HRAS mutations being found at a similar frequency in bladder cancer, and NRAS mutations being uncommon [37]. Both RAS and FGFR3 converge on the mitogen-activated protein kinases (MAPK) signaling pathway, and both have been associated with the Ta pathway of bladder cancer. In total, 85 % of Ta tumors have either the RAS or FGFR3 mutations. This suggests that some or all of the effects of activating mutations of FGFR3 occur through the RAS-MAPK pathway. RAS and FGFR3 mutations are mutually exclusive of each other, representing alternative means to confer the same phenotype of UCC cells. Prognostic data for RAS with respect to recurrence-free, progression-free, or disease-specific survival in bladder cancer are currently lacking.

4.4.5 PI3K Pathway

The phosphatidylinositol 3-kinase (PI3K) pathway, along with the RAS-MAPK pathway, are the two most important pathways involved in cell growth in UCC. The PI3K pathway is activated by several mechanisms, including by FGFR3 and Ras. In UCC, aside from the Ras and FGFR3 mutations, mutations within the PI3K pathway have been identified in PIK3CA, AKT1, and TSC1, as well as LOH, homozygous deletions, and inactivating mutations in PTEN. PTEN inactivation is generally associated with invasive disease, and will be described further below. PIK3CA is the alpha-catalytic subunit of PI3 kinase, and PIK3CA mutations are mainly associated with low-grade and low-stage tumors [38]. Though RAS and FGFR3 are mutually exclusive mutations, PIK3CA and FGFR3 mutations can co-occur. Together, they may have an additive oncogenic effect, and in one study recurrences of tumors harboring both mutations were higher in grade [37].

TSC1, as described above, is located on 9q and thus frequently has at least one allele deleted in UCC, with the other allele often mutated leading to loss of function. TSC1 encodes for hamartin, and it is an inhibitor of mammalian target of rapamycin (mTOR) activation. AKT, also known as protein kinase (PKB) is a key regulator in the PI3K pathway, and its downstream effects include the mTOR activation. Activating mutations in

AKT have been found in UCC, again suggesting one common pathway between loss of TSC1 and AKT mutation through activation of mTOR. Cellular work has suggested that PI3K pathway activation is needed for the invasive phenotype seen in PTEN defects, making PI3K inhibitors potential therapeutic agents [39]. Other potential therapeutic agents for UCC in the P13K pathway are AKT inhibitors and mTOR inhibitors, or a combination thereof. Of note, mTOR can be activated by both the MAPK and PI3K pathways, so direct inhibition of mTOR, such as with rapamycin, may be more effective than blockade of intermediary proteins in these pathways. The role of mTOR and the effect of its blockade in UCC are currently under investigation.

4.4.6 CDKN2A

Cyclin-dependent kinase inhibitor 2A (CDKN2A) located on 9p21 encodes two tumor suppressor proteins, P16(INK4a) and P14(ARF), involved in cell cycle arrest and senescence. TP16 is a negative regulator of RB, and TP14 is a negative regulator of TP53. CDKN2A is frequently inactivated by homozygous deletion in bladder cancer, though its exact role in tumor genesis in not clear. Rebouissou and colleagues investigated the role of CDKN2A as a function of FGFR3 and the Ta pathway [40]. A total of 288 bladder tumors were studied, with FGFR3 in 43 % and homozygous CDKN2A deletions in 19 %. CDKN2A deletions occurred more frequently in FGFR3-mutated tumors than in wild-type FGFR3 tumors. CDKN2A deletion was not associated with tumor stage when considering the entire cohort. However, when looking only at tumors with FGFR3 mutations, there was a stage correlation, with CDKN2A deletion found in 20 %, 27 %, and 79 % of Ta, T1, and T2-4 tumors respectively. The presence of CDKN2A deletion had no effect on disease recurrence, but was a significant predictor of progression independent of stage and grade. This suggests that homozygous CDKN2A loss plays a critical role in the progression to muscle invasive disease in the Ta pathway.

4.4.7 The CIS Pathway and Muscle Invasive Disease

Genetic changes associated with the CIS pathway result in invasion, in contrast to the changes of the Ta pathway that result in hyperplasia, or growth. TP53, PTEN, and RB1 pathways are the hallmarks of invasive disease, and alterations in more than one of these pathways carry increasingly worse prognosis [41]. While there is variance in data on the prevalence of genetic alterations in CIS, there is strong agreement that CIS has a high rate of TP53 (17p13) mutation and/or LOH of chromosome 17. Other frequent genetic alterations reported in CIS include LOH on 14q (70 %), 8p (65 %), 13q (56 %), 11p (54 %), and 4q (52 %) [42].

The reported frequency of chromosome 9 LOH in CIS is not consistent, which is likely related to the varied presentation of CIS. Primary CIS, which is not associated with a papillary or invasive lesion, has TP53 overexpression but lacks deletion of chromosome 9. In contrast, secondary CIS, which is associated with papillary lesions, can display alterations in chromosome 9. Chromosome 9 deletions are the most frequent abnormality in both low- and high-grade tumors, and the conversion of normal urothelium to dysplasia is associated with chromosome 9 deletions in 75 % of cases. Furthermore, secondary CIS will have the same molecular expression profiles as the adjacent papillary tumor [43] and morphologically normal urothelium in the same bladder [44]. This illustrates the overlapping of pathways to developing invasive disease, directly from flat CIS, versus the pathway of hyperplasia associated with high-grade disease (Fig. 4.1).

It should be noted that a high proportion of bladder tumors demonstrate a wild-type phenotype, having no mutations in FGFR-3 or TP53. This can be seen in 32 % of Ta, 40 % of T1, and 43 % of T2-4 tumors [25]. Thus, there is a high likelihood that mutations in other genes or changes in gene expression are involved in the development of bladder cancer.

4.4.8 TP53

TP53 is the hallmark of high-grade disease and invasiveness in urothelial cell cancer [23]. Located on chromosome 17p13, p53 tumor suppressor gene is one of the most well studied genes in cancer and is the most common genetic event in human malignancy, associated with over half of all tumors. This protein functions as a transcription factor that regulates expression of several downstream genes, its two major functions being cell cycle arrest and apoptosis. Since it is involved in checkpoint control after DNA damage, additional genetic changes can result when mutations to this gatekeeper gene occur. Over 50 % of high-grade disease has defects in TP53 [45]. TP53 mutations are generally not observed in Ta, found in approximately 20 % of T1, and 42 % of T2 disease. Approximately 5–20 % of low-grade tumors will progress to high-grade tumors, which requires the loss of P53 [46]. P53 mutations occur at the earliest stage of the CIS pathway compared to the late in the Ta pathway, at the muscle-invasive stage [25]. TP53 controls the proper function of TP21, another key protein in cell cycle regulation. Genetic malfunctions of TP53 and TP21 in concert have been associated with higher relapse rates and worse survival after recurrence compared to TP53 malfunction alone. Other alterations that affect function of the p53 pathway include those of overexpression of MDM2 and alteration of p14(ARF). MDM2 is a proto-oncogene that serves as the antagonist to TP53. The protein product of MDM2 binds to p53 and inhibits its transcriptional activity, targeting p53 for degradation. P14(ARF) blocks MDM2-induced p53 degradation, and as it is located on chromosome 9p, is frequently deleted in high-grade bladder cancer.

Measuring p53 overexpression by immuno-histochemistry is an accepted surrogate for the p53 mutation. Mutated p53 has a longer half-life compared to wild type, and positive staining for p53 in 10 % or more cells positively correlates with TP53 mutation. The use of p53 overexpression as a surrogate, and the simple classification of tumors being either wild-type or mutant has been challenged, citing evidence that different mutations of TP53 harbor distinct functional properties, and not all mutated forms of TP53 have a longer half-life. There is consensus, however, that p53 overexpression is strongly associated with bladder tumors of higher stage and grade and worse prognosis.

4.4.9 RB

Retinoblastoma (Rb) tumor suppressor gene is located on chromosome 13q and is altered in up to 50 % of invasive bladder cancers, however Rb alterations are infrequent in Ta tumors. Inactivation of this gene is more frequent in high-grade and advanced state bladder cancer, and its alteration has been associated with disease progression and decreased survival. Rb inactivation is also thought to be involved in genetic instability, a frequent hallmark of invasive disease. Loss of Rb function leads to aberrant control of the mitotic spindle and chromosome segregation resulting in aneuploidy. RB function is mediated by P16(INK4a), a cyclin-dependent kinase inhibitor, which is encoded by CDKN2A on chromosome 9p. While both p53 and Rb pathway alterations independently convey increased risk, the highest risk of progression and death after cystectomy is with alteration in both p53 and Rb pathways [21].

4.4.10 PTEN

PTEN (10q) protein is a multifunctional phosphatase whose target is PIP3 frequently inactivated in high-grade bladder cancer. De-phosphorylation of PIP3 results in inhibition of the PI3K signaling pathway, thus loss of PTEN allows for unregulated activity of this pathway. As noted above, activation of the PI3K pathway is necessary for the invasive phenotype associated with the loss of PTEN. Deletions of 10q are found in 24–58 % of invasive UC, but infrequent in low-grade NMIBC. Up to 41 % of tumors with altered p53 have down-regulation of PTEN, and in combination these alterations are associated with poor outcome [47].

4.5 Epigenetic Changes

The term epigenetic refers to mechanisms that permit the stable transmission of cellular traits without an alteration in DNA sequence or amount. Epigenetics encompasses many different phenomena, including DNA methylation, histone modifications, and post-transcriptional effects mediated by non-coding RNA transcripts, so called microRNAs (miRNAs). Epigenetic changes modulate gene expression to play a vital role in initiation of cancer and can alter aspects of tumor phenotypes, including invasion, angiogenesis, motility and proliferation. Epigenetic changes are among the earliest molecular events associated with transformation and could therefore precede morphologic alterations in cellular architecture.

DNA methylation is one of the most studied mechanisms of genetic change associated with cancer. This involves the methylation of cytosine bases in DNA which alters the capacity of transcription factors to bind DNA and initiate gene expression, resulting in transcriptional silencing. Methylation thus leads to repression of certain genes, and is used physiologically in development and differentiation to direct appropriate gene expression. In cancer, hypermethylation, particularly of promoter CpG (cytosine-phosphate-guanine) islands, is a mechanism utilized to initiate or promote carcinogenesis. A variety of genes have been demonstrated to be modulated in bladder cancer through hypermethylation, too numerous to review here. The functions of these genes include cell cycle control, differentiation, apoptosis, cellular adhesion, and migration [48]. In general, DNA methylation increases with increasing grade and stage [49, 50], suggesting hypermethylation promotes a more aggressive phenotype as with genetic instability. In addition, a recent genome-wide analysis of DNA methylation patterns revealed a distinct hypomethylation pattern only in non-invasive tumors relative to normal epithelium and invasive tumors, suggesting distinct epigenetics also differentiate the Ta and CIS pathways [49]. Lastly, the same study examined normal epithelia from bladders removed for cystectomy, and found hypermethylation at many loci that were shared with bladder tumors, particularly invasive bladder tumors (T2-4). This suggests DNA methylation is an early event in bladder carcinogenesis, as well as a source of the field effect seen in bladder UCC. Whether the normal bladder of patients with non-invasive tumors would more closely resemble the methylation patterns found in the Ta pathway could not be elucidated in this study. As DNA methylation is reversible and appears to be a crucial early event in bladder tumor development, DNA methyltransferase inhibitors may prove useful in both NMIBC and MIBC in the future.

Histones are involved in DNA packaging, and modification of histones through acetylation, phosphorylation or methylation can affect transcription of genes coiled around the histone complex. Studies on histone modification in bladder cancer are limited, however a recent study found that modification of histones through altering methylation and acetylation was responsible for a specific expression silencing profile (MRES) in bladder tumors and bladder cancer cell lines [51]. Furthermore, on clustering analysis, the MRES signature was associated with tumors and cells containing the CIS pathway expression signature, and was only rarely found in tumors with FGFR3 mutation, which is part of the Ta pathway. Thus, at least this portion of histone modification appears to be differentially utilized by the two pathways, and may signify a more aggressive phenotype.

Micro-RNAs are short, non-coding RNAs which can affect gene expression at the post-transcriptional level. Though they mainly function in silencing their target gene transcripts, either through impeding translation or targeting the transcripts for degradation, they may also cause increased expression of their target mRNAs in some circumstances. A variety of miRNAs differentially expressed in bladder cancer have been reported, also with a variety of targets including FGFR3, AKT, p53 and PTEN [48]. Expression profiling of miRNAs in bladder cancer has been performed [52, 53], each with interesting implications into the molecular pathways of bladder cancer. Catto found altered miRNA expression in normal urothelium of bladder cancer patients as compared to controls, suggesting another epigenetic mechanism occurring early in UCC development. They also found a pattern of decreased miRNA expression in low-grade tumors, including loss of miRNAs which normally suppress FGFR3 expression. In high-grade tumors they found up-regulation of a number of miRNAs, including one which affects p53. Dyrskjot similarly found expression differences between low-grade and high-grade tumors, and additionally identified miR-129, whose targets are GALNT1 and SOX4, as portending a poor prognosis. Others have also correlated miRNA expression patterns with recurrence and progression in low-grade and high-grade bladder cancers [54].

4.6 Recurrence and Prognosis

The clinical goal in bladder cancer management is to predict the fate of an individual tumor and to select the optimal individual treatment. Histopathologic features including tumor grade, depth of invasion, multiplicity, size, morphology, the presence of vascular or lymphatic invasion, and the presence or absence of CIS are currently used to predict relative risk of recurrence and progression. These features are all significant predictors of outcome in the bladder cancer population, but they do not provide accurate predictions for individual patients. The current amount of data available from high-throughput analysis like GWAS have led to investigations of specific clinical behavior based on a tumor's gene expression signature.

Using cDNA expression libraries, Dyrskjot et al. attempted to classify tumors as Ta versus T1 or T2. Eighty percent of Ta tumors were correctly classified, and Ta tumors that were falsely classified as T1 or T2 had a significantly worse prognosis [55]. Similarly, Wang et al. [56] developed a multiplex PCR assay using a 57-gene mRNA expression profile to predict Ta, T1, and T2 bladder cancer as high risk versus low risk of progression. At 2 years the tumors classified as high risk in each stage group had greater progression than those segregated as low risk. Such signatures may also be applicable to detection of cancer and predicting therapy response, though discussion of this is outside the scope of this chapter.

4.7 Conclusion

Bladder cancer is a multifactorial disease with well-established links to environmental factors and a clear demonstration of a genetic component in its development. Two separate pathways define the current model for bladder carcinogenesis, yet the exact genetic bases for the development of urothelial cell cancer is not well understood and will undoubtedly become more complex. Future research will focus toward furthering our understanding of the molecular basis for bladder carcinogenesis, along with development of risk prediction models that integrates genetic and environmental factors to predict individualized probability for bladder cancer development, prognosis, and guide treatment.

References

1. American Cancer Society. Cancer facts & figures 2013. Atlanta, GA: American Cancer Society; 2013.
2. Hayat MJ, Howlader N, Reichman ME, Edwards BK. Cancer statistics, trends, and multiple primary cancer analyses from the Surveillance, Epidemiology, and End Results (SEER) Program. Oncologist. 2007; 12(1):20–37.
3. Parkin DM. The global burden of urinary bladder cancer. Scand J Urol Nephrol Suppl. 2008;218:12–20.
4. Freedman ND, Silverman DT, Hollenbeck AR, Schatzkin A, Abnet CC. Association between smoking and risk of bladder cancer among men and women. JAMA. 2011;306(7):737–45.
5. Aben KK, Witjes JA, Schoenberg MP, Hulsbergen-van de Kaa C, Verbeek AL, Kiemeney LA. Familial aggregation of urothelial cell carcinoma. Int J Cancer. 2002;98(2):274–8.
6. Kiemeney LA, Schoenberg M. Familial transitional cell carcinoma. J Urol. 1996;156(3):867–72.
7. Mueller CM, Caporaso N, Greene MH. Familial and genetic risk of transitional cell carcinoma of the urinary tract. Urol Oncol. 2008;26(5):451–64.
8. Fletcher O, Easton D, Anderson K, Gilham C, Jay M, Peto J. Lifetime risks of common cancers among retinoblastoma survivors. J Natl Cancer Inst. 2004;96(5): 357–63.
9. Guo Z, Linn JF, Wu G, Anzick SL, Eisenberger CF, Halachmi S, et al. CDC91L1 (PIG-U) is a newly discovered oncogene in human bladder cancer. Nat Med. 2004;10(4):374–81.
10. Sijmons RH, Kiemeney LA, Witjes JA, Vasen HF. Urinary tract cancer and hereditary nonpolyposis

colorectal cancer: risks and screening options. J Urol. 1998;160(2):466–70.

11. Watson P, Lynch HT. The tumor spectrum in HNPCC. Anticancer Res. 1994;14(4B):1635–9.

12. Geary J, Sasieni P, Houlston R, Izatt L, Eeles R, Payne SJ, et al. Gene-related cancer spectrum in families with hereditary non-polyposis colorectal cancer (HNPCC). Fam Cancer. 2008;7(2):163–72.

13. van der Post RS, Kiemeney LA, Ligtenberg MJ, Witjes JA, Hulsbergen-van de Kaa CA, Bodmer D, et al. Risk of urothelial bladder cancer in Lynch syndrome is increased, in particular among MSH2 mutation carriers. J Med Genet. 2010;47(7):464–70.

14. Barrow PJ, Ingham S, O'Hara C, Green K, McIntyre I, Lalloo F, et al. The spectrum of urological malignancy in Lynch syndrome. Fam Cancer. 2013;12(1): 57–63.

15. Rothman N, Garcia-Closas M, Chatterjee N, Malats N, Wu X, Figueroa JD, et al. A multi-stage genome-wide association study of bladder cancer identifies multiple susceptibility loci. Nat Genet. 2010;42(11):978–84.

16. Kiemeney LA, Thorlacius S, Sulem P, Geller F, Aben KK, Stacey SN, et al. Sequence variant on 8q24 confers susceptibility to urinary bladder cancer. Nat Genet. 2008;40(11):1307–12.

17. Wu X, Ye Y, Kiemeney LA, Sulem P, Rafnar T, Matullo G, et al. Genetic variation in the prostate stem cell antigen gene PSCA confers susceptibility to urinary bladder cancer. Nat Genet. 2009;41(9):991–5.

18. Wu X, Hildebrandt MA, Chang DW. Genome-wide association studies of bladder cancer risk: a field synopsis of progress and potential applications. Cancer Metastasis Rev. 2009;28(3–4):269–80.

19. Kallioniemi A, Kallioniemi OP, Sudar D, Rutovitz D, Gray JW, Waldman F, et al. Comparative genomic hybridization for molecular cytogenetic analysis of solid tumors. Science. 1992;258(5083):818–21.

20. Chow NH, Cairns P, Eisenberger CF, Schoenberg MP, Taylor DC, Epstein JI, et al. Papillary urothelial hyperplasia is a clonal precursor to papillary transitional cell bladder cancer. Int J Cancer. 2000;89(6):514–8.

21. Cordon-Cardo C, Cote RJ, Sauter G. Genetic and molecular markers of urothelial premalignancy and malignancy. Scand J Urol Nephrol Suppl. 2000;205: 82–93.

22. Knowles MA. Bladder cancer subtypes defined by genomic alterations. Scand J Urol Nephrol Suppl. 2008;218:116–30.

23. Spruck 3rd CH, Ohneseit PF, Gonzalez-Zulueta M, Esrig D, Miyao N, Tsai YC, et al. Two molecular pathways to transitional cell carcinoma of the bladder. Cancer Res. 1994;54(3):784–8.

24. Bakkar AA, Wallerand H, Radvanyi F, Lahaye JB, Pissard S, Lecerf L, et al. FGFR3 and TP53 gene mutations define two distinct pathways in urothelial cell carcinoma of the bladder. Cancer Res. 2003;63(23):8108–12.

25. Neuzillet Y, Paoletti X, Ouerhani S, Mongiat-Artus P, Soliman H, de The H, et al. A meta-analysis of the relationship between FGFR3 and TP53 mutations in bladder cancer. PLoS One. 2012;7(12):e48993.

26. Knowles MA, Habuchi T, Kennedy W, Cuthbert-Heavens D. Mutation spectrum of the 9q34 tuberous sclerosis gene TSC1 in transitional cell carcinoma of the bladder. Cancer Res. 2003;63(22):7652–6.

27. Tomlinson DC, Baldo O, Harnden P, Knowles MA. FGFR3 protein expression and its relationship to mutation status and prognostic variables in bladder cancer. J Pathol. 2007;213(1):91–8.

28. Adar R, Monsonego-Ornan E, David P, Yayon A. Differential activation of cysteine-substitution mutants of fibroblast growth factor receptor 3 is determined by cysteine localization. J Bone Miner Res. 2002;17(5):860–8.

29. Gomez-Roman JJ, Saenz P, Molina M, Cuevas Gonzalez J, Escuredo K, Santa Cruz S, et al. Fibroblast growth factor receptor 3 is overexpressed in urinary tract carcinomas and modulates the neoplastic cell growth. Clin Cancer Res. 2005;11(2 Pt 1):459–65.

30. van Rhijn BW, Montironi R, Zwarthoff EC, Jobsis AC, van der Kwast TH. Frequent FGFR3 mutations in urothelial papilloma. J Pathol. 2002;198(2):245–51.

31. Obermann EC, Junker K, Stoehr R, Dietmaier W, Zaak D, Schubert J, et al. Frequent genetic alterations in flat urothelial hyperplasias and concomitant papillary bladder cancer as detected by CGH, LOH, and FISH analyses. J Pathol. 2003;199(1):50–7.

32. Pollard C, Smith SC, Theodorescu D. Molecular genesis of non-muscle-invasive urothelial carcinoma (NMIUC). Expert Rev Mol Med. 2010;12:e10.

33. Billerey C, Chopin D, Aubriot-Lorton MH, Ricol D, Gil Diez de Medina S, Van Rhijn B, et al. Frequent FGFR3 mutations in papillary non-invasive bladder (pTa) tumors. Am J Pathol. 2001;158(6):1955–9.

34. Bernard-Pierrot I, Brams A, Dunois-Larde C, Caillault A, Diez de Medina SG, Cappellen D, et al. Oncogenic properties of the mutated forms of fibroblast growth factor receptor 3b. Carcinogenesis. 2006;27(4):740–7.

35. Tomlinson DC, Hurst CD, Knowles MA. Knockdown by shRNA identifies S249C mutant FGFR3 as a potential therapeutic target in bladder cancer. Oncogene. 2007;26(40):5889–99.

36. Qing J, Du X, Chen Y, Chan P, Li H, Wu P, et al. Antibody-based targeting of FGFR3 in bladder carcinoma and t(4;14)-positive multiple myeloma in mice. J Clin Invest. 2009;119(5):1216–29.

37. Kompier LC, Lurkin I, van der Aa MN, van Rhijn BW, van der Kwast TH, Zwarthoff EC. FGFR3, HRAS, KRAS, NRAS and PIK3CA mutations in bladder cancer and their potential as biomarkers for surveillance and therapy. PLoS One. 2010;5(11):e13821.

38. Lopez-Knowles E, Hernandez S, Malats N, Kogevinas M, Lloreta J, Carrato A, et al. PIK3CA mutations are an early genetic alteration associated with FGFR3 mutations in superficial papillary bladder tumors. Cancer Res. 2006;66(15):7401–4.

39. Wu X, Obata T, Khan Q, Highshaw RA, De Vere WR, Sweeney C. The phosphatidylinositol-3 kinase pathway regulates bladder cancer cell invasion. BJU Int. 2004;93(1):143–50.

40. Rebouissou S, Herault A, Letouze E, Neuzillet Y, Laplanche A, Ofualuka K, et al. CDKN2A homozygous

deletion is associated with muscle invasion in FGFR3-mutated urothelial bladder carcinoma. J Pathol. 2012;227(3):315–24.

41. Chatterjee SJ, Datar R, Youssefzadeh D, George B, Goebell PJ, Stein JP, et al. Combined effects of p53, p21, and pRb expression in the progression of bladder transitional cell carcinoma. J Clin Oncol. 2004;22(6):1007–13.

42. Rosin MP, Cairns P, Epstein JI, Schoenberg MP, Sidransky D. Partial allelotype of carcinoma in situ of the human bladder. Cancer Res. 1995;55(22):5213–6.

43. Hopman AH, Kamps MA, Speel EJ, Schapers RF, Sauter G, Ramaekers FC. Identification of chromosome 9 alterations and p53 accumulation in isolated carcinoma in situ of the urinary bladder versus carcinoma in situ associated with carcinoma. Am J Pathol. 2002;161(4):1119–25.

44. Dyrskjot L, Kruhoffer M, Thykjaer T, Marcussen N, Jensen JL, Moller K, et al. Gene expression in the urinary bladder: a common carcinoma in situ gene expression signature exists disregarding histopathological classification. Cancer Res. 2004;64(11):4040–8.

45. Mallofre C, Castillo M, Morente V, Sole M. Immunohistochemical expression of CK20, p53, and Ki-67 as objective markers of urothelial dysplasia. Mod Pathol. 2003;16(3):187–91.

46. Han H, Wolff EM, Liang G. Epigenetic alterations in bladder cancer and their potential clinical implications. Adv Urol. 2012;2012:546917.

47. Puzio-Kuter AM, Castillo-Martin M, Kinkade CW, Wang X, Shen TH, Matos T, et al. Inactivation of p53 and Pten promotes invasive bladder cancer. Genes Dev. 2009;23(6):675–80.

48. Di Pierro GB, Gulia C, Cristini C, Fraietta G, Marini L, Grande P, et al. Bladder cancer: a simple model becomes complex. Curr Genomics. 2012;13(5):395–415.

49. Wolff EM, Chihara Y, Pan F, Weisenberger DJ, Siegmund KD, Sugano K, et al. Unique DNA methylation patterns distinguish noninvasive and invasive urothelial cancers and establish an epigenetic field defect in premalignant tissue. Cancer Res. 2010;70(20):8169–78.

50. Salem C, Liang G, Tsai YC, Coulter J, Knowles MA, Feng AC, et al. Progressive increases in de novo methylation of CpG islands in bladder cancer. Cancer Res. 2000;60(9):2473–6.

51. Vallot C, Stransky N, Bernard-Pierrot I, Herault A, Zucman-Rossi J, Chapeaublanc E, et al. A novel epigenetic phenotype associated with the most aggressive pathway of bladder tumor progression. J Natl Cancer Inst. 2011;103(1):47–60.

52. Dyrskjot L, Ostenfeld MS, Bramsen JB, Silahtaroglu AN, Lamy P, Ramanathan R, et al. Genomic profiling of microRNAs in bladder cancer: miR-129 is associated with poor outcome and promotes cell death in vitro. Cancer Res. 2009;69(11):4851–60.

53. Catto JW, Miah S, Owen HC, Bryant H, Myers K, Dudziec E, et al. Distinct microRNA alterations characterize high- and low-grade bladder cancer. Cancer Res. 2009;69(21):8472–81.

54. Dip N, Reis ST, Timoszczuk LS, Viana NI, Piantino CB, Morais DR, et al. Stage, grade and behavior of bladder urothelial carcinoma defined by the microRNA expression profile. J Urol. 2012;188(5):1951–6.

55. Dyrskjot L, Zieger K, Real FX, Malats N, Carrato A, Hurst C, et al. Gene expression signatures predict outcome in non-muscle-invasive bladder carcinoma: a multicenter validation study. Clin Cancer Res. 2007;13(12):3545–51.

56. Wang R, Morris DS, Tomlins SA, Lonigro RJ, Tsodikov A, Mehra R, et al. Development of a multiplex quantitative PCR signature to predict progression in non-muscle-invasive bladder cancer. Cancer Res. 2009;69(9):3810–8.

Timothy Kim, Joshua G. Griffin,
Jeffrey M. Holzbeierlein, and Wade J. Sexton

5.1 Introduction

Bladder cancer is the most common neoplasm of the urinary tract and the sixth most common malignancy in the United States [1]. While most are detected at the clinically localized stage, approximately 25 % of patients will initially present with regional or metastatic disease. Radiographic imaging is a vital part of the evaluation of both local and advanced bladder cancer as it assists the urologist in the determination of appropriate management. It furthermore plays an important role after definitive treatment for long-term cancer surveillance and in some cases management of surgical complications.

It is important to recognize that at the time of most patients having an established diagnosis of bladder cancer, they will have already undergone some form of imaging as part of a hematuria evaluation. In this chapter, we discuss the different imaging modalities used in diagnosis and staging in the context of both localized and advanced bladder cancer. We will also review the role of imaging in the setting of neoadjuvant chemotherapy and post-treatment cancer surveillance. Newer imaging techniques utilizing cystoscopy (narrow band imaging, confocal laser microendoscopy, and optimal coherence tomography) are not presently used in standard practice and will not be discussed.

5.2 Role of Imaging for Non-muscle Invasive Bladder Cancer (CIS, Ta, T1)

The majority of patients (approximately 75 %) presenting with urothelial cancers of the bladder are diagnosed with non-muscle invasive disease, that is, confined to the mucosal or lamina propria layers. Nonetheless, imaging is still an important part of this evaluation as it helps ensure accurate clinical staging while also evaluating the upper urothelial tracts for synchronous or metachronous lesions. There are several modalities that may be used in this evaluation including ultrasonography, contrast-enhanced radiography (i.e. intravenous pyelogram, retrograde pyelogram), computed tomography, and magnetic resonance imaging.

T. Kim, M.D. • W.J. Sexton, M.D. (✉)
Department of Genitourinary Oncology, Moffitt Cancer Center, 12902 Magnolia Drive, Tampa, FL 33612, USA
e-mail: timjkim@gmail.com; wade.sexton@moffitt.org

J.G. Griffin, M.D
Department of Urology, University of Kansas Medical Center, 3901 Rainbow Blvd, Mail Stop 3016, Kansas City, KS 66160, USA
e-mail: jggriffinmd@gmail.com

J.M. Holzbeierlein, M.D.
University of Kansas Hospital, 3901 Rainbow Blvd, Mail Stop 3016, Kansas City, KS 66160, USA
e-mail: jholzbeierlein@kumc.edu

B.R. Konety and S.S. Chang (eds.), *Management of Bladder Cancer: A Comprehensive Text With Clinical Scenarios*, DOI 10.1007/978-1-4939-1881-2_5,
© Springer Science+Business Media New York 2015

5.2.1 Radiography, Intravenous Pyelography, and Ultrasound

Plain radiography has no role in the evaluation of non-muscle invasive bladder cancer (NMIBC) given its lack of soft tissue contrast or definition. While there have been some case reports describing appearance of calcifications in the bladder showing up on plain x-ray, these are merely of historical perspective and will not be described. On the other hand, the addition of intravenous contrast to plain radiography (intravenous pyelography, IVP) has been used for many years in the field of urology. An IVP involves injection of intravenous contrast followed by serial radiographic and tomographic images obtained of the kidneys, ureter, and bladder as the contrast media moves through the urinary tract. For many years IVP was the study of choice along with cystoscopy in the evaluation of hematuria, however in the era of computed tomography and magnetic resonance imaging, this test has fallen out of favor. In the most recent version of the AUA Clinical Guidelines for asymptomatic microhematuria, IVP and ultrasound were considered less optimal imaging tests given their low sensitivity compared with magnetic resonance imaging (MRI) or computed tomography (CT) and high likelihood of missing a diagnosis [2]. When present on IVP, urothelial cancers may appear as a filling defect within the bladder or upper urinary tracts (Fig. 5.1) [3]. Papillary lesions, as often seen with non-invasive tumors, will have frond-like projections into the bladder lumen, giving the appearance of a poorly marginated filling defect within the bladder. A thickened bladder wall on the IVP may be seen in some cases of carcinoma in situ. One potential pitfall with IVP is that a large median lobe may be mistaken for a filling defect or bladder tumor.

Ultrasonography has several theoretical advantages as an imaging modality of the bladder and urinary tract. It is readily available, requires no patient preparation, is inexpensive, and not associated with radiation exposure. In addition, it allows for simultaneous evaluation of the upper tracts and may demonstrate hydronephrosis, renal calculi, or renal masses. The accuracy of ultrasound in visualizing bladder tumors depends

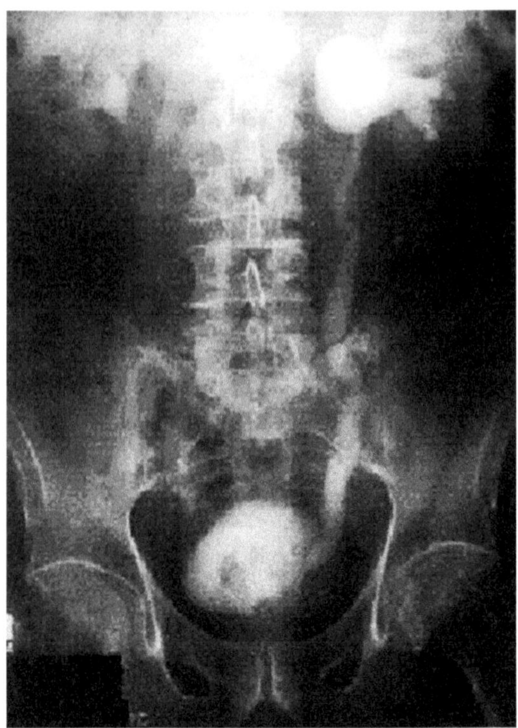

Fig. 5.1 Intravenous pyelogram demonstrating left hydroureteronephrosis and large filling defect within the bladder. *Reprinted with permission* [3]

on the degree of distention and tumor characteristics (size, morphology, and location) and is operator-dependent. Newer contrast-enhanced techniques show some promise for improving diagnostic accuracy in the imaging of bladder tumors for evaluation of hematuria. That being said, cystoscopy remains the gold standard diagnostic procedure and should be performed regardless of ultrasound findings.

Ultrasonography is a poor tool for staging of bladder cancer and it is rarely used after histologic confirmation. More commonly, ultrasound of the bladder is performed as part of the evaluation of the kidneys and an incidental lesion is noted. Bladder tumors on ultrasound typically appear as hypoechoic, plaque-like or polpypoid lesions projecting into the bladder lumen [4]. Doppler studies may demonstrate blood flow, especially in larger papillary lesions. Shadowing may also be present if there is calcification. Bladder wall thickening may also be apparent although this is a nonspecific finding.

The diagnostic accuracy of ultrasound for detection of bladder tumors is highly variable and dependent on size and location. Datta et al. showed that US had an overall sensitivity of 63 % and specificity of 99 % for detection of bladder cancer in a series of over 1,000 patients presenting with hematuria [5]. Smaller lesions are in particular more difficult to evaluate. For lesions less than 5 mm in diameter, Malone et al. found that US detected only 38 % of tumors compared to 82 % of those greater than 5 mm as confirmed by cystoscopy [6]. Several series have shown the importance of tumor location and sensitivity of US. The bladder neck, dome, and anterior bladder are all sites where US visualization is limited and may miss lesions [7, 8].

Contrast-enhanced ultrasonography (CEUS) is a newer form of ultrasonography that attempts to improve the diagnostic accuracy of ultrasound. This modality relies on intravenous microbubble contrast agents and a specialized ultrasound probe. The microbubbles are entirely intravascular and their properties result in high echogenicity when visualized on sonogram. This allows for evaluation of vasculature and neovascularity (i.e. tumors). It has been used for imaging of the spleen, liver, and kidneys [9]. Previous studies using CEUS of the bladder revealed that the mucosal and submucosal layers had early enhancement and the detrusor was relatively hypoechoic in comparison. Using CEUS of the bladder, the presence of a hypoechoic layer between the bladder tumor and bladder wall was predictive of non-invasive disease in a small study [10]. Most recently, Nicolau reported their experience using contrast-enhanced ultrasound in a cohort of 43 patients undergoing transurethral resection of bladder tumors. CEUS and routine US were performed the day prior to a transurethral resection of bladder tumor (TURBT). CEUS was more accurate than routine US in detection of bladder cancer (88.3 % vs. 72.09 %) and was particularly helpful in non-conclusive US cases. Sensitivity of CEUS was highest with lesions >5 mm (94.7 % vs. 20 % if <5 mm) [11]. More recently, three-dimensional ultrasound has been combined with CEUS in efforts to not only improve detection but also predict invasiveness. This new technique, as shown in Fig. 5.2, results in contrast-enhanced sonographic images in multiple planes allowing for a three-dimensional reconstruction of a bladder tumor. Of 60 bladder lesions evaluated with combined 3D US and CEUS prior to TURBT, all 16 muscle invasive tumors were correctly diagnosed. Inter-reader agreement was highest when these images were combined as compared to individual use (kappa = 0.914) [12].

Despite the advantages of ultrasound for bladder cancer imaging, it still lacks in diagnostic accuracy, especially for smaller lesions. Routine grey scale ultrasound is still considered inferior to other imaging modalities such as CT and MRI for evaluation and staging of bladder cancer. For the evaluation of hematuria, ultrasound is considered a suboptimal test based on the AUA guidelines [2]. With evolving technologies utilizing microbubble contrast and three-dimensional imaging, ultrasound imaging may play a more important role in imaging bladder tumors, but not without further refinement of the modality.

5.2.2 Computed Tomography and Urography for Non-invasive Disease

Multidetector row computed tomography (CT) is currently the most widely used imaging modality for bladder cancer. In practice many patients will have had some form of CT imaging prior to undergoing office cystoscopy or transurethral resection of a bladder tumor as this is usually performed as part of a hematuria evaluation. It is important to delineate the use of CT in the context of a hematuria evaluation versus staging after a confirmatory diagnosis of bladder cancer. In this section, we discuss the role of CT imaging as it relates to NMIBC. Later in this chapter, we will discuss CT imaging in the setting of invasive bladder cancer.

CT imaging for bladder cancer should be performed with intravenous contrast unless contraindicated due to renal insufficiency or allergy. Delayed images are essential and allow for assessment of the collecting system, ureters, and bladder. Advances in post-processing computerized technology now allow for reconstructed

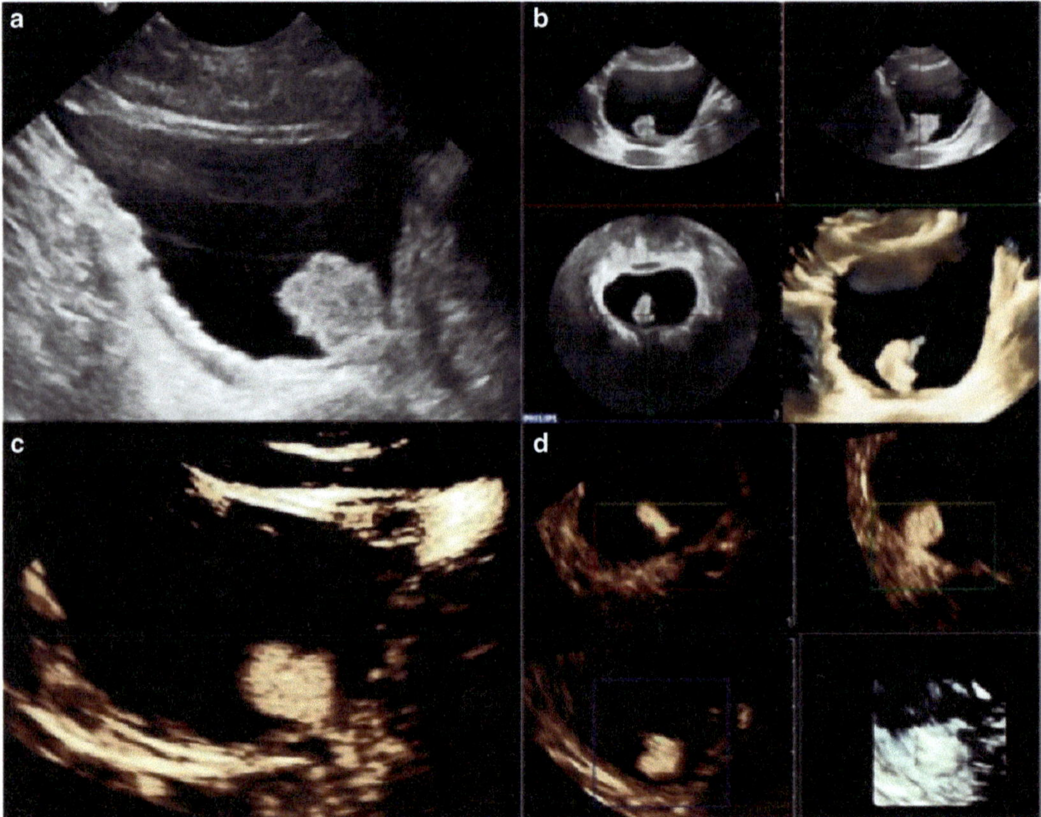

Fig. 5.2 Contrast-enhanced 3D ultrasound of patients with non-invasive bladder tumor. (**a**) Conventional 2D ultrasound; (**b**) 3D image from three rectangular planes; (**c**) Contrast enhanced 2D ultrasound with homogenous enhancement; (**d**) 3D contrast enhanced image. *Reprinted with permission* [12]

CT images in coronal and sagittal planes, which provide further improvements in evaluation of the urinary tract.

5.2.2.1 Low-Grade NMIBC

Most non-invasive bladder tumors are low grade and of papillary architecture. Malignant potential of these tumors is extremely low, with rates of progression less than 5 %. These tumors may vary in size, number, and characteristics. Papillary lesions may be seen as a focal filling defect projecting into the bladder or an area of asymmetric bladder wall thickening. Larger lesions may appear as an enhancing soft tissue density projecting into a relatively hypodense background of the urine filled bladder, or on delayed images as a filling defect (Fig. 5.3).

In the setting of non-invasive urothelial bladder cancer, ongoing surveillance after treatment is necessary to ensure there has been no disease recurrence. Cystoscopy is the mainstay of post-treatment cancer surveillance in low-grade non-invasive disease. Upper tract imaging should be performed every 1–2 years or more frequently in cases of high-grade recurrences, therefore CT urography continues to play a prominent role even at this stage.

5.2.2.2 High-Risk Non-invasive Disease

High-risk NMIBC includes carcinoma in situ, T1 (lamina propria invasion), and high-grade Ta. Morphologically the latter two may be indistinguishable from low-grade NMIBC on CT imaging while the former is virtually never seen on

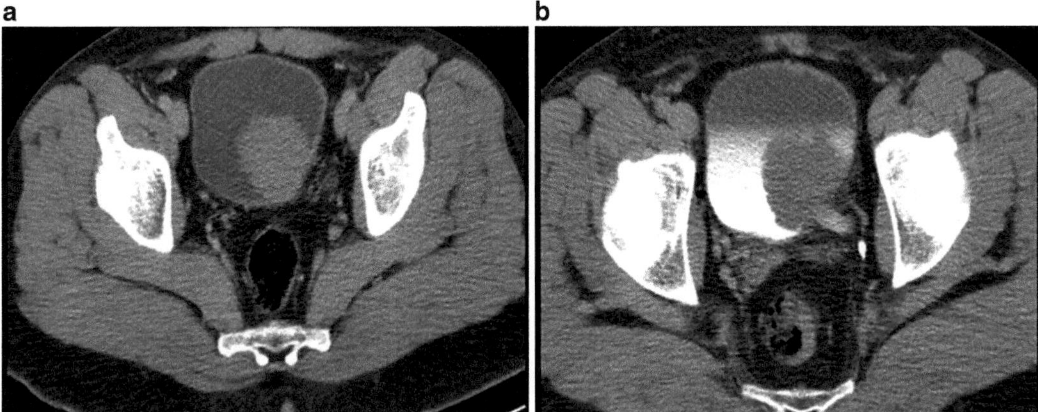

Fig. 5.3 Axial contrasted CT showing a large left-sided papillary bladder tumor. (**a**) Early contrast with enhancing tumor; (**b**) delayed images showing filling defects within the bladder and left ureter

imaging [13]. High-risk disease is associated with higher rates of recurrence and progression and adjuvant intravesical treatment after resection is recommended in order to reduce the chance of recurrence and progression. The role of imaging as part of surveillance after treatment is no different than that with low-grade NMIBC.

5.2.2.3 CT: Conclusion

Computed tomography urography (CTU) has become the imaging test of choice for NMIBC and is often performed prior to cystoscopy during hematuria evaluation. Contemporary sensitivity and specificity for bladder cancer detection using CTU range from 79 to 95 % and 83–99 %, respectively [14–16]. As will be discussed later, despite this diagnostic capability, CTU falls short when it comes to staging accuracy. Furthermore, CTU is unable to demonstrate carcinoma in situ and may miss small lesions, particularly when less than 1 cm [13]. Cystoscopic examination with transurethral resection therefore remains essential and to date cannot be replaced by CT.

5.2.3 Magnetic Resonance Imaging in NMIBC

Magnetic resonance imaging provides without question the best soft tissue contrast quality of all imaging modalities. This technique requires no radiation exposure but is more time-consuming and costly. The ability of MRI to produce images with such spatial resolution and detail rely on the effects of proton alignment within tissues when exposed to a magnetic field. In the most basic form, there are two phases in which images are constructed, T1 and T2. The contrast agent gadolinium is also used for better enhancement of tissues. As with computed tomography, multiplanar images in the axial, coronal, and sagittal planes can be constructed.

There are little data available in using MRI to evaluate the urinary bladder in NMIBC. However, MRI has been used to assess the urinary tract during a hematuria evaluation in patients who cannot tolerate iodinated contrast due to allergy. Magnetic resonance urography (MRU) is much similar to CTU, using gadolinium contrast to evaluate the urinary system in a delayed phase. On T1-weighted images, fluid (such as urine) is of low signal intensity and therefore the bladder appears hypointense. On T2-weighted images, fluid is of high signal intensity. On either of these phases, a bladder tumor may be demonstrated by an area of signal intensity contrasting that of urine and the bladder wall. For example, on T1-weighted imaging, a bladder tumor will likely appear as an area of intermediate intensity and on T2 phase the tumor will appear hypointense to the surrounding urine. The detrusor layer is of low signal intensity and should be intact for

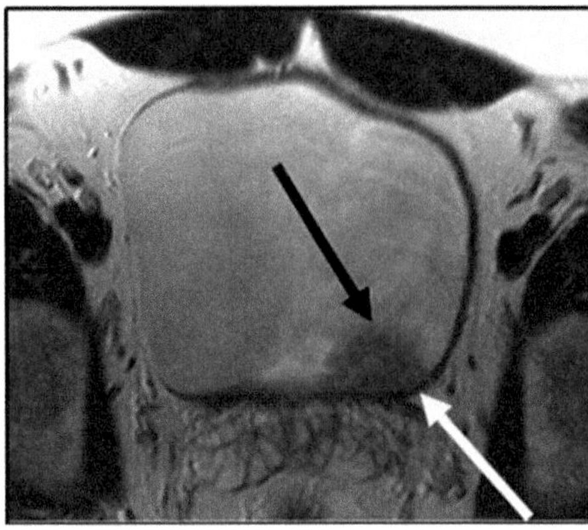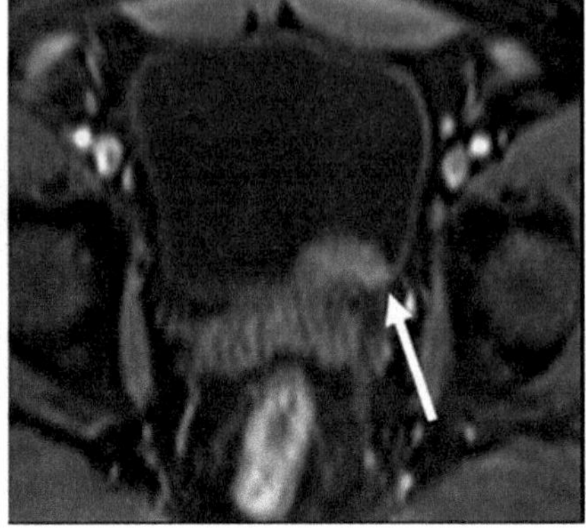

Fig. 5.4 (*Left*) T2 MRI showing non-invasive tumor with low signal intensity (*black arrow*). (*Right*) T1 MRI shows same tumor with high signal intensity compared to urine. *White arrows* denote intact detrusor layer. *Reprinted with permission* [17]

non-invasive tumors, as depicted in Fig. 5.4 [17]. With diffusion-weighted (DW) MRI (discussed later) the "inchworm sign," characterized as a low signal intensity stalk invaginating into a high signal intensity tumor, has shown to be highly accurate in predicting non-muscle invasive bladder cancer [18].

5.3 Role of Imaging in the Setting of Neoadjuvant Chemotherapy

The use of neoadjuvant systemic chemotherapy (NC) has been shown to result in improved overall survival [19]. However, controversy is still ongoing in regards to which patients should be initially managed with NC. For patients with organ confined disease ($\leq$clinical T2N0) radical cystectomy alone will likely cure most patients without the need for cytotoxic chemotherapy. On the other hand, clinical staging is notoriously inaccurate, with a discrepancy between clinical and pathologic staging in up to 50 % of cases [20]. Therefore, many of these patients will actually have more advanced disease after cystectomy and may require chemotherapy in an adjuvant setting. It has been our practice to treat patients with clinically advanced disease with neoadjuvant chemotherapy prior to radical cystectomy, although practice patterns and opinions vary on this matter. Nonetheless, radiographic imaging plays an important role in patient selection for neoadjuvant chemotherapy as well as monitoring response to treatment.

There are several findings on cross-sectional imaging with either CT or MRI that may suggest locally advanced disease. The most notable of these is hydronephrosis, which has been shown to be an independent predictor of both extravesical and node positive disease [18, 21]. Given this finding after staging one should give strong consideration to neoadjuvant chemotherapy prior to surgical resection. Hydronephrosis is apparent in both CT and MRI and is evident by dilation of the collecting system to varying degrees. Most commonly there is ureteral dilation to the level of the ureterovesical junction. It is important to evaluate the delayed images as hydroureteronephrosis may be seen as a result of upper tract TCC. If any of these findings are seen during staging of bladder cancer, one should strongly consider the use of neoadjuvant chemotherapy. Other findings suggestive of locally advanced disease include evidence of perivesical fat involvement and extension into other organs. Both of these radiographic findings are highly suspicious for T3 or T4 disease, although the lack of these findings does not necessarily rule out extravesical disease.

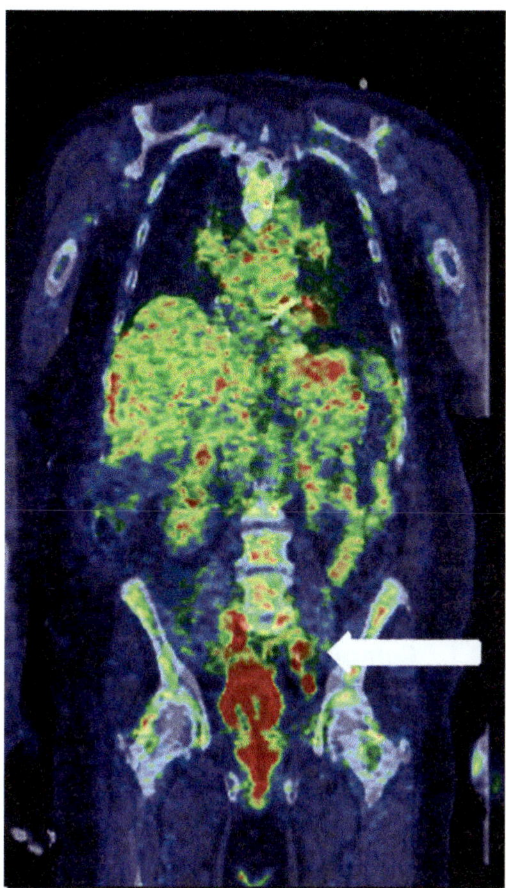

Fig. 5.5 FDG PET/CT in a 55-year-old male with T2 bladder cancer. Patient was found to have abnormal signal uptake in left iliac chain (*arrow*) and was treated with neoadjuvant chemotherapy

The use of positron emission tomography to better select patients who may benefit from NC has been evaluated in recent years. This functional study relies on the use of radio-labeled metabolic substrates to identify areas of abnormal uptake, which may suggest tumor metastasis (Fig. 5.5). To date, fludeoxyglucose (F 18) and [11C] choline have been the primary radiotracers used for bladder cancer staging with a diagnostic accuracy of 65–94 % in predicting lymph node metastasis. While it has been proposed that [11C] choline may be better for bladder cancer owing to lack of urinary excretion, no randomized controlled trials comparing the two have been conducted.

More recently, diffusion-weighted MRI has been added to conventional MRI to improve tumor staging in patients with bladder cancer. This technique relies on the relative movement of water through tissues, resulting in an apparent diffusion coefficient (ADC). It has previously been demonstrated that the ADC of bladder tumors is lower than that of the surrounding tissue [22]. Overall accuracy of predicting tumor stage was improved from 67 to 88 % with the addition of DW images to MRI T2 phase in one series [23]. Another single center experience found that use of DW-MRI with T1/T2-MRI reduced upstaging after cystectomy to 5 % [24]. While DW-MRI appears to improve diagnostic accuracy, to date most studies have been limited to small single institution experiences. Nonetheless, this newer technology holds promise in efforts to improve clinical staging to better select those patients who may benefit from NC.

Monitoring the response to neoadjuvant chemotherapy with imaging is important as well. Indeed, not all patients respond to NC and under those circumstances consideration should be given to proceeding with cystectomy. Furthermore, patients with nodal involvement who have an incomplete or no response to NC in particular have poor outcomes [25]. CT, MR, and positron emission tomography (PET) techniques have all been described as useful imaging studies during and after treatment with NC to evaluate for treatment response. At present there is no universally agreed upon strategy on how to best use imaging to monitor patients on NC. In our practices, we obtain imaging with CT or MRI after two cycles of treatment to evaluate for response. Patients in whom there appears to be objective response to chemotherapy receive 1–2 additional cycles, while those that show any signs of progression have chemotherapy interrupted and proceed to cystectomy as clinically indicated.

In efforts to better predict response of neoadjuvant chemotherapy in patients prior to cystectomy, newer modalities have been studied. Diffusion-weighted imaging (DWI) MRI had higher specificity and accuracy in predicting complete vs. partial response to chemoradiation prior to surgery when compared to T2-weighted and dynamic contrast-enhanced MRI phases in a small study of 20 patients with organ confined disease [26]. To date, this is the only experience using DWI in this setting. Martens and colleagues compared FDG-PET to conventional contrast-enhanced CT in a group of patients with lymph node positive bladder cancer undergoing NC. In this small cohort FDG-PET was no better than CT imaging in distinguishing responders from non-responders or complete vs. partial response [27].

5.4 Role of Imaging for Muscle Invasive Bladder Cancer (Clinical T2, T3, or T4)

While only about 25 % of urothelial carcinomas are found to be muscle invasive at the time of diagnosis, imaging plays a crucial role in the management of these patients. It is paramount to determine the presence of extravesical, nodal, and/or metastatic disease [28, 29] as these findings will affect treatment recommendations. This is particularly relevant as discussed previously; treatment paradigms are changing with increasing administration of neoadjuvant chemotherapy for locally advanced urothelial carcinoma [30–32].

Generally, plain radiography and ultrasound are not used routinely in the evaluation of muscle invasive urothelial carcinoma due to diminished sensitivity, the lack of high-resolution images and the absence of whole body imaging. While IVP has historically been used for detecting upper tract disease, it has a very limited role in the evaluation of locally advanced urothelial carcinoma. Like in NMIBC, CT and MRI have a predominant role in muscle invasive disease as these cross-sectional imaging modalities provide information on the overall clinical stage of the patient [33]. Additional imaging modalities include positron emission tomography (PET) and whole body bone scans. It is imperative that these studies be conducted prior to any radical extirpative surgery, as surgery may not be the initial treatment of choice for patients with advanced disease (non-organ confined extravesical tumor, regional node positive disease, or the presence of distant nodal or visceral metastases). Additionally, as most patients with muscle invasive disease will proceed to radical cystectomy, whole body imaging allows

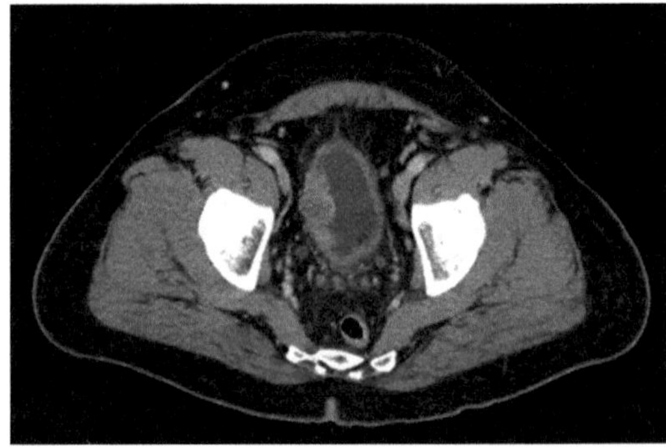

Fig. 5.6 CT demonstrating a right-sided bladder lesion that was found to be a pT3b bladder tumor

for surgical planning and facilitates the detection of anatomic variations such as duplicated ureters or ectopic kidneys.

5.4.1 Computed Tomography for Muscle Invasive Bladder Cancer

Although the primary method of in-situ clinical staging for urothelial carcinoma is with a transurethral resection, multidetector row computed tomography (CT) has become the most common modality for evaluating muscle invasive bladder cancers [34, 35]. This is due to its speed, widespread availability, and advantage of imaging multiple organs simultaneously. Considerations with the use of CT include radiation exposure and the need for an intravenous contrast agent which may be difficult in patients with contrast allergies or renal insufficiency.

Despite its widespread use, CT has a limited ability to accurately stage urothelial carcinoma. While complete intravesical lesions (stage T1) are usually apparent, there can be significant ambiguity in differentiating T2 from T3 disease [36] (Figs. 5.6 and 5.7). Several studies have demonstrated limited accuracy for CT in determining the depth of bladder invasion [37–39]. Paik et al. [40] reported an overall accuracy of 54.9 %, and under- and over-staging in 39 % and 6.1 % of patients respectively. Eight of their patients were found to have extravesical disease on CT, confirmed pathologically in only four.

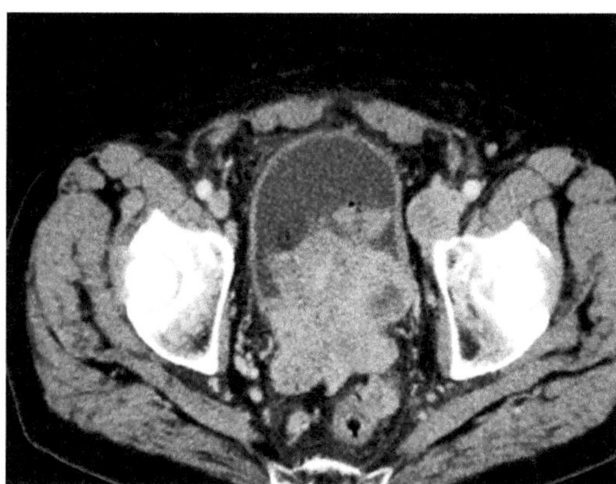

Fig. 5.7 CT demonstrating a bladder tumor easily identified as extravesical

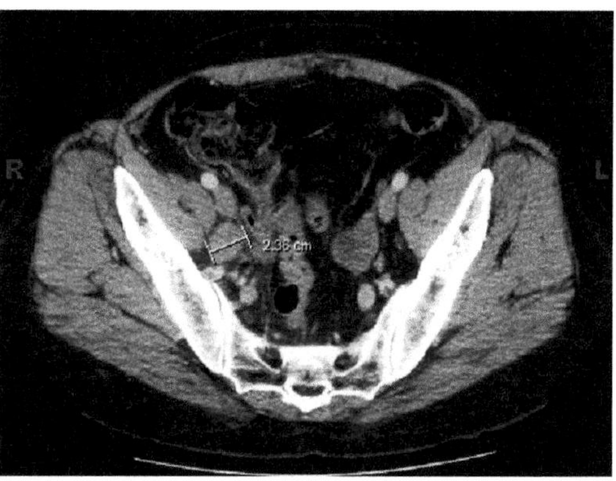

Fig. 5.8 CT demonstrates right obturator lymphadenopathy in a female patient with locally advanced bladder cancer. The node was positive for urothelial carcinoma at the time of radical cystectomy following neoadjuvant chemotherapy

More recently, Baltaci et al. [41] reported their series of 100 cases, in which only 22 of 57 (38.6 %) patients with extravesical invasion on CT were confirmed pathologically. Ambiguity of extravesical disease can be present after cystoscopic intervention and bladder tumor resection, which can cause perivesical fibrosis and mimic extravesical extension. To avoid this, imaging ideally should be obtained prior to any transurethral resection.

The presence of node positive disease is also an important prognostic factor in muscle invasive bladder cancer [42]. When examining nodal involvement with CT, it is purely an anatomic study without any functional assessment, thus lymph nodes are evaluated based on their anatomic architecture (Fig. 5.8). Size ≥ 10 mm in the short axis dimension is the most suggestive finding to determine nodal involvement. Lymph nodes also may become more rounded if involved with metastatic disease [36]. CT however, remains a poor predictor of lymph node involvement with accuracy between 5 and 50 % [42]. This poor predictive value is secondary to the inability to detect micrometastatic disease using CT.

5.4.2 Magnetic Resonance Imaging for Muscle Invasive Bladder Cancer

The role of MRI in muscle invasive bladder cancer is identical to CT: evaluation of extravesical, nodal, and metastatic disease. MRI is thought to be superior to CT in terms of local staging [34, 35, 43], however its slower speed, decreased availability, and discomfort for symptomatic patients and for those with claustrophobia make it a less accessible or optimal imaging modality for many. Despite the ability to more accurately evaluate soft tissue, there is no reported advantage in the staging of urothelial carcinoma. A recent study by Tekes et al. [44] reported on 67 patients with urothelial carcinoma staged using a dynamic MRI with gadolinium contrast and comparing results of clinical radiographic staging to pathologic stage. The overall accuracy of MRI was 62 %, with over-staging occurring in 32 % of patients. While this was found to be lower than previously published studies (72–95 % accuracy) [44], it is consistent with Vargas et al. [45] who in a prospective study found that MRI correctly staged 56 % of patients in their series while over-staging occurred in 38 % of cases.

With MRI, pelvic lymph nodes are more visible due to the surrounding adipose tissue, but this does not translate into higher accuracy in determining lymph node involvement [35]. Vargas et al. [45] report a sensitivity and specificity of only 50 % and 71 % respectively. As with CT, the determination of lymph node involvement is most reliant on a size criterion of ≥ 10 mm in shortest dimension. Normal and tumor bearing lymph nodes demonstrate similar enhancement on gadolinium-enhanced MRI.

5.4.3 Bone Scans for Muscle Invasive Bladder Cancer

Along with the lung and liver, bone is one of the more common sites of distant metastasis for urothelial carcinoma. Similar to PET scans, bone scans utilize an intravenous radio-isotope, which leads to "hot spots" or uptake seen on whole body scan. Not only metastatic disease, but also benign etiologies such as inflammation or previous trauma can create uptake noticeable on bone scan. Despite their high sensitivity for bone abnormalities, the low specificity of bone scans requires a skillful interpretation. Historically, preoperative bone scans were routinely ordered prior to radical cystectomy, which if positive would result in the patient's surgeon canceling the procedure. In contrast, Braendengen et al. [46] reviewed 91 patients following radical cystectomy who had undergone preoperative bone scans. The bone scans were scored on a scale indicating how likely it was the patient had bone metastases. They found no significant relationship between findings on preoperative bone scan and the development of subsequent bone metastases. Additionally, they evaluated 54 patients with muscle invasive urothelial carcinoma who underwent preoperative bone scan. Only three patients had positive studies that resulted in a change to their management strategy from primary surgery to primary systemic chemotherapy. Follow up revealed that one of these patients had a false-positive study, leaving only two patients who truly had metastatic bone progression. They concluded that preoperative bone scans were unnecessary as they did not contribute to the overall clinical decision making process. In today's practice, a bone scan should be ordered in the presence of symptoms such as new onset bone pain. An elevated serum alkaline phosphatase is another widely accepted indication for a bone scan, although this was not supported in the aforementioned study.

5.4.4 Positron Emission Tomography for Muscle Invasive Bladder Cancer

Positron emission tomography (PET) is a functional study with limited anatomic detail that detects the uptake of radio-isotopes by metabolically active cells in the body, such as tumor cells. In the initial diagnosis of urothelial carcinoma, the utility of PET scans is limited due to urinary excretion of the radio-isotope [43]. PET scans theoretically provide the ability to detect disease at an earlier stage, before any anatomic variation may be present. In practice however, PET scans have not routinely demonstrated superiority to detecting nodal involvement compared to CT, and may not be sensitive enough to detect node positivity unless the disease burden equates to a ≥ 10 mm lymph node [47]. There is a paucity of published data of the use of PET in urothelial carcinoma. One of the largest series published reported a sensitivity of 67 %, specificity of 86 %, and accuracy of 80 % [48] for staging of urothelial carcinoma.

Today, radiographic advancements have allowed PET scans to be fused with CT scans in order to create simultaneous anatomic and functional imagery (PET/CT). This combined image has allowed for greater accuracy than with either PET or CT alone. In their series, Kibel et al. [49] compared CT and bone scintigraphy vs. PET/CT in patients with urothelial carcinoma using [^{18}F] fluorodeoxyglucose (FDG) and found occult metastatic disease in 7 of 42 patients found to be negative on conventional CT scan. They reported a positive predictive value of 78 %, negative predictive value of 91 %, and sensitivity and specificity of 70 % and 94 % respectively for PET/CT, which is consistent with previously reported sensitivity and specificity of 60 % and 88 % respectively [47]. In addition, some authors have suggested that PET scans may provide prognostic information. Drieskens et al. [47] reported in their series a median overall survival of 32 months in patients with urothelial carcinoma and a negative PET/CT scan as opposed to 13.5 months with a positive PET/CT, which is reflective of the studies with a high positive predictive value.

One of the pitfalls of PET scans is the detection of false-positive lesions (Fig. 5.9). A false-positive evaluation can occur with intestinal uptake that mimics a metastatic lesion [47] or with areas of inflammation due to benign etiologies. Such findings must be clarified through clinical correlation and comparison or combination with CT scans or other diagnostic procedures.

In the post-treatment setting, PET scans can be utilized to detect disease response or progression after neoadjuvant chemotherapy (Fig. 5.10a, b). Post-cystectomy patients at risk for either locoregional or distant recurrence can be evaluated with PET if any suspicious or ambiguous lesions are found [50].

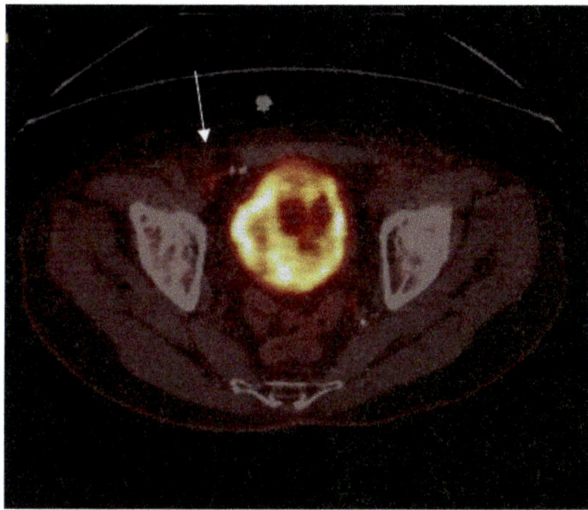

Fig. 5.9 PET/CT demonstrating a large hypermetabolic bladder tumor. Also appreciated is a right-sided mildy hypermetabolic region of soft tissue in the external iliac location, (*arrow*) which was found to be pathologically benign and attributed to granulomatous changes from prior inguinal hernia repair

5.5 Surveillance Imaging After Radical Surgery

Guidelines detailing a specific outline of follow up after radical cystectomy do not exist. Choice of imaging modality and timing is at the discretion of the surgeon, but should take into account the final pathologic tumor stage as more locally advanced disease warrants a stricter surveillance schedule. Generally, imaging of the chest, abdomen and pelvis should be performed every 3–12 months for at least 2 years with either CT or MRI [51]. A chest radiograph is considered a sufficient evaluation of the lungs; however, further work up with a CT Thorax needs to be obtained if there is a lesion of concern. Clinical suspicion should always prompt an evaluation with whole body imaging and additional studies as indicated including bone scintigraphy or PET/CT.

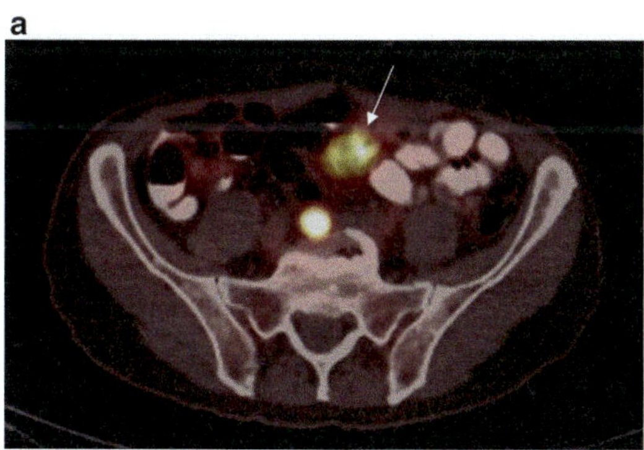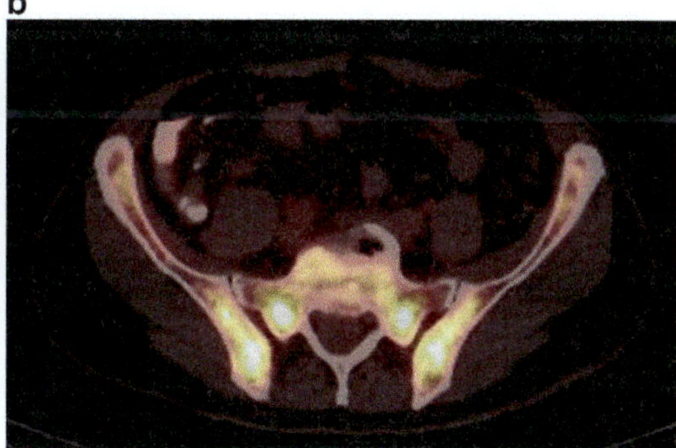

Fig. 5.10 (**a**) PET/CT reveals a large hypermetabolic pre-sacral lymph node in a male patient with muscle invasive urothelial carcinoma prior to neoadjuvant chemotherapy. Also apparent is a focus of false-positive uptake in the small intestine (*arrow*). (**b**) Resolution of the pre-sacral node after neoadjuvant chemotherapy as seen on PET/CT

References

1. Siegel R, Naishadham D, Jemal A. Cancer statistics, 2012. CA Cancer J Clin. 2012;2(1):10–29 [Comparative Study].
2. Davis R, Jones JS, Barocas DA, Castle EP, Lang EK, Leveillee RJ, et al. Diagnosis, evaluation and follow-up of asymptomatic microhematuria (AMH) in adults: AUA guideline. J Urol. 2012;188(6 Suppl):2473–81.
3. Amling CL. Diagnosis and management of superficial bladder cancer. Curr Probl Cancer. 2001;25(4):219–78.
4. Kundra V, Silverman PM. Imaging in oncology from the University of Texas M. D. Anderson Cancer Center. Imaging in the diagnosis, staging, and follow-up of cancer of the urinary bladder. Am J Roentgenol. 2003;180(4):1045–54.
5. Datta SN, Allen GM, Evans R, Vaughton KC, Lucas MG. Urinary tract ultrasonography in the evaluation of haematuria – a report of over 1,000 cases. Ann R Coll Surg Engl. 2002;84(3):203–5.
6. Malone PR, Weston-Underwood J, Aron PM, Wilkinson KW, Joseph AE, Riddle PR. The use of transabdominal ultrasound in the detection of early bladder tumours. Br J Urol. 1986;58(5):520–2.
7. Ozden E, Turgut AT, Turkolmez K, Resorlu B, Safak M. Effect of bladder carcinoma location on detection rates by ultrasonography and computed tomography. Urology. 2007;69(5):889–92.
8. Abu-Yousef MM, Narayana AS, Franken Jr EA, Brown RC. Urinary bladder tumors studied by cystosonography. Part I: detection. Radiology. 1984;153(1):223–6.
9. Quaia E. Microbubble ultrasound contrast agents: an update. Eur Radiol. 2007;17(8):1995–2008.
10. Caruso G, Salvaggio G, Campisi A, Melloni D, Midiri M, Bertolotto M, et al. Bladder tumor staging: comparison of contrast-enhanced and gray-scale ultrasound. Am J Roentgenol. 2010;194(1):151–6.
11. Nicolau C, Bunesch L, Peri L, Salvador R, Corral JM, Mallofre C, et al. Accuracy of contrast-enhanced ultrasound in the detection of bladder cancer. Br J Radiol. 2011;84(1008):1091–9.
12. Li QY, Tang J, He EH, Li YM, Zhou Y, Zhang X, et al. Clinical utility of three-dimensional contrast-enhanced ultrasound in the differentiation between noninvasive and invasive neoplasms of urinary bladder. Eur J Radiol. 2012;81(11):2936–42.
13. Wang LJ, Wong YC, Ng KF, Chuang CK, Lee SY, Wan YL. Tumor characteristics of urothelial carcinoma on multidetector computerized tomography urography. J Urol. 2010;183(6):2154–60.
14. Turney BW, Willatt JM, Nixon D, Crew JP, Cowan NC. Computed tomography urography for diagnosing bladder cancer. BJU Int. 2006;98(2):345–8.
15. Blick CG, Nazir SA, Mallett S, Turney BW, Onwu NN, Roberts IS, et al. Evaluation of diagnostic strategies for bladder cancer using computed tomography (CT) urography, flexible cystoscopy and voided urine cytology: results for 778 patients from a hospital haematuria clinic. BJU Int. 2012;110(1):84–94.
16. Sadow CA, Silverman SG, O'Leary MP, Signorovitch JE. Bladder cancer detection with CT urography in an Academic Medical Center. Radiology. 2008;249(1):195–202.
17. Rajesh A, Sokhi HK, Fung R, Mulcahy KA, Bankart MJ. Bladder cancer: evaluation of staging accuracy using dynamic MRI. Clin Radiol. 2011;66(12):1140–5.
18. Green DA, Rink M, Hansen J, Cha EK, Robinson B, Tian Z, et al. Accurate preoperative prediction of non-organ-confined bladder urothelial carcinoma at cystectomy. BJU Int. 2013;111(3):404–11.
19. Winquist E, Kirchner TS, Segal R, Chin J, Lukka H. Genitourinary Cancer Disease Site Group CCOPiE-bCPGI. Neoadjuvant chemotherapy for transitional cell carcinoma of the bladder: a systematic review and meta-analysis. J Urol. 2004;171(2 Pt 1):561–9.
20. Svatek RS, Shariat SF, Novara G, Skinner EC, Fradet Y, Bastian PJ, et al. Discrepancy between clinical and pathological stage: external validation of the impact on prognosis in an international radical cystectomy cohort. BJU Int. 2011;107(6):898–904.
21. Stimson CJ, Cookson MS, Barocas DA, Clark PE, Humphrey JE, Patel SG, et al. Preoperative hydronephrosis predicts extravesical and node positive disease in patients undergoing cystectomy for bladder cancer. J Urol. 2010;183(5):1732–7.
22. Matsuki M, Inada Y, Tatsugami F, Tanikake M, Narabayashi I, Katsuoka Y. Diffusion-weighted MR imaging for urinary bladder carcinoma: initial results. Eur Radiol. 2007;17(1):201–4.
23. Takeuchi M, Sasaki S, Ito M, Okada S, Takahashi S, Kawai T, et al. Urinary bladder cancer: diffusion-weighted MR imaging–accuracy for diagnosing T stage and estimating histologic grade. Radiology. 2009;251(1):112–21 [Evaluation Studies Research Support, Non-U.S. Gov't].
24. Watanabe H, Kanematsu M, Kondo H, Goshima S, Tsuge Y, Onozuka M, et al. Preoperative T staging of urinary bladder cancer: does diffusion-weighted MRI have supplementary value? Am J Roentgenol. 2009;192(5):1361–6.
25. Jensen JB, Ulhoi BP, Jensen KM. Prognostic value of lymph-node dissection in patients undergoing radical cystectomy following previous oncological treatment for bladder cancer. Scand J Urol Nephrol. 2011;45(6):436–43.
26. Yoshida S, Koga F, Kawakami S, Ishii C, Tanaka H, Numao N, et al. Initial experience of diffusion-weighted magnetic resonance imaging to assess therapeutic response to induction chemoradiotherapy against muscle-invasive bladder cancer. Urology. 2010;75(2):387–91.
27. Mertens LS, Fioole-Bruining A, van Rhijn BW, Kerst JM, Bergman AM, Vogel WV, et al. FDG-positron emission tomography/computerized tomography for monitoring the response of pelvic lymph node metastasis to neoadjuvant chemotherapy for bladder cancer. J Urol. 2013;189(5):1687–91.
28. Dighe MK, Bhargava P, Wright J. Urinary bladder masses: techniques, imaging spectrum, and staging. J Comput Assist Tomogr. 2011;35(4):411–24 [Review].

29. Ficarra V, Dalpiaz O, Alrabi N, Novara G, Galfano A, Artibani W. Correlation between clinical and pathological staging in a series of radical cystectomies for bladder carcinoma. BJU Int. 2005;95(6):786–90.
30. Grossman HB, Natale RB, Tangen CM, Speights VO, Vogelzang NJ, Trump DL, et al. Neoadjuvant chemotherapy plus cystectomy compared with cystectomy alone for locally advanced bladder cancer. N Engl J Med. 2003;349(9):859–66.
31. Sherif A, Holmberg L, Rintala E, Mestad O, Nilsson J, Nilsson S, et al. Neoadjuvant cisplatinum based combination chemotherapy in patients with invasive bladder cancer: a combined analysis of two Nordic studies. Eur Urol. 2004;45(3):297–303 [Research Support, Non-U.S. Gov't].
32. Malmstrom PU, Rintala E, Wahlqvist R, Hellstrom P, Hellsten S, Hannisdal E. Five-year followup of a prospective trial of radical cystectomy and neoadjuvant chemotherapy: nordic cystectomy trial I. The Nordic Cooperative Bladder Cancer Study Group. J Urol. 1996;155(6):1903–6.
33. Husband JE. Computer tomography and magnetic resonance imaging in the evaluation of bladder cancer. J Belge Radiol. 1995;78(6):350–5 [Research Support, Non-U.S. Gov't Review].
34. Beyersdorff D, Zhang J, Schoder H, Bochner B, Hricak H. Bladder cancer: can imaging change patient management? Curr Opin Urol. 2008;18(1):98–104 [Review].
35. Cowan NC, Crew JP. Imaging bladder cancer. Curr Opin Urol. 2010;20(5):409–13 [Review].
36. Setty BN, Holalkere NS, Sahani DV, Uppot RN, Harisinghani M, Blake MA. State-of-the-art cross-sectional imaging in bladder cancer. Curr Probl Diagn Radiol. 2007;36(2):83–96 [Review].
37. Voges GE, Tauschke E, Stockle M, Alken P, Hohenfellner R. Computerized tomography: an unreliable method for accurate staging of bladder tumors in patients who are candidates for radical cystectomy. J Urol. 1989;142(4):972–4 [Comparative Study].
38. Bryan PJ, Butler HE, LiPuma JP, Resnick MI, Kursh ED. CT and MR imaging in staging bladder neoplasms. J Comput Assist Tomogr. 1987;11(1):96–101 [Comparative Study].
39. Yaman O, Baltaci S, Arikan N, Yilmaz E, Gogus O. Staging with computed tomography, transrectal ultrasonography and transurethral resection of bladder tumour: comparison with final pathological stage in invasive bladder carcinoma. Br J Urol. 1996;78(2):197–200 [Comparative Study].
40. Paik ML, Scolieri MJ, Brown SL, Spirnak JP, Resnick MI. Limitations of computerized tomography in staging invasive bladder cancer before radical cystectomy. J Urol. 2000;163(6):1693–6 [Research Support, Non-U.S. Gov't].
41. Baltaci S, Resorlu B, Yagci C, Turkolmez K, Gogus C, Beduk Y. Computerized tomography for detecting perivesical infiltration and lymph node metastasis in invasive bladder carcinoma. Urol Int. 2008;81(4):399–402.
42. Tilki D, Brausi M, Colombo R, Evans CP, Fradet Y, Fritsche HM, et al. Lymphadenectomy for bladder cancer at the time of radical cystectomy. Eur Urol. 2013;64(2):266–76.
43. Verma S, Rajesh A, Prasad SR, Gaitonde K, Lall CG, Mouraviev V, et al. Urinary bladder cancer: role of MR imaging. Radiographics. 2012;32(2):371–87 [Research Support, Non-U.S. Gov't Review].
44. Tekes A, Kamel I, Imam K, Szarf G, Schoenberg M, Nasir K, et al. Dynamic MRI of bladder cancer: evaluation of staging accuracy. Am J Roentgenol. 2005;184(1):121–7.
45. Vargas HA, Akin O, Schoder H, Olgac S, Dalbagni G, Hricak H, et al. Prospective evaluation of MRI, (1)(1) C-acetate PET/CT and contrast-enhanced CT for staging of bladder cancer. Eur J Radiol. 2012;81(12):4131–7 [Comparative Study].
46. Braendengen M, Winderen M, Fossa SD. Clinical significance of routine pre-cystectomy bone scans in patients with muscle-invasive bladder cancer. Br J Urol. 1996;77(1):36–40.
47. Drieskens O, Oyen R, Van Poppel H, Vankan Y, Flamen P, Mortelmans L. FDG-PET for preoperative staging of bladder cancer. Eur J Nucl Med Mol Imaging. 2005;32(12):1412–7 [Clinical Trial].
48. Bachor R, Kotzerke J, Reske SN, Hautmann R. Lymph node staging of bladder neck carcinoma with positron emission tomography. Urologe A. 1999;38(1):46–50.
49. Kibel AS, Dehdashti F, Katz MD, Klim AP, Grubb RL, Humphrey PA, et al. Prospective study of [18F] fluorodeoxyglucose positron emission tomography/ computed tomography for staging of muscle-invasive bladder carcinoma. J Clin Oncol. 2009;27(26):4314–20.
50. Schoder H, Larson SM. Positron emission tomography for prostate, bladder, and renal cancer. Semin Nucl Med. 2004;34(4):274–92 [Review].
51. Network NCC. Bladder cancer. Fort Washington, PA, Version I. 2013 [cited 2013 September 1]; Available from: www.nccn.org

New Imaging Techniques in the Staging of Urothelial Carcinoma of the Bladder

Ramdev Konijeti and Adam S. Kibel

6.1 Introduction

The management of urothelial carcinoma of the bladder (UCB) is highly dependent on stage. Tumors confined to the mucosa can be safely managed with local resection with or without intravesical agents. In contrast, locally advanced UCB is managed more aggressively with radical cystectomy, often with systemic chemotherapy administered either in the neoadjuvant or adjuvant setting. Lastly, metastatic disease is managed with systemic chemotherapy alone. Accordingly, accurate pre-treatment staging of UCB is an essential component of effective care, in that it affords appropriate selection of patients for optimal intervention.

Unfortunately, current standard imaging modalities do not effectively identify local extent of tumor or micrometastatic disease [1–7]. Historically, when compared to transurethral resection or radical cystectomy for assessment of depth of invasion, the overall accuracy of computed tomography (CT) ranges from 55 to 92 % [4]. The accuracy of magnetic resonance imaging (MRI) for assessing depth of invasion into muscle is better than CT, ranging from 73 to 96 % [3]. Overall, the results of CT and MRI for the detection of lymph node metastases are similar, as they are both based on size criteria with sensitivities for detection of disease confirmed on histology ranging from 48 to 87 % [3]. This unfortunately limits the ability to detect up to approximately half of patients with metastatic disease who would potentially benefit from earlier institution of systemic therapy. Current algorithms for identification of visceral, bone and pulmonary metastatic disease are fraught with similarly poor sensitivity and specificity.

This chapter aims to address the newer imaging techniques used in the setting of staging of UCB. When considering treatment for UCB, determination of the extent of local disease and/or nodal involvement is of utmost importance to assess which patients are best suited for conservative management versus a single or multimodal therapy. While conventional imaging techniques clearly play a central role in the assessment of bladder cancer, the focus of this chapter will be to highlight the current state-of-the-art with respect to use of newer magnetic resonance (e.g. diffusion-weighted MRI (DW MRI), dynamic contrast enhanced MRI (DCE MRI), and MRI lymphography) and nuclear medicine (positron emission tomography (PET) and PET/CT) techniques for these purposes.

R. Konijeti, M.D. • A.S. Kibel, M.D. (✉)
Division of Urology, Department of Surgery,
Brigham and Women's Hospital, Harvard Medical School, 45 Francis Street, Boston, MA 02115, USA
e-mail: akibel@partners.org

B.R. Konety and S.S. Chang (eds.), *Management of Bladder Cancer:
A Comprehensive Text With Clinical Scenarios*, DOI 10.1007/978-1-4939-1881-2_6,
© Springer Science+Business Media New York 2015

6.2 Assessment of Local Disease Extent

The accurate assessment of depth of invasion is a significant problem in the management of bladder carcinoma. While inaccurate staging rarely occurs for low-grade disease, high-grade disease is more aggressive than initially appreciated. Herr et al. demonstrated that 28 % of patients with high-grade pathologic (pT1) UCB on initial resection were found to have residual T1 disease at re-resection [8]. Furthermore, up to 40 % of patients with clinical T1 (cT1) disease demonstrate muscle invasion in the final cystectomy specimen [9]. In addition, even after re-resection, cT1 tumors still have a very high rate of progression indicating that many will or have already developed invasive disease, even if it cannot be identified [8].

The clinical utility of assessing depth of invasion is not limited simply to identification of patients in need of extirpative surgery, but also to identification of those in need of neoadjuvant systemic chemotherapy. Since approximately 50 % of patients with extravesical extension develop metastatic disease [10] and neoadjuvant chemotherapy has been demonstrated to be most effective in patients with increased depth of invasion into the bladder wall [11], more accurate assessment of depth of invasion will steer patients most in need of aggressive therapy in that direction.

6.2.1 Conventional MRI

Advantages of conventional MRI when compared to CT are improved soft tissue contrast resolution and the lack of ionizing radiation. On T1-weighted (T1W) images, the bladder tumor typically has low-to-intermediate signal intensity similar to that of the bladder wall. However, on T2-weighted (T2W) images, the tumor tends to be more appreciable, as it contrasts with adjacent structures (i.e. its signal intensity is between that of the darker bladder wall and the brighter urine), thus facilitating tumor assessment [12]. In studies performed prior to the advent of multidetector row CT, MRI was reported to be up to 33 % more accurate than conventional CT for assessment of depth of invasion [3]. A final advantage is that MRI does not utilize ionizing radiation, therefore making it more favorable in populations that might need repeat examinations due to concerns about cancer risk from repeat radiation exposure [13].

However, as mentioned previously, conventional MRI with T1W/T2W imaging does not accurately assess if a bladder mass is actually cancer, assess the extent of local wall invasion, or assess microscopic invasion. To help address this challenge, MRI has evolved and functional pulse sequences (DW MRI and DCE MRI) have been developed to determine both grade and stage of the local lesion.

6.2.2 Diffusion-Weighted MRI (DW MRI)

DW MRI produces in vivo images of biological tissues weighted with the local microstructural characteristics of water diffusion. Essentially, this provides an indication of how far a water molecule can move. Malignant tissues have been shown to have more restricted diffusion, also known as an Apparent Diffusion Coefficient (ADC), when compared with normal tissues. This is due to the fact that cancer cells are smaller and therefore water cannot move as far [12].

Early work in DW MRI focused on cancer detection, rather than local staging. One of the earliest reports demonstrating the potential utility of DW MRI for imaging of bladder carcinoma was by Matsuki et al. [14]. They reported the sensitivity and positive predictive value (PPV) for detection of bladder tumors at 100 % in 17 urinary bladder carcinomas. All lesions, compared to cystoscopy as the gold standard, demonstrated high signal intensity relative to surrounding tissue and a significantly lower ADC value. Abou-El-Ghar et al. compared conventional T2W MRI to DW MRI in 130 patients with gross hematuria for the detection of UCB [15]. They reported the sensitivity/specificity of DW MRI and T2W MRI for local UCB detection to be 98 %/92 % and 96 %/86 %, respectively, in comparison to cystoscopy. However, this difference was not statistically significant. Avcu et al. reported a sensitivity and specificity of 100 % and 77 %, respectively, for DW MRI in the detection of 46 malignant bladder lesions [16]. These studies focus on detection rates of malignant bladder lesions, compared to cystoscopy, and although DW MRI is less invasive, it has yet to be found to be equivalent or superior to the gold standard of cystoscopy for UCB detection and has significantly higher cost.

The potential advantage of DW MRI lies with the ability to assess local depth of tumor invasion, as well as histologic grade. Although it demonstrated inferior sensitivity compared to unenhanced and gadolinium-enhanced images, Watanabe et al. reported that DW MRI demonstrated superior specificity of 93 % (compared to 79 % for both unenhanced and enhanced images) in the identification of tumors $\geq$T2. Furthermore, they demonstrated that the correlation between the radiologic and pathologic stages was greater with DW MRI, in comparison to unenhanced and enhanced sequences ($p=0.044$ and $p=0.031$, respectively) [17].

Another study evaluating the ability of DW MRI to assess depth of invasion is a prospective study of 106 patients conducted by El-Assmy et al. They noted a local staging accuracy with DW MRI of 63.6 % (21/33), 75.7 % (25/33), 93.7 % (30/32), and 87.5 % (7/8) for stages T1, T2, T3, and T4, respectively, compared to an overall staging accuracy of only 39.6 % for T2W MRI, both of which were compared to the gold standard of histopathology following tumor resection or radical cystectomy. They demonstrated that the accuracy of DW MRI in differentiating superficial from invasive tumors and organ-confined from non-organ-confined tumors was 63.6 % and 69.6 %, respectively. This was in comparison to respective accuracies of 6.1 % and 15.1 % for conventional T2W MRI [18].

In addition to prospectively evaluating its ability to determine T stage of UCB, grade can be assessed using ADC values. Takeuchi et al. correlated ADC values in DW MRI to histological grade of 52 bladder tumors in 40 patients. The accuracy for assessment of T stage of T2W MRI versus combined T2W MRI with DW MRI was improved from 67 to 88 %. The overall accuracy for diagnosing $\geq$T2 bladder carcinoma was significantly improved by adding diffusion-weighted images ($p<0.01$). Additionally, the mean ADC of grade 3 (G3) tumors was significantly lower than that of grade 1 and 2 tumors ($p<0.01$) [19].

6.2.3 Dynamic Contrast-Enhanced MRI (DCE MRI)

An MRI technique that can be used either as an alternative or a supplement to DW MRI is dynamic contrast-enhanced MRI (DCE MRI). DCE MRI provides an index of tumor vascularity compared to normal bladder wall vascularity. With this modality, Fast Gradient Recalled Echo (GRE) T1W images are obtained before, during, and after intravenous injection of gadolinium. Since malignant bladder lesions have more blood vessels, they tend to enhance earlier and with more intensity than the remainder of the bladder wall [20]. A study by Tuncbilek et al. in which 24 patients were examined using DCE MRI to investigate its ability to measure bladder cancer angiogenesis, noted a correlation between DCE MRI parameters and microvessel density (assessed by immunostaining), and histologic grade. Furthermore, a significant difference ($p<0.05$) was seen between groups of patients with and without local recurrence with regard to two of the DCE MRI parameters (peak time enhancement in the first and second minute after contrast administration (E(max/1) and E(max/2))) [21], providing evidence that DCE MRI may be used to noninvasively assess histopathologic characteristics and to predict local recurrence.

In an effort to evaluate DCE MRI in tumor and node staging and differentiation of urinary bladder cancer from postbiopsy effects, Barentz et al. prospectively evaluated 61 consecutive patients with histologically proven urinary bladder cancer. Patients underwent unenhanced and DCE MRI 1–4 weeks after undergoing transurethral resection or biopsy. With the DCE technique, they were able to demonstrate that malignant bladder lesions enhanced earlier than normal bladder wall in comparison to unenhanced images [22].

To evaluate the utility of DCE MRI in the staging of superficial tumors, Scattoni et al. correlated histopathologic findings to imaging findings in unenhanced and DCE MRI. The overall accuracy of DCE MRI compared to T1W and T2W MRI in assessment of depth of invasion of UCB in 48 patients was reported to be 81 % compared to 58 % and 71 %, respectively. With respect to superficial involvement of the bladder wall (Ta-T1 disease), DCE MRI correctly assessed 84 % of cases and muscular infiltration ($\geq$T2 disease) in 63 % of cases [23].

6.2.4 Positron Emission Tomography/Computed Tomography (PET/CT)

Positron emission tomography (PET) imaging leverages a core characteristic of cancer cells: increased metabolism. PET affords the opportunity to use a systemically administered, radiolabeled tracer that can be followed as it is metabolized. These tracers are preferentially consumed by metabolically active cells, including cancer cells. Tracers that have been investigated for utility in bladder cancer imaging include ^{18}F-fluorodeoxyglucose (^{18}F-FDG), ^{11}C-choline, ^{11}C-methionine, and ^{11}C-acetate.

While these tracers share an affinity for rapidly dividing cells, they leverage different metabolic processes. The most commonly used is ^{18}F-FDG, a radiolabeled glucose analog that enters tumor cells via glucose transporters and undergoes limited metabolism once inside, thus resulting in intracellular accumulation [24]. ^{11}C-choline depends on a different cellular process. It is eventually synthesized into ^{11}C-phosphatidylcholine, which is a major constituent of the cell membrane. The uptake of choline by cells is, therefore, enhanced during tumor proliferation [25]. A significant limitation to ^{11}C-choline is its short half-life, limiting its use to institutions with an on-site cyclotron [20]. ^{11}C-methionine is proportional to the amino acid transport within cells. Methionine is used for protein synthesis, as it is used to convert S-adenosylmethionine, which acts as a donor of methyl groups in various biologic processes; it is a precursor in polyamine synthesis and the transsulfuration pathway. Cancer cells are dependent on the external supply of methionine because the transmethylation rate is high in tumor cells. As such, increased methionine uptake can be considered a marker of malignant tissue [26]. In contrast, ^{11}C acetate uptake depends on lipid synthesis. It is metabolized and incorporated into the cellular lipid pool, mostly for the purpose of cell membrane synthesis. Increased incorporation of acetate into cells is a marker of increased fatty acid synthesis. ^{11}C-acetate has a very short half-life and, as a result, requires the presence of an on-site cyclotron, similar to ^{11}C-choline [25]. While ^{11}C-choline, ^{11}C-methionine, and ^{11}C-acetate have minimal excretion in the urine, a significant limitation of ^{18}F-FDG is its urinary excretion thus obscuring the ability to visualize and assess the wall of the bladder [20].

Despite the potential for intravesical tracer accumulation to interfere with images of the bladder, PET/CT with ^{18}F-FDG has been explored in the assessment of localized disease. To overcome the limitation of the mode of elimination of this tracer, investigators have used forced diuresis and bladder drainage. Anjos et al. examined a total of 17 patients with UCB (6 who subsequently underwent a cystectomy and 11 who did not) using ^{18}F-FDG PET/CT. They obtained initial imaging, but also additional pelvic images obtained 1 h after intravenous furosemide and oral hydration. Of the total group of 17 patients, the delayed images using diuresis and hydration changed the final PET/CT reading in seven patients. Additionally, 41 % of patients were upstaged on the basis of the delayed pelvic images alone [27].

Another method that facilitates use of ^{18}F-FDG PET/CT to identify local disease was use of Foley catheter drainage by Kibel et al. [28]. To facilitate clearance of urinary activity, a Foley catheter was placed before injection of FDG, followed by intravenous furosemide approximately 20 min later, with hydration administered throughout the study. Of 34 patients in whom a primary tumor focus was identified at the time of cystectomy, 28 (82 %) demonstrated increased FDG uptake on preoperative ^{18}F-FDG PET/CT.

Conventional CT has been compared to ^{18}F-FDG PET/CT in assessment of local disease. Lodde et al. compared conventional CT to ^{18}F-FDG PET/CT with forced diuresis in 70 patients of whom 44 patients had known muscle-invasive disease prior to radical cystectomy. Of these 44 patients, four had no residual cancer in the bladder at definitive pathology, leaving 40 for sensitivity calculations. Conventional CT had a sensitivity of 77 %, which was lower than that for ^{18}F-FDG PET/CT, which was 85 %. However the specificity of ^{18}F-FDG PET/CT was 25 %, compared to 50 % for conventional CT, meaning that ^{18}F-FDG PET/CT more frequently incorrectly identified tumor in bladder. CT missed six residual muscle-invasive UCBs, compared to four missed by ^{18}F-FDG PET/CT. ^{18}F-FDG PET/CT detected one cancer in a bladder diverticulum and detected 2 of 13 prostate invasions (pT4a) [29].

This mixed data limit the role of ^{18}F-FDG PET/CT to appropriately assess local disease in a reliable manner. The above data demonstrated that, although it is feasible, ^{18}F-FDG PET/CT does not appear to add additional information to the gold standard of transurethral resection in assessment of depth of invasion of local UCB.

[11]C-choline has also been investigated in the assessment of localized disease. Gofrit et al. evaluated 16 patients who underwent ^{11}C-choline PET/CTfollowed by radical surgery in comparison with histopathologic findings. ^{11}C-choline uptake was found in all primary tumors. The series included three patients with refractory bladder carcinoma in situ, which was visualized in all three. They were able to demonstrate not only excellent sensitivity for use of ^{11}C-choline PET/CT, but the potential ability to identify CIS [30]. Picchio et al. compared the diagnostic accuracy of preoperative contrast-enhanced CT and ^{11}C-choline PET for the staging of 27 patients who underwent radical cystectomy. The presence of residual bladder cancer (pTa-pT4) was correctly detected in 84 % and 96 % of histologically tumor-positive patients by CT and ^{11}C-choline PET, respectively. They concluded that ^{11}C-choline PET is comparable to CT for detecting residual cancer after transurethral resection [31]. These studies raise the possibility that ^{11}C-choline PET could identify occult CIS or cancer in patients with positive cytologies or local response to chemotherapy prior to surgery or radiation therapy. This remains to be proven and the short half-life of the tracer limits its use to selected centers.

Two other less extensively studied tracers, ^{11}C-methionine and ^{11}C-acetate, have been explored but not found to be superior to conventional imaging. Ahlstrom et al. examined ^{11}C-methionine in the diagnosis and staging of UCB in patients with biopsy-proven disease prior to treatment with resection or cystectomy. Eighteen out of twenty-three primary tumors were detected, but this modality was not superior to CT or MRI [32]. ^{11}C-acetate PET/CT has also failed to demonstrate superiority. In a prospective comparison of ^{11}C-acetate PET/CT, MRI, and contrast-enhanced CT for staging of local UCB, all three imaging modalities were found to have similar accuracy (50 %, 56 %, and 75 %, respectively) in 16 patients with histologically confirmed bladder cancer prior to radical cystectomy. For all modalities, staging accuracy was reduced in patients with a history of prior intravesical and/or systemic chemotherapy [33].

PET/CT, although feasible, is limited with respect to detection and staging of local UCB, due to tracer accumulation within the urinary bladder, in the case of ^{18}F-FDG, and limited data and short half-life, in the case of ^{11}C-choline, ^{11}C-methionine, and ^{11}C-acetate. However, early reports demonstrate promise with respect to non-invasive detection of carcinoma in situ and re-staging of the primary tumor following transurethral resection and prior to radical cystectomy.

6.3 Assessment of Metastatic Disease

The current standard of detection for nodal involvement of UCB is based on size (positive findings if pelvic nodes are greater than 8 mm and abdominal nodes are greater than 10 mm in maximum short-axis diameter) on cross-sectional imaging [3]. Since metastatic disease does exist in lymph nodes smaller than the aforementioned size criteria, this definition will miss up to 50 % of metastatic disease [3]. In addition, patients have enlarged lymph nodes for reasons other than metastatic cancer and may be incorrectly characterized as having metastatic cancer.

Furthermore, improved identification of bone metastatic disease is clearly needed. Current National Comprehensive Cancer Network (NCCN) guidelines advocate the use of bone scintigraphy only in the setting of an abnormal serum alkaline phosphatase (AP) [34]. However, Abbosh et al. demonstrated that although serum AP demonstrated reasonable specificity (86 %) and negative predictive value (86 %), up to half of patients with bone metastases have normal serum AP levels [35].

Appropriate staging of patients, with respect to the presence and location of metastatic disease, is crucial for risk stratification and most importantly for appropriate treatment selection. The pattern of UCB recurrence at distant sites indicates that the predominant cause is occult micrometastases present at the time of cystectomy. Grossman et al. demonstrated that neoadjuvant chemotherapy followed by radical cystectomy improved survival compared to radical cystectomy alone, indicating that micrometastatic disease could be effectively treated [11]. Because of physical limitations that might arise after radical cystectomy, fewer candidates can tolerate postoperative chemotherapy [36]. The effectiveness of neoadjuvant chemotherapy and the poor tolerability of adjuvant chemotherapy are perhaps the most compelling reasons to correctly identify patients with micrometastatic disease preoperatively.

6.4 MRI Lymphography

One modality that might address our current barriers to detection of micrometastatic nodal disease is the use of ultra small superparamagnetic iron oxide (USPIO) particles. USPIO nanoparticles are composed of iron oxide crystals coated with polymers to avoid uncontrolled aggregation of the magnetic crystals. They preferentially accumulate in the normal lymphatic tissue of the lymph nodes.

Metastatic disease leaves a defect in the signal which is detected by MRI [37].

The initial clinical experience with USPIO particles was published by Bellin et al. who studied 30 adults suspected of having lymph node metastases in a variety of malignancies who underwent MR imaging before and 22–26 h after intravenous infusion of USPIO particles. Subsequently, suspicious lymph nodes were biopsies or resected. The MRI images demonstrated 100 % sensitivity and 80 % specificity in detection of lymph node metastases [38].

USPIO particles in bladder cancer were first studied by Deserno et al. who demonstrated selective decrease in signal intensity on T2W images in nodal metastases, when compared to normal nodal tissue. In 58 patients with proven UCB on biopsy or transurethral resection and no other prior imaging, 172 nodes imaged prior to surgical excision or image-guided biopsy with the use of the particles revealed 50 malignant nodes. This translated to a sensitivity and specificity of 92 % and 76 % for detection of nodal metastatic disease, respectively. Additionally, of 12 normal-sized lymph nodes found eventually to harbor metastatic disease on histopathologic analysis, this technique accurately identified ten [39].

A second study attempted to prove that USPIO particles were superior to DW MRI by performing preoperative 3-T MRI before and after administration of the USPIO particles in 21 patients prior to radical cystectomy with extended lymphadenectomy. Diagnostic accuracy was similar for both conventional MRI and MRI with USPIO particles. The only improvement was time of analysis, which was significantly shorter with USPIO-DW MRI compared to conventional MR (13 min versus 80 min, respectively; $p < 0.0001$) [40], which is of limited clinical benefit. Additional potential of this imaging modality continues to be explored.

6.4.1 Positron Emission Tomography/Computed Tomography (PET/CT)

PET/CT is emerging as the best novel modality to detect micrometastatic disease. A clear advantage of PET/CT over cross-sectional imaging,

MRI lymphography, and bone scintigraphy is that nodal, visceral, and bony metastatic disease can be identified with a single imaging modality. When combined with CT, PET allows for the combination of the optimal functional imaging of PET with the anatomic characterization of CT. As discussed previously, tracers that have been investigated for utility in UCB staging include ^{18}F-fluorodeoxyglucose (^{18}F-FDG), ^{11}C-choline, ^{11}C-methionine, and ^{11}C-acetate.

Detection of metastatic disease with ^{18}F-FDG PET/CT has shown more promise than its use in detection of local disease. Drieskens et al. evaluated the utility of preoperative ^{18}F-FDG PET and CT done separately, followed by correlative imaging leading to a PET/CT result, in 40 patients with histology-proven bladder cancer and compared their results to histopathology (via lymphadenectomy or biopsy) and clinical follow-up for 12 months. They reported a sensitivity and specificity of 60 % and 88 %, respectively, for detection of nodal and/or metastatic disease with ^{18}F-FDG PET/CT. Diagnostic discordances between PET/CT and CT alone were found in 9 out of 40 (approximately 23 %), among whom PET was correct in 6 patients (3 with true-positive and 1 with true-negative distant metastases, and 2 with true-negative lymph nodes). PET/CT, compared to conventional CT, enabled true upstaging of distant metastatic disease and true downstaging of NM-negative disease [41].

Kibel et al. evaluated the ability of preoperative ^{18}F-FDG PET/CT to identify metastatic disease. They prospectively evaluated 43 chemotherapy-naïve patients with clinical stage T2-T3N0M0 urothelial carcinoma of the bladder preoperatively with ^{18}F-FDG PET/CT, all of whom had negative conventional CT and bone scintigraphy. Positive findings were confirmed with percutaneous biopsy or open lymphadenectomy, whereas patients with negative findings were subjected to complete lymphadenectomy. ^{18}F-FDG PET/CT demonstrated a sensitivity and specificity of 70 % and 94 %, respectively. Most importantly, negative ^{18}F-FDG PET/CT findings correlated significantly with recurrence-free survival, disease-specific survival, and overall survival. Of note, two patients with positive PET/CT had an altered treatment approach following

biopsy confirmation of nodal disease. One underwent neoadjuvant chemotherapy followed by cystectomy and remained disease-free at 24 months post-cystectomy. Another was found to have widespread metastatic disease, obviating the need for surgery, and ultimately died of metastatic disease 5 months following the PET/CT [28].

Conventional cross-sectional imaging, with CT or MRI, was compared to ^{18}F-FDG PET/CT by Apolo et al. They analyzed findings in 47 patients who underwent ^{18}F-FDG PET/CT after conventional CT or MRI. Findings were then compared to biopsy, obtained at the discretion of the practicing oncologist, or serial CT or MRI. They demonstrated an overall sensitivity and specificity of 87 % and 88 %, respectively, for ^{18}F-FDG PET/CT in 135 lesions in 47 patients. ^{18}F-FDG PET/CT detected additional metastatic deposits in 40 % of patients. Furthermore, clinicians changed their planned management in 68 % of patients based on the ^{18}F-FDG PET/CT results. Physicians reported that additional imaging tests were avoided with the use of FDG-PET/CT, and the need for biopsy was negated in 21 % of patients, thus avoiding an invasive procedure. In patients planned for treatment of organ-confined muscle-invasive disease, 19 % were found to have metastatic disease on FDG-PET/CT and thus required systemic chemotherapy. In some instances, surveillance was changed to treatment, and local treatment with radiation therapy was changed to systemic chemotherapy for more advanced disease in one patient. Within the group with a change of treatment, eight patients had a biopsy, and one patient had additional imaging (MRI) because of the findings on PET/CT [42].

Lodde et al. also compared conventional CT to ^{18}F-FDG PET/CT for evaluation of metastatic disease in 70 patients with a variety of clinical stages of disease. Some underwent preoperative imaging and others who underwent postoperative imaging or imaging after chemotherapy. The overall sensitivity of ^{18}F-FDG PET/CT for detection of pelvic node metastasis was 57 % compared to only 33 % for conventional CT. Furthermore, to evaluate extrapelvic metastasis, they considered 36 patients who had $\geq$6 months of imaging follow-up. Extrapelvic suspicious areas on ^{18}F-FDG PET/CT images at the beginning of the study were assessed and were found in a total of 20 patients. Suspicious areas on ^{18}F-FDG PET/CT were in the retroperitoneum in 8 patients, in the mediastinum in 5, and in the lungs in 13. Other areas with positive images were in bone (three patients), supraclavicular cervical nodes (six), thyroid (one), left adrenal gland (one), and right renal pelvis (one). Of these 20 patients, 10 had multiple synchronous lesions including lymph nodes in the retroperitoneum or mediastinum. UCB progressed in nine of the ten patients and six died of their disease. In the other ten patients with extrapelvic positive images and no pelvic or retroperitoneal lymph nodes, nine had lesions in the lung. While some of these may have represented metastatic UCB, none were confirmed. This was due to the fact that some of these patients progressed and died prior to biopsy of their lung lesions and others were found to have primary carcinoma of the lung [29]. Therefore, lung lesions identified on ^{18}F-FDG PET/CT should be confirmed to be related to UCB, as they might be due to other processes.

In addition to assessing lymphatic and visceral metastases, Lodde et al. also examined ^{18}F-FDG PET/CT to detect bone metastasis. They compared 36 bone scintigraphy results with ^{18}F-FDG PET/CT. Both techniques detected three patients with bone metastasis. In one case, however, additional pelvic and vertebral bone metastases were detected by ^{18}F-FDG PET/CT only [29]. Abbosh et al. recently corroborated this finding by demonstrating that bone scan and ^{18}F-FDG PET/CT were able to identify a similar proportion of patients with skeletal metastasis, but bone scan failed to identify additional lesions seen on PET [43].

The above studies have demonstrated the utility of ^{18}F-FDG PET/CT in the preoperative evaluation of individuals with invasive bladder cancer. Furthermore, they underscore the utility of a single imaging modality to obviate the need for multiple, separate, modalities to identify visceral, pulmonary and bone disease in patients suffering from UCB.

Additional agents have been explored as tracers for use in PET/CT for identification of metastatic UCB. In a study of 27 patients with UCB prior to radical cystectomy and lymphadenec-

tomy, Picchio et al. demonstrated that ^{11}C-choline PET had a significantly higher accuracy than CT for demonstrating lymph node involvement [31]. In a study of 18 patients with transitional cell carcinoma, all of whom had prior negative CT of the chest, abdomen, and pelvis. Gofrit et al. noted three out of six patients with evidence of ^{11}C-choline uptake in lymph nodes that were ultimately positive for disease on histopathology at the time of radical cystectomy. Furthermore, this study reported the ability to visualize bone metastases not previously noted on CT [30]. Maurer et al. assessed the accuracy of ^{11}C-choline PET/CT compared with CT for lymph node staging in 44 patients with localized bladder cancer prior to radical cystectomy. The sensitivity/specificity of ^{11}C-choline PET/CT and conventional CT were 58 %/66 % and 75 %/56 %, respectively; thus, the authors concluded that ^{11}C-choline PET/CT did not offer added diagnostic efficacy over conventional CT [44].

[11]C-choline was compared to ^{18}F-FDG in a study by Golan et al. The two tracers were compared for the evaluation of both local and metastatic disease in 20 consecutive patients. The positive predictive value of ^{11}C-choline PET/CT versus ^{18}F-FDG PET/CT was 79.4 % versus 88.2 %, respectively, for detection of extravesical lesions. Interestingly, ^{18}F-FDG PET/CT correctly identified four extravesical metastases missed by choline PET. The authors concluded that ^{11}C-choline PET/CT carried no appreciable advantage to ^{18}F-FDG PET/CT [45].

Other tracers used in PET, such as ^{11}C-methionine and ^{11}C-acetate, have also shown promise with respect to detection of distant disease in UCB in small pilot studies. PET with ^{11}C-methionine was employed by Letocha et al. in 44 separate examinations involving 29 patients with localized or metastatic transitional cell carcinoma of the urinary bladder. In four patients, PET was performed at three different time points: before chemotherapy, after one course, and after three courses. They noted that the overall diagnostic accuracy of ^{11}C-methionine PET was poor in this study, but showed some promise for monitoring patients with poor response to systemic therapy [46].

[11]C-acetate has also been investigated for the purpose of the detection of metastatic UCB. Schoder et al. investigated the utility of ^{11}C-acetate PET/CT for staging of bladder cancer and response assessment after neoadjuvant chemotherapy. Seventeen patients underwent ^{11}C-acetate PET/CT $\leq$1 month before planned radical cystectomy and pelvic lymph node dissection, ten of whom underwent neoadjuvant chemotherapy prior to PET. Histopathology from surgery served as the gold standard. A total of 494 lymph nodes (108 nodal regions) were removed in the 16 patients who underwent cystectomy (one patient did not ultimately undergo radical cystectomy). Two ^{11}C-acetate positive nodal regions from two patients, and the biopsied retroperitoneal region from a third contained metastases, all of which were negative on conventional CT. Overall, this study demonstrated that ^{11}C-acetate PET/CT had good sensitivity (100 %) and specificity (87 %) for correct identification of metastatic nodal regions [47].

PET/CT, particularly with ^{18}F-FDG, carries with it the potential to identify metastatic disease not otherwise seen on conventional cross-sectional imaging, with the added benefit of identification of visceral and bony metastases with one imaging study. Further research is needed to elucidate the utility and efficacy of imaging with other tracers.

6.5 Conclusions

Emerging MR techniques enable improved visualization of the bladder wall, for better assessment of local tumor extent. Patients with occult invasion of the muscle can undergo earlier definitive treatment with radical cystectomy. Although PET/CT has been explored in the assessment of local disease, the appropriate tracer and technique for achieving adequate local assessment remains undetermined.

Recent major advances with respect to staging of bladder cancer have been in the realm of extravesical metastatic disease. The advent of

unique radiotracers, particularly ^{18}F-FDG and ^{11}C-choline, afford the opportunity to detect early metastatic disease, as well as the ability to identify visceral and bone metastases, all with one imaging study. Patients with metastatic disease could be guided to earlier systemic chemotherapy and possibly away from needless radical surgery.

References

1. Baltaci S, et al. Computerized tomography for detecting perivesical infiltration and lymph node metastasis in invasive bladder carcinoma. Urol Int. 2008;81(4): 399–402.
2. Caterino M, et al. Primary cancer of the urinary bladder: CT evaluation of the T parameter with different techniques. Abdom Imaging. 2001;26(4):433–8.
3. Cowan NC, Crew JP. Imaging bladder cancer. Curr Opin Urol. 2010;20(5):409–13.
4. Kundra V, Silverman PM. Imaging in oncology from the University of Texas M. D. Anderson Cancer Center. Imaging in the diagnosis, staging, and follow-up of cancer of the urinary bladder. AJR Am J Roentgenol. 2003;180(4):1045–54.
5. Paik ML, et al. Limitations of computerized tomography in staging invasive bladder cancer before radical cystectomy. J Urol. 2000;163(6):1693–6.
6. Voges GE, et al. Computerized tomography: an unreliable method for accurate staging of bladder tumors in patients who are candidates for radical cystectomy. J Urol. 1989;142(4):972–4.
7. Yaman O, et al. Staging with computed tomography, transrectal ultrasonography and transurethral resection of bladder tumour: comparison with final pathological stage in invasive bladder carcinoma. Br J Urol. 1996;78(2):197–200.
8. Herr HW, Donat SM, Dalbagni G. Can restaging transurethral resection of T1 bladder cancer select patients for immediate cystectomy? J Urol. 2007; 177(1):75–9. discussion 79.
9. Dutta SC, et al. Clinical under staging of high risk nonmuscle invasive urothelial carcinoma treated with radical cystectomy. J Urol. 2001;166(2):490–3.
10. Stein JP, et al. Radical cystectomy in the treatment of invasive bladder cancer: long-term results in 1,054 patients. J Clin Oncol. 2001;19(3):666–75.
11. Grossman HB, et al. Neoadjuvant chemotherapy plus cystectomy compared with cystectomy alone for locally advanced bladder cancer. N Engl J Med. 2003; 349(9):859–66.
12. Moses KA, et al. Bladder cancer imaging: an update. Curr Opin Urol. 2011;21(5):393–7.
13. Silverman SG, Leyendecker JR, Amis Jr ES. What is the current role of CT urography and MR urography

in the evaluation of the urinary tract? Radiology. 2009;250(2):309–23.

14. Matsuki M, et al. Diffusion-weighted MR imaging for urinary bladder carcinoma: initial results. Eur Radiol. 2007;17(1):201–4.

15. Abou-El-Ghar ME, et al. Bladder cancer: diagnosis with diffusion-weighted MR imaging in patients with gross hematuria. Radiology. 2009;251(2):415–21.

16. Avcu S, et al. The value of diffusion-weighted MRI in the diagnosis of malignant and benign urinary bladder lesions. Br J Radiol. 2011;84(1006):875–82.

17. Watanabe H, et al. Preoperative T staging of urinary bladder cancer: does diffusion-weighted MRI have supplementary value? AJR Am J Roentgenol. 2009;192(5):1361–6.

18. El-Assmy A, et al. Bladder tumour staging: comparison of diffusion- and T2-weighted MR imaging. Eur Radiol. 2009;19(7):1575–81.

19. Takeuchi M, et al. Urinary bladder cancer: diffusion-weighted MR imaging–accuracy for diagnosing T stage and estimating histologic grade. Radiology. 2009;251(1):112–21.

20. Bouchelouche KB, Turkbey, Choyke PL. PET/CT and MRI in bladder cancer. J Cancer Sci Ther 2012;S14(1).

21. Tuncbilek N, et al. Value of dynamic contrast-enhanced MRI and correlation with tumor angiogenesis in bladder cancer. AJR Am J Roentgenol. 2009;192(4):949–55.

22. Barentsz JO, et al. Staging urinary bladder cancer after transurethral biopsy: value of fast dynamic contrast-enhanced MR imaging. Radiology. 1996; 201(1):185–93.

23. Scattoni V, et al. Dynamic gadolinium-enhanced magnetic resonance imaging in staging of superficial bladder cancer. J Urol. 1996;155(5):1594–9.

24. Ak I, Stokkel MP, Pauwels EK. Positron emission tomography with 2-[18F]fluoro-2-deoxy-D-glucose in oncology. Part II. The clinical value in detecting and staging primary tumours. J Cancer Res Clin Oncol. 2000;126(10):560–74.

25. Jana S, Blaufox MD. Nuclear medicine studies of the prostate, testes, and bladder. Semin Nucl Med. 2006;36(1):51–72.

26. Leskinen-Kallio S, et al. Uptake of carbon-11-methionine and fluorodeoxyglucose in non-Hodgkin's lymphoma: a PET study. J Nucl Med. 1991;32(6): 1211–8.

27. Anjos DA, et al. 18F-FDG PET/CT delayed images after diuretic for restaging invasive bladder cancer. J Nucl Med. 2007;48(5):764–70.

28. Kibel AS, et al. Prospective study of [18F]fluorodeoxyglucose positron emission tomography/computed tomography for staging of muscle-invasive bladder carcinoma. J Clin Oncol. 2009;27(26):4314–20.

29. Lodde M, et al. Evaluation of fluorodeoxyglucose positron-emission tomography with computed tomography for staging of urothelial carcinoma. BJU Int. 2010;106(5):658–63.

30. Gofrit ON, et al. Contribution of 11C-choline positron emission tomography/computerized tomography to preoperative staging of advanced transitional cell carcinoma. J Urol. 2006;176(3):940–4. discussion 944.

31. Picchio M, et al. Value of 11C-choline PET and contrast-enhanced CT for staging of bladder cancer: correlation with histopathologic findings. J Nucl Med. 2006;47(6):938–44.

32. Ahlstrom H, et al. Positron emission tomography in the diagnosis and staging of urinary bladder cancer. Acta Radiol. 1996;37(2):180–5.

33. Vargas HA, et al. Prospective evaluation of MRI, (1)(1)C-acetate PET/CT and contrast-enhanced CT for staging of bladder cancer. Eur J Radiol. 2012;81(12): 4131–7.

34. National Comprehensive Cancer Network. NCCN Guidelines Version 1. 2013 bladder cancer. 2013 [cited 2013 September 3]; Available from: http://www.nccn.org/professionals/physician_gls/pdf/bladder.pdf

35. Abbosh P, et al. Evaluation of alkaline phosphatase as a marker for bone metastasis in patients with muscle-invasive bladder cancer. J Urol. 2013;189(4 Suppl):e770.

36. Millikan R, et al. Integrated therapy for locally advanced bladder cancer: final report of a randomized trial of cystectomy plus adjuvant M-VAC versus cystectomy with both preoperative and postoperative M-VAC. J Clin Oncol. 2001;19(20):4005–13.

37. Bellin MF, Roy C. Magnetic resonance lymphography. Curr Opin Urol. 2007;17(1):65–9.

38. Bellin MF, et al. Lymph node metastases: safety and effectiveness of MR imaging with ultrasmall superparamagnetic iron oxide particles–initial clinical experience. Radiology. 1998;207(3):799–808.

39. Deserno WM, et al. Urinary bladder cancer: preoperative nodal staging with ferumoxtran-10-enhanced MR imaging. Radiology. 2004;233(2):449–56.

40. Thoeny HC, et al. Combined ultrasmall superparamagnetic particles of iron oxide-enhanced and diffusion-weighted magnetic resonance imaging reliably detect pelvic lymph node metastases in normal-sized nodes of bladder and prostate cancer patients. Eur Urol. 2009;55(4):761–9.

41. Drieskens O, et al. FDG-PET for preoperative staging of bladder cancer. Eur J Nucl Med Mol Imaging. 2005;32(12):1412–7.

42. Apolo AB, et al. Clinical value of fluorine-18 2-fluoro-2-deoxy-D-glucose positron emission tomography/computed tomography in bladder cancer. J Clin Oncol. 2010;28(25):3973–8.

43. Abbosh P, et al. Utility of FDG-PET/CT in identifying bone metastasis in patients with bladder cancer. J Urol. 2013;189(4 Suppl):e903.

44. Maurer T, et al. Diagnostic efficacy of [11C]choline positron emission tomography/computed tomography compared with conventional computed tomography in lymph node staging of patients with bladder cancer prior to radical cystectomy. Eur Urol. 2012;61(5):1031–8.

45. Golan S, et al. Comparison of 11C-choline with 18F-FDG in positron emission tomography/computerized tomography for staging urothelial carcinoma: a prospective study. J Urol. 2011;186(2):436–41.

46. Letocha H, et al. Positron emission tomography with L-methyl-11C-methionine in the monitoring of therapy response in muscle-invasive transitional cell carcinoma of the urinary bladder. Br J Urol. 1994;74(6):767–74.

47. Schoder H, et al. Initial results with (11)C-acetate positron emission tomography/computed tomography (PET/CT) in the staging of urinary bladder cancer. Mol Imaging Biol. 2012;14(2):245–51.

John L. Gore

Abbreviations

NMIBC	Non-muscle-invasive bladder cancer
TURBT	Transurethral resection of bladder tumor
SEER	Surveillance Epidemiology, and End Results
NCCN	National Comprehensive Cancer Network
MMC	Mitomycin C
BCG	Bacillus Calmette-Guérin
USQC	Urological Surgery Quality Collaborative
SCOAP	Surgical Care and Outcomes Assessment Program
PQRS	Physicians Quality Reporting System
CMS	Centers for Medicare & Medicaid Services

7.1 Socioeconomic Status and Bladder Cancer

Bladder cancer is a disease that predominantly affects elderly individuals with a history of tobacco use. Compared with other urologic cancers, bladder cancer has an older peak incidence (Fig. 7.1), with few newly diagnosed bladder cancer patients being younger than 65 years old, irrespective of patient gender or race/ethnicity (Fig. 7.2). Age correlates with comorbidity [1], and the preponderance of smoking history or active tobacco use among newly diagnosed bladder cancer patients means that many incident bladder cancer cases will be complicated by chronic lung disease and cardiovascular disease [2]. Race/ethnicity appears to be associated with bladder cancer risk as well. Whites have more than twice the odds of developing bladder cancer than African American and Hispanic men and women. Bladder cancer also has a gender predisposition: men are more likely to be diagnosed with bladder cancer than women. Fewer than one-third of cystectomy patients in Medicare claims data are women [3]. Thus, the profile of the average bladder cancer patient is an elderly white male with at least two comorbid conditions [4].

The risk factors that predispose patients to developing bladder cancer include tobacco consumption and environmental exposures to carcinogens such as those found in dyes and cleaning solvents [4]. Professions associated with these exposures include workers in the rubber, leather, and textile industries. Painters, truck drivers, and hairdressers similarly experience higher risks of developing bladder cancer. The nature of the professions that predispose to bladder cancer means that most patients newly diagnosed with bladder cancer are of lower socioeconomic status.

J.L. Gore, M.D., M.S., F.A.C.S (✉)
Department of Urology, University of Washington,
1959 NE Pacific St, Box 356510, Seattle, WA
98195-6510, USA

Fred Hutchinson Cancer Research Center,
Seattle, WA, USA
e-mail: jlgore@u.washington.edu

B.R. Konety and S.S. Chang (eds.), *Management of Bladder Cancer:*
A Comprehensive Text With Clinical Scenarios, DOI 10.1007/978-1-4939-1881-2_7,
© Springer Science+Business Media New York 2015

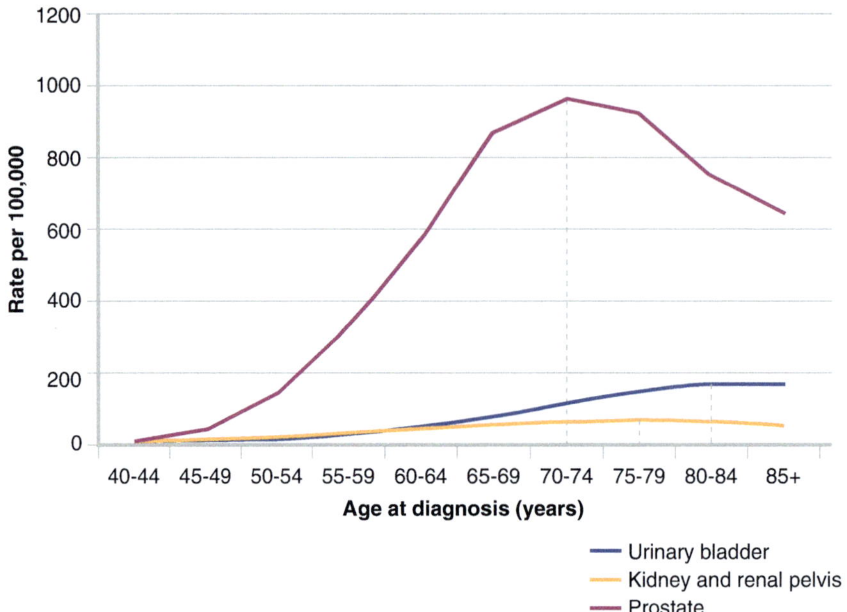

Fig. 7.1 Age-specific incidence of prostate, kidney, and bladder cancer

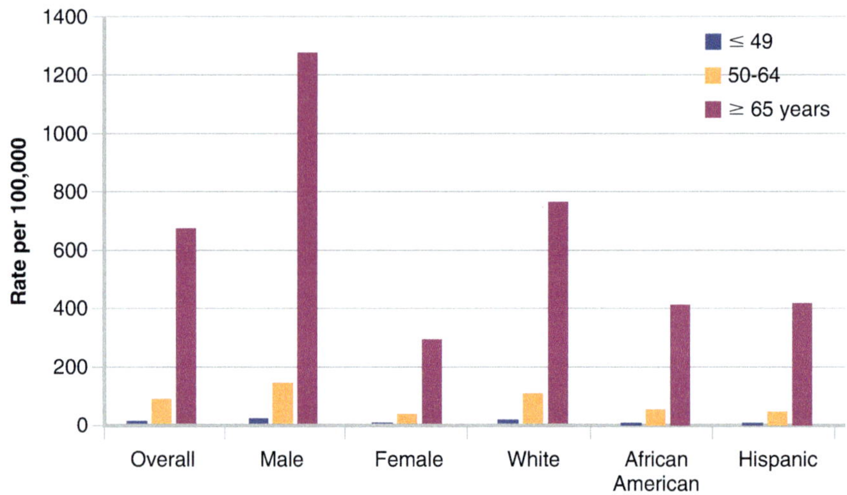

Fig. 7.2 Bladder cancer incidence by age stratified by gender and race/ethnicity

In addition to disproportionately affecting blue-collar careers [5], tobacco use is more common among less educated, lower income individuals [6]. Men and women living below the poverty line are more likely to smoke than higher income individuals [7]. As the predominant risk factor for bladder cancer, tobacco use patterns in the US further contribute to the socioeconomic "profiling" of the average bladder cancer patient.

7.2 Disparities in Bladder Cancer Care

The socioeconomic characteristics of the typical bladder cancer patient partly explain many of the health care disparities that have been identified in bladder cancer. Bladder cancer is a remarkably heterogeneous disease wherein most non-muscle-invasive bladder cancer (NMIBC) cases are more analogous to a chronic disease with low risk of cancer-specific death, yet muscle-invasive bladder cancer, even when clinically localized, confers high risk for progression to metastases and bladder cancer mortality. Thus, stage at presentation is an important determinant of survival in bladder cancer [8].

Access to health care services is often described using the conceptual framework of the Anderson Behavioral Model [9]. Under this model, factors that influence the receipt of health care services include predisposing, enabling, need-based, and contextual determinants. Predisposing factors are immutable personal characteristics that are associated with likelihood of health care delivery, such as gender, age, or race/ethnicity. In bladder cancer, women experience worse survival outcomes possibly as a result of delays in diagnosis imposed by provider practice patterns [10, 11]. Women with hematuria, the symptom that induces most bladder cancer diagnoses, are more likely to receive a course of antibiotics and delayed urologic referral [12].

Race/ethnicity has been shown to impact treatment and health outcomes in bladder cancer. African American men and women suffer inequities in the diagnosis and treatment of bladder cancer. Cancer grade, an important prognostic indicator in NMIBC, and cancer stage, which is closely associated with bladder cancer-specific survival, are both higher among African Americans than among whites [13–15]. Stage at presentation may vary as a result of delays in realizing care for symptoms indicative of a new bladder cancer diagnosis. However, once diagnosed, African Americans may experience disparities in treatment. For grade and stage-matched cancers, African Americans are less likely than whites to undergo surgery [16, 17].

Among clinically localized muscle-invasive bladder cancer patients, African Americans are more likely to undergo alternative treatments to the gold standard of management with radical cystectomy. Radiation, combination radiation with chemotherapy, and—most concerning—no further treatment beyond the initial diagnostic transurethral resection of bladder tumor (TURBT), are all more common among African Americans compared with whites [16, 18]. For African Americans that undergo radical cystectomy, the predisposition of racial-ethnic minorities to receive care at urban underserved hospitals may explain worse postoperative survival outcomes compared with whites [19].

Enabling factors are patient characteristics that either facilitate or encumber access to health care services. In the US health care system, insurance status is an important determinant of access; other factors in this category include education level, occupation, and income. Americans are either adequately insured, underinsured, or uninsured. In 2011, 55 % of Americans had employer-based health insurance, 15 % were covered by Medicare (some of which were dually covered with employer-based insurance), 17 % had Medicaid coverage, and 16 %—or more than 48 million individuals—were uninsured [20]. Because most insurance in the US derives from employment, having commercial insurance is an indicator of higher socioeconomic status [21].

Most population-based analyses of bladder cancer care have employed Medicare-based data, which limits conclusions about the influence of insurance on access. However, in general, uninsured and underinsured patients experience delays in care and are found to have later-stage cancers once diagnosed [22, 23]. Among patients in the National Cancer Database, those with Medicaid coverage and uninsured patients with muscle-invasive bladder cancer were less likely to undergo radical cystectomy [17]. As a result, the survival outcomes of underinsured and insured bladder cancer patient may suffer, compared with better-insured patients [15].

Insurance status may explain or further exacerbate racial/ethnic and socioeconomic disparities in bladder cancer outcomes. The majority of African Americans have government-sponsored health insurance or are uninsured [24]. Furthermore, more than 70 % of Medicaid patients live in US census tracts in the lowest 2 quartiles of household income. Bladder cancer patients with Medicaid likely experience delays in care and have decreased access to needed services such as radical cystectomy for locally advanced bladder cancer [25].

Socioeconomic status has been shown to correlate with cancer survival in general [7]. Specific to bladder cancer, men and women in executive or managerial professions have better survival outcomes than blue collar workers, although this finding has not been corroborated with more contemporary data [26]. Income and education, which are linked, may enable better health outcomes in bladder cancer through facilitation of access to expert providers beyond those locally available.

Lastly, contextual factors, which refer to determinants peripheral to the patient that influence the care they receive. For many conditions, the local health care environment in which patients require care is as important as the predisposing and enabling factors that influence access [27]. For urologic conditions, the availability of a trained urologist has been shown to affect the likelihood that a patient receives needed surgery. For muscle-invasive bladder cancer, the travel distance between a patient's residence and a urologist that performs radical cystectomy is strongly associated with the odds that a stage II bladder cancer patient undergoes radical cystectomy [3]. Contextual factors explain differential access to health care among rural Americans, but also apply to urban underserved areas.

7.3 Quality of Bladder Cancer Care

Nationally, patients receive just over half of the health care services that are recommended by guidelines for common general medical conditions [28]. Physicians appear to more comprehensively care for cancer and surgical conditions, but quality of care deficiencies remain. The Dartmouth Atlas describes supply-sensitive care, susceptible to overuse, as health care services that depend on local resources, but for which evidence is lacking [27]. Preference-sensitive care, subject to both patient and provider preferences, is a common source of variation in the delivery of health care services. Effective care practices are evidence-driven, but they are often underused as a result of resource discrepancies such as the availability of trained surgeons.

Value is the product of health care quality and health care costs. High value health care services provide high quality care at low cost. Both components are receiving attention by payers and legislators. Bladder cancer is a potential target for this attention given that economic analyses have demonstrated that, per capita, bladder cancer is the costliest cancer in the US [29]. Sources of the increased expenditure for bladder cancer include the need for invasive procedures to conduct bladder cancer surveillance, the high frequency of interval surveillance recommended by national guidelines, and the high cost of the index admission for patients undergoing radical cystectomy for muscle-invasive bladder cancer.

Radical cystectomy is an example of effective care according to the Dartmouth Atlas categories. Guidelines recommend radical cystectomy and urinary diversion for the management of muscle-invasive bladder cancer, yet review of population-based data suggests that few patients with stage II bladder cancer undergo cystectomy [3]. From data that links Medicare claims with the Surveillance, Epidemiology, and End Results (SEER) national cancer registry, only 21 % of patients with muscle-invasive bladder cancer were treated with radical cystectomy, compared with 28 % who underwent chemotherapy and/or radiation and 51 % who received no further intervention following the diagnostic TURBT. However, most of the bladder cancer guidelines are based upon expert opinion rather than high-level evidence derived from clinical trials, which may explain why bladder cancer care is subject to substantial variation in the US. For example, although radical cystectomy is recommended by several guidelines as standard of care therapy for muscle-invasive bladder cancer, the comparative effectiveness of radical cystectomy versus alternative treatments such as bladder-sparing combination chemotherapy and radiation has not been rigorously evaluated in a clinical trial.

Clinical trials have evaluated the efficacy of neoadjuvant chemotherapy in anticipation of planned exenterative surgery for muscle-invasive bladder cancer. Based upon documented survival benefit among patients randomized to neoadjuvant chemotherapy with cisplatin-based regimens [30], the National Comprehensive Cancer Network (NCCN) recommends that neoadjuvant chemotherapy be strongly considered for cystectomy candidates [31]. Many of these patients have occult metastases that confer high risk for bladder cancer-specific mortality [8]. Yet, administrative claims demonstrated marked underuse of chemotherapy in the neoadjuvant setting [32, 33].

Consideration of chemotherapy and optimization of comorbid conditions can impose delays in care for patients with muscle-invasive bladder cancer. Providers experienced in the care of stage II and higher bladder cancers, especially those working in multidisciplinary teams, may be able to manage these concerns more efficiently. This is critical to health outcomes in this population as delays in care for patients that require cystectomy can impact cancer-specific survival. Patients for whom the period between the diagnosis of muscle-invasive disease and extirpative treatment with radical cystectomy exceeds 3 months have higher rates of pathologic upstaging [34] and worse overall and cancer-specific survival outcomes [35, 36]. These delays occur in more than one-third of cases [36].

Other surgical factors may further impact survival from muscle-invasive bladder cancer. Candidates for partial cystectomy are typically older patients with greater burden of comorbid conditions for whom radical cystectomy may be too high risk and in whom the tumor is in an appropriate location for partial resection [8]. In most academic, high-volume bladder cancer centers, fewer than 5 % of patients are considered eligible for partial cystectomy. Yet review of nationally representative hospital discharge claims suggests that 20 % of patients undergoing surgical extirpation of locally advanced bladder cancers with either radical cystectomy or partial cystectomy receive the more limited partial cystectomy [37]. Similarly, despite more broad acceptance of the importance of extended lymphadenectomy in muscle-invasive bladder cancer, most surgeons nationwide appear to perform a more limited lymphadenectomy [38]. These important findings may indicate that the health outcomes of locally advanced bladder cancer patients are being compromised by sub-standard surgical practices.

Patients with NMIBC generally have low risk for bladder cancer mortality; however, a fraction of NMIBC patients progress to having more aggressive cancers. For these men and women, rigorous adherence to a regimen of intravesical treatments may be associated with reduced risk for tumor recurrence and disease progression. Following TURBT, a meta-analysis demonstrated that an immediate instillation of Mitomycin C (MMC) reduces the risk of bladder cancer recurrence by nearly 40 % [39]. Yet this may occur rarely in general urologic practice. Analysis of SEER-Medicare linked claims demonstrated that fewer than 5 % of patients receive an instillation of intravesical chemotherapy following TURBT [40]. Billing claims from a commercial payer corroborated these results [41].

Following this initial NMIBC care episode, NCCN guidelines recommend an induction course of intravesical immunotherapy, vigilant surveillance with regular cystoscopies and cytologies, and maintenance intravesical immunotherapy [31]. Whether due to provider variation or patient factors possibly related to the invasive nature of cystoscopy and intravesical immunotherapy, Medicare beneficiaries appear to receive only a fraction of this recommended care. A patient with high-grade NMIBC should receive quarterly surveillance cystoscopies in the 2 years following their initial diagnosis. Yet Schrag et al. demonstrated that fewer than half of patients undergo the requisite cystocopic surveillance [42].

More contemporary analyses of linked SEER-Medicare data have evaluated compliance with cystoscopy, cytology, and intravesical therapy in high-grade NMIBC and identified substantial gaps between NCCN guidelines and community bladder cancer clinical practice [40, 43]. Fewer than one-third of patients receive induction courses of intravesical Bacillus Calmette–Guérin (BCG) [40]. Following initial management of high-grade NMIBC with induction BCG, maintenance BCG has been shown to reduce rates of recurrence and progression [44]. However, maintenance BCG may be rarely used in clinical practice [40, 45]; the variation in compliance with recommendations and clinical trial evidence for BCG may be attributable to surgeon practices rather than patient characteristics. The surgeon diagnosing and treating an initial high-grade NMIBC was found to explain a large proportion of the variation in receipt of these therapies. Thus, the person diagnosing a new bladder cancer has a substantial impact on the sequence of therapies that may be given. As a result, the survival outcomes of bladder cancer patients may be compromised: Chamie et al. demonstrated poorer bladder cancer-specific survival among patients with lower compliance with guideline-recommended NMIBC care [43].

7.4 Quality Improvement in Bladder Cancer

These variations may represent quality of care concerns that reflect low value health care delivery. Certainly, these data suggest that an opportunity exists to improve the clinical outcomes of bladder cancer patients through greater attention to the quality of health care they receive. Importantly, the administrative data used to identify quality concerns in bladder cancer may lack the granularity required to accurately capture detailed elements of care such as intravesical MMC. Through a multicenter quality improvement collaborative, Barocas et al. evaluated the quality improvement potential of efforts to increase appropriate use of post-TURBT MMC [46]. Contrary to the findings from administrative claims, the authors found high levels of what they termed "judicious use" of MMC. Judicious use referred to the fact that provider decisions to *not* give MMC may represent appropriate decision-making. Combining appropriate non-use with appropriate use results in compliance with judicious MMC utilization in over 80 % of cases. Addressing bladder cancer quality will require this mode of transparent reporting of provider-specific outcomes with a greater level of data detail than can be abstracted from sources such as Medicare claims.

The MMC data derive from the first clinician-led quality collaborative in urology, the Urological Surgery Quality Collaborative (USQC) [47]. General surgery quality collaboratives have previously demonstrated substantial cost savings associated with collaborative participation [48, 49]. A Michigan general surgery collaborative was associated with reductions in complications rates that increased over time yielding a $20 million cost savings to the health care system [50]. The Washington State Surgical Care and Outcomes Assessment Program (SCOAP) has produced similar results in colorectal and bariatric surgery [51].

The USQC is a multicenter effort linking academic urologic practices with large urology group practices in which clinicians develop abstraction tools that can be used to collect data that is relevant to health care quality. Through these efforts, the USQC has implemented feedback reports to reduce overuse of advanced imaging in the staging of low-risk clinically localized prostate cancer [52]. Although MMC use was deemed appropriate, the methods by which the USQC measured these outcomes could facilitate identification of processes of perioperative care around radical cystectomy and urinary diversion that would improve outcomes or decrease surgical morbidity. Yet broadening collaborative-type efforts would require tremendous resources for data abstraction and feedback reporting that may limit application of these exciting results to a larger population.

Directing patients to high quality providers may address quality concerns in bladder cancer care. Surgical outcomes may be better when patients are cared for at high volume centers [53]. To some degree, patients in need of cystectomy are already being directed toward high volume providers. Hollenbeck et al. identified a natural regionalization of cystectomy care over the 1990s to high volume, urban academic centers [54]. Data suggesting a relationship between travel distance and receipt of radical cystectomy suggest that few providers are available that offer radical cystectomy [3], and thus care is being directed to select centers. As a result, hospital-specific cystectomy volumes are increasing, and the number of hospitals performing cystectomies are declining [55]. This concentration of complex bladder cancer surgery to high volume centers may explain observed declines in postoperative mortality [55, 56].

Payers have taken note. The Leapfrog Group unites private and public health care payers to implement purchasing principles that direct patients to providers based on their safety and quality ratings [57]. The Leapfrog Criteria may not have impacted risk for inpatient mortality [58], but the Leapfrog Group has raised public awareness about health care quality concerns. Similarly, Blue Cross Blue Shield of America implemented a regionalization model for medical care including surgical care for complex and rare cancers. Identified centers of excellence, based on volume and other processes of care, are decreed Blue Distinction Centers and patients are routed to these facilities. Patients cared for at Blue Distinction Centers have been shown to have superior outcomes than patients treated by other providers [59].

Regionalization models have caveats. For patients without employer-based health insurance, policy-based regionalization efforts would be needed to ensure that disparities in care by insurance status are not further compounded by exclusion of access to centers of excellence for radical cystectomy care. Currently, underinsured and uninsured patients are more likely to receive care at hospitals in lower volume quartiles for complex surgical conditions such as radical cystectomy [55]. Restriction from opportunities to access high volume cystectomy providers could further exacerbate disparities by socioeconomic status and race/ethnicity. Regionalization can also saturate high volume centers, leading to delays in care known to confer adverse health outcomes in muscle-invasive bladder cancer [34–36].

At the national level, efforts are emerging to incentivize high quality care, which have variable relevance to bladder cancer care. Partly as a result of the efforts of the Leapfrog Group, the Medicare Modernization Act of 2003 and later the Tax Relief and Health Care Act of 2006 created the Physician Quality Reporting System (PQRS) [60]. Now the nation's largest pay-for-performance initiative, PQRS began as a voluntary program, but became permanent with the Medicare Improvements for Patients and Providers Act of 2008 (MIPPA). PQRS began as an incentive, but noncompliance with the requirement to report

will lead to penalties by 2015. However, no PQRS measures specifically apply to bladder cancer care. According to the American Urological Association, as of 2012, only 15 PQRS measures applied to urologic care, with the only disease-specific measures referring to prostate cancer care and urinary incontinence [61]. Generation of bladder cancer-specific PQRS measures could target identified quality of care concerns and improve compliance with guideline-recommended bladder cancer care. A more direct financial incentive would be increased payment for cystectomy, for which reimbursement has lagged remarkably behind inflation rates [62], yet this is unlikely to occur.

An initiative with potential to impact bladder cancer care is the concept of bundled payments for inpatient episodes of surgical care. Under a bundled payment system, providers receive a defined total reimbursement for all care related to a surgery and discrete postoperative global period, including readmissions [63]. The Centers for Medicare and Medicaid Services (CMS) are evaluating bundled payments with the Acute Care Episode Demonstration Project in cardiovascular and orthopedic procedures [64]. Miller et al. analyzed Medicare data and identified substantial variation in the costs of post-discharge care following major inpatient surgical procedures suggesting that these demonstration projects are likely to achieve cost savings [65]. Given the high cost of the index radical cystectomy admission and the high rates of readmissions following radical cystectomy for bladder cancer [66–70], bundling payments for cystectomy care could induce practice changes that improve health care quality and health outcomes for bladder cancer patients.

Other policy initiatives that might influence bladder cancer incidence and mortality include addressing tobacco use in America. Public health legislation on tobacco can support cancer control. The rigorous tobacco laws enacted in California in 1995 that restricted smoking in public venues were shown to be associated with reduced incidence of lung cancer over time compared with lung cancer rates in states with less restrictive tobacco control programs [7]. A trend was observed toward decreasing incidence of bladder cancer, although this was not statistically significant. As of April 2013, there only 10 states with no form of legislation covering smoking in public places [71]. In 28 states, bans limit smoking in all enclosed public places, affecting 49 % of the US population [71]. With increasing implementation of these bans or consideration of a federal ban, we may witness further declines in bladder cancer incidence.

Lastly, increasing the quality of the evidence underlying guideline recommendations for bladder cancer care may address the identified variation in the delivery of bladder cancer services. The NCCN guidelines for bladder cancer care derive mainly from expert opinion due to the paucity of high quality clinical trials in bladder cancer care [31]. Advocacy could direct funding for bladder cancer research, including clinical trials.

7.5   Conclusions

Bladder cancer is a costly condition for which health care delivery is susceptible to marked variation and possible quality of care deficiencies. Quality of care concerns can relate to health care disparities which may disproportionately affect bladder cancer patients, given the preponderance of low socioeconomic status among bladder cancer survivors due to its associated risk factors. Quality improvement may derive from local efforts such as clinician-led urologic collaboratives, as well as national efforts through policy changes.

References

1. Anderson G, Horvath J. The growing burden of chronic disease in America. Public Health Rep. 2004;119(3):263–70.
2. Megwalu II, Vlahiotis A, Radwan M, Piccirillo JF, Kibel AS. Prognostic impact of comorbidity in patients with bladder cancer. Eur Urol. 2008;53(3): 581–9.
3. Gore JL, Litwin MS, Lai J, Yano EM, Madison R, Setodji C, et al. Use of radical cystectomy for patients with invasive bladder cancer. J Natl Cancer Inst. 2010;102(11):802–11.
4. Wood DP. Urothelial tumors of the bladder. In: Wein AJ, Kavoussi LR, Novick AC, Partin AW, Peters CA, editors. Campbell-Walsh urology. 10th ed. Philadelphia: Saunders; 2012. p. 2309–34.
5. Leppert JT, Shvarts O, Kawaoka K, Lieberman R, Belldegrun AS, Pantuck AJ. Prevention of bladder cancer: a review. Eur Urol. 2006;49(2):226–34.
6. Goy J, Rosenberg MW, King WD. Health risk behaviors: examining social inequalities in bladder and colorectal cancers. Ann Epidemiol. 2008;18(2): 156–62.
7. Ward E, Jemal A, Cokkinides V, Singh GK, Cardinez C, Ghafoor A, et al. Cancer disparities by race/ethnicity and socioeconomic status. CA Cancer J Clin. 2004;54(2):78–93.
8. Schoenberg MP, Gonzalgo ML. Management of invasive and metastatic bladder cancer. In: Wein AJ, Kavoussi LR, Novick AC, Partin AW, Peters CA, editors. Campbell-Walsh urology. 9th ed. Philadelphia: Saunders; 2006. p. 2468–78.
9. Andersen R, Rice TH, Kominski GF. Changing the U.S. health care system: key issues in health services policy and management. 3rd ed. San Francisco: Jossey-Bass; 2007.
10. Mungan NA, Aben KK, Schoenberg MP, Visser O, Coebergh JW, Witjes JA, et al. Gender differences in stage-adjusted bladder cancer survival. Urology. 2000;55(6):876–80.
11. Brookfield KF, Cheung MC, Gomez C, Yang R, Nieder AM, Lee DJ, et al. Survival disparities among African American women with invasive bladder cancer in Florida. Cancer. 2009;115(18):4196–209.
12. Johnson EK, Daignault S, Zhang Y, Lee CT. Patterns of hematuria referral to urologists: does a gender disparity exist? Urology. 2008;72(3):498–502.
13. Lee CT, Dunn RL, Williams C, Underwood 3rd W. Racial disparity in bladder cancer: trends in tumor presentation at diagnosis. J Urol. 2006;176(3):927–33.
14. Scosyrev E, Noyes K, Feng C, Messing E. Sex and racial differences in bladder cancer presentation and mortality in the US. Cancer. 2009;115(1):68–74.
15. Mallin K, David KA, Carroll PR, Milowsky MI, Nanus DM. Transitional cell carcinoma of the bladder: racial and gender disparities in survival (1993 to 2002), stage and grade (1993 to 2007). J Urol. 2011;185(5):1631–6.
16. Konety BR, Joslyn SA. Factors influencing aggressive therapy for bladder cancer: an analysis of data from the SEER program. J Urol. 2003;170(5):1765–71.
17. Fedeli U, Fedewa SA, Ward EM. Treatment of muscle invasive bladder cancer: evidence from the National Cancer Database, 2003 to 2007. J Urol. 2011;185(1): 72–8.
18. Jacobs BL, Montgomery JS, Zhang Y, Skolarus TA, Weizer AZ, Hollenbeck BK. Disparities in bladder cancer. Urol Oncol. 2012;30(1):81–8.
19. Taub DA, Hollenbeck BK, Cooper KL, Dunn RL, Miller DC, Taylor JM, et al. Racial disparities in resource utilization for cystectomy. Urology. 2006; 67(2):288–93.

20. Todd SR, Sommers BD. Overview of the uninsured in the United States: a summary of the 2012 Current Population Survey Report. Washington, DC: U.S. Department of Health and Human Services; 2012. Available from: http://aspe.hhs.gov/health/reports/2012/UninsuredInTheUS/ib.shtml. Accessed 4 Dec 2012.

21. Emanuel EJ. Healthcare, guaranteed: a simple, secure solution for America. 1st ed. New York: PublicAffairs; 2008.

22. Halpern MT, Ward EM, Pavluck AL, Schrag NM, Bian J, Chen AY. Association of insurance status and ethnicity with cancer stage at diagnosis for 12 cancer sites: a retrospective analysis. Lancet Oncol. 2008;9(3):222–31.

23. Ward EM, Fedewa SA, Cokkinides V, Virgo K. The association of insurance and stage at diagnosis among patients aged 55 to 74 years in the national cancer database. Cancer J. 2010;16(6):614–21.

24. Ward E, Halpern M, Schrag N, Cokkinides V, DeSantis C, Bandi P, et al. Association of insurance with cancer care utilization and outcomes. CA Cancer J Clin. 2008;58(1):9–31.

25. Koroukian SM, Bakaki PM, Raghavan D. Survival disparities by Medicaid status: an analysis of 8 cancers. Cancer. 2012;118(17):4271–9.

26. Vagero D, Persson G. Cancer survival and social class in Sweden. J Epidemiol Community Health. 1987;41(3):204–9.

27. The Dartmouth atlas of health care, 1999. Chicago IL: American Hospital Publishing; 1999.

28. McGlynn EA, Asch SM, Adams J, Keesey J, Hicks J, DeCristofaro A, et al. The quality of health care delivered to adults in the United States. N Engl J Med. 2003;348(26):2635–45.

29. Botteman MF, Pashos CL, Redaelli A, Laskin B, Hauser R. The health economics of bladder cancer: a comprehensive review of the published literature. Pharmacoeconomics. 2003;21(18):1315–30.

30. Grossman HB, Natale RB, Tangen CM, Speights VO, Vogelzang NJ, Trump DL, et al. Neoadjuvant chemotherapy plus cystectomy compared with cystectomy alone for locally advanced bladder cancer. N Engl J Med. 2003;349(9):859–66.

31. Montie JE, Clark PE, Eisenberger MA, El-Galley R, Greenberg RE, Herr HW, et al. Bladder cancer. J Natl Compr Canc Netw. 2009;7(1):8–39.

32. David KA, Milowsky MI, Ritchey J, Carroll PR, Nanus DM. Low incidence of perioperative chemotherapy for stage III bladder cancer 1998 to 2003: a report from the National Cancer Data Base. J Urol. 2007;178(2):451–4.

33. Porter MP, Kerrigan MC, Donato BM, Ramsey SD. Patterns of use of systemic chemotherapy for Medicare beneficiaries with urothelial bladder cancer. Urol Oncol. 2011;29(3):252–8.

34. Chang SS, Hassan JM, Cookson MS, Wells N, Smith Jr JA. Delaying radical cystectomy for muscle invasive bladder cancer results in worse pathological stage. J Urol. 2003;170(4 Pt 1):1085–7.

35. Sanchez-Ortiz RF, Huang WC, Mick R, Van Arsdalen KN, Wein AJ, Malkowicz SB. An interval longer than 12 weeks between the diagnosis of muscle invasion and cystectomy is associated with worse outcome in bladder carcinoma. J Urol. 2003;169(1):110–5.

36. Gore JL, Lai J, Setodji CM, Litwin MS, Saigal CS. Mortality increases when radical cystectomy is delayed more than 12 weeks: results from a Surveillance, Epidemiology, and End Results-Medicare analysis. Cancer. 2009;115(5):988–96.

37. Hollenbeck BK, Taub DA, Dunn RL, Wei JT. Quality of care: partial cystectomy for bladder cancer—a case of inappropriate use? J Urol. 2005;174(3):1050–4.

38. Hedgepeth RC, Zhang Y, Skolarus TA, Hollenbeck BK. Variation in use of lymph node dissection during radical cystectomy for bladder cancer. Urology. 2011;77(2):385–90.

39. Sylvester RJ, Oosterlinck W, van der Meijden AP. A single immediate postoperative instillation of chemotherapy decreases the risk of recurrence in patients with stage Ta T1 bladder cancer: a meta-analysis of published results of randomized clinical trials. J Urol. 2004;171(6 Pt 1):2186–90.

40. Chamie K, Saigal CS, Lai J, Hanley JM, Setodji CM, Konety BR, et al. Compliance with guidelines for patients with bladder cancer: variation in the delivery of care. Cancer. 2011;117(23):5392–401.

41. Madeb R, Golijanin D, Noyes K, Fisher S, Stephenson JJ, Long SR, et al. Treatment of nonmuscle invading bladder cancer: do physicians in the United States practice evidence based medicine? The use and economic implications of intravesical chemotherapy after transurethral resection of bladder tumors. Cancer. 2009;115(12):2660–70.

42. Schrag D, Hsieh LJ, Rabbani F, Bach PB, Herr H, Begg CB. Adherence to surveillance among patients with superficial bladder cancer. J Natl Cancer Inst. 2003;95(8):588–97.

43. Chamie K, Saigal CS, Lai J, Hanley JM, Setodji CM, Konety BR, et al. Quality of care in patients with bladder cancer: a case report? Cancer. 2012;118(5):1412–21.

44. Lamm DL, Blumenstein BA, Crissman JD, Montie JE, Gottesman JE, Lowe BA, et al. Maintenance bacillus Calmette-Guerin immunotherapy for recurrent TA, T1 and carcinoma in situ transitional cell carcinoma of the bladder: a randomized Southwest Oncology Group Study. J Urol. 2000;163(4):1124–9.

45. Huang GJ, Hamilton AS, Lo M, Stein JP, Penson DF. Predictors of intravesical therapy for nonmuscle invasive bladder cancer: results from the surveillance, epidemiology and end results program 2003 patterns of care project. J Urol. 2008;180(2):520–4.

46. Barocas DA, Liu A, Burks FN, Suh RS, Schuster TG, Bradford T, et al. Practice-based collaboration to improve the use of immediate intravesical therapy after resection for non-muscle-invasive bladder cancer. J Urol. 2013;190(6):2011–6.

47. Miller DC, Murtagh DS, Suh RS, Knapp PM, Dunn RL, Montie JE. Establishment of a urological surgery quality collaborative. J Urol. 2010;184(6):2485–90.

48. Birkmeyer NJ, Share D, Campbell Jr DA, Prager RL, Moscucci M, Birkmeyer JD. Partnering with payers to improve surgical quality: the Michigan plan. Surgery. 2005;138(5):815–20.

49. Flum DR, Fisher N, Thompson J, Marcus-Smith M, Florence M, Pellegrini CA. Washington State's approach to variability in surgical processes/outcomes: Surgical Clinical Outcomes Assessment Program (SCOAP). Surgery. 2005;138(5):821–8.

50. Share DA, Campbell DA, Birkmeyer N, Prager RL, Gurm HS, Moscucci M, et al. How a regional collaborative of hospitals and physicians in Michigan cut costs and improved the quality of care. Health Aff (Millwood). 2011;30(4):636–45.

51. Kwon S, Florence M, Grigas P, Horton M, Horvath K, Johnson M, et al. Creating a learning healthcare system in surgery: Washington State's Surgical Care and Outcomes Assessment Program (SCOAP) at 5 years. Surgery. 2012;151(2):146–52.

52. Miller DC, Murtagh DS, Suh RS, Knapp PM, Schuster TG, Dunn RL, et al. Regional collaboration to improve radiographic staging practices among men with early stage prostate cancer. J Urol. 2011;186(3):844–9.

53. Birkmeyer JD, Stukel TA, Siewers AE, Goodney PP, Wennberg DE, Lucas FL. Surgeon volume and operative mortality in the United States. N Engl J Med. 2003;349(22):2117–27.

54. Hollenbeck BK, Taub DA, Miller DC, Dunn RL, Montie JE, Wei JT. The regionalization of radical cystectomy to specific medical centers. J Urol. 2005; 174(4 Pt 1):1385–9.

55. Finks JF, Osborne NH, Birkmeyer JD. Trends in hospital volume and operative mortality for high-risk surgery. N Engl J Med. 2011;364(22):2128–37.

56. Hollenbeck BK, Dunn RL, Miller DC, Daignault S, Taub DA, Wei JT. Volume-based referral for cancer surgery: informing the debate. J Clin Oncol. 2007; 25(1):91–6.

57. The Leapfrog Group Fact Sheet. Washington, DC: The Leapfrog Group; 2012. Available from: http://www.leapfroggroup.org/about_us/leapfrog-factsheet. Accessed 29 Oct 2012

58. Kernisan LP, Lee SJ, Boscardin WJ, Landefeld CS, Dudley RA. Association between hospital-reported Leapfrog Safe Practices Scores and inpatient mortality. JAMA. 2009;301(13):1341–8.

59. FACT SHEET: Blue Distinction®. 2012. Available from: http://www.bcbs.com/why-bcbs/blue-distinction/blue-distinction-fact-sheet.pdf. Accessed Oct 15 2012.

60. Physician Quality Reporting System. Baltimore, MD: Centers for Medicare & Medicaid Services; 2012. Available from: http://www.cms.gov/Medicare/Quality-Initiatives-Patient-Assessment-Instruments/PQRS/index.html?redirect=/PQRS. Accessed 22 Oct 2012.

61. PQRS Toolkit. Linthicum, MD: American Urological Association; 2012. Available from: http://www.aua-net.org/content/health-policy/regulation-and-reimbursement/payor-information/pqrs-toolkit.cfm. Accessed Jun 2013.

62. Lotan Y, Cadeddu JA, Roehrborn CG, Stage KH. The value of your time: evaluation of effects of changes in medicare reimbursement rates on the practice of urology. J Urol. 2004;172(5 Pt 1):1958–62.

63. Hussey PS, Sorbero ME, Mehrotra A, Liu H, Damberg CL. Episode-based performance measurement and payment: making it a reality. Health Aff (Millwood). 2009;28(5):1406–17.

64. Hernandez V, De La Pena E, Martin MD, Blazquez C, Diaz FJ, Llorente C. External validation and applicability of the EORTC risk tables for non-muscle-invasive bladder cancer. World J Urol. 2011;29(4):409–14.

65. Miller DC, Gust C, Dimick JB, Birkmeyer N, Skinner J, Birkmeyer JD. Large variations in Medicare payments for surgery highlight savings potential from bundled payment programs. Health Aff (Millwood). 2011;30(11):2107–15.

66. Chang SS, Cookson MS, Baumgartner RG, Wells N, Smith Jr JA. Analysis of early complications after radical cystectomy: results of a collaborative care pathway. J Urol. 2002;167(5):2012–6.

67. Hollenbeck BK, Miller DC, Taub D, Dunn RL, Khuri SF, Henderson WG, et al. Identifying risk factors for potentially avoidable complications following radical cystectomy. J Urol. 2005;174(4 Pt 1):1231–7.

68. Konety BR, Allareddy V, Herr H. Complications after radical cystectomy: analysis of population-based data. Urology. 2006;68(1):58–64.

69. Gilbert SM, Dunn RL, Miller DC, Daignault S, Ye Z, Hollenbeck BK. Mortality after urologic cancer surgery: impact of non-index case volume. Urology. 2008;71(5):906–10.

70. Stimson CJ, Chang SS, Barocas DA, Humphrey JE, Patel SG, Clark PE, et al. Early and late perioperative outcomes following radical cystectomy: 90-day readmissions, morbidity and mortality in a contemporary series. J Urol. 2010;184(4):1296–300.

71. Overview list—how many smokefree laws? Berkeley, CA: American Nonsmokers' Rights Foundation; 2013. Available from: http://www.no-smoke.org/pdf/mediaordlist.pdf. Accessed Jun 2013.

Christopher B. Anderson, David F. Penson, and Daniel A. Barocas

Everything that can be counted does not necessarily count; everything that counts cannot necessarily be counted

—Albert Einstein

8.1 Introduction: The Cost of Survival

Therapeutic endpoints for cancer treatments were historically measured by quantitative outcomes, such as disease-specific, recurrence-free and overall survival, and achieved at any cost, namely short-term morbidity and mortality [1]. Yet, these treatment goals and costs are not always in line with patient goals, preferences and values, and may not be acceptable to the patient [2, 3]. Any disease or treatment can result in varying amounts of short- and long-term physical (pain, creation of an ostomy), functional (urinary, sexual, bowel), psychosocial (depression, adapting to a new health state), emotional (fulfilling family roles), and occupational (professional or domestic) impairment. These represent different types of treatment costs that we know to be important factors in cancer treatment. The fundamental consideration in modern cancer care is: what is the cost of survival? [4]

In 2013, many cancers, including urothelial carcinoma, have become chronic diseases as a result of an improvement in our knowledge and treatment of the disease. Although patients now live for years with their diseases and the consequences of treatment, they have made it clear that there is more to life than simply "not dying" [5]. As a result, the objectives of treating cancer have broadened from quantitative measures (if a patient survives) to qualitative measures (how a patient survives) with an emphasis on patient-centered care [6, 7].

This is particularly true for the treatment of bladder cancer. Some patients require radical cystectomy (RC) with urinary diversion, which is associated with significant morbidity and alterations in patient body image, functionality, sexual function and urinary continence with a nearly 40 % mortality rate at 5 years [8–10]. Others are managed endoscopically and are subject to multiple uncomfortable intravesical treatments and bothersome urinary symptoms. Unfortunately, traditional quantitative outcomes do not completely capture the impact of bladder cancer or its treatment.

C.B. Anderson, M.D. (✉)
Memorial Sloan Kettering Cancer Center,
Department of Surgery, Urology Service,
1275 York Avenue, New York, NY 10065, USA

Department of Urologic Surgery, Vanderbilt
University Medical Center,
Nashville, TN 37232-2765, USA
e-mail: andersc3@mskcc.org

D.F. Penson, M.D., M.P.H.
Department of Urologic Surgery,
Center for Surgical Quality and Outcomes Research,
Vanderbilt University Medical Center,
2525 West End Avenue, Suite 1200, Nashville,
TN 37203, USA
e-mail: david.penson@vanderbilt.edu

D.A. Barocas, M.D., M.P.H.
Department of Urologic Surgery, Center for Surgical
Quality and Outcomes Research, Vanderbilt
University Medical Center, A-1302 Medical Center
North, Nashville, TN 37232-2765, USA
e-mail: dan.barocas@vanderbilt.edu

B.R. Konety and S.S. Chang (eds.), *Management of Bladder Cancer:
A Comprehensive Text With Clinical Scenarios*, DOI 10.1007/978-1-4939-1881-2_8,
© Springer Science+Business Media New York 2015

One way of providing a more complete evaluation of the subjective impact of a disease or its treatment is to measure patient quality of life (QOL). This measure captures many of the physical and psychological effects of treatment that patients consider important. Interest in QOL has grown over the past 40 years and today plays a central role in cancer treatment. The goal of this chapter is to describe the significance of QOL in the treatment of bladder cancer and how to measure and incorporate QOL into clinical practice.

8.2   Defining Quality of Life: Counting the Uncountable

It has long been recognized that the state of health is "not merely the absence of disease" but also the presence of "physical, mental, and social well-being," and as surgeons it is our goal to not only treat disease, but also to improve our patient's well-being [11]. In essence, quality of life is the presence and amount of patient well-being and encompasses multiple domains, including health status, functional capacity, financial stability, job security, amount of independence, spirituality, and social relationships. Health-related quality of life (HRQOL) refers specifically to the elements in a patient's life that are affected by their health status. HRQOL is a multidimensional construct that includes general health domains such as physical, emotional and psychological functioning, presence of symptoms, social and familial support, and satisfaction with healthcare delivery, as well as disease-specific domains such as urinary and bowel function, body image and sexuality for bladder cancer patients [12]. Importantly, HRQOL also includes amount of bother related to each domain.

Due to the broad nature of the concept, no standard definition of HRQOL exists. It has been described as a "patient's appraisal of and satisfaction with their current level of functioning as compared to what they perceive to be possible or ideal," and the extent to which "medical interventions impact the functional, psychological, social and economic life" of a patient [12, 13]. Calman simply defines HRQOL as the gap between a patient's expectations and experiences (Fig. 8.1a) [14]. The most vital element of HRQOL is that it is a patient-centric assessment that cannot be assigned or assumed, but only measured by patient report [14].

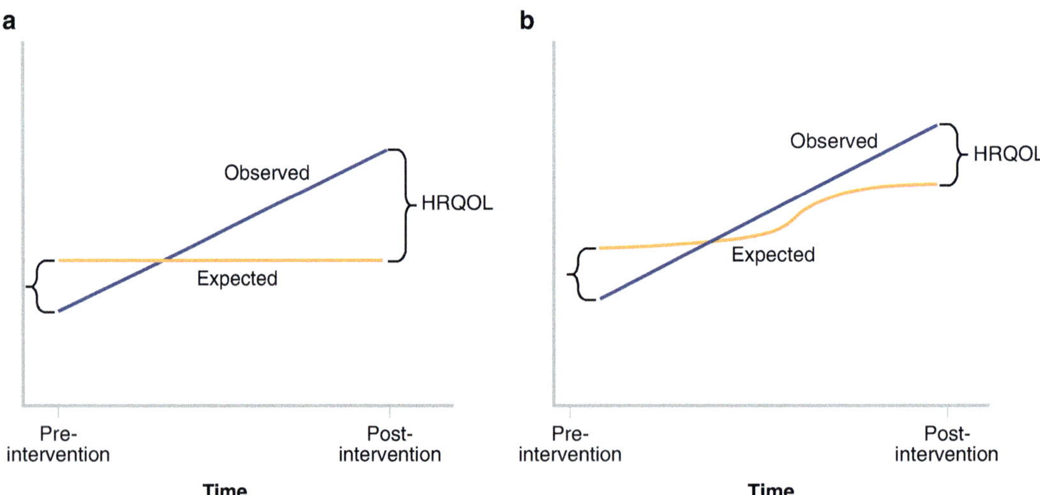

Fig. 8.1 (**a**) HRQOL before and after an intervention represented as the gap between patient expectation and actual experience. Since the observed (*solid line*) is below expected (*dashed line*), pre-intervention HRQOL is low while it is high post-intervention. (**b**) HRQOL accounting for changing expectations with time (response shift). Post-intervention HRQOL is lower than estimated in (**a**) [14]

There is a critical distinction between HRQOL and health status. Whereas health status refers primarily to the direct physical and functional effects of disease, HRQOL also encompasses how patients perceive and react to their health status [15]. Such a distinction must be made because patients with impaired "objective" health states, such as those with severe disabilities or in hospice care, may have outstanding coping mechanisms and different expectations around their condition and report surprisingly high HRQOL [16, 17]. Thus, it is inaccurate to make assumptions on HRQOL based on health status alone.

HRQOL is predicated strongly on the patient's preference, or *relative* desirability, of a given health status [18]. Given the subjectivity of HRQOL, it is heavily influenced by a patient's values, goals, experiences and opinions, and may change with interventions, differing expectations or ongoing experience. It may also vary between patients who have different judgments of similar health states [19]. Because HRQOL is highly personal, it has proven difficult to define, measure and gain acceptance in the clinical setting. However, with improved understanding of what constitutes HRQOL and how it is quantified, its role in the care of cancer patients has become essential.

8.3 Assessing Quality of Life: The Importance of a Subjective Metric

Measuring and utilizing HRQOL in the patient care and research settings is important for several reasons. Patients thirst for information about their diagnosis, prognosis and what to expect during their treatment, and rely on their physician for this type of counseling [20]. By measuring HRQOL and quantifying the physical, emotional, psychosocial and functional impacts of a disease or treatment, physicians can more accurately counsel their patients. Patients fear the implications of a cancer diagnosis, the consequences of a radical operation, and the possibility of death, which can often be allayed through honest discussion [21]. Well-informed patients may also have better psychological outcomes and increased treatment satisfaction [21, 22].

Counseling not only helps educate patients, but maximizes future HRQOL by enabling surgeons to become an "honest broker" and set realistic expectations [23, 24]. Discussing HRQOL concerns may improve communication and screen for important problems not regularly discussed at clinic visits. For instance, cancer patients are known to be at substantial risk for depression, sometimes long after their treatment [25–27]. Symptoms of depression detected during QOL assessment may prompt specialist referral and failure to do so may result in untreated diagnoses that exacerbate disease trajectory or prolong recovery. Patients tend to be grateful for discussions of HQROL topics, indicating the importance of HRQOL in their disease, treatment and physician relationship [28]. And as the primary purpose for measuring any health outcome is to improve it, physicians can identify unrecognized problems with their treatment plans or patient support mechanisms through the analysis of HRQOL [29].

Quality of life data may also improve shared clinical decision making. There are many factors to consider when treating a cancer patient, and surgeons must tailor their treatment to a patient's value system [7, 24]. For instance, if social continence is more important to a patient with invasive bladder cancer than the risk of urinary retention, they may be better suited with an orthotopic neobladder (ONB) rather than an ileal conduit (IC). With information on how different treatments normally impact HRQOL, physicians may be better able to individualize treatment plans. Interestingly, QOL may impact prognosis [30–32]. Palapattu measured the amount of psychological distress prior to RC and found that preoperative somatic distress was associated with disease progression [32]. Mansson demonstrated that certain types of defense strategies impacted how well patients adapted to their new health status after RC [33].

HRQOL is an increasingly important measurement in clinical trials and has already been used as a clinically relevant outcome [34, 35]. There are several circumstances when measuring HRQOL is absolutely necessary in the clinical trial setting [36]:

- When measuring the benefit of adjuvant therapy with a moderate risk of disease recurrence.
- If survival is expected to be similar between treatment arms.
- If the treatment is performed for palliation.
- When comparing surgical techniques expected to have similar oncologic outcomes.

In each of these circumstances, as well as many others, patient HRQOL should be measured as it may be the only difference between treatment arms. In fact, HRQOL has become such an important metric that clinical trial groups such as the European Organization for Research and Treatment of Cancer (EORTC) have emphasized routinely including HRQOL measurements in clinical trials [37]. The Patient-Centered Outcomes Research Institute (PCORI) was established by the United States government in 2010 to promote research initiatives that investigate the "relative health outcomes, clinical effectiveness, and appropriateness" of medical interventions, emphasizing the central role of patient-reported outcomes and HRQOL in treatment decision-making [38]. With an emphasis on improving healthcare quality, treatment outcomes, including morbidity, survival and quality of life, have become surrogates for quality of care [39]. Since HRQOL is a priority in comprehensive cancer treatment, it will be an increasingly important endpoint in measuring quality of care [6, 40].

Finally, HRQOL has also gained importance in health policy decisions through its role in the calculation of quality-adjusted life years (QALYs). A QALY is an outcome used to compare the relative value of different treatments by contrasting their cost, or effectiveness, per year of quality life gained and requires measurement of patient HRQOL. QALYs have already been used in large-scale healthcare change and will likely continue to be an important outcome in policy decisions [41].

In all, measuring and utilizing HRQOL in the clinical and research setting is a valuable practice with increasing importance. Some even consider failure to measure and utilize HRQOL to be "neither good science nor good medicine" [21].

8.4 HRQOL in Bladder Cancer Patients: Scope of the Issue

In most early clinical trials, including those in bladder cancer, HRQOL was not assessed [19, 42]. In addition to coping with a new cancer diagnosis, patients with bladder cancer are subject to an array of treatment- and disease-related issues that cause significant anxiety and distress. Patients being managed endoscopically may require multiple painful operations and intravesical instillations, experience bothersome urinary symptoms and be at risk for disease recurrence and progression [43–46]. RC patients undergo a procedure associated with significant morbidity, psychological distress and life-changing consequences, such as urinary incontinence, sexual dysfunction, impaired functional status and changes in body image [8, 47–51]. Even after treatment, bladder cancer survivors may be at risk for diminished HRQOL secondary to ongoing lifestyle factors, such as diet, exercise and smoking [52, 53].

With the popularization of the ONB, urologists assumed it would be associated with improved HRQOL in comparison to incontinent urinary diversions given the avoidance of an external appliance and replication of physiologic voiding. Multiple studies, including a Cochrane review [54], attempted to demonstrate an improvement in HRQOL with ONB, however this has proven difficult [19, 47, 55]. One explanation is that there is no real difference in HRQOL between diversion types. Alternatively, the available methods to assess HRQOL in bladder cancer patients may not be sufficiently sensitive to detect nuanced differences between treatment types. Many HRQOL studies in bladder cancer patients did not use validated, disease-specific questionnaires, but instead used suboptimal techniques for measuring HRQOL such as "homemade" questionnaires or patient interviews [24]. Lastly, weaknesses in study design may lead to difficulties in demonstrating any differences if they are present. In general, HRQOL studies in bladder cancer have been small, single institution, retrospective studies with significant methodological flaws [56].

Many investigators fail to collaborate with experts in QOL study design, such as statisticians and psychologists, and studies often lack pre-intervention and longitudinal assessments [56]. There are very few prospective studies and no level I evidence supporting HRQOL differences between diversion types or between any other treatments for bladder cancer.

Thus, bladder cancer patients are at risk for a reduction in HRQOL, yet much is still unknown about and the true impact of the disease and its treatment [57]. To date, most HRQOL research in bladder cancer has been in the RC population with a paucity in the native bladder population. Any attempt to identify real differences in HRQOL across diversion or treatment types would require a large, high-quality prospective study that controls for patient and decision-making confounders, although randomization to diversion type is probably not feasible.

8.5 Response Shift: Adaptation to Health States

While HRQOL can change secondary to an outcome or intervention, it can also change due to variation in expectation (Fig. 8.1a) [14]. As patients adapt to new disease states, HRQOL can change as they recalibrate their point of reference (their expected health status), reprioritize the relative importance of the aspects of their life that constitute HRQOL or reconceptualize their very definition of HRQOL [58]. This variation in HRQOL secondary to changing expectations is known as response shift (Fig. 8.1b) [19]. Response shift is either an inherent property of how HRQOL is defined or measured and may confound the interpretation of HRQOL differences.

Response shift may explain unexpected HRQOL differences or lack thereof, such as the similar QOL between lottery winners and non-winners and high HRQOL among patients with declining health states [16, 18, 59]. Similarly, most RC patients are "generally satisfied" and have similar HRQOL to the general population and to other RC patients despite differences in functional outcomes and diversion type, reflecting their ability to adapt similarly to different health states [19, 49, 55, 60]. Recall bias is another example of response shift. As patients adapt to new health states and change their perspective, any assessment of prior HRQOL may be inaccurate (Fig. 8.1b) [18, 61, 62].

Response shift can make the measurement of HRQOL challenging and must be accounted for when designing a study and interpreting study findings. Going forward, methods for adjusting for response shift will improve the fidelity of HRQOL assessments.

8.6 Measuring Health-Related Quality of Life: Instruments

In order to generate useful and generalizable HRQOL data, there are numerous important study design considerations, including who should measure it, what to measure and when and how it should be measured [63].

8.6.1 Who

Although physicians may accurately assess health status, they lack insight into how it impacts patient's daily lives. For example, the Karnofsky Performance Status (KPS), a well-known assessment, is a physician's evaluation of a patient's functional status [64]. Although the KPS has been used extensively in clinical trials, it has been criticized for accuracy, completeness and reliance on the physician's assessment rather than patient report [65, 66]. Indeed, we now understand that it is neither appropriate nor accurate for a physician to define patient HRQOL [67]. Similarly, patient proxies such as spouses, friends and family members lack the perspective to accurately assess patient HRQOL and should not be queried unless the patient is unable to be directly assessed [18, 68]. HRQOL is a patient-centric concept that is best measured through direct patient assessment.

8.6.2 How

The simplest way to determine subjective outcome is to ask patients if a treatment improved their life. While most people can articulate the quality of their experience such communication cannot be quantified, necessitating the standardization and quantification of HRQOL. There are generally two methods for measuring HRQOL: patient-completed questionnaires and researcher-administered interviews. Because interviews are time and labor-intensive, questionnaires, also known as instruments, are typically preferred. Instruments are inexpensive, practical and easy to administer. HRQOL instruments are complex tools that require a rigorous process of development and implementation.

Instrument development is a multistep process that begins by determining what aspects of HRQOL are to be measured, then generating and assembling questions into a single instrument and finally performing a psychometric analysis [69]. Question, or item, development ideally involves input from multiple perspectives, such as physicians, patients, epidemiologists and psychologists. First, candidate items are developed through a review of the literature to ascertain previously identified important HRQOL issues, as well as through patient focus groups to help identify domains of interest. The item list is then refined by expert analysis and patient feedback from semi-structured interviews.

Item responses are either recorded on a Likert scale, in which several answer options are presented in a categorical fashion, or a visual analog scale, where patients mark their answer along a continuum between two ends of a spectrum. Most instruments use Likert scales due to easier data capture and simplicity of answering. There are several factors to consider in instrument development. Each item must be written below an eighth grade reading level, free of abbreviations and complex terms, and contain only one question to ensure patient comprehension [70]. Furthermore, items must not include any language perceived to be offensive, which is typically detected during pilot and cross-cultural testing. Also, there is generally a trade-off between breadth (number of domains) and depth (number of items) of assessment. In order to minimize patient burden, there must be a balance between the two, with a possible bias toward breadth given the uncertainty of the impact of a disease or treatment [5].

Once an instrument has been created, it must undergo psychometric analysis to verify its measurement properties [71]. Involvement by statisticians or psychometricians in this step is mandatory. First, an instrument is tested for reliability, which evaluates its precision, or freedom from measurement error. The two most common measures of reliability are internal consistency and test–retest. Internal consistency reliability is the amount of internal agreement among items. For instance, all items intended to measure functional status should score similarly and correlate highly. Internal consistency reliability is quantified with Crohnbach's coefficient alpha. A value of >0.7 indicates good reliability, however if it is too high (>0.9) the instrument may have excessive homogeneity suggesting item redundancy. Test–retest reliability is how well an instrument's results are reproducible, and is measured by administering the instrument to the same subject within a relatively short time span, often a matter of weeks. Test–retest reliability is quantified by correlation coefficients, with >0.7 considered highly reliable [23].

Still, a highly precise instrument is not necessarily accurate. Hence, an instrument must be tested for validity, which is its ability to measure the truth. Because validity varies based on the context and population for which it is used, an instrument must be validated separately for different clinical scenarios. For example, an instrument validated to measure incontinence symptoms in neurogenic bladder patients does not mean it can evaluate the same symptoms in prostate cancer patients. There are three types of validity: face, construct and criterion. Face validity, also known as content validity, is a subjective assessment of how well the instrument measures HRQOL. It represents an "enlightened common sense" impression by experts in the field as to whether the instrument includes necessary items and does not include irrelevant ones [72]. Criterion validity is the correlation between the instrument and a "gold standard" instrument when administered concurrently. An instrument is highly valid if it scores similarly and correlates highly ($r > 0.7$) with the gold standard. For example, if an instrument designed to measure bother from urinary incontinence correlated highly with daily pad use, it would have high criterion validity. If a gold standard does not exist, criterion validity cannot be measured. Lastly, construct validity is a retrospective assessment of how well an instrument measures what it was designed to measure. Construct validity can be difficult to assess and often takes years of instrument use before establishing. Two methods for evaluating construct validity are convergent and divergent validity [73]. Convergent validity is established when different instruments designed to theoretically measure the same concept converge on the same results. Alternatively, divergent validity is established when instruments measuring unrelated concepts have opposite results. Construct validity is quantified with correlation coefficients, with >0.7 considered highly valid.

Once reliability and validity are established, an instrument should be evaluated for responsiveness, or how well it detects change over time. For instance, the American Urological Association-Symptom Index (AUA-SI) is expected to change as a man receives treatment for lower urinary tract symptoms. A highly responsive instrument is able to detect even small changes in HRQOL. A common question is what amount change in HRQOL is considered clinically meaningful. For example, what difference in AUA-SI is clinically relevant? While there is no number universally regarded as meaningful, at least half the instrument's standard deviation is often a good rule [74]. Once each of these properties has been explored, the final step is to implement the instrument into clinical practice.

8.6.3 When

Measuring HRQOL should be a seamless part of clinic visits and included in most clinical trials, much like obtaining a vital sign. Given its subjectivity, HRQOL can be easily influenced by the context in which it is measured, necessitating standardization of the schedule and setting of instrument administration. Since HRQOL is constantly in flux, patients must be asked to evaluate their HRQOL within a specific time frame, such as within the past week or month. One must also determine at which points during the course of disease or treatment measurements should be taken. A baseline assessment is always indicated, as are regular assessments thereafter in a longitudinal fashion. After RC, HRQOL may return to near baseline levels within 1 year, thus evaluations within the first year are likely responsive to disease-specific changes [75]. In addition to timing, it is important to standardize where patients complete instruments. For instance, if one patient is assessed at home and another in the hospital, it would be unclear if HRQOL differences were real or due to the setting in which the instrument was completed.

Thus, validated instruments are the most appropriate method for evaluating HRQOL in bladder cancer patients, and they should be commonplace in both the clinic and in clinical trials [13, 63].

8.7 Selecting an Instrument: Finding the Best Fit

There are a multitude of standardized instruments to measure HRQOL including general, cancer-specific, disease-specific, utility and treatment-specific instruments [19]. General instruments can be applied to larger populations and compared across different disease states and treatment modalities, however they are less sensitive to disease- or treatment-specific changes. On the other hand, disease-specific instruments are more sensitive to changes in a particular disease state, but lack generalizability across different patient groups.

There are several factors into selecting the best instrument (Table 8.1). The first and most important step in selecting the appropriate HRQOL instrument is to ask a specific research question and determine which aspects of HRQOL are most important to assess. One must also consider the

Table 8.1 Factors in instrument selection

Is it valid and reliable?
Are norms available?
Is it suitable for the targeted population?
Are questions easy to read and understand?
Is scoring easy or complex?
Is the layout of the questions clear?
What is the format of the questions?
Is it comprehensive but brief as possible?
Does it ask socially loaded questions?
Who will complete the questions?

[21]

characteristics of the study population, as well as the instrument itself. Only established instruments with known psychometric properties that have been validated in the intended study population should be used. To select a non-validated instrument without known psychometric properties or an ad hoc questionnaire is unacceptable in any high-quality clinical research.

As HRQOL is a multidimensional construct, any instrument should measure multiple general and disease-specific domains [76]. This is commonly achieved using a modular instrument that consists of a set of general HRQOL questions and set of disease-specific items known as a module [69]. Furthermore, it is often useful to assess a patient's overall satisfaction, in order to determine the clinical relevance of HRQOL changes.

8.7.1 General HRQOL Instruments

Most general instruments assess several basic HRQOL areas including physical, psychosocial and emotional functioning, mobility, self-care activities, energy, cognitive function, general health and pain [13]. The three most commonly used general HRQOL instruments for cancer patients are the SF-36, FACT-G, and EORTC QLQ-30. Each is designed to be completed by the patient. Other well-known general HRQOL instruments are the Sickness Impact Profile and Nottingham Health Profile [77, 78]. While many general instruments have been used to measure

HRQOL in bladder cancer patients, none have been validated in this population.

1. *Medical Outcomes Short Form Health Survey (SF-36)*: The SF-36 is a well-known, widely used general HRQOL instrument developed by the RAND Institute [79]. It has been used in a variety of disease states, including bladder cancer, and is considered by many the gold standard for measuring general HRQOL [80–83]. The SF-36 consists of 36 items organized into eight domains (role limitations-physical, role limitations-emotional, social functioning, physical functioning, mental health, energy/vitality, pain, and general health) grouped into two scales (physical and mental). Each item is scored on a Likert scale. There are shorter versions of the SF-36 with 8 (SF-8) or 12 (SF-12) items, which have been produced to reduce respondent burden and are psychometrically validated [84].

2. *Functional Assessment of Cancer Therapy—General (FACT-G)*: Unlike the SF-36, the FACT-G is an instrument designed to measure cancer-specific general HRQOL. It is a validated 28-item instrument that consists of four domains (physical, functional, social, and emotional well-being) with each item scored on a Likert scale [85]. The FACT-G has been used in bladder cancer patients [80, 86, 87].

3. *European Organization for the Research and Treatment of Cancer Quality of Life Core Questionnaire (EORTC QLQ-30)*: Similar to the FACT-G, the EORTC QLQ-30 is designed to measure cancer-specific general HRQOL. It is a 30-item instrument that consists of six functional subscales (physical, role, cognitive, emotional, social, and global) and three symptom scales (pain, fatigue, and emesis) [88]. Each item is scored on a Likert scale. This instrument has been used to study HRQOL in bladder cancer patients [89, 90].

There are also a variety of instruments designed to assess specific aspects of general HRQOL such as pain, body image, mental health, and functionality. For a comprehensive list of HRQOL instruments refer to www.proqolid.com.

8.7.2 Disease-Specific HRQOL Instruments

General HRQOL instruments lack the ability to capture important disease-specific issues experienced by patients with bladder cancer, such as continence, body image and bowel problems. As is often demonstrated by psychometric analysis of disease-specific instruments, there can be low correlation between disease-specific and general HRQOL items, suggesting disease-specific items measure concepts not captured with generic ones, and vice versa [91, 92]. Historically, instruments assessing HRQOL in bladder cancer patients were either general HRQOL instruments or invalidated homemade questionnaires [47, 82, 93–95]. Several bladder cancer-specific HRQOL instruments have since been developed, and two have thus far been validated [91, 92].

1. *FACT-Vanderbilt Cystectomy Index (FACT-VCI)*: The FACT-VCI is a modular instrument composed of the 28-item FACT-G and a novel 17-item module [96]. Each item is scored on a 4-point Likert scale. The FACT-VCI was specifically developed to measure HRQOL in bladder cancer patients undergoing radical cystectomy. It was validated in RC patients and has good reliability, validity and responsiveness [91]. It is scored as a simple summary of all 15 gender-neutral questions (items 1–15) with a separate score for sexual function (items 16 and 17). The FACT-VCI is highly specific for detecting RC-related problems and also measures general HRQOL changes. It has been used to assess HRQOL in RC patients [97, 98] and is currently being used in large prospective studies [99].

2. *Bladder Cancer Index (BCI)*: The BCI was also developed to measure HRQOL in bladder cancer patients [100]. It consists of 34 items, each scored on a Likert scale, organized into three domains (urinary, bowel, and sexual) with function and bother measured in each domain. Unlike the FACT-VCI, the BCI measures HRQOL in both RC and non-RC patients and is reliable, valid and responsive in these populations [49, 92]. Its main advantage is its generalizability across all patients with bladder cancer. However, some items may be inapplicable to certain patients, which may limit its face validity. For instance, a patient being managed endoscopically may be unable to answer questions about urine leakage causing skin irritation, whereas this would be highly applicable to a patient with an IC. Notably, the BCI fails to measure important emotional, functional and psychosocial domains of HRQOL requiring the co-administration of a supplemental instrument for complete HRQOL assessment.

3. *FACT-Bladder (FACT-BL)*: The FACT-BL is also a modular instrument designed to measure HRQOL in bladder cancer patients [101, 102]. It is based on the FACT-G with a 13-item module. Although the FACT-BL has been used clinically [57, 87, 103], it has not yet been validated in bladder cancer patients.

4. *EORTC QLQ-BLM-30*: The QLQ-BLM-30 is a modular instrument designed to measure HRQOL in patients with muscle-invasive bladder cancer. It is based off of the EORTC QLQ-30 and has a bladder-cancer specific module [104]. Although it has been used clinically [89], it has not yet been validated in patients with muscle-invasive bladder cancer and studies with this instrument are ongoing [105].

5. *EORTC QLQ-BLS-24*: The QLQ-BLS-24 is a modular instrument designed to measure HRQOL in patients with non-muscle-invasive bladder cancer. Similar to the BLM-30, it is based off of the EORTC QLQ-30, but instead has a non-muscle-invasive-specific module [104]. It has not been validated in patients with non-muscle-invasive bladder cancer and studies with this instrument are ongoing [106].

8.7.3 Health Utility Instruments

Utility instruments measure patient preferences for different health states which are used to compare the relative effectiveness or cost of treatments [107]. Measuring health utilities begins by defining particular health states and then determining patient valuations of each state, where 1 is equivalent to perfect health and 0 is death.

The outcome is expressed in QALYs, which is a preference-weighted measure combined with a survival estimate. Utility instruments include the EQ-5D [108], SF-6D [109], Health Utilities Index [110] and Quality of Well Being-Self Administered [111]. Utility instruments typically use different types of response scales. The standard gamble asks patients with impaired health how much they would risk for an intervention that could either cure them or kill them, while time-tradeoff asks patients how much life they would be willing to give up to achieve perfect health.

8.8 HRQOL in Bladder Cancer Patients: The "Hard" Data

Since the inception of HRQOL in bladder cancer, well over 50 studies have been published using over a dozen instruments, most of which attempt to identify differences between types of urinary diversion in RC patients. There are several large and well-performed reviews that nicely summarize studies to date, none of which have demonstrated consistent superiority of any single diversion type [19, 47, 54–56, 95, 112, 113]. They have, however, confirmed a consistent decrease in HRQOL after RC with gradual improvement over the first 12 months for most patients. Although the literature on HRQOL after RC is extensive, its scientific quality is relatively poor, contributing to its inability to demonstrate a HRQOL difference between diversion types [113]. Although HRQOL has been studied for nearly every diversion type, ONB and IC are the most common.

In one of the longest prospective studies, Hedgepeth reported HRQOL differences in 226 RC patients using the BCI [49]. With 8 years of follow-up, IC patients had gradual improvement in their body image to near baseline, while ONB patients had persistently decreased body image scores. Ileal conduit patients had higher postoperative urinary function, but similar levels of urinary bother, bowel and sexual domains as ONB patients. Hardt prospectively evaluated patients undergoing continent and incontinent diversions and found similar HRQOL between diversion types and that over 75 % of patients would choose the same diversion again [114]. Allareddy mailed the FACT-BL to 259 bladder cancer patients, 82 of whom had undergone RC and 177 had native bladders [57]. In this cross-sectional study, there was no difference in HRQOL between RC and native bladder patients or IC and continent diversion patients.

Still, some *have* demonstrated relevant differences in diversion types. In the validation study of the FACT-VCI, IC patients had significantly higher HRQOL than ONB patients 1 year after surgery, although this study was not powered nor designed to explore differences between diversion types [91]. Conversely, Hobisch sent the EORTC-QLQ-30 and a self-designed questionnaire to 102 patients after RC, and reported ONB patients had superior HRQOL outcomes to IC patients and would almost uniformly recommend their diversion type to another patient, while only a third of IC patients would do the same [90]. Although not a comparative study, women with ONB were found to have a surprisingly high rate of voiding dysfunction, including hypercontinence and incontinence [115]. In general, while IC patients tend to have more problems with leakage, skin irritation and are less likely to travel, ONB patients may experience problems with incontinence and hypercontinence [55, 116]. Interestingly, the associated bother with these two diversions is almost identical in many studies and both sets of patients have similarly high levels of satisfaction, oftentimes comparable to population norms.

While the majority of emphasis on HRQOL after RC and urinary diversion focus on urinary problems, sexual function is also an important issue. Although many men and women will have substantial sexual dysfunction prior to surgery, there are still many patients for whom maintenance of sexual function is a priority. Men are at risk for erectile dysfunction and women may be left with a foreshortened and denervated vagina resulting in substantial sexual dysfunction. Zippe administered the Index of Female Sexual Function to 27 sexually active women before and after RC and found significant reductions in vaginal lubrication, ability to achieve orgasm, sexual desire and increased dyspareunia, with about half unable to have successful vaginal intercourse postoperatively [117]. Zippe similarly administered the Sexual Health Inventory for Men (SHIM) to 49 sexually active men and found substantial decreases in SHIM scores after RC, with 86 % of men unable to produce an erection sufficient for vaginal penetration, particularly those that underwent non-nerve sparing RC [118].

Another area of study in RC patients has been in the potential HRQOL benefits of robotic-assisted laparoscopic RC (RARC). RARC is associated with less intraoperative blood loss and analgesic requirement, and a shorter hospital stay and time to regular diet at the cost of an increased operating room time and equipment expenses [119]. RARC appears to have a similar rate of complications and short-term oncologic efficacy. Yuh administered the FACT-BL to 57 patients undergoing RARC and identified significant HRQOL reductions in several domains with return to baseline at 6 months [103]. In another study out of Roswell Park, the CARE instrument was administered pre- and postoperatively to 91 patients undergoing RARC [120]. The overall score decreased by nearly 50 % at 1 week with near complete recovery at 10 weeks. Specifically, both pain and cognition scores demonstrated a fairly rapid recovery to near baseline by approximately 1 month, but gastrointestinal and activity scores did not recover until at least 3 months. Although these single-armed analyses demonstrate promising HRQOL results with RARC, no publications to date have compared HRQOL between open RC and RARC although preliminary, unpublished data suggest no difference between the two approaches [99, 121].

Approximately 75 % of patients with bladder cancer have non-muscle-invasive disease and are treated endoscopically. While this treatment is significantly less morbid than RC, it is still associated with HRQOL changes and patient distress. Muezzingolu demonstrated high pain scores among patients undergoing surveillance cystoscopy, which seemed to worsen with each subsequent procedure [45]. Yoshimura administered the SF-36 to 133 patients undergoing transurethral resection of a bladder tumor (TURBT) and found significant decreases in nearly every general HRQOL domain as compared to population norms [46]. Although non-muscle-invasive bladder cancer is rarely lethal, cystoscopy and TURBT are associated with pain, patient distress and impaired HRQOL. Given the frequent use of endoscopy in bladder cancer patients, finding ways to improve this experience is needed.

Thus, despite the abundance of HRQOL studies in bladder cancer there are many unanswered questions about which type of urinary diversion is superior. Even with high-quality data supporting a particular diversion, higher postoperative HRQOL will always be achieved by extensive preoperative counseling, setting realistic expectations and matching the right patient to the right diversion.

8.9 Conclusion

HRQOL is a vital component when counseling and treating bladder cancer patients, and is also an important comparative-effectiveness research outcome. Although there is no gold-standard method for measuring HRQOL in bladder cancer, the use of reliable, valid and responsive disease-specific instruments is mandatory. Furthermore, HRQOL studies should include input from statisticians or other specialists in study design, and account for known difficulties with HRQOL measurement, such as response shift. Although studies to date have not consistently demonstrated the superiority of any diversion type, with proper patient selection and preoperative counseling, postoperative HRQOL can be comparable between diversions. With ongoing study of HRQOL in bladder cancer, we will continue to improve cancer survivorship and refine patient treatment.

References

1. Greer S. The psychological dimension in cancer treatment. Soc Sci Med. 1984;18(4):345–9. Epub 1984/01/01.
2. Tannock IF. Management of breast and prostate cancer: how does quality of life enter the equation?

Oncology (Williston Park). 1990;4(5):149–56. discussion 71. Epub 1990/05/01.

3. Burns L, Chase D, Goodwin Jr WJ. Treatment of patients with stage IV cancer: do the ends justify the means? Otolaryngol Head Neck Surg. 1987;97(1): 8–14.

4. Izsak FC, Medalie JH. Comprehensive follow-up of carcinoma patients. J Chronic Dis. 1971;24(2):179–91. Epub 1971/07/01.

5. Ware Jr JE. Methodology in behavioral and psychosocial cancer research. Conceptualizing disease impact and treatment outcomes. Cancer. 1984;53(10 Suppl):2316–26. Epub 1984/05/15.

6. Outcomes of cancer treatment for technology assessment and cancer treatment guidelines. American Society of Clinical Oncology. J Clin Oncol. 1996;14(2):671–9. Epub 1996/02/01

7. Lee CT. Quality of life following incontinent cutaneous and orthotopic urinary diversions. Curr Treat Options Oncol. 2009;10(3–4):275–86. Epub 2009/09/19.

8. Shabsigh A, Korets R, Vora KC, Brooks CM, Cronin AM, Savage C, et al. Defining early morbidity of radical cystectomy for patients with bladder cancer using a standardized reporting methodology. Eur Urol. 2009;55(1):164–74. Epub 2008/08/05.

9. Whitmore Jr WF, Marshall VF. Radical total cystectomy for cancer of the bladder: 230 consecutive cases five years later. J Urol. 1962;87:853–68. Epub 1962/06/01.

10. Stein JP, Lieskovsky G, Cote R, Groshen S, Feng AC, Boyd S, et al. Radical cystectomy in the treatment of invasive bladder cancer: long-term results in 1,054 patients. J Clin Oncol. 2001;19(3):666–75. Epub 2001/02/07.

11. CONSTITUTION of the World Health Organization. Chron World Health Organ. 1947;1(1–2):29–43. Epub 1947/01/01.

12. Cella DF, Tulsky DS. Quality of life in cancer: definition, purpose, and method of measurement. Cancer Invest. 1993;11(3):327–36. Epub 1993/01/01.

13. Aaronson NK, Calais da Silva F, Yoshida O, van Dam FS, Fossa SD, Miyakawa M, et al. Quality of life assessment in bladder cancer clinical trials: conceptual, methodological and practical issues. Prog Clin Biol Res. 1986;221:149–70. Epub 1986/01/01.

14. Calman KC. Quality of life in cancer patients—an hypothesis. J Med Ethics. 1984;10(3):124–7. Epub 1984/09/01.

15. Weymuller E, Deleyiannis FW-B, Yueh B. Quality of life in patients with head and neck cancer. In: Meyers E, Suen J, Meyers J, EYN H, editors. Cancer of the head and neck. 4th ed. Philadelphia: Saunders; 2003.

16. Temel JS, Greer JA, Muzikansky A, Gallagher ER, Admane S, Jackson VA, et al. Early palliative care for patients with metastatic non-small-cell lung cancer. N Engl J Med. 2010;363(8):733–42. Epub 2010/09/08.

17. Lule D, Zickler C, Hacker S, Bruno MA, Demertzi A, Pellas F, et al. Life can be worth living in locked-in syndrome. Prog Brain Res. 2009;177:339–51. Epub 2009/10/13.

18. Postulart D, Adang EM. Response shift and adaptation in chronically ill patients. Med Decis Making. 2000;20(2):186–93. Epub 2000/04/20.

19. van der Veen JH, van Andel G, Kurth KH. Quality-of-life assessment in bladder cancer. World J Urol. 1999;17(4):219–24. Epub 1999/08/25.

20. D'Angelica M, Hirsch K, Ross H, Passik S, Brennan MF. Surgeon-patient communication in the treatment of pancreatic cancer. Arch Surg. 1998;133(9):962–6. Epub 1998/09/28.

21. Fallowfield L. The quality of life: the missing measurement in health care. London: Souvenir Press; 1990.

22. Fallowfield LJ, Baum M, Maguire GP. Effects of breast conservation on psychological morbidity associated with diagnosis and treatment of early breast cancer. Br Med J (Clin Res Ed). 1986;293(6558):1331–4. Epub 1986/11/22.

23. Buck D, Jacoby A. Health outcomes and quality of life. In: Dyck P, editor. Peripheral neuropathy. 4th ed. Philadelphia: Elsevier; 2005.

24. Evans B, Montie JE, Gilbert SM. Incontinent or continent urinary diversion: how to make the right choice. Curr Opin Urol. 2010;20(5):421–5. Epub 2010/07/10.

25. Mitchell AJ, Chan M, Bhatti H, Halton M, Grassi L, Johansen C, et al. Prevalence of depression, anxiety, and adjustment disorder in oncological, haematological, and palliative-care settings: a meta-analysis of 94 interview-based studies. Lancet Oncol. 2011;12(2):160–74. Epub 2011/01/22.

26. Werner A, Stenner C, Schuz J. Patient versus clinician symptom reporting: how accurate is the detection of distress in the oncologic after-care? Psychooncology. 2011. Epub 2011/05/06

27. Fobair P, Hoppe RT, Bloom J, Cox R, Varghese A, Spiegel D. Psychosocial problems among survivors of Hodgkin's disease. J Clin Oncol. 1986;4(5):805–14. Epub 1986/05/01.

28. Litwin MS, Hays RD, Fink A, Ganz PA, Leake B, Brook RH. The UCLA Prostate Cancer Index: development, reliability, and validity of a health-related quality of life measure. Med Care. 1998;36(7):1002–12. Epub 1998/07/23.

29. Church J. Outcomes analysis and measurement of quality of life. In: Fazio V, Church J, Delaney C, editors. Current therapy in colon and rectal surgery. 2nd ed. Elsevier Mosby: Philadelphia; 2005.

30. de Graeff A, de Leeuw JR, Ros WJ, Hordijk GJ, Blijham GH, Winnubst JA. Sociodemographic factors and quality of life as prognostic indicators in head and neck cancer. Eur J Cancer. 2001;37(3): 332–9. Epub 2001/03/10.

31. Pompili C, Salati M, Refai M, Berardi R, Onofri A, Mazzanti P, et al. Preoperative quality of life predicts survival following pulmonary resection in stage I non-small-cell lung cancer. Eur J Cardiothorac Surg. 2012;43(5):905–10.

32. Palapattu GS, Bastian PJ, Slavney PR, Haisfield-Wolfe ME, Walker JM, Brintzenhofeszoc K, et al. Preoperative somatic symptoms are associated with disease progression in patients with bladder carcinoma after cystectomy. Cancer. 2004;101(10):2209–13. Epub 2004/10/12.
33. Mansson A, Christensson P, Johnson G, Colleen S. Can preoperative psychological defensive strategies, mood and type of lower urinary tract reconstruction predict psychosocial adjustment after cystectomy in patients with bladder cancer? Br J Urol. 1998;82(3):348–56. Epub 1998/10/17.
34. Burris 3rd HA, Moore MJ, Andersen J, Green MR, Rothenberg ML, Modiano MR, et al. Improvements in survival and clinical benefit with gemcitabine as first-line therapy for patients with advanced pancreas cancer: a randomized trial. J Clin Oncol. 1997;15(6):2403–13. Epub 1997/06/01.
35. Moore MJ, Osoba D, Murphy K, Tannock IF, Armitage A, Findlay B, et al. Use of palliative end points to evaluate the effects of mitoxantrone and low-dose prednisone in patients with hormonally resistant prostate cancer. J Clin Oncol. 1994;12(4):689–94. Epub 1994/04/01.
36. Whalen GF, Ferrans CE. Quality of life as an outcome in clinical trials and cancer care: a primer for surgeons. J Surg Oncol. 2001;77(4):270–6. Epub 2001/07/27.
37. EORTC Quality of Life. Available from: http://groups.eortc.be/qol/. Accessed 21 Apr 2013.
38. Patient-Centered Outcomes Research Institute. Available from: http://www.pcori.org. Accessed 21 Apr 2013.
39. Donabedian A. Evaluating the quality of medical care. Milbank Mem Fund Q. 1966;44(3 Suppl):166–206. Epub 1966/07/01.
40. Sheldon A, Ryser CP, Krant MJ. An integrated family orientated cancer care program: the report of a pilot project in the socio-emotional management of chronic disease. J Chronic Dis. 1970;22(11):743–55. Epub 1970/04/01.
41. Hadorn DC. Setting health care priorities in Oregon. Cost-effectiveness meets the rule of rescue. JAMA. 1991;265(17):2218–25. Epub 1991/05/01.
42. O'Young J, McPeek B. Quality of life variables in surgical trials. J Chronic Dis. 1987;40(6):513–22. Epub 1987/01/01.
43. Abbona A, Morabito F, Rossi R, Billia M, Liberale F, Ferrando U. Quality of life in patients undergone oncopreventive intravesical treatment for superficial bladder cancer. Arch Ital Urol Androl. 2007;79(4):143–6. Epub 2008/02/29.
44. Mack D, Frick J. Quality of life in patients undergoing bacille Calmette-Guerin therapy for superficial bladder cancer. Br J Urol. 1996;78(3):369–71. Epub 1996/09/01.
45. Muezzinoglu T, Ceylan Y, Temeltas G, Lekili M, Buyuksu C. Evaluation of pain caused by urethrocystoscopy in patients with superficial bladder cancer: a perspective of quality of life. Onkologie. 2005;28(5):260–4. Epub 2005/05/04.
46. Yoshimura K, Utsunomiya N, Ichioka K, Matsui Y, Terai A, Arai Y. Impact of superficial bladder cancer and transurethral resection on general health-related quality of life: an SF-36 survey. Urology. 2005;65(2):290–4. Epub 2005/02/15.
47. Gerharz EW, Mansson A, Hunt S, Skinner EC, Mansson W. Quality of life after cystectomy and urinary diversion: an evidence based analysis. J Urol. 2005;174(5):1729–36. Epub 2005/10/12.
48. Hautmann RE, de Petriconi RC, Volkmer BG. 25 years of experience with 1,000 neobladders: long-term complications. J Urol. 2011;185(6):2207–12. Epub 2011/04/19.
49. Hedgepeth RC, Gilbert SM, He C, Lee CT, Wood Jr DP. Body image and bladder cancer specific quality of life in patients with ileal conduit and neobladder urinary diversions. Urology. 2010;76(3):671–5. Epub 2010/05/11.
50. Palapattu GS, Haisfield-Wolfe ME, Walker JM, BrintzenhofeSzoc K, Trock B, Zabora J, et al. Assessment of perioperative psychological distress in patients undergoing radical cystectomy for bladder cancer. J Urol. 2004;172(5 Pt 1):1814–7. Epub 2004/11/16.
51. Shimko MS, Tollefson MK, Umbreit EC, Farmer SA, Blute ML, Frank I. Long-term complications of conduit urinary diversion. J Urol. 2011;185(2):562–7. Epub 2010/12/21.
52. Blanchard CM, Courneya KS, Stein K. Cancer survivors' adherence to lifestyle behavior recommendations and associations with health-related quality of life: results from the American Cancer Society's SCS-II. J Clin Oncol. 2008;26(13):2198–204. Epub 2008/05/01.
53. Karvinen KH, Courneya KS, North S, Venner P. Associations between exercise and quality of life in bladder cancer survivors: a population-based study. Cancer Epidemiol Biomarkers Prev. 2007;16(5):984–90. Epub 2007/05/18.
54. Cody JD, Nabi G, Dublin N, McClinton S, Neal DE, Pickard R, et al. Urinary diversion and bladder reconstruction/replacement using intestinal segments for intractable incontinence or following cystectomy. Cochrane Database Syst Rev. 2012;2, CD003306. Epub 2012/02/18.
55. Porter MP, Penson DF. Health related quality of life after radical cystectomy and urinary diversion for bladder cancer: a systematic review and critical analysis of the literature. J Urol. 2005;173(4):1318–22. Epub 2005/03/11.
56. Wright JL, Porter MP. Quality-of-life assessment in patients with bladder cancer. Nat Clin Pract Urol. 2007;4(3):147–54. Epub 2007/03/10.
57. Allareddy V, Kennedy J, West MM, Konety BR. Quality of life in long-term survivors of bladder cancer. Cancer. 2006;106(11):2355–62. Epub 2006/05/02.
58. Visser MR, Oort FJ, van Lanschot JJ, van der Velden J, Kloek JJ, Gouma DJ, et al. The role of recalibration response shift in explaining bodily pain in cancer patients undergoing invasive surgery: an empirical investigation of the Sprangers and Schwartz model. Psychooncology. 2013;22(3):515–22. Epub 2012/01/17.

59. Brickman P, Coates D, Janoff-Bulman R. Lottery winners and accident victims: is happiness relative? J Pers Soc Psychol. 1978;36(8):917–27. Epub 1978/08/01.

60. McGuire MS, Grimaldi G, Grotas J, Russo P. The type of urinary diversion after radical cystectomy significantly impacts on the patient's quality of life. Ann Surg Oncol. 2000;7(1):4–8. Epub 2000/02/16.

61. Adang EM, Kootstra G, Engel GL, van Hooff JP, Merckelbach HL. Do retrospective and prospective quality of life assessments differ for pancreas-kidney transplant recipients? Transpl Int. 1998;11(1):11–5. Epub 1998/03/21.

62. Adang EM, Kootstra G, Baeten CG, Engel GL. Quality-of-life ratings in patients with chronic illnesses. JAMA. 1997;277(13):1038. Epub 1997/04/02.

63. Aaronson NK. Quality of life assessment in clinical trials: methodologic issues. Control Clin Trials. 1989;10(4 Suppl):195S–208. Epub 1989/12/01.

64. Karnofsky DA, Burchenal J. The clinical evaluation of chemotheraputic agents in cancer. In: MacLeod C, editor. Evaluation of chemotheraputic agents. New York: Colombia University Press; 1949. p. 196.

65. Hutchinson TA, Boyd NF, Feinstein AR, Gonda A, Hollomby D, Rowat B. Scientific problems in clinical scales, as demonstrated in the Karnofsky index of performance status. J Chronic Dis. 1979;32(9–10):661–6. Epub 1979/01/01.

66. Schag CC, Heinrich RL, Ganz PA. Karnofsky performance status revisited: reliability, validity, and guidelines. J Clin Oncol. 1984;2(3):187–93. Epub 1984/03/01.

67. Slevin ML, Plant H, Lynch D, Drinkwater J, Gregory WM. Who should measure quality of life, the doctor or the patient? Br J Cancer. 1988;57(1):109–12. Epub 1988/01/01.

68. Dinglas VD, Gifford JM, Husain N, Colantuoni E, Needham DM. Quality of life before intensive care using EQ-5D: patient versus proxy responses. Crit Care Med. 2013;41(1):9–14. Epub 2012/12/13.

69. Vickery CW, Blazeby JM, Conroy T, Arraras J, Sezer O, Koller M, et al. Development of an EORTC disease-specific quality of life module for use in patients with gastric cancer. Eur J Cancer. 2001;37(8):966–71. Epub 2001/05/04.

70. Paasche-Orlow MK, Taylor HA, Brancati FL. Readability standards for informed-consent forms as compared with actual readability. N Engl J Med. 2003;348(8):721–6. Epub 2003/02/21.

71. Terwee CB, Bot SD, de Boer MR, van der Windt DA, Knol DL, Dekker J, et al. Quality criteria were proposed for measurement properties of health status questionnaires. J Clin Epidemiol. 2007;60(1):34–42. Epub 2006/12/13.

72. Gill TM, Feinstein AR. A critical appraisal of the quality of quality-of-life measurements. JAMA. 1994;272(8):619–26. Epub 1994/08/24.

73. Parkinson JP, Konety BR. Health related quality of life assessments for patients with bladder cancer. J Urol. 2004;172(6 Pt 1):2130–6. Epub 2004/11/13.

74. Norman GR, Sloan JA, Wyrwich KW. Interpretation of changes in health-related quality of life: the remarkable universality of half a standard deviation. Med Care. 2003;41(5):582–92. Epub 2003/04/30.

75. Kulaksizoglu H, Toktas G, Kulaksizoglu IB, Aglamis E, Unluer E. When should quality of life be measured after radical cystectomy? Eur Urol. 2002;42(4):350–5. Epub 2002/10/04.

76. Guyatt GH, Naylor CD, Juniper E, Heyland DK, Jaeschke R, Cook DJ. Users' guides to the medical literature. XII. How to use articles about health-related quality of life. Evidence-Based Medicine Working Group. JAMA. 1997;277(15):1232–7. Epub 1997/04/16.

77. Bergner M, Bobbitt RA, Carter WB, Gilson BS. The Sickness Impact Profile: development and final revision of a health status measure. Med Care. 1981;19(8):787–805. Epub 1981/08/01.

78. Hunt SM, McEwen J, McKenna SP. Measuring health status: a new tool for clinicians and epidemiologists. J R Coll Gen Pract. 1985;35(273):185–8. Epub 1985/04/01.

79. Ware Jr JE, Sherbourne CD. The MOS 36-item short-form health survey (SF-36). I. Conceptual framework and item selection. Med Care. 1992;30(6):473–83. Epub 1992/06/11.

80. Dutta SC, Chang SC, Coffey CS, Smith Jr JA, Jack G, Cookson MS. Health related quality of life assessment after radical cystectomy: comparison of ileal conduit with continent orthotopic neobladder. J Urol. 2002;168(1):164–7. Epub 2002/06/07.

81. Harano M, Eto M, Nakamura M, Hasegawa Y, Kano M, Yamaguchi A, et al. A pilot study of the assessment of the quality of life, functional results, and complications in patients with an ileal neobladder for invasive bladder cancer. Int J Urol. 2007;14(2):112–7. Epub 2007/02/17.

82. Hara I, Miyake H, Hara S, Gotoh A, Nakamura I, Okada H, et al. Health-related quality of life after radical cystectomy for bladder cancer: a comparison of ileal conduit and orthotopic bladder replacement. BJU Int. 2002;89(1):10–3. Epub 2002/02/19.

83. Autorino R, Quarto G, Di Lorenzo G, De Sio M, Perdona S, Giannarini G, et al. Health related quality of life after radical cystectomy: comparison of ileal conduit to continent orthotopic neobladder. Eur J Surg Oncol. 2009;35(8):858–64. Epub 2008/10/01.

84. Quality Metric. Available from: http://www.qualitymetric.com/WhatWeDo/SFHealthSurveys/tabid/184/Default.aspx. Accessed 21 Apr 2013.

85. Cella DF, Tulsky DS, Gray G, Sarafian B, Linn E, Bonomi A, et al. The Functional Assessment of Cancer Therapy scale: development and validation of the general measure. J Clin Oncol. 1993;11(3):570–9. Epub 1993/03/01.

86. Kikuchi E, Horiguchi Y, Nakashima J, Ohigashi T, Oya M, Nakagawa K, et al. Assessment of long-term quality of life using the FACT-BL questionnaire in patients with an ileal conduit, continent reservoir, or

orthotopic neobladder. Jpn J Clin Oncol. 2006; 36(11):712–6. Epub 2006/10/05.

87. Mansson A, Al Amin M, Malmstrom PU, Wijkstrom H, Abol Enein H, Mansson W. Patient-assessed outcomes in Swedish and Egyptian men undergoing radical cystectomy and orthotopic bladder substitution—a prospective comparative study. Urology. 2007;70(6):1086–90. Epub 2007/12/26.

88. Aaronson NK, Ahmedzai S, Bergman B, Bullinger M, Cull A, Duez NJ, et al. The European Organization for Research and Treatment of Cancer QLQ-C30: a quality-of-life instrument for use in international clinical trials in oncology. J Natl Cancer Inst. 1993;85(5):365–76. Epub 1993/03/03.

89. Sogni F, Brausi M, Frea B, Martinengo C, Faggiano F, Tizzani A, et al. Morbidity and quality of life in elderly patients receiving ileal conduit or orthotopic neobladder after radical cystectomy for invasive bladder cancer. Urology. 2008;71(5):919–23. Epub 2008/03/22.

90. Hobisch A, Tosun K, Kinzl J, Kemmler G, Bartsch G, Holtl L, et al. Quality of life after cystectomy and orthotopic neobladder versus ileal conduit urinary diversion. World J Urol. 2000;18(5):338–44. Epub 2000/12/29.

91. Anderson CB, Feurer ID, Large MC, Steinberg GD, Barocas DA, Cookson MS, et al. Psychometric characteristics of a condition-specific, health-related quality-of-life survey: the FACT-Vanderbilt Cystectomy Index. Urology. 2012;80(1):77–83. Epub 2012/05/23.

92. Gilbert SM, Dunn RL, Hollenbeck BK, Montie JE, Lee CT, Wood DP, et al. Development and validation of the Bladder Cancer Index: a comprehensive, disease specific measure of health related quality of life in patients with localized bladder cancer. J Urol. 2010;183(5):1764–9. Epub 2010/03/20.

93. Bjerre BD, Johansen C, Steven K. Health-related quality of life after cystectomy: bladder substitution compared with ileal conduit diversion. A questionnaire survey. Br J Urol. 1995;75(2):200–5. Epub 1995/02/01.

94. Protogerou V, Moschou M, Antoniou N, Varkarakis J, Bamias A, Deliveliotis C. Modified S-pouch neobladder vs ileal conduit and a matched control population: a quality-of-life survey. BJU Int. 2004;94(3):350–4. Epub 2004/08/05.

95. Somani BK, Gimlin D, Fayers P, N'Dow J. Quality of life and body image for bladder cancer patients undergoing radical cystectomy and urinary diversion—a prospective cohort study with a systematic review of literature. Urology. 2009;74(5):1138–43. Epub 2009/09/24.

96. Cookson MS, Dutta SC, Chang SS, Clark T, Smith Jr JA, Wells N. Health related quality of life in patients treated with radical cystectomy and urinary diversion for urothelial carcinoma of the bladder: development and validation of a new disease specific questionnaire. J Urol. 2003;170(5):1926–30. Epub 2003/10/09.

97. Large MC, Katz MH, Shikanov S, Eggener SE, Steinberg GD. Orthotopic neobladder versus Indiana pouch in women: a comparison of health related quality of life outcomes. J Urol. 2010;183(1):201–6. Epub 2009/11/17.

98. Vakalopoulos I, Dimitriadis G, Anastasiadis A, Gkotsos G, Radopoulos D. Does intubated uretero-ureterocutaneostomy provide better health-related quality of life than orthotopic neobladder in patients after radical cystectomy for invasive bladder cancer? Int Urol Nephrol. 2011;43(3):743–8. Epub 2011/02/22.

99. Parekh DJ, Messer J, Fitzgerald J, Ercole B, Svatek R. Perioperative outcomes and oncologic efficacy from a pilot prospective randomized clinical trial of open versus robotic assisted radical cystectomy. J Urol. 2013;189(2):474–9. Epub 2012/09/29.

100. Gilbert SM, Wood DP, Dunn RL, Weizer AZ, Lee CT, Montie JE, et al. Measuring health-related quality of life outcomes in bladder cancer patients using the Bladder Cancer Index (BCI). Cancer. 2007;109(9):1756–62. Epub 2007/03/17.

101. FACT-BL. Available from: http://www.facit.org/FACITOrg/Questionnaires. Accessed 10 Mar 2013.

102. Mansson A, Davidsson T, Hunt S, Mansson W. The quality of life in men after radical cystectomy with a continent cutaneous diversion or orthotopic bladder substitution: is there a difference? BJU Int. 2002;90(4):386–90. Epub 2002/08/15.

103. Yuh B, Butt Z, Fazili A, Piacente P, Tan W, Wilding G, et al. Short-term quality-of-life assessed after robot-assisted radical cystectomy: a prospective analysis. BJU Int. 2009;103(6):800–4. Epub 2008/11/22.

104. Pavone-Macaluso M, Corselli G, Ingargiola GB, Serretta V. The Urologic Cooperative Group of the EORTC. Structure, scope, research, results. Arch Ital Urol Androl. 1997;69(4):209–15. Epub 1998/01/07. Il gruppo cooperativo urologico dell'EORTC. Struttura, scopi, ricerche, risultati.

105. EORTC QLQ-BLM-30. Available from: http://groups.eortc.be/qol/bladder-cancer-eortc-qlq-bls24-eortc-qlq-blm30. Accessed 10 Mar 2013.

106. EORTC QLQ-BLS-24. Available from: http://groups.eortc.be/qol/bladder-cancer-eortc-qlq-bls24-eortc-qlq-blm30. Accessed 10 Mar 2013.

107. Kaplan RM. Quality of life assessment for cost/utility studies in cancer. Cancer Treat Rev. 1993;19 Suppl A:85–96. Epub 1993/01/01.

108. Brooks R. EuroQol: the current state of play. Health Policy. 1996;37(1):53–72. Epub 1996/06/06.

109. Brazier J, Roberts J, Deverill M. The estimation of a preference-based measure of health from the SF-36. J Health Econ. 2002;21(2):271–92. Epub 2002/04/10.

110. Furlong WJ, Feeny DH, Torrance GW, Barr RD. The Health Utilities Index (HUI) system for assessing health-related quality of life in clinical studies. Ann Med. 2001;33(5):375–84. Epub 2001/08/09.

111. Andresen EM, Rothenberg BM, Kaplan RM. Performance of a self-administered mailed version

of the Quality of Well-Being (QWB-SA) questionnaire among older adults. Med Care. 1998;36(9):1349–60. Epub 1998/09/28.

112. Somani B, MacLennan S, N'Dow J. Quality of life with urinary diversion. Eur Urol Suppl. 2010;9(10):763–71.

113. Hautmann RE, Abol-Enein H, Hafez K, Haro I, Mansson W, Mills RD, et al. Urinary diversion. Urology. 2007;69(1 Suppl):17–49. Epub 2007/02/07.

114. Hardt J, Filipas D, Hohenfellner R, Egle UT. Quality of life in patients with bladder carcinoma after cystectomy: first results of a prospective study. Qual Life Res. 2000;9(1):1–12. Epub 2000/09/12.

115. Anderson CB, Cookson MS, Chang SS, Clark PE, Smith Jr JA, Kaufman MR. Voiding function in women with orthotopic neobladder urinary diversion. J Urol. 2012;188(1):200–4. Epub 2012/05/18.

116. Ahmadi H, Skinner EC, Simma-Chiang V, Miranda G, Cai J, Penson DF, et al. Urinary functional outcome following radical cystoprostatectomy and ileal neobladder reconstruction in male patients. J Urol. 2013;189(5):1782–8. Epub 2012/11/20.

117. Zippe CD, Raina R, Shah AD, Massanyi EZ, Agarwal A, Ulchaker J, et al. Female sexual dysfunction after radical cystectomy: a new outcome measure. Urology. 2004;63(6):1153–7. Epub 2004/06/09.

118. Zippe CD, Raina R, Massanyi EZ, Agarwal A, Jones JS, Ulchaker J, et al. Sexual function after male radical cystectomy in a sexually active population. Urology. 2004;64(4):682–5. discussion 5–6. Epub 2004/10/20.

119. Orvieto MA, DeCastro GJ, Trinh QD, Jeldres C, Katz MH, Patel VR, et al. Oncological and functional outcomes after robot-assisted radical cystectomy: critical review of current status. Urology. 2011;78(5):977–84. Epub 2011/09/06.

120. Stegemann A, Rehman S, Brewer K, Kesavadas T, Hussain A, Chandrasekhar R, et al. Short-term patient-reported quality of life after robot-assisted radical cystectomy using the Convalescence and Recovery Evaluation. Urology. 2012;79(6):1274–9. Epub 2012/04/24.

121. Tallman C, Aboumohamed A, Weizer AZ, Dailey S, Khan A, Din R, et al. Health related quality of life outcomes after robotic-assisted and open radical cystectomy: a Multi-Institutional Study. American Urological Association Annual Meeting 2013, Abstract #1625.

Luis A. Kluth, Bernard H. Bochner,
and Shahrokh F. Shariat

9.1 Introduction

9.1.1 Prognostic Factors

Prognostication and risk assessment are essential for treatment decision-making, patient counseling, and determination of eligibility for clinical trials.

L.A. Kluth, M.D.
Department of Urology, New York Presbyterian
Hospital, Weill Cornell Medical College,
525 East 68th Street, Starr 900, New York,
NY 10065, USA

Department of Urology, University Medical-Center
Hamburg-Eppendorf, Martinistr. 52, 20246
Hamburg, Germany
e-mail: L.Kluth@uke.de

B.H. Bochner, M.D., F.A.C.S.
Department of Urology, Memorial Sloan-Kettering
Cancer Center, Kimmel Center for Prostate and
Urologic Tumors, 353 E. 68th Street, New York,
NY 10065, USA
e-mail: bochnerb@mskcc.org

S.F. Shariat, M.D. (✉)
Department of Urology, New York Presbyterian
Hospital, Weill Cornell Medical College,
525 East 68th Street, Starr 900, New York,
NY 10065, USA

Division of Medical Oncology, New York
Presbyterian Hospital, Weill Cornell Medical
College, New York, NY, USA

Department of Urology, Medical University of
Vienna, Währinger Gürtel 18-20,
1090 Vienna, Austria
e-mail: sfshariat@gmail.com

More than most other malignancies, urothelial carcinoma of the bladder cancer (UCB) is a highly aggressive and heterogeneous disease with high prevalence and recurrence rates. In patients with non-muscle invasive bladder cancer (NMIBC), predictors of outcomes could help in the decision-making regarding follow-up scheduling, administration of intravesical instillation therapies (immediate postoperative instillation of chemotherapy (IPOP) and/or adjuvant) [1], and/or early radical cystectomy (RC). In patients with muscle-invasive bladder cancer (MIBC) who underwent RC, an accurate prediction of the presence of lymph node metastasis and the probability of disease recurrence is essential for selecting patients who might benefit from neoadjuvant and/or adjuvant systemic chemotherapy [2].

Anatomical staging systems present the simplest examples of a prediction tool by categorizing the disease based on stage-adjusted outcome. The American Joint Committee on Cancer TNM staging system has been validated and used universally to predict the risk of disease recurrence in patients after RC [3]. These staging systems provide useful estimates of survival outcome; however, the inherent heterogeneity of tumor biology, patient characteristics, and variability in the thoroughness of surgical staging lead to significant variation in outcomes within each stage category. Furthermore, current staging systems for UCB do not incorporate important clinical, pathological, and molecular markers of disease outcome. That said, many patients with UCB are

B.R. Konety and S.S. Chang (eds.), *Management of Bladder Cancer:
A Comprehensive Text With Clinical Scenarios*, DOI 10.1007/978-1-4939-1881-2_9,
© Springer Science+Business Media New York 2015

elderly and have significant comorbidities, thus competing risks are important in evaluating outcomes and choosing personalized therapies.

9.1.2 Prediction Tools

Recent significant advances have been made in the development of predictive tools including risk stratifications, nomograms, and staging scores, that provide useful risk estimates for patients with UCB [4–8]. Among the available prediction tools, nomograms currently represent the most accurate and widely used tools for prediction of outcomes in patients with cancer [6, 9, 10].

Accuracy represents an important consideration of a prognostic model and should ideally be validated in an external cohort. However, internal validation is a commonly used alternative; the bootstrapping-derived accuracy estimates represent the closest to external validity-derived estimates [11, 12]. That is, no model is perfect and generally accepted accuracy for a model to be clinically useful ranges from 70 to 80 %. While a nomogram may contribute to a better distribution between study arms, a higher accuracy will be achieved when using it for risk stratification within a clinical protocol or to interpret treatment outcomes based on a more accurate description of the patient population under study. It is therefore crucial to assess the performance characteristics of a predictive model, which is also called calibration. Calibration plots demonstrate the relationship between predicted and observed probabilities of the outcome of interest. For clinicians, it is essential to know the performance characteristics of the model they routinely use in clinical practice as some predictive models may perform substantially worse in an external cohort.

The general applicability of a predictive model is important because patient and model characteristics may vary and thereby undermine the performance of the model. The ability to generalize a prediction model may be limited by differences in disease and population characteristics, as well as stage and/or grade migration. For example, a model that has been developed on patients in the pre-PSA era may not be relevant to patients in the post-PSA era due to the biomarker itself, but also due to possible shifts in stage based on changes in care pathways. Thus it is critical to understand the population from which a risk model was developed, as this should then be applied to similar populations for use.

For clinicians the level of complexity represents an important consideration of prediction tools, as excessively complex models are clearly not user-friendly in busy clinical practice. Predictive models that require computational infrastructure might cause problems for general applicability in certain environments [6, 10, 13].

In this chapter, we aimed to give an overview of the prognostic factors and currently available prediction tools associated with UCB recurrence, progression, and mortality. We stratified the chapter by disease states: NMIBC, MIBC, and metastatic UCB. We present the prediction tools by recording predictor variables, the number of patients used for their development, tool-specific features, predictive accuracy estimates, and whether internal and/or external validation has been performed.

9.2 Non-muscle Invasive Bladder Cancer

9.2.1 Prognostic Factors

9.2.1.1 Clinical Factors

9.2.1.1.1 Age
Age at diagnosis has been shown to be associated with disease recurrence, disease progression [14, 15], cancer-specific mortality [15], and response to Bacille Calmette-Guérin (BCG) (Table 9.1) [16–20]. These worse outcomes in elderly patients could be attributed to changes in the biologic potential of the tumor and host as well as to differences in quality of care (i.e., greater reluctance to recommend aggressive treatment in the elderly) [19, 21].

9.2.1.1.2 Race
In a study using the SEER data, 5-year cancer-specific survival was consistently worse in Afro-Americans than in other ethnic groups, even after adjusting for the effect of tumor stage and grade [22]. Moreover, these worse outcomes were persistent over time (1975–2005). To better

Table 9.1 Summary of the preoperative/clinical and pathologic prognostic factors in patients with non-muscle invasive bladder cancer

	Comments	References
Age	Advanced age is an independent predictor of DR, DP, and CSM	[14–21]
Race	Afro-Americans are at higher risk of CSM compared to other racial groups	[22]
Gender	Female gender is an independent predictor of worse DR, DP, and CSM	[14, 23–26]
Obesity	Body mass index ≥ 30 kg/m^2 is an independent predictor of DR, DP, and CSM	[15]
Smoking	Smokers are more likely to be diagnosed with UCB and at higher risk of DR, DP, and CSM	[27–31]
Prior recurrence	Recurrent tumors are at higher risk of DP	[25, 32–35]
Tumor size	Larger tumor size is an independent predictor of DR and DP	[25, 36, 37]
Multifocality	Multifocality is an independent predictor of DR	[25, 36, 37]
Pathologic tumor stage	Advanced pathologic T-stage is an independent predictor of DR, DP, and CSM. The depth of invasion of the muscularis mucosae is also associated with worse outcomes (DR, DP, and CSM)	[14, 25, 37, 39–41]
Pathologic tumor grade	Higher tumor grade (Grade 3 or high grade) is an independent predictor of worse outcomes (DR, DP, and CSM) (both the 1973 and the 2004 World Health Organization classifications)	[38, 42–48]
Concomitant carcinoma in situ	Concomitant carcinoma in situ is associated with advanced tumor stage and grade and is an independent predictor of worse outcomes (DR and DP)	[26, 37, 49, 50]
Lymphovascular invasion	The presence of lymphovascular invasion is an independent predictor of worse outcomes (DP and CSM)	[48, 51–55]
Histologic variants	The presence of a micropapillary variant is an independent predictor of understaging and occurrence of distant metastasis	[56–58]
Delay of cystectomy	Delay of RC >3 months after initial diagnosis is associated with extravesical or node-positive disease, and worse oncologic outcome. Controversial findings	[59–62]

DR disease recurrence, *DP* disease progression, *CSM* cancer-specific mortality

understand these race disparities, as well as the disparities in socioeconomic status and their effect on outcomes of NMIBC, further studies on access to care, quality of care, exposure history, molecular characteristics, and treatment strategies are needed.

9.2.1.1.3 Gender

UCB is more common in men than in women. Data supporting a worse outcome in female patients have been inconsistent. Some studies have demonstrated that female gender is associated with worse oncologic outcomes compared to male gender in NMIBC [14, 23, 24]. However, Sylvester et al. did not find any prognostic value to gender in seven randomized EORTC trials with a total of 2,596 patients with Ta or T1 NMIBC who received different regimens of intravesical therapy after TURB [25]. In a recent retrospective study of 146 patients with primary T1HG UCB [26], female gender was associated with higher risk of disease recurrence in univariable analysis, and disease progression and any-cause mortality in multivariable analyses. In a large multi-institutional cohort of 916 T1HG UCB patients, female gender was an independent predictor of disease recurrence [24]. Additional studies are needed to clarify the gender risk for NMIBC.

9.2.1.1.4 Obesity

In NMIBC, Kluth et al. reported recently that obese patients diagnosed with clinical T1HG were at higher risk of disease recurrence, disease progression, and cancer-specific mortality compared to their non-obese counterparts [15]. In this study, patients with a body mass index ≥ 30 kg/m^2

were considered as obese. The authors hypothesized that this could be due to change in the underlying biologic potential of the tumor, the host's defense mechanisms, differences in the transurethral resection and intravesical therapy efficacy, comorbidities, as well as possibly socioeconomic factors. Further work is needed to improve our understanding of UCB outcomes in this growing population and to modify its impact on outcomes.

9.2.1.1.5　Smoking

Smoking exposure is the best-established causative agent for UCB [27]. Recently, smoking status (current vs. never) and cumulative exposure have been associated with disease recurrence [28], disease progression and response to BCG, both in primary [29, 30] and recurrent NMIBC [30, 31]. Interestingly, it has been shown that smoking cessation >10 years prior to disease might mitigate this detrimental effect suggesting a potential benefit of smoking cessation on prognosis of NMIBC [30, 31]. These data suggest that smoking cessation could help improve outcomes in patients with NMIBC.

9.2.1.2　Pathologic Factors
9.2.1.2.1　Prior Recurrence

The impact of prior recurrences on outcomes of patients with NMIBC has been assessed by several studies [25]. The CUETO group, in a prospective randomized study comparing the standard 81 mg dose of BCG with 27 mg, reported that prior UCB was a significant factor affecting disease progression in multivariable analysis [32]. In a study comparing primary and recurrent tumors, Alkhateeb et al. have shown that recurrent tumors were at higher risk of disease progression [33]. These findings were confirmed and extended by the association of high-risk patients with cancer-specific mortality [34]. Notably, failure to achieve a complete response to induction BCG therapy resulting in disease recurrence has been shown to be associated with worse cancer-specific mortality [35].

9.2.1.2.2　Tumor Size and Multifocality

Tumor size has been shown to be associated with disease recurrence and progression, with the most commonly used cut-off being 3 cm [25, 36, 37]. Multifocality represents a more controversial prognostic factor, which correlates with disease recurrence rather than disease progression [37].

9.2.1.2.3　Tumor Stage

The pathologic stage from TUR specimen has been correlated with outcomes [38]. T1 tumors have higher rates of disease recurrence, disease progression, and cancer-specific mortality compared to Ta tumors [14, 25, 37]. Furthermore, several studies have reported on the prognostic interest of substaging according to invasion in T1 tumors above (T1a), in (T1b), or beyond the muscularis mucosae (T1c) [39, 40]. However, this T1 substage has not been adopted in clinical guidelines due to the lack of consensus among pathologists regarding the identification of the muscularis mucosae and independent prognostic value. Therefore, a new reproducible substaging system in order to discern T1-microinvasive (T1m) and T1-extensive-invasive (T1e) tumors has been proposed and is currently being validated [41].

9.2.1.2.4　Tumor Grade

Historically, the initial grading system of 1973 had a high interobserver variation due to the lack of clear definitions for the three pathologic grades and on increasingly high percentage of tumors classified as grade 2 [38, 42–44]. A new classification was adopted by the World Health Organization and the International Society of Urological Pathology (ISUP) in 1998, and published in 2004. This new grading system introduced detailed histologic criteria to decrease the interobserver variability. Finally, the intermediate grade (grade 2), which was the subject of controversies has been eliminated [38, 42–44]. To date, though the prognostic value of both grading systems has been validated, the published comparisons of these two grading systems, however, have not clearly confirmed that the new one is superior in terms of reproducibility [38, 45, 46]. It has been shown that patients with grade 3 and high-grade tumors are at highest risk of disease recurrence and progression; that said, grade 3 seems to have worse outcomes than high-grade tumors due to the heterogeneity in the subgroup of high-grade tumors [38, 44, 47]. The EAU guidelines recommend using both grading systems as long as the prognostic role of the WHO 2004 is not validated in prospective trials [48].

9.2.1.2.5 Concomitant Carcinoma In Situ

Concomitant carcinoma in situ (CIS) is a validated prognostic factor for both disease recurrence and disease progression in NMIBC [37, 49]. In 2000, the SWOG has shown that CIS generally responds favorably to BCG [50]. Palou et al. have recently evaluated the incidence of CIS in the prostatic urethra (routinely evaluated by biopsy) in 146 patients with primary T1G3 NMIBC treated with BCG [26]. The authors reported an incidence of 10 % in the prostatic urethra, which was associated with both disease recurrence and progression. These findings suggest that prostatic urethra involvement should be evaluated routinely in all patients suspected of having high-grade tumor or in case of presence of CIS in the bladder.

9.2.1.2.6 Lymphovascular Invasion

Several studies have shown that the presence of lymphovascular invasion (LVI), defined as the presence of carcinoma in the endothelial lining or in the vascular wall, predicts disease progression and cancer-specific mortality [51–54]. The major drawback is the reproducibility among pathologists [55]. However, the EAU guidelines recommend that the presence (or not) of LVI must be reported in pathologic reports [48].

9.2.1.2.7 Histologic Variants

Histologic variants such as micropapillary variant of UCB represent a poor prognostic factor in patients with NMIBC [56–58]. From a pathologic point of view, it remains critical to differentiate whether micropapillary urothelial carcinoma is invasive or non-invasive [57]. While some cases of non-invasive micropapillary UC are not necessarily associated with an adverse outcome, invasive micropapillary UC is an aggressive disease, thereby suggesting it to be an important risk of understaging and occurrence of distant metastasis in these patients [56–58]. In addition, Kamat et al. reported intravesical BCG therapy to be

ineffective against micropapillary UC, thus suggesting RC as the optimal treatment strategy for non-muscle invasive micropapillary UC before disease progression [56].

Other sections to consider would be prior response to therapy: progression is exceedingly high in those that recur/do not respond to BCG. Also we could include the data on pathology of the restaging TURBT and outcome. Particular in T1 patients those without invasive changes on the second TUR are more likely to respond to BCG whereas residual T1 on the restaging predicts strongly for progression despite BCG.

9.2.1.3 Surgical Factors
9.2.1.3.1 Delay of Radical Cystectomy

Recently, in several studies the time from diagnosis to treatment has been evaluated and shown that patients who were treated with RC later than 3 months after initial diagnosis were of increased risk of extravesical stage, node-positive disease and worse outcomes compared to those treated within 3 months [59, 60]. However, another recent study could not confirm these findings [61]. Interestingly, the time to RC does not only affect outcomes but also the type of urinary diversion [62], thereby reflecting general health status.

9.2.2 Predictive Tools

9.2.2.1 Prediction of Disease Recurrence and Progression in NMIBC

In the study of 1,529 patients with NMIBC, Millan-Rodriguez et al. assessed predictors of disease recurrence, progression, and mortality and developed a different risk groups based on multifocality, tumor size, intravesical BCG therapy, and presence of concomitant CIS [63]. Tumor grade was the most powerful predictor of disease progression and disease-specific mortality.

In 2006, the European Organization for Research and Treatment of Cancer (EORTC) Genitourinary (GU) group developed a scoring system and risk tables [25], based on data from 2,596 patients diagnosed with Ta/T1 tumors, who were randomized in seven previous EORTC-GU group trials. The scoring system was built on the six most relevant clinical and pathologic predictors of outcomes such as tumor stage and grade, number of tumors, tumor size, concomitant CIS, and prior recurrence rate (Table 9.2). However, the study was limited by the low number of patients treated with BCG, the high rate of IPOP, and the fact that no Re-TUR was performed.

Therefore, the Club Urológico Español de Tratamiento Oncológico (CUETO) developed a scoring model, which predicts the short- and long-term probability of disease recurrence and progression in 1,062 patients with NMIBC from four CUETO trials that compared the efficacy of different intravesical BCG treatments [14]. These patients received 12 instillations during 5–6 months; however, neither immediate postoperative instillation nor re-TUR was performed. The scoring system was based on seven factors including age, gender, prior recurrence status, number of tumors, tumor stage, tumor grade, and the presence of concomitant CIS.

Though many clinicians are using these scoring systems in daily practice, to date, only few studies have externally validated both these models [64–66]. Furthermore, these validation studies have reported an overestimation of both the risks of disease recurrence and progression, especially in the high-risk group of patients [64–66]. One possible explanation is the high rate of intravesical chemotherapy in the EORTC trials.

Xylinas et al. recently evaluated the discrimination of the EORTC risk tables and the CUETO scoring model in a large retrospective multicenter study of 4,689 NMIBC patients [66]. Therefore, the authors created Cox regression models for time to disease recurrence and progression, thus incorporated the patients' calculated risk score as a predictor into both of these models and then calculated their discrimination. The EORTC risk tables and the CUETO scoring system exhibited a poor discrimination and overestimated the risk for both disease recurrence and progression in NMIBC patients.

The first nomogram in UCB was published in 2005 and estimated the risk of disease recurrence and progression based on a multi-institutional cohort of 2,681 patients with Ta, T1, or Tis UCB [67]. All patients had previous histologically confirmed NMIBC and provided voided urine samples for cytologic and NMP22 analyses before undergoing cystoscopy. In case of suspicious cystoscopy or cytology, patients were further investigated with transurethral biopsies. Overall, 898 patients had a recurrent UCB: 24 % had grade 1, 43 % grade 2, and 33 % grade 3 tumors; 45 % had Ta, 32 % T1 or CIS, and 23 % T2 tumors. In uni- and multivariable analyses, age, urine cytology status, and urinary NMP22 level were associated with outcomes ($p<0.001$). The predictive accuracy of a model based on patient age, gender, and urine cytology significantly increased for all three endpoints when NMP22 level was included as a variable.

Whereas the nomogram from Shariat et al. takes into account age, gender, pre-cystoscopy cytology, and NMP22 to predict recurrence and progression during the follow up of patients with a previous history of NMIBC [67], the EORTC [25] and CUETO [14] tables predict a patient's future short- and long-term probabilities of recurrence and progression at the time of the initial diagnosis or at the time of a recurrence based on the clinical and pathologic characteristics. Thus, these two prediction tools serve different and complimentary purposes.

9.2.2.2 Preoperative Prediction of Pathologic Features and Outcomes at Radical Cystectomy

In the pre-cystectomy setting, the clinical staging is often inaccurate; however, remains a major determinant of treatment decision-making [68]. Accurate preoperative risk-assessment models could help to predict (1) non-organ-confined disease, thus enabling a better selection of patients who may benefit from neoadjuvant chemotherapy; (2) which T1HG patients should undergo early RC; and (3) prediction of lymph node metastasis and thereby provide guidance for the indication and extent of lymph node dissection.

Karakiewicz et al. developed a preoperative nomogram which can predict advanced pathologic stage (pT3–4) and presence of lymph node metastasis based on a multicenter cohort of 731 patients with available clinical and pathologic staging data [69]. When patient age, clinical tumor stage and grade, and presence of carcinoma in situ were integrated within the nomogram, a 76 % accuracy

Table 9.2 Available predictive models in bladder cancer before radical cystectomy

Pre-cystectomy tools

Reference	Prediction form	Patient population	Outcome	No. of pts.	Variables	Accuracy	Validation
Qureshi et al. [193]	Artificial neural network	Ta T1	Recurrence-free survival (RFS) within 6 months	56	EGFR, c-erbB2, p53, tumor stage, tumor grade, tumor size, number of tumors, gender, smoking status, histology of mucosal biopsies, carcinoma in situ (CIS), metaplasia, architecture, tumor location	75 % (RFS)	Internal
		Ta T1	Progression-free survival (PFS) within 1 year	105		80 % (PFS)	
		T2–T4	Cancer-specific free survival (CSS)	56		82 % (CSS)	
Catto et al. [192]	Neuro-fuzzy modeling	Ta-T4	RFS	109	P53, mismatch repair proteins, tumor stage, tumor grade, age, smoking, previous cancer	88–95 %	Internal
Millan-Rodriguez et al. [63]	Risk stratification	NMIBC	RFS, PFS, and CCS	1,529	Number of tumors, tumor size, tumor stage, tumor grade, CIS, intravesical Bacillus Calmette-Guerrin (BCG)	Not reported	Not performed
Sylvester et al. [25]	Look-up table	NMIBC	RFS and PFS	2,596	Number of tumors, tumor size, prior recurrence rate, tumor stage, tumor grade, concomitant CIS	Not reported	Internal and external
Fernandez-Gomez [14]	Look-up table	NMIBC	RFS and PFS	1,062	Age, gender, tumor stage, tumor grade, prior recurrence rate, multiplicity and concomitant CIS	CCI: 0.69	Internal
Shariat et al. [67]	Probability nomogram	NMIBC	RFS and PFS	2,681	Age, gender, urine cytology, dichotomized NMP22 level (and institution)	84 % for RFS of any UCB 87 % for RFS of high-grade UCB or T1 and higher stage 86 % for RFS of stage ≥ T2 UCB	Internal
Karakiewicz et al. [69]	Probability nomogram	NMIBC and MIBC	Cystectomy T and N stage	731	Age, TUR stage, TUR grade, CIS	76 % T stage 63 % N stage	Internal
Green et al. [55]	Probability nomogram	NMIBC and MIBC	Non-organ-confined disease at radical cystectomy (pT3/Nany or pTany/N+)	201	Tumor stage, presence of LVI, radiographic evidence of non-organ-confined UCB or hydronephrosis	83 %	Internal
Shariat et al. [70]	Nodal Staging Score	NMIBC and MIBC	Lymph node metastasis at radical cystectomy	4,335	Tumor stage, number of lymph nodes removed, number of positive lymph nodes		Internal

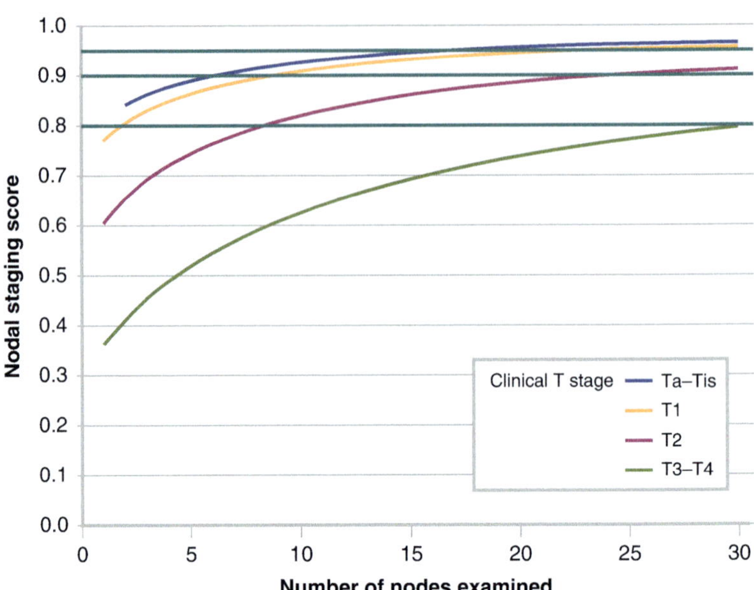

Fig. 9.1 Sensitivity of the pathologic evaluation of nodal disease stratified by clinical tumor stage in 4,335 patients who were treated with radical cystectomy with pelvic lymphadenectomy. Vertical axis is the probability of missing nodal disease (1 − sensitivity) and horizontal axis is the number of examined nodes. Adapted from Shariat et al. Eur Urol 2012;61:237–242

was recorded in predicting advance pathologic stage vs. 71 % when TUR stage alone was used. In predicting lymph node metastasis, the nomogram showed an accuracy of 63 % when TUR stage and grade were used compared to 61 % of patients using TUR stage alone. Heterogeneity in lymph node staging in this multicenter series likely contributed to the lower accuracy of the model.

In a similar fashion and a more contemporary cohort, Green et al. developed a nomogram which predicts non-organ confined UCB based on a single-institution cohort of 201 patients with clinically organ-confined disease who underwent RC with pelvic lymph node dissection without neoadjuvant chemotherapy [55]. The authors found that clinical tumor stage, presence of LVI, and radiographic evidence of non-organ-confined UCB or hydronephrosis were independently associated with pT3/Nany UCB. Furthermore, clinical tumor stage and presence of LVI remained independent predictors of pT3/Nany or pTany/N + UCB, for which the final nomogram showed a predictive accuracy of 83 %.

Recently, Shariat et al. developed a preoperative clinical Nodal Staging Score, which estimates the number of lymph nodes needed to be removed to ensure that a node-negative patient is indeed without lymph node metastasis, based on the numbers of lymph nodes examined and clinical tumor stage (Fig. 9.1) [70].

Pre-cystectomy nomograms provide only a modest increase in accuracy and reasons for this may include differences in TUR technique, non-standardized use of restaging biopsies, inaccuracy and variable use of preoperative imaging, and variability in the pathologic evaluation. The integration of other pathologic prognostic markers, for example LVI in addition to molecular markers of disease, possibly will enhance predictive accuracy of pre-cystectomy nomograms [71]. Nevertheless, they demonstrate that the combined use of clinical and pathologic variables, which cannot always be integrated within look-up tables, results in more accurate predictions than the use of a single variable.

9.3 Muscle-Invasive Bladder Cancer

9.3.1 Prognostic Factors

9.3.1.1 Preoperative/Clinical Factors

9.3.1.1.1 Age

The extent to which advanced chronologic age impacts the indications for and outcomes of RC is controversial. Though it has been reported in small surgical series that older patients fare well compared to their younger counterparts in terms of complications and perioperative outcomes [72, 73],

Nielsen et al. have shown in a study of 888 patients who underwent RC for UCB, that higher age at RC is associated with extravesical disease, pathologic upstaging, and higher cancer-specific mortality. These findings have been subsequently validated in several studies [74, 75]. The impact of age on treatment tolerability and tumor biology may relate to cancer outcomes but remains to be clarified.

9.3.1.1.2 Gender

The influence of gender on the incidence, staging, prognosis, and survival in UCB has been poorly investigated and understood [76]. Recent epidemiologic [77–80] and translational research [81, 82] has shed some light on the complex relationship between gender and UCB. A growing body of evidence has shown that despite UCB being more common in men, women with bladder cancer have worse survival than men in both non-muscle invasive [14, 24] and muscle-invasive bladder cancer [83, 84].

Hormonal differences have been discussed as a possible explanation for discrepancy in UCB biology [81, 82, 85]. Another reason for gender-specific discrepancies in UCB outcomes may be inequalities in health care and treatment delay. That is, for example, among patients treated with RC for UCB, female patients have been found to have significantly longer operative times, higher blood loss, higher transfusion rates, and a greater rate of perioperative complications than males [86–88]. Interestingly, it has been reported that women were more likely to present with more advanced bladder cancer than men in a retrospective study of the Netherlands Cancer Registry between 1989 and 1994 which provided data of more than 20,000 UCB patients [89]. One reason for this might be that women who present with initial macrohematuria are treated for urinary tract infection by their gynecologist or general practitioner, thus primary treatment is delayed [90]. Finally, differences in stage distribution have been suggested to be an alternative etiology for the disproportionally higher cancer-specific mortality among female UCB patients [91, 92]. However, large collaborative studies have demonstrated that even after adjustment for the effect of tumor stage, female patients experience worse outcomes after RC [93, 94]. Kluth et al. recently

reported in a multi-institutional study of 8,102 (6,497 (80%) males and 1,605 (20%) females) patients treated with RC for UCB, that female gender was associated with disease recurrence in univariable, but not multivariable analysis [211]. Interestingly, although female gender was an independent predictor for cancer-specific mortality, there was no significant interaction between gender and either stage, nodal metastasis or LVI.

9.3.1.1.3 Performance Status and Comorbidity

Patients with poor performance status and higher comorbidity have been shown to have a higher mortality. In a single-center experience, Boorjian et al. evaluated five different comorbidity indices of 891 patients who underwent RC: the American Society of Anesthesiologists (ASA) score, Charlson comorbidity index (CCI), Elixhauser index (EI), and Eastern Cooperative Oncology Group performance status (ECOG) [95]. The authors found that EI, ASA, and ECOG were significantly associated with 90-day perioperative mortality. Moreover, within a median follow-up of 10 years, CCI, EI, ASA, and ECOG were independent predictors of 5-year cancer-specific survival. These findings are in line with recent studies that reported a higher comorbidity to be associated with a higher risk of postoperative and any-cause mortality [96].

9.3.1.1.4 Laboratory Values

Several studies suggest that different laboratory markers assessed at the time of RC are associated with oncologic outcomes. In a recent published single-center study of 246 consecutive patients who underwent RC for UCB, it has been found that CRP evaluated at the time of RC was independently associated with a higher risk of cancer-specific mortality [97]. These findings are in line with a recent screening study among healthy individuals in which elevated CRP concentrations indicated a higher risk of developing UCB [98]. Furthermore, Yoshida et al. found in a study of 88 MIBC patients treated with chemoradiotherapy only, an association of elevated CRP and adverse outcome [99]. Leukocytosis (higher WBC) is a sensitive, non-specific marker of inflammation associated with systemic progress such as cancer metastasis [100]. Elevated platelet count is frequently observed in patients with cancer and has been reported as a prognostic factor in several tumors such as renal cancer [101]. In a recent published retrospective study of 258 patients who underwent RC, the presence of thrombocytosis at RC was associated with higher cancer-specific mortality [102]. Hypoalbuminemia is controversial as a nutritional marker due to its long half-time and the potential impact of systemic factors such as inflammation and stress on serum albumin [103]. However, it has been shown that preoperative albumin is associated with a higher risk of overall survival in UCB patients after RC [104].

9.3.1.1.5 Obesity

In MIBC, Chromecki et al. have recently shown that obesity (defined as BMI ≥ 30 kg/m^2) is associated with a higher risk of disease recurrence, cancer-specific mortality, and overall mortality in a study cohort of 4,118 patients who underwent RC and lymphadenectomy for UCB [105]. These findings suggest that metabolic syndrome is an important area of investigation and therapy in patients with UCB. In contrast, Hafron et al. reported no significant association between higher BMI and disease-specific survival in RC patients [106]. However, this study was limited by its small sample size and a high rate of preoperative therapies.

9.3.1.1.6 Smoking

Recently, Rink et al. found that current smokers were at a significantly higher risk of experiencing disease recurrence after RC compared with former and never smokers, who had a similar risk [107]. These findings are in line with previous studies in NMIBC [29–31] and MIBC, in which smoking duration and quantity have been shown to be associated with higher tumor stage and grade in patients with newly diagnosed UCB [108, 109]. Similarly to previous studies in NMIBC [110], patients who stopped smoking more than 10 years before RC had less aggressive tumor stages and improved prognosis compared to those who stopped less than 10 years before RC or were current smokers at RC.

9.3.1.2 Intraoperative/Surgical Factors
9.3.1.2.1 Lymph Node Dissection and Invasion

Recently, several localization studies in UCB patients with regards to lymph node dissection demonstrated that no metastatic lymph nodes are found outside the pelvis if the pelvic lymph nodes are negative [111, 112]. In contrast, a multicenter study by Leissner et al. has shown that there may be a low rate of "skip" metastases to higher lymph nodes [113]. However, the extent and impact on survival of lymph node dissection in UCB is highly controversial [113–122].

Therefore, many studies have tried to establish a minimum number of lymph nodes needed to be taken at the time of RC in an effort to reduce understaging and maximize survival [121, 123]. In node-positive patients, one of the largest single-center reports of patients treated with RC, the recurrence-free survival at 10 years for patients with eight or fewer positive lymph nodes was significantly higher than in those with more than eight positive lymph nodes (40 % vs 10 %, respectively) [124]. In pathologic node-negative patients, increasing the number of LNs has also been suggested to result in better survival [115, 119]. In a recent multi-institutional study of 4,188 pN0 patients after RC, a lymph node removal over 20 nodes resulted in a survival benefit [125]. Many of these retrospective studies may however represent stage migration with more thorough pelvic lymph node dissections and not a therapeutic effect.

9.3.1.3 Postoperative/Pathologic Factors
9.3.1.3.1 Pathologic Tumor Stage

Tumor stage has been clearly established as one of the most important predictors of cancer-specific and overall mortality in patients after RC (Table 9.3) [124, 126]. The clinical TNM staging system combines a pathologic evaluation of the TUR specimen with findings from an examination under anesthesia and preoperative radiographic imaging. Unfortunately, inaccuracies in clinical staging are highlighted in that up to 40 % of patients are up-staged and about 25 % are down-

Table 9.3 Summary of the preoperative/clinical, intraoperative, and pathologic prognostic factors in patients with muscle invasive bladder cancer

	Comments	References
Age	Advanced age is an independent predictor of extravesical disease, pathologic upstaging, and CSM	[1–4]
Gender	Female gender is an independent predictor of worse DR and CSM	[5–25]
Performance status and comorbidity	Poor performance status and higher comorbidity are independent predictor of 90-day perioperative mortality, CSM, and any-cause mortality	[26, 27, 211]
Laboratory values	Elevated CRP, leukocytosis (higher WBC), thrombocytosis (elevated platelet count) are independent predictors of CSM. Hypoalbuminemia is associated with perioperative and overall mortality	[28–35]
Obesity	Body mass index ≥ 30 kg/m^2 is an independent predictor of DR, CSM, and overall mortality	[36, 37]
Smoking	Smokers are more likely to experience DR. Smoking cessation >10 years is associated with improved diagnosis	[38–44]
Lymph node dissection/invasion	Lymph node metastasis is an independent predictor of DR and CSM	[45–59]
Pathologic tumor stage	Advanced pathologic T-stage is an independent predictor of CSM and overall mortality	[58, 60–62]
Pathologic tumor grade	While tumor grade is one of the most important predictors of disease recurrence and progression after TUR and/or intravesical immunotherapy, the predictive power after RC is limited	[58, 60, 63, 64]
Lymph node invasion	Lymph node metastasis is the most important pathologic prognostic factor after RC and is associated with higher risk of DR and survival	[50, 51, 60, 65–67]
Soft tissue surgical margin	Soft tissue surgical margin is an independent predictor of DR and CSM	[68, 69]
Tumor size	Larger tumor size is an independent predictor of CSM	[69–71]
Lymphovascular invasion	The presence of lymphovascular invasion is an independent predictor of DP and CSM. That is also true in lymph node negative patients	[72–79]
Histologic variants	Studies have failed to show significant differences in outcomes between UC and squamous histology. Non-UC/non-squamous histology is an independent predictor of DP and CSM. Previous studies failed to show significant association between histologic variants and outcomes	[80–84]

DR disease recurrence, *DP* disease progression, *CSM* cancer-specific mortality

staged after pathologic assessment of the RC specimen, thus limiting the prognostic accuracy of clinical staging system [68]. The problem of understaging has significant implications such as in counseling patients for neoadjuvant chemotherapy [2]. After RC and lymph node dissection, the pathologic evaluation of the specimen provides a more accurate stratification of cancer-specific outcome. The 5-year bladder cancer-specific survival in patients with $\leq$pT1, pT2, pT3, and pT4 is reported as 80–90 %, 50–70 %, 30–45 % and 20–35 %, respectively [124, 126].

9.3.1.3.2 Pathologic Tumor Grade
Tumor grading systems are designed to reflect the degree of tumor cell anaplasia. Recently, members of the WHO and the International Society of Urological Pathologists (ISUP) published the WHO/ISUP consensus classification of urothelial neoplasms of the urinary bladder. That is, there is no uniformly accepted grading system for UCB. The WHO/ISUP system classifies bladder tumors into papillary urothelial neoplasms of low malignant potential, or papillary carcinomas of low or high grade [127]. While tumor grade is one of the most important predictors of disease recurrence and progression after TUR and/or intravesical immunotherapy, the predictive power after RC is limited [128]. One of the reasons may be because most patients undergoing RC have high-grade disease [124, 126].

9.3.1.3.3 Lymph Node Invasion

The presence of lymph node metastasis is the most important pathologic prognostic factor after RC, with associated 15–30 % 5-year survival rates [4, 116, 117]. Multi-institutional series of patients treated with RC have shown that approximately 70–80 % of patients with pathologic node-positive disease experience disease recurrence compared to 30–40 % of patients with extravesical disease and pathologically negative lymph nodes within 5 years of surgery [4, 5, 126]. Tarin et al. have recently investigated impact of lymph node involvement by location on disease outcomes using the 2010 TNM staging system [129]. Of 591 patients treated with radical cystectomy with mapping pelvic lymph node dissection, 114 patients (19 %) had lymph node involvement and 42 patients (7 %) had pN3 disease. The authors could demonstrate that lymph node location was not associated with outcomes; however, the number of positive lymph nodes was associated with worse oncologic outcomes. Interestingly, a similar disease recurrence-free survival for patients with pN3 disease compared to pN1 or pN2 tumors has been shown.

9.3.1.3.4 Soft Tissue Surgical Margin

The positive soft tissue surgical margin rate (STSM) is usually rare after RC (2–10 %); however, it is a strong independent predictor of local disease recurrence and cancer-specific mortality. The finding of a positive STSM correlates with tumor stage, previous pelvic radiation, extent of lymph node dissection, and surgeon experience [130]. The Southwest Oncology Group 8710 trial reported a 100 % local disease recurrence, and 0 % 5-year cancer-specific rate among 25 patients with a positive STSM after RC [130].

Xylinas et al. identified 231 patients with positive STSM of a multi-institutional cohort of 4,335 patients (5.3 %) treated with RC and lymphadenectomy. Actuarial cancer-specific survival estimates at 2 and 5 years after RC were 33 ± 3 and 25 ± 4 %, respectively [131]. Moreover, it has been shown that higher body mass index, higher tumor stage, presence of grade 3 disease, lymphovascular invasion (LVI), and lymph node involvement were all independently associated with disease recurrence (all p values <0.05). Furthermore, higher tumor stage, LVI, and lymph node involvement were independently associated with cancer specific mortality, while location and multifocality of STSM were not associated with outcomes.

9.3.1.3.5 Tumor Size

The current pathologic TNM classification of bladder cancer relies on the depth of tissue invasion, but does not consider the size of the index tumor. However, in several recent reports, tumor size was identified as an independent predictor of cancer-specific mortality [131, 132]. It has been shown that the 10-year cancer-specific mortality was 94 % for patients with pT2 tumors of ≤ 3 cm and only 68 % for pT2 tumors of >3 cm ($p < 0.001$) [133] While published proposed size threshold criteria have varied, there is a strong rationale to include tumor size as an important risk stratification variable for patients treated with RC.

9.3.1.3.6 Lymphovascular Invasion

LVI is an important step in systemic cancer cell dissemination [134, 135]. LVI is an established independent predictor of disease recurrence and cancer-specific mortality, thus help identifying patients without lymph node metastasis who are at increased risk of disease recurrence and mortality despite RC [136–138]. LVI has been identified in 30–50 % of RC specimens, and positively correlates with adverse pathologic features. Several previous studies found that LVI is an independent predictor of disease recurrence and cancer-specific mortality in lymph node-negative, non-metastatic patients treated with RC [139–141]. This is an important distinction, as node-positive patients are usually recommended to receive adjuvant chemotherapy regardless of LVI status. Knowing that patients with negative nodes and positive LVI are at higher risk of recurrence might change the treatment in these patients.

9.3.1.3.7 Histologic Subtype/Variants

In Western countries, the most common histologic subtype of bladder cancer is UC, comprising >90 % of cases [142]. Histologic subtypes of non-UC of the bladder include mesenchymal and epithelial tumors of other histologic types. Epithelial cancers include squamous cell, adenocarcinoma, and small cell/neuroendocrine carcinoma.

Several previous studies failed to show a significant difference in cancer-specific mortality when comparing squamous and UC histology [142–144]. Conversely, non-UC/non-squamous histology (i.e. adenocarcinoma, small cell carcinoma, carcinosarcoma, etc.) was identified as an independent predictor of disease recurrence and cancer-specific mortality [142].

Recently, Xylinas et al. analyzed differences between pure UCB and UCB with variant histology in 1,984 treated with RC [145]. The authors reported one-fourth of UCB patients treated with RC harbored histologic UCB variants, which were associated with features of biologically aggressive disease. While variant UCB histology was associated with worse outcomes in univariable analyses, this effect did not remain significant in multivariable analyses.

The nested variant of UC has recently shown to be associated with a high rate of locally advanced disease at RC [146]. However, when stage was matched in this analysis with a median follow up of 10.8 years, no significant differences on disease recurrence or survival were observed between patients with pure UC and those with the nested variant.

9.3.1.4 Tissue-Based Molecular Markers

9.3.1.4.1 Cell Cycle

p53 (gene and protein) is known as the "guardian of the genome," because it plays important roles in the regulation of the cell cycle, DNA repair, and apoptosis (Table 9.4) [147, 148]. It presents one of the most commonly mutated genes in humans; its expression reflects chromosome 17p abnormalities. Previous studies support the view that p53 nuclear accumulation is predictive of the outcome in patients treated with RC [149–152]. In these studies it has been shown that the proportion of specimens with altered p53 expression progressively increases from normal urothelium to NMIBC, to MIBC and finally to metastatic lymph node UCB. Moreover, retrospective studies demonstrate that p53 is associated with a greater risk of disease recurrence and cancer-specific mortality [147, 153–156]. There is evidence however for and against the prognostic role of p53. A prospective randomized study demonstrated no prognostic significance to p53 status in a series of muscle invasive lesions. Reasons for the discrepancies between studies may be related to the choice of antibody used in p53 assays, variability in interpretation and stratification criteria, and inconsistencies in specimen handling and other technical procedures [157]. Recent meta-analysis found that immunohistochemistry was the most commonly (96 % of the 117 studies) used approach to assess p53 status, with molecular analysis being used in the other five studies [150]. Interestingly, the p53 status was a stronger predictor of UCB outcomes in patients treated with RC than chromosomal alterations or expression patterns of p21, pRB, p27, p16, cyclin E1, or cyclin D1 [158].

The retinoblastoma gene is the prototype tumor-suppressor gene that encodes a nuclear protein (pRb) which is an important cell cycle regulator [147]. Recent evidence suggests that the predictive power of pRB may be inferior to that of other cell cycle regulators in both NMIBC and MIBC [147, 155, 159, 160]. However, pRb as part of a biomarker panel improved the predictive accuracy of a base model for disease recurrence and cancer-specific mortality after RC in MIBC [155]. Nevertheless, to date, the clinical utility of pRB in UCB prognostication seems limited and remains to be validated.

Ki-67 is a nuclear protein expressed by proliferating cells that regulates all phases of the cell cycle. Ki-67 overexpression has been shown to be independently associated with disease recurrence and stage-adjusted cancer-specific mortality in RC patients [161, 162]. Though Ki67 seems to be the most convincing biomarker for prognostication in MIBC, its impact in NMIBC is still controversial [158, 159, 163].

p21 binds to and inhibits the activity of cyclin-dependent kinase complexes, and thus functions as a regulator of cell cycle progression at G1 [164]. In MIBC patients, p21 was an independent predictor of both disease recurrence and cancer-specific mortality [155, 165]. In patients with organ-confined disease, p21 remained independently associated with outcomes when combined in a multivariable model with p27 and p53 [153].

Table 9.4 Selection of tissue-based biomarkers for staging and prognostication of bladder cancer

Biomarker	Function	Relevant studies (year of publication)	N	Findings
Cell-cycle				
p53	Inhibits G1-S progression	Schrier et al. (2006)	80	Altered expression of p53 associated with DR and CSM in pT1N0
		Esuvaranthan et al. (2007)	80	Altered p53 not associated with response to intravesical BCG, DR, DP, and CSM in NMIBC
		Moonen et al. (2007)	105	No additional value for p53 mutation analysis for high-risk NMIBC
		Shariat et al. (2009)	324	Incorporating p53 expression into clinico-pathologic predictive model improved accuracy in RC patients with organ-confined disease
		Shariat et al. (2010)	692	p53 as part of biomarker panel improved predictive accuracy for DR and CSM in patients with locally advanced disease after RC
		Shariat et al. (2010)	692	Incorporating p53 expression into clinico-pathologic predictive model does not improve accuracy in RC patients with locally advanced disease
		Goebell et al. (2011)	3,421	Altered p53 associated with DP in patients with $\geq$ T1 disease
		Stadler et al. (2011)	499	p53 status has no association to DR, OS, or adjuvant chemotherapy benefit in Phase III trial of targeted chemotherapy for pT1/T2 patients based on p53 positivity
		Mitra et al. (2013)	212	p53 associated with DR and CSM after RC p53 as part of 9 biomarker panel with smoking intensity improved predictive accuracy for DR and CSM after RC
pRB	Cell cycle regulator Sequesters E2F Inhibitor of cell-cycle progression	Shariat et al. (2010)	692	pRB as part of biomarker panel improved predictive accuracy for DR and CSM in patients with locally advanced disease
		Park et al. (2011)	61	No predictive value for pRb expression on IVR or DP in BCG-treated high-grade T1 NMIBC
Ki-67	Marker of cell proliferation	Margulis et al. (2009)	713	High Ki-67 labeling index independently associated with DR and CSM in RC patients and improved predictive model for these outcomes
		Shariat et al. (2009)	80	Altered Ki-67 predictive of DR and CSM in pT1 UCB patients at RC
		Behnsawy et al. (2009)	161	No predictive value for Ki-67 expression on IVR in newly diagnosed NMIBC
		Park et al. (2011)	61	No predictive value for Ki-67 expression on IVR and DP in BCG-treated high-grade T1 patients

p21	Cyclin-dependent kinase inhibitor Regulator at G1 checkpoint	Stein et al. (1998)	242	p21 status was an independent predictor of DR and CSM after RC
		Shariat et al. (2003)	49	Altered p21 expression independently associated with DR and DP in patient with Cis
		Shariat et al. (2007)	74	Combination of p21 with p53, pRB, and p27 stratified patients into statistically significantly different risk groups for DR and DP in patients with NMIBC
		Shariat et al. (2007)	300	p21 has cooperative/synergistic action with p53, p27, and pRB
		Shariat et al. (2009)	80	Altered p21 not predictive of DR and CSM in pT1 UCB patients at RC
		Shariat et al. (2010)	692	p21 as part of biomarker panel improved predictive accuracy for DR and CSM in patients with locally advanced disease
p27	Cyclin-dependent kinase inhibitor	Shariat et al. (2009)	80	Altered p27 predictive of DR and CSM in pT1 UCB patients at RC
Cyclins	Deregulation of the G1/S transition	Del Pizzo et al. (1999)	50	Decreased expression of cyclin E1 significantly associated with advanced pathologic stage, LVI, LNM, and CSM
		Shariat et al. (2006)	235	Cyclin D1 immunoreactivity elevated in UCB patients compared to controls, but not associated with clinical or pathologic characteristics
Apoptosis				
Caspase-3	Protease that acts as an apoptosis effector	Karam et al. (2007)	226	49 % of the patients had loss of caspase-3 expression, which was associated with higher pathologic grade and stage, and presence of LNM Loss of caspase-3 independent predictor of CSM after RC
		Karam et al. (2007)	226	Overexpression of bcl-2 found in 32 % of RC specimens, and correlated with higher pathologic stage, DR and CSM
Survivin	Acts as inhibitor of apoptosis by blocking downstream caspase activity	Shultz et al. (2004)	37	Protein and mRNA level associated with cancer presence, higher tumor grade, and advanced pathologic stage
		Karam et al. (2007)	226	Survivin overexpression present in 63 % of UCB specimens, and associated with higher pathologic stage, presence of LVI, LNM, DR and CSM in 219 patients treated with RC
		Shariat et al. (2007)	231	The proportion of specimens with survivin overexpression increased gradually from NMIBC to advanced bladder cancer and to LNM
		Shariat et al. (2009)	726	Altered survivin status added to standard clinico-pathologic predictive model improved accuracy for prediction of DR and CSM in T1-3 N0 subgroup
		Xi et al. (2012)	72	Survivin overexpression associated with DR in NMIBC

(continued)

Table 9.4 (continued)

Biomarker	Function	Relevant studies (year of publication)	N	Findings
Angiogenesis				
MVD	Traditional histologic marker of angiogenesis	Bochner et al. (1995)	164	Patients with high microvessel density (>100 microvessels per hpf) were at highest risk of DR and CSM
		Jaeger et al. (1995)	41	Higher MVD in the primary tumor if LNM
		Shariat et al. (2010)	204	Failed to detect an association between MVD and prognosis, but MVD higher in patients with LNM Higher relative MVD in LNM
		Ajili et al. (2012)	28	MVD associated with DR in patients with T1HG NMIBC treated with BCG
Thrombospondin-1	Component of the extracellular matrix Implicated in the regulation of cell growth and proliferation Inhibitor of angiogenesis	Grossfeld et al. (1997)	163	Altered thrombospondin-1 expression independently associated with increased risk of DR and CSM in 163 patients treated with RC
		Shariat et al. (2010)	204	Decreased thrombospondin-1 independently associated with DR and CSM Loss of thrombospondin-1 expression associated with alterations in other cell cycle regulators such as p21 and p27

N number of patients, *MVD* microvessel density, *RC* radical cystectomy, *DR* disease recurrence, *DP* disease progression, *OM* overall mortality, *CSM* cancer-specific mortality, *NMIBC* non-muscle invasive bladder cancer, *MIBC* muscle invasive bladder cancer, *UCB* urothelial carcinoma of bladder, *LNM* lymph node metastasis

Conversely, p21 expression alone was not an independent predictor of outcomes in the subgroup of patients with pT1 disease [158], suggesting that p21 does not predict outcomes in NMIBC.

The product of the p27, a member of the Cip/Kip family of Cdk inhibitors, prolongs cell cycle arrest in the G1 phase. Though in NMIBC, p27 has been found to have only limited predictive value, in patients with MIBC treated with RC, p27 significantly improved prediction of disease recurrence and cancer-specific mortality [158]. No prospective validation however has confirmed the ability of this marker to improve prediction of disease status after RC.

Cyclin E1 is the predominant regulatory protein determining rates of cell-cycle transition from the G1 to S phase, thereby thus affecting oncogenesis [166, 167]. Cyclin E1 expression was significantly decreased in patients with advanced pathologic stage, LVI, metastases to regional lymph nodes, and cancer-specific mortality in both TUR and RC specimens. The role of cyclins is currently evaluated in prospective multicenter studies.

9.3.1.4.2 Apoptosis

Apoptosis, or programmed cell death, is a complex and highly regulated process comprising a series of coordinated steps resulting in cell death [168].

Activated caspase-3 is a protease that constitutes an important downstream step in both the intrinsic and extrinsic apoptotic pathways and promotes apoptosis by cleaving multiple cellular components [169]. The prognostic value of this biomarker is controversial [170–172]. In a most recent study evaluating the combined effect of apoptotic markers on oncologic outcomes in 226 patients treated with RC, Karam et al. demonstrated that altered caspase-3 expression was associated with features of biologically and clinically aggressive disease and independently predicted cancer-specific mortality after RC [172].

Survivin is a member of the Inhibitor of Apoptosis family, and its overexpression inhibits extrinsic and intrinsic pathways of apoptosis, by blocking downstream caspase activity [173]. Survivin represents a promising marker in UCB outcome prediction since it has been shown that overexpression is associated with cancer presence and features of aggressive disease [174–176], as well as disease recurrence and cancer-specific mortality [177, 178]. Survivin is an attractive target for therapy in UCB [168], because of its selective and substantial upregulation in UCB and its causal role in cancer progression [179]. In addition, recently, survivin expression has been associated with disease recurrence in NMIBC [180].

9.3.1.4.3 Angiogenesis

Angiogenesis is a critical event in the initiation and progression of solid malignancies. Traditionally, angiogenesis has been quantified by microvessel density (MVD: >100 microvessels per hpf) [181]. Bochner et al. reported that high MVD were associated with higher disease recurrence and cancer-specific mortality after RC [182]; however, others did not confirm these results [183–185]. Reasons for that may be found in differences in staining and scoring protocols as well as variability in MVD due to tumor heterogeneity.

Thrombospondin-1 is a glycoprotein of the extracellular matrix that has been implicated in the regulation of cell growth and proliferation, thus a potent inhibitor of angiogenesis. Altered thrombospondin-1 expression was independently associated with an increased risk of disease recurrence and all-cause mortality [186]. However, the prognostic value of thrombospondin-1 was not independent of p53 expression status [185].

Due to the complexity of the molecular abnormalities in UCB, it is unlikely that a single biomarker can accurately differentiate tumors of similar clinicopathologic phenotypes into precise prognostic categories. Therefore, combinations of independent, complementary biomarkers may provide a more accurate prediction of outcome compared to any single biomarker [155, 158, 187, 188]. Recently, Lotan et al. investigated prospectively a panel of biomarkers in 216 patients with high-grade UCB treated with RC between 2007 and 2012 [189]. Expression of p53, p21, p27, cyclin E1, and Ki-67 was altered in 54 %, 26 %, 46 %, 15 %, and 75 % patients, respectively. In a multivariable analysis, the number of altered biomarkers remained an independent predictor of disease recurrence and cancer-specific mortality. Future investigations should focus on promising biomarker combinations that encompass a variety of different pathways in order to increase the predictive value and possibility for targeted therapy. Critical to the adoption of any marker/marker panel will be prospective validation that clarifies the clinical usefulness in predicting postoperative behavior.

9.3.2 Prediction Tools

9.3.2.1 Postoperative Prediction Tools for Disease Recurrence and Survival After Radical Cystectomy

9.3.2.1.1 Nomograms

Several nomograms after RC have been developed to predict the natural history of surgically treated UCB and thus to help in the decision-making process regarding the use of adjuvant therapy (Table 9.5) [4–6]. The Bladder Cancer Research Consortium (BCRC) developed three nomograms to determine the probabilities of disease recurrence, cancer-specific and all-cause mortality at 2, 5 and 8 years after RC (Fig. 9.2; available at www.nomogram.org) [5, 6]. The disease recurrence nomogram showed a 78 % accuracy and comprised pathologic features such as T and N stages, pathologic grade, presence of LVI and CIS at RC, as well as the administration of chemotherapy (either neoadjuvant, adjuvant or both), and/or radiation. The predictive accuracy of the nomograms for cancer-specific and all-cause mortality nomogram were 78 % in 73 %, respectively.

In the same year, the International Bladder Cancer Nomogram Consortium (IBCNC) published a postoperative nomogram predicting the 5-year risk of disease recurrence following RC and pelvic lymph node dissection (available at www.nomograms.org) based on the data of more than 9,000 patients from 12 centers (including the BCRC) [4]. The nomogram included significant features such as age, gender, grade, pathologic stage, histologic type, lymph node status, and time from diagnosis to surgery. The predictive accuracy of the nomogram was 75 % and statistically superior to the AJCC TNM staging (68 %) or the standard pathologic grouping models (62 %). Interestingly, based on the same patient data, Vickers et al. have demonstrated in a decision analysis approach that a nomogram cutoff outperformed pathologic stage for decision-making regarding chemotherapy. Thus the authors concluded that referring patients to adjuvant chemotherapy on the basis of a multivariate model is likely to lead to better patient outcomes than the use of pathologic groups.

Recently, Xylinas et al. developed competing-risk, probability nomograms that predict disease recurrence and cancer-specific survival of chemotherapy-naive pT1-3 N0 UCB patients ($n=2,145$). With a median follow-up of 45 months, the 5-year disease recurrence-free and cancer-specific survival estimates were 68 and 73 %, respectively.

In contrast, Rink et al. developed two nomograms predicting disease recurrence and cancer-specific mortality based on 381 patients with nodal metastases from a multi-institutional cohort of 4,335 patients with UCB treated with RC and lymphadenectomy without preoperative chemo- or radiotherapy. Including gender, tumor stage, STSM, lymph node density, and administration of adjuvant chemotherapy, the model showed a predictive accuracy for disease recurrence-free and cancer-specific survival of 63 and 66 %, respectively.

9.3.2.1.2 Other Prediction Tools

Bassi et al. developed an ANN utilizing gender, several pathologic features, and history of upper tract UC as input variables for prediction of 5-year all-cause survival after RC [190]. In a single institution cohort of 369 patients, the prognostic accuracy of the ANN (76 %; based on 12 variables) was slightly superior to the logistic regression model that was based on only two statistically significant variables (75 %; stage and grade). Unfortunately, the comparison of the accuracy of both models was performed on the same population.

A promising Artificial Intelligence model, a neurofuzzymodel (NFM), to predict disease recurrence following RC and PLND was elegantly developed by Catto et al. Therefore, 609 patients with organ-confined disease and no lymph node metastases were identified. Two NFM were trained, tested, and validated to predict the risk of

Table 9.5 Available prediction tools in bladder cancer after radical cystectomy

Post-cystectomy tools

Reference	Prediction form	Patient population	Endpoint/Outcome	No. of pts.	Variables	Accuracy	Validation
Karakiewicz et al. [5]	Probability nomogram	Radical cystectomy	2, 5 and 8 year RFS	731	Age, T-stage, N-stage, pathologic grade, LVI, CIS, adjuvant radiotherapy, adjuvant chemotherapy, neoadjuvant chemotherapy	78 %	External
Shariat et al. [126]	Probability nomogram	Radical cystectomy	2, 5, 8 year CSM and overall survival	731	Age, T-stage, N-stage, pathologic grade, LVI, adjuvant radiotherapy, adjuvant chemotherapy, neoadjuvant chemotherapy	79 % (ACS) 73 % (CSS)	External
Bochner et al. [4]	Probability nomogram	Radical Cystectomy	5 year RFS	9,064	Age, gender, tumor stage, Nodal status, grade, histology, time from diagnosis to surgery	75 %	External
Shariat et al. [188]	Probability nomogram	Radical cystectomy pTa-3N0M0	2, 5, 8 year RFS and CSM	191	p53, p21, pRB, p27, cyclin E1, gender, age, pathologic stage, grade, LVI, concomitant carcinoma in situ	83.4 % (RFS) 86.9 % (CSS)	Internal
Xylinas et al. [7]	Probability nomogram	Radical cystectomy pT1-3 pN0	2, 5 and 7 year RFS and CSM	2,145	T-stage, STSM, and LVI	2, 5 and 7-year RFS: 67 %, 65 % and 64 %, respectively 2, 5 and 7-year CSS: 69 %, 66 % and 66 %, respectively	External
Rink et al. [195]	Probability nomogram	Radical cystectomy with pN1.	2 year RFS and CSM	381	Gender, tumor stage, STSM, lymph node density, adjuvant chemotherapy	63 % (RFS) 66 % (CSS)	Internal
Bassi et al. [190]	Artificial neural network	Radical cystectomy	5 year all cause survival	369	Age, gender, T stage, N stage, grade, LVI, grade, concomitant prostate cancer, history of upper tract UC	76 %	Internal
Catto et al. [191]	Neuro-fuzzy modeling	Radical cystectomy	2 and 5 year RFS	609	Gender, tumor stage, tumor grade, concomitant CIS, lymphovascular invasion (LVI), margin status, administration of chemotherapy	84 %	Internal
Sonpavde et al. [212]	Risk stratification	Radical cystectomy	5 year RFS and all cause survival	707	Gender, grade, LVI, number of lymph nodes, age	68 %	Internal
Sonpavde et al. [213]	Risk stratification	Radical cystectomy	5 year RFS and all cause survival	578	Age, grade, gender, LVI, STSM, number of lymph nodes, decade	66 %	External

(continued)

Table 9.5 (continued)

Post-cystectomy tools

Reference	Prediction form	Patient population	Endpoint/Outcome	No. of pts.	Variables	Accuracy	Validation
Gakis et al. [97]	Risk stratification	Radical cystectomy	3 year CSM	246	T-stage, lymph node density, STSM, CRP level	79 %	Internal
Todenhoefer et al. [199]	Risk stratification	Radical cystectomy	3 year CSM	258	T-stage, STSM, thrombocytosis	75 % (CSS)	Internal
Shariat et al. [70]	Nodal Staging Score	Radical cystectomy	Lymph node metastasis at radical cystectomy	4,335	Number of lymph nodes removed, number of positive lymph nodes, T-stage, LVI		Internal

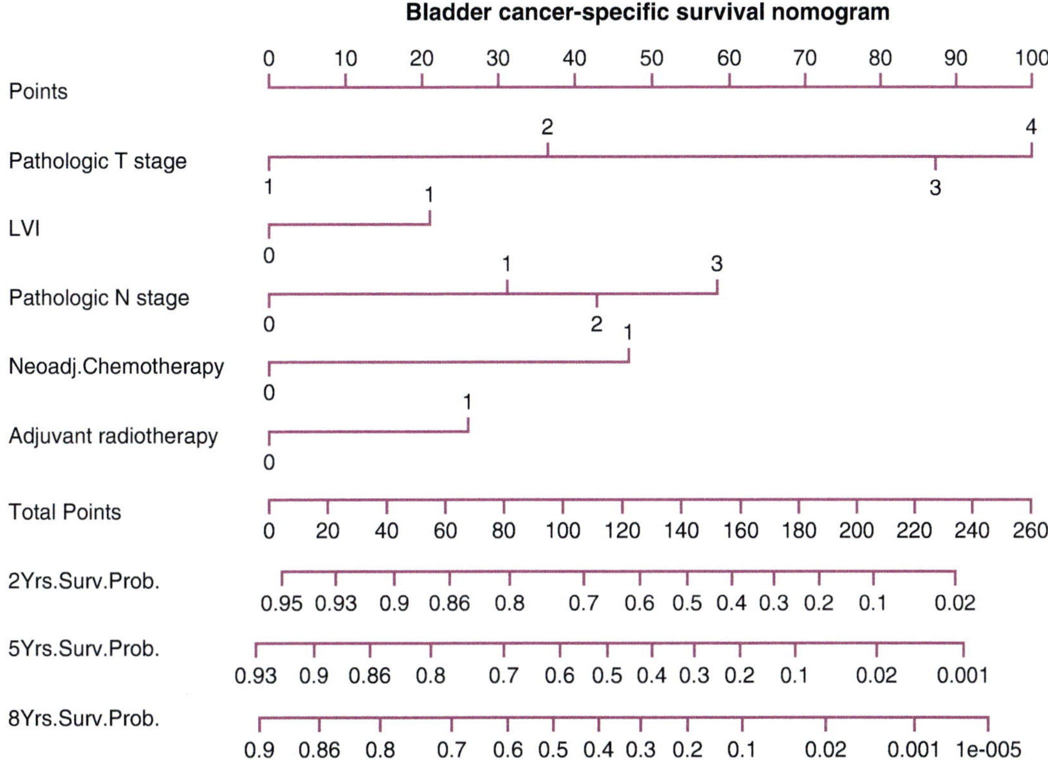

Fig. 9.2 Bladder cancer-specific survival nomogram in 731 patients treated with radical cystectomy and bilateral lymphadenectomy for urothelial carcinoma of the bladder. Instructions for nomogram use: Locate patient values at each axis. Draw a vertical line to the "Point" axis to determine how many points are attributed for each variable value. Sum the points for all variables. Locate the sum on the "Total Points" line. Draw a vertical line toward the "2Yrs.Surv.Prob.," "5Yrs.Surv.Prob.," and "8Yrs.Surv. Prob." axes to determine, respectively, the 2-year, 5-year, and 8-year survival probabilities. Adapted from Shariat et al. Clin Cancer Res 2006;12:6663

disease recurrence after RC, thus the model showed a predictive accuracy of 84 % [191].

Gakis et al. developed a risk-score model predicting the 3-year cancer-specific survival by including significant pathologic features such as higher tumor stage, positive STSM, higher lymph node density, and elevated CRP levels [97]. The accuracy of this model was 79 %. The same study group developed a similar risk-score predicting the 3-year cancer-specific survival based on pathologic features (tumor stage, STSM) and thrombocytosis with a 75 % accuracy [102].

Recently, Shariat et al. developed a model (pathologic Nodal Staging Score) to estimate the probability that a pathologic node-negative UCB patient is indeed free of lymph node metastasis. To this end, the authors analyzed data of 4,335 patients treated with RC and bilat- eral lymph node dissection. Based on the number of lymph nodes examined and pathologic features, they demonstrated that the probability of missing a positive node decreases with the increasing number of nodes examined. Furthermore, the probability of having a positive node increased proportionally with advancing pathologic T stage and LVI.

9.3.2.1.3 Nomograms Including Novel Biomarkers

Only few studies have demonstrated a significant improvement in predictive accuracy, when biomarkers were added to established predictors in the predictive tool setting [172, 188, 192, 193]. One of these studies, for example, demonstrated in 191 pTa-3N0M0 patients following RC that the addition of a panel of five well-established cell cycle regulatory biomarkers (p53, pRB, p21, p27, and cyclin E1) improved the predictive accuracy of competing-risk nomograms and survival in these patients. In comparison, two smaller studies have added biomarkers to standard clinico-pathologic features using pre-cystectomy prediction tools (ANN and neuro-fuzzy modeling) [192, 193]. Prediction tools such as these that incorporate pathologic and molecular information could form the basis for counseling patients regarding their risk of disease recurrence following surgery and for designing clinical trials to test adjuvant treatment strategies in high-risk patients.

Several limitations of nomograms and other prediction tools to patient risk stratification should be noted. First, and foremost, their retrospective nature of data accrual and the fact that all currently available predictive tools in UCB are not perfectly accurate. Furthermore, all available nomograms and predictive tools were derived and are applicable to centers of excellence for bladder surgery, thus the general applicability requires additional validation. The fundamental issue raised by opponents of predictive tools is regarding their utility. Indeed, to date, there are no prospective randomized studies that clearly demonstrate improving patient care by using prediction tools. However, despite these limitations, nomograms and prediction tools provide optimum accuracy for individualized evidence-based decision-making process of UCB.

9.3.2.1.4 Prediction models using genomic data

Recently, there have been published studies on using genomic data sets. It is likely that future prediction models will rely on biology from these types of cellular interrogations.

Developed a gene expression model predicting the response to M-VAC chemotherapy based on TUR tumor biopsy materials from 27 patients with T2a-T3bN0M0 UCB who were expected to undergo RC as a primary treatment using a cDNA microarray comprising of 27,648 genes [212] .

The authors found 14 genes that were expressed differently between nine responder (downstaging after 2 courses of MVAC, ≤pT1 or ≤T1) and 9 non-responders (upstaging after 2 courses of MVAC, ≥pT2 or ≥T2). Based on these gene expression profiles a prediction scoring system for chemosensitivity was established. The study is limited by the small dataset and needs to be prospectively validated. Further refinement is needed in the clinical laboratory setting to bring this test to routine clinical use.

Smith et al. developed a 20-genes model based on the expression of TUR- tumor tissue to predict the risk of lymph node invasion in clinically lymph node negative MIBC patients prior to RC [213]. A training dataset of 156 patients from two independent centers was used to develop the gene expression model and determine cutoffs for lymph node metastasis. External validation was performed on 185 patients from a prospective randomized phase 3 trial evaluating two different adjuvant chemotherapy regimens. The gene expression model demonstrated 67% (AUC) discrimination for discriminating lymph node negative and positive patients in the validation cohort. Although the gene model was externally validated on a prospective cohort, the clinical assay has not undergone analytic validation yet.

9.4 Metastatic and Recurrent Bladder Cancer

9.4.1 Prognostic Factors

Patients with UCB who experience disease recurrence after RC and those with metastatic disease have very poor outcomes. Despite advances in surgical techniques and systemic chemotherapies [124, 126, 194], the majority of patients will die from UCB within 1 year after disease recurrence and only few patients survive beyond 2 years after disease recurrence [195]. Modern salvage chemotherapies may prolong survival if a patient responds; however, cure is very rare [196, 197], thus underscoring the lethal nature of UCB once the disease recurs and becomes systemic [124, 126, 194]. While the natural history of UCB from RC to disease recurrence has been intensively investigated [4–6], that of patients who experience disease recurrence after RC and/or have metastatic disease is still poorly understood. Accurate prediction of clinical outcomes after disease recurrence could help in patient counseling and clinical trial design and analysis. There are only a few studies that analyzed prognostic factors for outcomes in UCB patients with disease recurrence after RC and/or metastatic disease.

9.4.1.1 Time from Radical Cystectomy to Disease Recurrence

Recently, several study groups found that in patients who experience disease recurrence, the median time from RC to disease recurrence was less than 12 months [198–200]. Mitra et al. reported that a time to disease recurrence <12 months is associated with worse outcomes in patients with UCB [198]. Rink et al. confirmed that time from RC to disease recurrence is a strong predictor of survival after disease recurrence [195]. The shorter the time from surgery to disease recurrence, the shorter is the survival time. Interestingly, the 1-year risk of cancer-specific mortality after disease recurrence disproportionately improved in patients experiencing disease recurrence after 12 months. In other words, while even after 12 months it remained true that the shorter the time to disease recurrence the faster the mortality, the change in rate becomes less significant if the time to disease recurrence is more than 12 months.

The time to disease recurrence may be considered as a surrogate for the burden of disease thus suggesting that patients with a shorter time to disease recurrence had occult metastatic disease that became clinically evident faster. Therefore, the time to recurrence should be considered as a valuable predictor for outcome prognostication in patients treated with RC and experienced disease recurrence.

9.4.1.2 Pathologic Factors

Several established pathologic characteristics such as non-organ-confined pathologic stage, lymph node metastasis and positive soft tissue surgical margin as well as the clinical factors such as advanced age and female gender have previously been shown to be significantly associated with survival outcomes in patients treated with RC and LND [4, 76, 124, 126, 131, 194, 201]. Moreover, a recent study has found these factors to predict cancer-specific mortality even after disease recurrence [195]. That said, it seems

reasonable that the more biologically aggressive the disease, the faster the disease may recur.

Pathologic stage and nodal status are still the most well established independent predictors for outcomes [202, 203]. Notably, these factors cannot only help in outcome prediction after RC, but should also be taken into consideration for decision-making in regards of patient counseling and risk stratification after disease recurrence. Unfortunately, most studies investigating metastatic UC patients [204–207], fail to evaluate pathologic factors and/or are unable to assess time to disease recurrence. They are inherent to the multicenter and retrospective design including a lack of data regarding a possible delay between diagnosis and surgery due to patient preferences and comorbidities.

9.4.2 Prediction Tools

Bajorin et al. reported that two risk factors, a poor Karnofsky performance status (KPS) and the presence of visceral metastases (Bajorin criteria), can stratify patients with non-resectable or metastatic urothelial carcinoma into separate risk groups with regards to overall mortality [204]. This and other studies [96, 205] suggest that comorbidities are important and should be taken into account for predicting survival in both localized and metastatic UCB. Recent studies confirmed that not only the presence, but the number [199, 200] and location [199] of visceral metastasis can predict outcomes in patients who experienced disease recurrence after RC.

Though the Bajorin risk grouping has been validated in the setting of prospective randomized trials [205, 206], since then in 1999, this risk stratification has been the only prediction model available for patients with metastatic UCB. In addition, Bajorin et al.'s and the following studies included a selected group of patients who were eligible for inclusion in these trials (i.e., receiving chemotherapy), possibly introducing a selection bias. Moreover, the patients included in these studies present a heterogeneous cohort with unresectable and/or metastatic UC at presentation of both the lower and upper urinary tract.

Recently, Apolo et al. developed a model that predicts overall survival in 308 metastatic UC patients receiving a cisplatin-based chemotherapy on seven prospective phase II trials and compared this model with the Bajorin risk model [207]. The final model included four variables, namely the presence of visceral metastases, KPS, albumin, and hemoglobin. Comparison of both models to the patient cohort resulted in a favorable discrimination for the new developed model with four variables (c-index: 0.67 vs. 0.63). The objective of the developed nomogram was to predict the 1-, 2-, and 5-year overall survival and to improve accuracy over the prognostic MSKCC (Bajorin) prediction model. That said, the two additional markers are controversially discussed. Hypoalbuminemia is controversial due to its long half-time and the potential impact of systemic factors such as inflammation and stress on serum albumin [103]. However, preoperative albumin is associated with a higher risk of overall survival in UCB patients after RC [104]. Though anemia is a variable associated with cancer-specific survival [208], hemoglobin levels of cancer patients may be confounded by administration of blood transfusions or erythropoietin substitution [209]. However, the authors could not control for these factors due to the study's retrospective character. Galsky et al. recently published a similar pretreatment nomogram based on 399 UC patients who received a first-line cisplatin-based chemotherapy [210]. However, in both studies, all patients were receiving a cisplatin-based chemotherapy and had a larger burden of metastasis compared to our study.

Nakagawa et al. have recently developed a risk model to predict survival in patients with disease recurrence after RC which was based on four factors: time to recurrence, symptoms of recurrence, number of metastatic organs, and CRP level. However, this study was clearly limited by its small number of patients ($n = 114$) and single-center character. The 1-year cancer-specific free survival of this cohort was 89 %, 30 %, and 12 % for patients with favorable (0–1 risk factors), intermediate (2 risk factors) and poor risk (3–4 risk factors). The clinical benefit of this risk stratification needs to be assessed using c-index and longer datasets.

References

1. Sylvester RJ, Oosterlinck W, van der Meijden AP. A single immediate postoperative instillation of chemotherapy decreases the risk of recurrence in patients with stage Ta T1 bladder cancer: a meta-analysis of published results of randomized clinical trials. J Urol. 2004;171(6 Pt 1):2186–90. quiz 2435.
2. Meeks JJ, Bellmunt J, Bochner BH, Clarke NW, Daneshmand S, Galsky MD, Hahn NM, Lerner SP, Mason M, Powles T, et al. A systematic review of neoadjuvant and adjuvant chemotherapy for muscle-invasive bladder cancer. Eur Urol. 2012;62(3): 523–33.
3. Edge SB, Compton CC. The American Joint Committee on Cancer: the 7th edition of the AJCC cancer staging manual and the future of TNM. Ann Surg Oncol. 2010;17(6):1471–4.
4. Bochner BH, Kattan MW, Vora KC. Postoperative nomogram predicting risk of recurrence after radical cystectomy for bladder cancer. J Clin Oncol. 2006;24(24):3967–72.
5. Karakiewicz PI, Shariat SF, Palapattu GS, Gilad AE, Lotan Y, Rogers CG, Vazina A, Gupta A, Bastian PJ, Perrotte P, et al. Nomogram for predicting disease recurrence after radical cystectomy for transitional cell carcinoma of the bladder. J Urol. 2006;176(4 Pt 1):1354–61. discussion 1361–1352.
6. Shariat SF, Karakiewicz PI, Palapattu GS, Amiel GE, Lotan Y, Rogers CG, Vazina A, Bastian PJ, Gupta A, Sagalowsky AI, et al. Nomograms provide improved accuracy for predicting survival after radical cystectomy. Clin Cancer Res. 2006;12(22): 6663–76.
7. Xylinas E, Cha EK, Sun M, Rink M, Trinh QD, Novara G, Green DA, Pycha A, Fradet Y, Daneshmand S, et al. Risk stratification of pT1-3N0 patients after radical cystectomy for adjuvant chemotherapy counselling. Br J Cancer. 2012;107(11):1826–32.
8. Shariat SF, Rink M, Ehdaie B, Xylinas E, Babjuk M, Merseburger AS, Svatek RS, Cha EK, Tagawa ST, Fajkovic H, et al. Pathologic nodal staging score for bladder cancer: a decision tool for adjuvant therapy after radical cystectomy. Eur Urol. 2013;63(2):371–8.
9. Shariat SF, Kattan MW, Vickers AJ, Karakiewicz PI, Scardino PT. Critical review of prostate cancer predictive tools. Future Oncol. 2009;5(10):1555–84.
10. Shariat SF, Capitanio U, Jeldres C, Karakiewicz PI. Can nomograms be superior to other prediction tools? BJU Int. 2009;103(4):492–5. discussion 495–497.
11. Kattan MW. Nomograms. Introduction. Semin Urol Oncol. 2002;20(2):79–81.
12. Kattan MW. J Urol. 2003;170(6 Pt 2):S6–9. discussion S10.
13. Kattan MW. Nomograms are superior to staging and risk grouping systems for identifying high-risk patients: preoperative application in prostate cancer. Curr Opin Urol. 2003;13(2):111–6.

14. Fernandez-Gomez J, Madero R, Solsona E, Unda M, Martinez-Pineiro L, Gonzalez M, Portillo J, Ojea A, Pertusa C, Rodriguez-Molina J, et al. Predicting nonmuscle invasive bladder cancer recurrence and progression in patients treated with bacillus Calmette-Guerin: the CUETO scoring model. J Urol. 2009;182(5):2195–203.

15. Kluth LA, Xylinas E, Crivelli JJ, Passoni N, Comploj E, Pycha A, Chrystal J, Sun M, Karakiewicz PI, Gontero P, et al. Obesity is associated with worse outcomes in patients with T1 high grade urothelial carcinoma of the bladder. J Urol. 2013;190(2): 480–6.

16. Saint F, Salomon L, Quintela R, Cicco A, Hoznek A, Abbou CC, Chopin DK. Do prognostic parameters of remission versus relapse after Bacillus Calmette-Guerin (BCG) immunotherapy exist? Analysis of a quarter century of literature. Eur Urol. 2003;43(4): 351–60. discussion 360–351.

17. Joudi FN, Smith BJ, O'Donnell MA, Konety BR. The impact of age on the response of patients with superficial bladder cancer to intravesical immunotherapy. J Urol. 2006;175(5):1634–9. discussion 1639–1640.

18. Herr HW. Age and outcome of superficial bladder cancer treated with bacille Calmette-Guerin therapy. Urology. 2007;70(1):65–8.

19. Shariat SF, Sfakianos JP, Droller MJ, Karakiewicz PI, Meryn S, Bochner BH. The effect of age and gender on bladder cancer: a critical review of the literature. BJU Int. 2010;105(3):300–8.

20. Rosevear HM, Lightfoot AJ, Birusingh KK, Maymi JL, Nepple KG, O'Donnell MA. Factors affecting response to bacillus Calmette-Guerin plus interferon for urothelial carcinoma in situ. J Urol. 2011;186(3): 817–23.

21. Gray PJ, Fedewa SA, Shipley WU, Efstathiou JA, Lin CC, Zietman AL, Virgo KS. Use of potentially curative therapies for muscle-invasive bladder cancer in the United States: results from the National Cancer Data Base. Eur Urol. 2013;63(5):823–9.

22. Yee DS, Ishill NM, Lowrance WT, Herr HW, Elkin EB. Ethnic differences in bladder cancer survival. Urology. 2011;78(3):544–9.

23. Puente D, Malats N, Cecchini L, Tardon A, Garcia-Closas R, Serra C, Carrato A, Sala M, Boixeda R, Dosemeci M, et al. Gender-related differences in clinical and pathological characteristics and therapy of bladder cancer. Eur Urol. 2003;43(1):53–62.

24. Kluth LA, Fajkovic H, Xylinas E, Crivelli JJ, Passoni N, Roupret M, Becker A, Comploj E, Pycha A, Holmang S, et al. Female gender is associated with higher risk of disease recurrence in patients with primary T1 high-grade urothelial carcinoma of the bladder. World J Urol. 2013;31(5):1029–36.

25. Sylvester RJ, van der Meijden AP, Oosterlinck W, Witjes JA, Bouffioux C, Denis L, Newling DW, Kurth K. Predicting recurrence and progression in individual patients with stage Ta T1 bladder cancer using EORTC risk tables: a combined analysis of 2596 patients from seven EORTC trials. Eur Urol. 2006;49(3):466–75. discussion 475–467.

26. Palou J, Sylvester RJ, Faba OR, Parada R, Pena JA, Algaba F, Villavicencio H. Female gender and carcinoma in situ in the prostatic urethra are prognostic factors for recurrence, progression, and disease-specific mortality in T1G3 bladder cancer patients treated with bacillus Calmette-Guerin. Eur Urol. 2012;62(1):118–25.

27. Freedman ND, Silverman DT, Hollenbeck AR, Schatzkin A, Abnet CC. Association between smoking and risk of bladder cancer among men and women. JAMA. 2011;306(7):737–45.

28. Lammers RJ, Witjes WP, Hendricksen K, Caris CT, Janzing-Pastors MH, Witjes JA. Smoking status is a risk factor for recurrence after transurethral resection of non-muscle-invasive bladder cancer. Eur Urol. 2011;60(4):713–20.

29. Rink M, Xylinas E, Babjuk M, Pycha A, Karakiewicz PI, Novara G, Dahlem R, Shariat SF. Smoking reduces the efficacy of intravesical bacillus Calmette-Guerin immunotherapy in non-muscle-invasive bladder cancer. Eur Urol. 2012;62(6):1204–6.

30. Rink M, Furberg H, Zabor EC, Xylinas E, Babjuk M, Pycha A, Lotan Y, Karakiewicz PI, Novara G, Robinson BD, et al. Impact of smoking and smoking cessation on oncologic outcomes in primary non-muscle-invasive bladder cancer. Eur Urol. 2013;63(4):724–32.

31. Rink M, Xylinas E, Babjuk M, Hansen J, Pycha A, Comploj E, Lotan Y, Sun M, Karakiewicz PI, Abdennabi J, et al. Impact of smoking on outcomes of patients with a history of recurrent nonmuscle invasive bladder cancer. J Urol. 2012;188(6): 2120–7.

32. Martinez-Pineiro JA, Flores N, Isorna S, Solsona E, Sebastian JL, Pertusa C, Rioja LA, Martinez-Pineiro L, Vela R, Camacho JE, et al. Long-term follow-up of a randomized prospective trial comparing a standard 81 mg dose of intravesical bacille Calmette-Guerin with a reduced dose of 27 mg in superficial bladder cancer. BJU Int. 2002;89(7):671–80.

33. Alkhateeb SS, Van Rhijn BW, Finelli A, van der Kwast T, Evans A, Hanna S, Vajpeyi R, Fleshner NE, Jewett MA, Zlotta AR. Nonprimary pT1 nonmuscle invasive bladder cancer treated with bacillus Calmette-Guerin is associated with higher risk of progression compared to primary T1 tumors. J Urol. 2010;184(1):81–6.

34. Thomas F, Noon AP, Rubin N, Goepel JR, Catto JW. Comparative outcomes of primary, recurrent, and progressive high-risk non-muscle-invasive bladder cancer. Eur Urol. 2013;63(1):145–54.

35. Lerner SP, Tangen CM, Sucharew H, Wood D, Crawford ED. Failure to achieve a complete response to induction BCG therapy is associated with increased risk of disease worsening and death in patients with high risk non-muscle invasive bladder cancer. Urol Oncol. 2009;27(2):155–9.

36. Denzinger S, Otto W, Fritsche HM, Roessler W, Wieland WF, Hartmann A, Burger M. Bladder sparing approach for initial T1G3 bladder cancer: do multifocality, size of tumor or concomitant carcinoma in situ matter? A long-term analysis of 132 patients. Int J Urol. 2007;14(11):995–9. discussion 999.

37. Fernandez-Gomez J, Solsona E, Unda M, Martinez-Pineiro L, Gonzalez M, Hernandez R, Madero R, Ojea A, Pertusa C, Rodriguez-Molina J, et al. Prognostic factors in patients with non-muscle-invasive bladder cancer treated with bacillus Calmette-Guerin: multivariate analysis of data from four randomized CUETO trials. Eur Urol. 2008; 53(5):992–1001.

38. Amin MB, McKenney JK, Paner GP, Hansel DE, Grignon DJ, Montironi R, Lin O, Jorda M, Jenkins LC, Soloway M, et al. ICUD-EAU International Consultation on Bladder Cancer 2012: pathology. Eur Urol. 2013;63(1):16–35.

39. Chang WC, Chang YH, Pan CC. Prognostic significance in substaging of T1 urinary bladder urothelial carcinoma on transurethral resection. Am J Surg Pathol. 2012;36(3):454–61.

40. Orsola A, Trias I, Raventos CX, Espanol I, Cecchini L, Bucar S, Salinas D, Orsola I. Initial high-grade T1 urothelial cell carcinoma: feasibility and prognostic significance of lamina propria invasion microstaging (T1a/b/c) in BCG-treated and BCG-non-treated patients. Eur Urol. 2005;48(2):231–8. discussion 238.

41. van Rhijn BW, van der Kwast TH, Alkhateeb SS, Fleshner NE, van Leenders GJ, Bostrom PJ, van der Aa MN, Kakiashvili DM, Bangma CH, Jewett MA, et al. A new and highly prognostic system to discern T1 bladder cancer substage. Eur Urol. 2012;61(2): 378–84.

42. Pan CC, Chang YH, Chen KK, Yu HJ, Sun CH, Ho DM. Prognostic significance of the 2004 WHO/ISUP classification for prediction of recurrence, progression, and cancer-specific mortality of non-muscle-invasive urothelial tumors of the urinary bladder: a clinicopathologic study of 1,515 cases. Am J Clin Pathol. 2010;133(5):788–95.

43. Burger M, van der Aa MN, van Oers JM, Brinkmann A, van der Kwast TH, Steyerberg EC, Stoehr R, Kirkels WJ, Denzinger S, Wild PJ, et al. Prediction of progression of non-muscle-invasive bladder cancer by WHO 1973 and 2004 grading and by FGFR3 mutation status: a prospective study. Eur Urol. 2008;54(4):835–43.

44. MacLennan GT, Kirkali Z, Cheng L. Histologic grading of noninvasive papillary urothelial neoplasms. Eur Urol. 2007;51(4):889–97. discussion 897–888.

45. May M, Brookman-Amissah S, Roigas J, Hartmann A, Storkel S, Kristiansen G, Gilfrich C, Borchardt R, Hoschke B, Kaufmann O, et al. Prognostic accuracy of individual uropathologists in noninvasive urinary bladder carcinoma: a multicentre study comparing the 1973 and 2004 World Health Organisation classifications. Eur Urol. 2010;57(5):850–8.

46. van Rhijn BW, van Leenders GJ, Ooms BC, Kirkels WJ, Zlotta AR, Boeve ER, Jobsis AC, van der Kwast TH. The pathologist's mean grade is constant and individualizes the prognostic value of bladder cancer grading. Eur Urol. 2010;57(6):1052–7.

47. Lopez-Beltran A, Montironi R. Non-invasive urothelial neoplasms: according to the most recent WHO classification. Eur Urol. 2004;46(2):170–6.

48. Babjuk M, Oosterlinck W, Sylvester R, Kaasinen E, Bohle A, Palou-Redorta J. EAU guidelines on non-muscle-invasive urothelial carcinoma of the bladder. Eur Urol. 2008;54(2):303–14.

49. Kakiashvili DM, van Rhijn BW, Trottier G, Jewett MA, Fleshner NE, Finelli A, Azuero J, Bangma CH, Vajpeyi R, Alkhateeb S, et al. Long-term follow-up of T1 high-grade bladder cancer after intravesical bacille Calmette-Guerin treatment. BJU Int. 2011;107(4):540–6.

50. Lamm DL, Blumenstein BA, Crissman JD, Montie JE, Gottesman JE, Lowe BA, Sarosdy MF, Bohl RD, Grossman HB, Beck TM, et al. Maintenance bacillus Calmette-Guerin immunotherapy for recurrent TA, T1 and carcinoma in situ transitional cell carcinoma of the bladder: a randomized Southwest Oncology Group Study. J Urol. 2000;163(4):1124–9.

51. Kunju LP, You L, Zhang Y, Daignault S, Montie JE, Lee CT. Lymphovascular invasion of urothelial cancer in matched transurethral bladder tumor resection and radical cystectomy specimens. J Urol. 2008;180(5):1928–32. discussion 1932.

52. Cho KS, Seo HK, Joung JY, Park WS, Ro JY, Han KS, Chung J, Lee KH. Lymphovascular invasion in transurethral resection specimens as predictor of progression and metastasis in patients with newly diagnosed T1 bladder urothelial cancer. J Urol. 2009;182(6):2625–30.

53. Streeper NM, Simons CM, Konety BR, Muirhead DM, Williams RD, O'Donnell MA, Joudi FN. The significance of lymphovascular invasion in transurethral resection of bladder tumour and cystectomy specimens on the survival of patients with urothelial bladder cancer. BJU Int. 2009;103(4):475–9.

54. Resnick MJ, Bergey M, Magerfleisch L, Tomaszewski JE, Malkowicz SB, Guzzo TJ. Longitudinal evaluation of the concordance and prognostic value of lymphovascular invasion in transurethral resection and radical cystectomy specimens. BJU Int. 2011;107(1):46–52.

55. Green DA, Rink M, Hansen J, Cha EK, Robinson B, Tian Z, Chun FK, Tagawa S, Karakiewicz PI, Fisch M, et al. Accurate preoperative prediction of non-organ-confined bladder urothelial carcinoma at cystectomy. BJU Int. 2013;111(3):404–11.

56. Kamat AM, Gee JR, Dinney CP, Grossman HB, Swanson DA, Millikan RE, Detry MA, Robinson TL, Pisters LL. The case for early cystectomy in the

treatment of nonmuscle invasive micropapillary bladder carcinoma. J Urol. 2006;175(3 Pt 1):881–5.

57. Amin A, Epstein JI. Noninvasive micropapillary urothelial carcinoma: a clinicopathologic study of 18 cases. Hum Pathol. 2012;43(12):2124–8.

58. Gaya JM, Palou J, Algaba F, Arce J, Rodriguez-Faba O, Villavicencio H. The case for conservative management in the treatment of patients with non-muscle-invasive micropapillary bladder carcinoma without carcinoma in situ. Can J Urol. 2010;17(5): 5370–6.

59. Chang SS, Hassan JM, Cookson MS, Wells N, Smith Jr JA. Delaying radical cystectomy for muscle invasive bladder cancer results in worse pathological stage. J Urol. 2003;170(4 Pt 1):1085–7.

60. Lee CT, Madii R, Daignault S, Dunn RL, Zhang Y, Montie JE, Wood Jr DP. Cystectomy delay more than 3 months from initial bladder cancer diagnosis results in decreased disease specific and overall survival. J Urol. 2006;175(4):1262–7. discussion 1267.

61. Nielsen ME, Palapattu GS, Karakiewicz PI, Lotan Y, Bastian PJ, Lerner SP, Sagalowsky AI, Schoenberg MP, Shariat SF. A delay in radical cystectomy of >3 months is not associated with a worse clinical outcome. BJU Int. 2007;100(5):1015–20.

62. Hautmann RE, Paiss T. Does the option of the ileal neobladder stimulate patient and physician decision toward earlier cystectomy? J Urol. 1998;159(6): 1845–50.

63. Millan-Rodriguez F, Chechile-Toniolo G, Salvador-Bayarri J, Palou J, Algaba F, Vicente-Rodriguez J. Primary superficial bladder cancer risk groups according to progression, mortality and recurrence. J Urol. 2000;164(3 Pt 1):680–4.

64. Fernandez-Gomez J, Madero R, Solsona E, Unda M, Martinez-Pineiro L, Ojea A, Portillo J, Montesinos M, Gonzalez M, Pertusa C, et al. The EORTC tables overestimate the risk of recurrence and progression in patients with non-muscle-invasive bladder cancer treated with bacillus Calmette-Guerin: external validation of the EORTC risk tables. Eur Urol. 2011;60(3):423–30.

65. Hernandez V, De La Pena E, Martin MD, Blazquez C, Diaz FJ, Llorente C. External validation and applicability of the EORTC risk tables for non-muscle-invasive bladder cancer. World J Urol. 2011;29(4):409–14.

66. Xylinas E, Kent M, Kluth L, Pycha A, Comploj E, Svatek RS, Lotan Y, Trinh QD, Karakiewicz PI, Holmang S, et al. Accuracy of the EORTC risk tables and of the CUETO scoring model to predict outcomes in non-muscle-invasive urothelial carcinoma of the bladder. Br J Cancer. 2013;109(6): 1460–6.

67. Shariat SF, Zippe C, Ludecke G, Boman H, Sanchez-Carbayo M, Casella R, Mian C, Friedrich MG, Eissa S, Akaza H, et al. Nomograms including nuclear matrix protein 22 for prediction of disease recurrence and progression in patients with Ta, T1 or CIS transitional cell carcinoma of the bladder. J Urol. 2005;173(5):1518–25.

68. Shariat SF, Palapattu GS, Karakiewicz PI, Rogers CG, Vazina A, Bastian PJ, Schoenberg MP, Lerner SP, Sagalowsky AI, Lotan Y. Discrepancy between clinical and pathologic stage: impact on prognosis after radical cystectomy. Eur Urol. 2007;51(1):137–49. discussion 149–151.

69. Karakiewicz PI, Shariat SF, Palapattu GS, Perrotte P, Lotan Y, Rogers CG, Amiel GE, Vazina A, Gupta A, Bastian PJ, et al. Precystectomy nomogram for prediction of advanced bladder cancer stage. Eur Urol. 2006;50(6):1254–60. discussion 1261–1252.

70. Shariat SF, Ehdaie B, Rink M, Cha EK, Svatek RS, Chromecki TF, Fajkovic H, Novara G, David SG, Daneshmand S, et al. Clinical nodal staging scores for bladder cancer: a proposal for preoperative risk assessment. Eur Urol. 2012;61(2):237–42.

71. Shariat SF, Karam JA, Lerner SP. Molecular markers in bladder cancer. Curr Opin Urol. 2008;18(1):1–8.

72. Soulie M, Straub M, Game X, Seguin P, De Petriconi R, Plante P, Hautmann RE. A multicenter study of the morbidity of radical cystectomy in select elderly patients with bladder cancer. J Urol. 2002;167(3): 1325–8.

73. Chang SS, Alberts G, Cookson MS, Smith Jr JA. Radical cystectomy is safe in elderly patients at high risk. J Urol. 2001;166(3):938–41.

74. Thrasher JB, Frazier HA, Robertson JE, Dodge RK, Paulson DF. Clinical variables which serve as predictors of cancer-specific survival among patients treated with radical cystectomy for transitional cell carcinoma of the bladder and prostate. Cancer. 1994;73(6):1708–15.

75. Clark PE, Stein JP, Groshen SG, Cai J, Miranda G, Lieskovsky G, Skinner DG. Radical cystectomy in the elderly: comparison of survival between younger and older patients. Cancer. 2005;103(3):546–52.

76. Fajkovic H, Halpern JA, Cha EK, Bahadori A, Chromecki TF, Karakiewicz PI, Breinl E, Merseburger AS, Shariat SF. Impact of gender on bladder cancer incidence, staging, and prognosis. World J Urol. 2011;29(4):457–63.

77. Boorjian SA, Zhu F, Herr HW. The effect of gender on response to bacillus Calmette-Guerin therapy for patients with non-muscle-invasive urothelial carcinoma of the bladder. BJU Int. 2010;106(3):357–61.

78. McGrath M, Michaud DS, De Vivo I. Hormonal and reproductive factors and the risk of bladder cancer in women. Am J Epidemiol. 2006;163(3):236–44.

79. Donsky H, Coyle S, Scosyrev E, Messing EM. Sex differences in incidence and mortality of bladder and kidney cancers: national estimates from 49 countries. Urol Oncol. 2014;32(1):40.e23–31.

80. Scosyrev E, Golijanin D, Wu G, Messing E. The burden of bladder cancer in men and women: analysis of the years of life lost. BJU Int. 2012;109(1):57–62.

81. Shen SS, Smith CL, Hsieh JT, Yu J, Kim IY, Jian W, Sonpavde G, Ayala GE, Younes M, Lerner SP. Expression of estrogen receptors-alpha and -beta in bladder cancer cell lines and human bladder tumor tissue. Cancer. 2006;106(12):2610–6.

82. Boorjian S, Ugras S, Mongan NP, Gudas LJ, You X, Tickoo SK, Scherr DS. Androgen receptor expression is inversely correlated with pathologic tumor stage in bladder cancer. Urology. 2004;64(2):383–8.

83. May M, Bastian PJ, Brookman-May S, Fritsche HM, Tilki D, Otto W, Bolenz C, Gilfrich C, Trojan L, Herrmann E, et al. Gender-specific differences in cancer-specific survival after radical cystectomy for patients with urothelial carcinoma of the urinary bladder in pathologic tumor stage T4a. Urol Oncol. 2013;31(7):1141–7.

84. Otto W, May M, Fritsche HM, Dragun D, Aziz A, Gierth M, Trojan L, Herrmann E, Moritz R, Ellinger J, et al. Analysis of sex differences in cancer-specific survival and perioperative mortality following radical cystectomy: results of a large German multicenter study of nearly 2500 patients with urothelial carcinoma of the bladder. Gend Med. 2012;9(6):481–9.

85. Zhuang YH, Blauer M, Tammela T, Tuohimaa P. Immunodetection of androgen receptor in human urinary bladder cancer. Histopathology. 1997;30(6): 556–62.

86. Siegrist T, Savage C, Shabsigh A, Cronin A, Donat SM. Analysis of gender differences in early perioperative complications following radical cystectomy at a tertiary cancer center using a standardized reporting methodology. Urol Oncol. 2010;28(1):112–7.

87. Liberman D, Lughezzani G, Sun M, Alasker A, Thuret R, Abdollah F, Budaus L, Widmer H, Graefen M, Montorsi F, et al. Perioperative mortality is significantly greater in septuagenarian and octogenarian patients treated with radical cystectomy for urothelial carcinoma of the bladder. Urology. 2011;77(3):660–6.

88. Taub DA, Hollenbeck BK, Cooper KL, Dunn RL, Miller DC, Taylor JM, Wei JT. Racial disparities in resource utilization for cystectomy. Urology. 2006;67(2):288–93.

89. Mungan NA, Kiemeney LA, van Dijck JA, van der Poel HG, Witjes JA. Gender differences in stage distribution of bladder cancer. Urology. 2000;55(3): 368–71.

90. Johnson EK, Daignault S, Zhang Y, Lee CT. Patterns of hematuria referral to urologists: does a gender disparity exist? Urology. 2008;72(3):498–502. discussion 502–493.

91. Kiemeney LA, Coebergh JW, Koper NP, van der Heijden LH, Pauwels RP, Schapers RF, Verbeek AL. Bladder cancer incidence and survival in the south-eastern part of The Netherlands, 1975–1989. Eur J Cancer. 1994;30A(8):1134–7.

92. Micheli A, Mariotto A, Giorgi Rossi A, Gatta G, Muti P. The prognostic role of gender in survival of adult cancer patients. EUROCARE Working Group. Eur J Cancer. 1998;34(14 Spec No):2271–8.

93. Mungan NA, Aben KK, Schoenberg MP, Visser O, Coebergh JW, Witjes JA, Kiemeney LA. Gender differences in stage-adjusted bladder cancer survival. Urology. 2000;55(6):876–80.

94. Fleshner NE, Herr HW, Stewart AK, Murphy GP, Mettlin C, Menck HR. The National Cancer Data Base report on bladder carcinoma. The American College of Surgeons Commission on Cancer and the American Cancer Society. Cancer. 1996;78(7):1505–13.

95. Boorjian SA, Kim SP, Tollefson MK, Carrasco A, Cheville JC, Thompson RH, Thapa P, Frank I. Comparative performance of comorbidity indices for estimating perioperative and 5-year all cause mortality following radical cystectomy for bladder cancer. J Urol. 2013;190(1):55–60.

96. Mayr R, May M, Martini T, Lodde M, Comploj E, Pycha A, Strobel J, Denzinger S, Otto W, Wieland W, et al. Comorbidity and performance indices as predictors of cancer-independent mortality but not of cancer-specific mortality after radical cystectomy for urothelial carcinoma of the bladder. Eur Urol. 2012;62(4):662–70.

97. Gakis G, Todenhofer T, Renninger M, Schilling D, Sievert KD, Schwentner C, Stenzl A. Development of a new outcome prediction model in carcinoma invading the bladder based on preoperative serum C-reactive protein and standard pathological risk factors: the TNR-C score. BJU Int. 2011;108(11):1800–5.

98. Trichopoulos D, Psaltopoulou T, Orfanos P, Trichopoulou A, Boffetta P. Plasma C-reactive protein and risk of cancer: a prospective study from Greece. Cancer Epidemiol Biomarkers Prev. 2006;15(2):381–4.

99. Yoshida S, Saito K, Koga F, Yokoyama M, Kageyama Y, Masuda H, Kobayashi T, Kawakami S, Kihara K. C-reactive protein level predicts prognosis in patients with muscle-invasive bladder cancer treated with chemoradiotherapy. BJU Int. 2008;101(8): 978–81.

100. Ripamonti CI, Farina G, Garassino MC. Predictive models in palliative care. Cancer. 2009;115(13 Suppl):3128–34.

101. Inoue K, Kohashikawa K, Suzuki S, Shimada M, Yoshida H. Prognostic significance of thrombocytosis in renal cell carcinoma patients. Int J Urol. 2004;11(6):364–7.

102. Todenhofer T, Renninger M, Schwentner C, Stenzl A, Gakis G. A new prognostic model for cancer-specific survival after radical cystectomy including pretreatment thrombocytosis and standard pathological risk factors. BJU Int. 2012;110(11 Pt B): E533–40.

103. Gibbs J, Cull W, Henderson W, Daley J, Hur K, Khuri SF. Preoperative serum albumin level as a predictor of operative mortality and morbidity: results from the National VA Surgical Risk Study. Arch Surg. 1999;134(1):36–42.

104. Gregg JR, Cookson MS, Phillips S, Salem S, Chang SS, Clark PE, Davis R, Stimson Jr CJ, Aghazadeh

M, Smith Jr JA, et al. Effect of preoperative nutritional deficiency on mortality after radical cystectomy for bladder cancer. J Urol. 2011;185(1):90–6.

105. Chromecki TF, Cha EK, Fajkovic H, Rink M, Ehdaie B, Svatek RS, Karakiewicz PI, Lotan Y, Tilki D, Bastian PJ, et al. Obesity is associated with worse oncological outcomes in patients treated with radical cystectomy. BJU Int. 2013;111(2):249–55.

106. Hafron J, Mitra N, Dalbagni G, Bochner B, Herr H, Donat SM. Does body mass index affect survival of patients undergoing radical or partial cystectomy for bladder cancer? J Urol. 2005;173(5):1513–7.

107. Rink M, Zabor EC, Furberg H, Xylinas E, Ehdaie B, Novara G, Babjuk M, Pycha A, Lotan Y, Trinh QD, et al. Impact of smoking and smoking cessation on outcomes in bladder cancer patients treated with radical cystectomy. Eur Urol. 2013;64(3):456–64.

108. Sturgeon SR, Hartge P, Silverman DT, Kantor AF, Linehan WM, Lynch C, Hoover RN. Associations between bladder cancer risk factors and tumor stage and grade at diagnosis. Epidemiology. 1994;5(2):218–25.

109. Jiang X, Castelao JE, Yuan JM, Stern MC, Conti DV, Cortessis VK, Pike MC, Gago-Dominguez M. Cigarette smoking and subtypes of bladder cancer. Int J Cancer. 2012;130(4):896–901.

110. Chen CH, Shun CT, Huang KH, Huang CY, Tsai YC, Yu HJ, Pu YS. Stopping smoking might reduce tumour recurrence in nonmuscle-invasive bladder cancer. BJU Int. 2007;100(2):281–6. discussion 286.

111. Roth B, Wissmeyer MP, Zehnder P, Birkhauser FD, Thalmann GN, Krause TM, Studer UE. A new multimodality technique accurately maps the primary lymphatic landing sites of the bladder. Eur Urol. 2010;57(2):205–11.

112. Jensen JB, Ulhoi BP, Jensen KM. Lymph node mapping in patients with bladder cancer undergoing radical cystectomy and lymph node dissection to the level of the inferior mesenteric artery. BJU Int. 2010;106(2):199–205.

113. Leissner J, Ghoneim MA, Abol-Enein H, Thuroff JW, Franzaring L, Fisch M, Schulze H, Managadze G, Allhoff EP, Managadze G, el-Baz MA, et al. Extended radical lymphadenectomy in patients with urothelial bladder cancer: results of a prospective multicenter study. J Urol. 2004;171(1):139–44.

114. Wright JL, Lin DW, Porter MP. The association between extent of lymphadenectomy and survival among patients with lymph node metastases undergoing radical cystectomy. Cancer. 2008;112(11):2401–8.

115. May M, Herrmann E, Bolenz C, Brookman-May S, Tiemann A, Moritz R, Fritsche HM, Burger M, Trojan L, Michel MS, et al. Association between the number of dissected lymph nodes during pelvic lymphadenectomy and cancer-specific survival in patients with lymph node-negative urothelial carcinoma of the bladder undergoing radical cystectomy. Ann Surg Oncol. 2011;18(7):2018–25.

116. Stein JP. The role of lymphadenectomy in patients undergoing radical cystectomy for bladder cancer. Curr Oncol Rep. 2007;9(3):213–21.

117. Herr HW, Faulkner JR, Grossman HB, Natale RB, deVere White R, Sarosdy MF, Crawford ED. Surgical factors influence bladder cancer outcomes: a cooperative group report. J Clin Oncol. 2004;22(14):2781–9.

118. Poulsen AL, Horn T, Steven K. Radical cystectomy: extending the limits of pelvic lymph node dissection improves survival for patients with bladder cancer confined to the bladder wall. J Urol. 1998;160(6 Pt 1):2015–9. discussion 2020.

119. Herr HW, Bochner BH, Dalbagni G, Donat SM, Reuter VE, Bajorin DF. Impact of the number of lymph nodes retrieved on outcome in patients with muscle invasive bladder cancer. J Urol. 2002;167(3):1295–8.

120. Lerner SP, Skinner DG, Lieskovsky G, Boyd SD, Groshen SL, Ziogas A, Skinner E, Nichols P, Hopwood B. The rationale for en bloc pelvic lymph node dissection for bladder cancer patients with nodal metastases: long-term results. J Urol. 1993;149(4):758–64. discussion 764–755.

121. Koppie TM, Vickers AJ, Vora K, Dalbagni G, Bochner BH. Standardization of pelvic lymphadenectomy performed at radical cystectomy: can we establish a minimum number of lymph nodes that should be removed? Cancer. 2006;107(10):2368–74.

122. Zehnder P, Studer UE, Skinner EC, Dorin RP, Cai J, Roth B, Miranda G, Birkhauser F, Stein J, Burkhard FC, et al. Super extended versus extended pelvic lymph node dissection in patients undergoing radical cystectomy for bladder cancer: a comparative study. J Urol. 2011;186(4):1261–8.

123. Konety BR, Joslyn SA, O'Donnell MA. Extent of pelvic lymphadenectomy and its impact on outcome in patients diagnosed with bladder cancer: analysis of data from the Surveillance, Epidemiology and End Results Program data base. J Urol. 2003;169(3):946–50.

124. Stein JP, Lieskovsky G, Cote R, Groshen S, Feng AC, Boyd S, Skinner E, Bochner B, Thangathurai D, Mikhail M, et al. Radical cystectomy in the treatment of invasive bladder cancer: long-term results in 1,054 patients. J Clin Oncol. 2001;19(3):666–75.

125. Rink M, Shariat SF, Xylinas E, Fitzgerald JP, Hansen J, Green DA, Kamat AM, Novara G, Daneshmand S, Fradet Y, et al. Does increasing the nodal yield improve outcomes in patients without nodal metastasis at radical cystectomy? World J Urol. 2012;30(6):807–14.

126. Shariat SF, Karakiewicz PI, Palapattu GS, Lotan Y, Rogers CG, Amiel GE, Vazina A, Gupta A, Bastian PJ, Sagalowsky AI, et al. Outcomes of radical cystectomy for transitional cell carcinoma of the bladder: a contemporary series from the Bladder Cancer Research Consortium. J Urol. 2006;176(6 Pt 1):2414–22. discussion 2422.

127. Epstein JI, Amin MB, Reuter VR, Mostofi FK. The World Health Organization/International Society of Urological Pathology consensus classification of urothelial (transitional cell) neoplasms of the urinary

bladder. Bladder Consensus Conference Committee. Am J Surg Pathol. 1998;22(12):1435–48.

128. Kirkali Z, Chan T, Manoharan M, Algaba F, Busch C, Cheng L, Kiemeney L, Kriegmair M, Montironi R, Murphy WM, et al. Bladder cancer: epidemiology, staging and grading, and diagnosis. Urology. 2005;66(6 Suppl 1):4–34.

129. Tarin TV, Power NE, Ehdaie B, Sfakianos JP, Silberstein JL, Savage CJ, Sjoberg D, Dalbagni G, Bochner BH. Lymph node-positive bladder cancer treated with radical cystectomy and lymphadenectomy: effect of the level of node positivity. Eur Urol. 2012;61(5):1025–30.

130. Herr HW. Surgical factors in the treatment of superficial and invasive bladder cancer. Urol Clin North Am. 2005;32(2):157–64.

131. Xylinas E, Rink M, Novara G, Green DA, Clozel T, Fritsche HM, Guillonneau B, Lotan Y, Kassouf W, Tilki D, et al. Predictors of survival in patients with soft tissue surgical margin involvement at radical cystectomy. Ann Surg Oncol. 2013;20(3):1027–34.

132. Fung CY, Shipley WU, Young RH, Griffin PP, Convery KM, Kaufman DS, Althausen AF, Heney NM, Prout Jr GR. Prognostic factors in invasive bladder carcinoma in a prospective trial of preoperative adjuvant chemotherapy and radiotherapy. J Clin Oncol. 1991;9(9):1533–42.

133. Cheng L, Weaver AL, Leibovich BC, Ramnani DM, Neumann RM, Scherer BG, Nehra A, Zincke H, Bostwick DG. Predicting the survival of bladder carcinoma patients treated with radical cystectomy. Cancer. 2000;88(10):2326–32.

134. Alitalo K, Mohla S, Ruoslahti E. Lymphangiogenesis and cancer: meeting report. Cancer Res. 2004; 64(24):9225–9.

135. Padera TP, Kadambi A, di Tomaso E, Carreira CM, Brown EB, Boucher Y, Choi NC, Mathisen D, Wain J, Mark EJ, et al. Lymphatic metastasis in the absence of functional intratumor lymphatics. Science. 2002;296(5574):1883–6.

136. Algaba F. Lymphovascular invasion as a prognostic tool for advanced bladder cancer. Curr Opin Urol. 2006;16(5):367–71.

137. Shariat SF, Svatek RS, Tilki D, Skinner E, Karakiewicz PI, Capitanio U, Bastian PJ, Volkmer BG, Kassouf W, Novara G, et al. International validation of the prognostic value of lymphovascular invasion in patients treated with radical cystectomy. BJU Int. 2010;105(10):1402–12.

138. Fritsche HM, May M, Denzinger S, Otto W, Siegert S, Giedl C, Giedl J, Eder F, Agaimy A, Novotny V, et al. Prognostic value of perinodal lymphovascular invasion following radical cystectomy for lymph node-positive urothelial carcinoma. Eur Urol. 2013; 63(4):739–44.

139. Lotan Y, Gupta A, Shariat SF, Palapattu GS, Vazina A, Karakiewicz PI, Bastian PJ, Rogers CG, Amiel G, Perotte P, et al. Lymphovascular invasion is independently associated with overall survival, cause-specific survival, and local and distant recurrence in patients with negative lymph nodes at radical cystectomy. J Clin Oncol. 2005;23(27):6533–9.

140. Tilki D, Shariat SF, Lotan Y, Rink M, Karakiewicz PI, Schoenberg MP, Lerner SP, Sonpavde G, Sagalowsky AI, Gupta A. Lymphovascular invasion is independently associated with bladder cancer recurrence and survival in patients with final stage T1 disease and negative lymph nodes after radical cystectomy. BJU Int. 2013;111(8):1215–21.

141. Quek ML, Stein JP, Nichols PW, Cai J, Miranda G, Groshen S, Daneshmand S, Skinner EC, Skinner DG. Prognostic significance of lymphovascular invasion of bladder cancer treated with radical cystectomy. J Urol. 2005;174(1):103–6.

142. Rogers CG, Palapattu GS, Shariat SF, Karakiewicz PI, Bastian PJ, Lotan Y, Gupta A, Vazina A, Gilad A, Sagalowsky AI, et al. Clinical outcomes following radical cystectomy for primary nontransitional cell carcinoma of the bladder compared to transitional cell carcinoma of the bladder. J Urol. 2006;175(6):2048–53. discussion 2053.

143. Mitra AP, Bartsch CC, Bartsch Jr G, Miranda G, Skinner EC, Daneshmand S. Does presence of squamous and glandular differentiation in urothelial carcinoma of the bladder at cystectomy portend poor prognosis? An intensive case-control analysis. Urol Oncol. 2014;32(2):117–27.

144. Kim SP, Frank I, Cheville JC, Thompson RH, Weight CJ, Thapa P, Boorjian SA. The impact of squamous and glandular differentiation on survival after radical cystectomy for urothelial carcinoma. J Urol. 2012;188(2):405–9.

145. Xylinas E, Rink M, Robinson BD, Lotan Y, Babjuk M, Brisuda A, Green DA, Kluth LA, Pycha A, Fradet Y, et al. Impact of histological variants on oncological outcomes of patients with urothelial carcinoma of the bladder treated with radical cystectomy. Eur J Cancer. 2013;49(8):1889–97.

146. Linder BJ, Frank I, Cheville JC, Thompson RH, Thapa P, Tarrell RF, Boorjian SA. Outcomes following radical cystectomy for nested variant of urothelial carcinoma: a matched cohort analysis. J Urol. 2013;189(5):1670–5.

147. Matsushita K, Cha EK, Matsumoto K, Baba S, Chromecki TF, Fajkovic H, Sun M, Karakiewicz PI, Scherr DS, Shariat SF. Immunohistochemical biomarkers for bladder cancer prognosis. Int J Urol. 2011;18(9):616–29.

148. Vogelstein B, Lane D, Levine AJ. Surfing the p53 network. Nature. 2000;408(6810):307–10.

149. Chatterjee SJ, Datar R, Youssefzadeh D, George B, Goebell PJ, Stein JP, Young L, Shi SR, Gee C, Groshen S, et al. Combined effects of p53, p21, and pRb expression in the progression of bladder transitional cell carcinoma. J Clin Oncol. 2004;22(6): 1007–13.

150. Malats N, Bustos A, Nascimento CM, Fernandez F, Rivas M, Puente D, Kogevinas M, Real FX. P53 as a prognostic marker for bladder cancer: a meta-analysis and review. Lancet Oncol. 2005;6(9):678–86.

151. Shariat SF, Lotan Y, Karakiewicz PI, Ashfaq R, Isbarn H, Fradet Y, Bastian PJ, Nielsen ME, Capitanio U, Jeldres C, et al. p53 predictive value for pT1-2 N0 disease at radical cystectomy. J Urol. 2009;182(3):907–13.

152. Shariat SF, Tokunaga H, Zhou J, Kim J, Ayala GE, Benedict WF, Lerner SP. p53, p21, pRB, and p16 expression predict clinical outcome in cystectomy with bladder cancer. J Clin Oncol. 2004;22(6):1014–24.

153. Shariat SF, Zlotta AR, Ashfaq R, Sagalowsky AI, Lotan Y. Cooperative effect of cell-cycle regulators expression on bladder cancer development and biologic aggressiveness. Mod Pathol. 2007;20(4):445–59.

154. Shariat SF, Bolenz C, Karakiewicz PI, Fradet Y, Ashfaq R, Bastian PJ, Nielsen ME, Capitanio U, Jeldres C, Rigaud J, et al. p53 expression in patients with advanced urothelial cancer of the urinary bladder. BJU Int. 2010;105(4):489–95.

155. Shariat SF, Chade DC, Karakiewicz PI, Ashfaq R, Isbarn H, Fradet Y, Bastian PJ, Nielsen ME, Capitanio U, Jeldres C, et al. Combination of multiple molecular markers can improve prognostication in patients with locally advanced and lymph node positive bladder cancer. J Urol. 2010;183(1):68–75.

156. Neuzillet Y, Paoletti X, Ouerhani S, Mongiat-Artus P, Soliman H, de The H, Sibony M, Denoux Y, Molinie V, Herault A, et al. A meta-analysis of the relationship between FGFR3 and TP53 mutations in bladder cancer. PLoS One. 2012;7(12):e48993.

157. Stadler WM, Lerner SP, Groshen S, Stein JP, Shi SR, Raghavan D, Esrig D, Steinberg G, Wood D, Klotz L, et al. Phase III study of molecularly targeted adjuvant therapy in locally advanced urothelial cancer of the bladder based on p53 status. J Clin Oncol. 2011;29(25):3443–9.

158. Shariat SF, Bolenz C, Godoy G, Fradet Y, Ashfaq R, Karakiewicz PI, Isbarn H, Jeldres C, Rigaud J, Sagalowsky AI, et al. Predictive value of combined immunohistochemical markers in patients with pT1 urothelial carcinoma at radical cystectomy. J Urol. 2009;182(1):78–84. discussion 84.

159. Park J, Song C, Shin E, Hong JH, Kim CS, Ahn H. Do molecular biomarkers have prognostic value in primary T1G3 bladder cancer treated with bacillus Calmette-Guerin intravesical therapy? Urol Oncol. 2013;31(6):849–56.

160. Lenz P, Pfeiffer R, Baris D, Schned AR, Takikita M, Poscablo MC, Schwenn M, Johnson A, Jones M, Kida M, et al. Cell-cycle control in urothelial carcinoma: large-scale tissue array analysis of tumor tissue from Maine and Vermont. Cancer Epidemiol Biomarkers Prev. 2012;21(9):1555–64.

161. Margulis V, Shariat SF, Ashfaq R, Sagalowsky AI, Lotan Y. Ki-67 is an independent predictor of bladder cancer outcome in patients treated with radical cystectomy for organ-confined disease. Clin Cancer Res. 2006;12(24):7369–73.

162. Margulis V, Lotan Y, Karakiewicz PI, Fradet Y, Ashfaq R, Capitanio U, Montorsi F, Bastian PJ, Nielsen ME, Muller SC, et al. Multi-institutional validation of the predictive value of Ki-67 labeling index in patients with urinary bladder cancer. J Natl Cancer Inst. 2009;101(2):114–9.

163. Behnsawy HM, Miyake H, Abdalla MA, Sayed MA, Ahmed AE, Fujisawa M. Expression of cell cycle-associated proteins in non-muscle-invasive bladder cancer: correlation with intravesical recurrence following transurethral resection. Urol Oncol. 2011;29(5):495–501.

164. Harada K, Ogden GR. An overview of the cell cycle arrest protein, p21(WAF1). Oral Oncol. 2000;36(1):3–7.

165. Mitra AP, Castelao JE, Hawes D, Tsao-Wei DD, Jiang X, Shi SR, Datar RH, Skinner EC, Stein JP, Groshen S, et al. Combination of molecular alterations and smoking intensity predicts bladder cancer outcome: a report from the Los Angeles Cancer Surveillance Program. Cancer. 2013;119(4):756–65.

166. Shariat SF, Ashfaq R, Sagalowsky AI, Lotan Y. Correlation of cyclin D1 and E1 expression with bladder cancer presence, invasion, progression, and metastasis. Hum Pathol. 2006;37(12):1568–76.

167. Del Pizzo JJ, Borkowski A, Jacobs SC, Kyprianou N. Loss of cell cycle regulators p27(Kip1) and cyclin E in transitional cell carcinoma of the bladder correlates with tumor grade and patient survival. Am J Pathol. 1999;155(4):1129–36.

168. Margulis V, Lotan Y, Shariat SF. Survivin: a promising biomarker for detection and prognosis of bladder cancer. World J Urol. 2008;26(1):59–65.

169. Arai M, Sasaki A, Saito N, Nakazato Y. Immunohistochemical analysis of cleaved caspase-3 detects high level of apoptosis frequently in diffuse large B-cell lymphomas of the central nervous system. Pathol Int. 2005;55(3):122–9.

170. Burton PB, Anderson CJ, Corbishly CM. Caspase 3 and p27 as predictors of invasive bladder cancer. N Engl J Med. 2000;343(19):1418–20.

171. Giannopoulou I, Nakopoulou L, Zervas A, Lazaris AC, Stravodimos C, Giannopoulos A, Davaris PS. Immunohistochemical study of pro-apoptotic factors Bax, Fas and CPP32 in urinary bladder cancer: prognostic implications. Urol Res. 2002;30(5):342–5.

172. Karam JA, Lotan Y, Karakiewicz PI, Ashfaq R, Sagalowsky AI, Roehrborn CG, Shariat SF. Use of combined apoptosis biomarkers for prediction of bladder cancer recurrence and mortality after radical cystectomy. Lancet Oncol. 2007;8(2):128–36.

173. Altieri DC. Survivin, versatile modulation of cell division and apoptosis in cancer. Oncogene. 2003;22(53):8581–9.

174. Schultz IJ, Kiemeney LA, Karthaus HF, Witjes JA, Willems JL, Swinkels DW, Gunnewiek JM, de Kok JB. Survivin mRNA copy number in bladder washings predicts tumor recurrence in patients with superficial urothelial cell carcinomas. Clin Chem. 2004;50(8):1425–8.

175. Shariat SF, Casella R, Khoddami SM, Hernandez G, Sulser T, Gasser TC, Lerner SP. Urine detection of

survivin is a sensitive marker for the noninvasive diagnosis of bladder cancer. J Urol. 2004;171(2 Pt 1):626–30.

176. Smith SD, Wheeler MA, Plescia J, Colberg JW, Weiss RM, Alterieri DC. Urine detection of survivin and diagnosis of bladder cancer. JAMA. 2001;285(3): 324–8.

177. Shariat SF, Ashfaq R, Karakiewicz PI, Saeedi O, Sagalowsky AI, Lotan Y. Survivin expression is associated with bladder cancer presence, stage, progression, and mortality. Cancer. 2007;109(6):1106–13.

178. Shariat SF, Karakiewicz PI, Godoy G, Karam JA, Ashfaq R, Fradet Y, Isbarn H, Montorsi F, Jeldres C, Bastian PJ, et al. Survivin as a prognostic marker for urothelial carcinoma of the bladder: a multicenter external validation study. Clin Cancer Res. 2009; 15(22):7012–9.

179. Salz W, Eisenberg D, Plescia J, Garlick DS, Weiss RM, Wu XR, Sun TT, Altieri DC. A survivin gene signature predicts aggressive tumor behavior. Cancer Res. 2005;65(9):3531–4.

180. Xi RC, Sheng YR, Chen WH, Sheng L, Gang JJ, Tong Z, Shan Z, Ying GH, Dong LC. Expression of survivin and livin predicts early recurrence in non-muscle invasive bladder cancer. J Surg Oncol. 2013; 107(5):550–4.

181. Barbieri CE, Lotan Y, Lee RK, Sonpavde G, Karakiewicz PI, Robinson B, Scherr DS, Shariat SF. Tissue-based molecular markers for bladder cancer. Minerva Urol Nefrol. 2010;62(3):241–58.

182. Bochner BH, Cote RJ, Weidner N, Groshen S, Chen SC, Skinner DG, Nichols PW. Angiogenesis in bladder cancer: relationship between microvessel density and tumor prognosis. J Natl Cancer Inst. 1995;87(21): 1603–12.

183. Jaeger TM, Weidner N, Chew K, Moore DH, Kerschmann RL, Waldman FM, Carroll PR. Tumor angiogenesis correlates with lymph node metastases in invasive bladder cancer. J Urol. 1995;154(1):69–71.

184. Inoue K, Slaton JW, Karashima T, Yoshikawa C, Shuin T, Sweeney P, Millikan R, Dinney CP. The prognostic value of angiogenesis factor expression for predicting recurrence and metastasis of bladder cancer after neoadjuvant chemotherapy and radical cystectomy. Clin Cancer Res. 2000;6(12):4866–73.

185. Shariat SF, Youssef RF, Gupta A, Chade DC, Karakiewicz PI, Isbarn H, Jeldres C, Sagalowsky AI, Ashfaq R, Lotan Y. Association of angiogenesis related markers with bladder cancer outcomes and other molecular markers. J Urol. 2010;183(5):1744–50.

186. Grossfeld GD, Ginsberg DA, Stein JP, Bochner BH, Esrig D, Groshen S, Dunn M, Nichols PW, Taylor CR, Skinner DG, et al. Thrombospondin-1 expression in bladder cancer: association with p53 alterations, tumor angiogenesis, and tumor progression. J Natl Cancer Inst. 1997;89(3):219–27.

187. Shariat SF, Karakiewicz PI, Ashfaq R, Isbarn H, Fradet Y, Bastian PJ, Nielsen ME, Capitanio U, Jeldres C, Montorsi F, et al. Combination of cell cycle regulating bio-markers improves prognosis in

patients with organ-confined urothelial carcinoma at radical cystectomy. J Urol. 2008;179(4):578.

188. Shariat SF, Karakiewicz PI, Ashfaq R, Lerner SP, Palapattu GS, Cote RJ, Sagalowsky AI, Lotan Y. Multiple biomarkers improve prediction of bladder cancer recurrence and mortality in patients undergoing cystectomy. Cancer. 2008;112(2):315–25.

189. Lotan Y, Bagrodia A, Passoni N, Rachakonda V, Kapur P, Arriaga Y, Bolenz C, Margulis V, Raj GV, Sagalowsky AI, et al. Prospective evaluation of a molecular marker panel for prediction of recurrence and cancer-specific survival after radical cystectomy. Eur Urol. 2013;64(3):465–71.

190. Bassi P, Sacco E, De Marco V, Aragona M, Volpe A. Prognostic accuracy of an artificial neural network in patients undergoing radical cystectomy for bladder cancer: a comparison with logistic regression analysis. BJU Int. 2007;99(5):1007–12.

191. Catto JW, Abbod MF, Linkens DA, Larre S, Rosario DJ, Hamdy FC. Neurofuzzy modeling to determine recurrence risk following radical cystectomy for nonmetastatic urothelial carcinoma of the bladder. Clin Cancer Res. 2009;15(9):3150–5.

192. Catto JW, Linkens DA, Abbod MF, Chen M, Burton JL, Feeley KM, Hamdy FC. Artificial intelligence in predicting bladder cancer outcome: a comparison of neuro-fuzzy modeling and artificial neural networks. Clin Cancer Res. 2003;9(11): 4172–7.

193. Qureshi KN, Naguib RN, Hamdy FC, Neal DE, Mellon JK. Neural network analysis of clinicopathological and molecular markers in bladder cancer. J Urol. 2000;163(2):630–3.

194. Stenzl A, Cowan NC, De Santis M, Kuczyk MA, Merseburger AS, Ribal MJ, Sherif A, Witjes JA. Treatment of muscle-invasive and metastatic bladder cancer: update of the EAU guidelines. Eur Urol. 2011;59(6):1009–18.

195. Rink M, Lee DJ, Kent M, Xylinas E, Fritsche HM, Babjuk M, Brisuda A, Hansen J, Green DA, Aziz A, et al. Predictors of cancer-specific mortality after disease recurrence following radical cystectomy. BJU Int. 2013;111(3 Pt B):E30–6.

196. von der Maase H, Sengelov L, Roberts JT, Ricci S, Dogliotti L, Oliver T, Moore MJ, Zimmermann A, Arning M. Long-term survival results of a randomized trial comparing gemcitabine plus cisplatin, with methotrexate, vinblastine, doxorubicin, plus cisplatin in patients with bladder cancer. J Clin Oncol. 2005;23(21):4602–8.

197. Sternberg CN, Donat SM, Bellmunt J, Millikan RE, Stadler W, De Mulder P, Sherif A, von der Maase H, Tsukamoto T, Soloway MS. Chemotherapy for bladder cancer: treatment guidelines for neoadjuvant chemotherapy, bladder preservation, adjuvant chemotherapy, and metastatic cancer. Urology. 2007; 69(1 Suppl):62–79.

198. Mitra AP, Quinn DI, Dorff TB, Skinner EC, Schuckman AK, Miranda G, Gill IS, Daneshmand S. Factors influencing post-recurrence survival in

bladder cancer following radical cystectomy. BJU Int. 2012;109(6):846–54.

199. Ploeg M, Kums AC, Aben KK, van Lin EN, Smits G, Vergunst H, Viddeleer AC, Geboers AD, van Berkel H, van Boven E, et al. Prognostic factors for survival in patients with recurrence of muscle invasive bladder cancer after treatment with curative intent. Clin Genitourin Cancer. 2011;9(1):14–21.

200. Nakagawa T, Hara T, Kawahara T, Ogata Y, Nakanishi H, Komiyama M, Arai E, Kanai Y, Fujimoto H. Prognostic risk stratification of patients with urothelial carcinoma of the bladder with recurrence after radical cystectomy. J Urol. 2013; 189(4):1275–81.

201. Chromecki TF, Mauermann J, Cha EK, Svatek RS, Fajkovic H, Karakiewicz PI, Lotan Y, Tilki D, Bastian PJ, Volkmer BG, et al. Multicenter validation of the prognostic value of patient age in patients treated with radical cystectomy. World J Urol. 2012;30(6):753–9.

202. Nuhn P, May M, Sun M, Fritsche HM, Brookman-May S, Buchner A, Bolenz C, Moritz R, Herrmann E, Burger M, et al. External validation of postoperative nomograms for prediction of all-cause mortality, cancer-specific mortality, and recurrence in patients with urothelial carcinoma of the bladder. Eur Urol. 2012;61(1):58–64.

203. Rink M, Shariat SF. Can we apply nomograms derived in the United States to European patients? Yes, we can! Eur Urol. 2012;61(1):65–6.

204. Bajorin DF, Dodd PM, Mazumdar M, Fazzari M, McCaffrey JA, Scher HI, Herr H, Higgins G, Boyle MG. Long-term survival in metastatic transitional-cell carcinoma and prognostic factors predicting outcome of therapy. J Clin Oncol. 1999;17(10):3173–81.

205. Bellmunt J, von der Maase H, Mead GM, Skoneczna I, De Santis M, Daugaard G, Boehle A, Chevreau C, Paz-Ares L, Laufman LR, et al. Randomized phase III study comparing paclitaxel/cisplatin/gemcitabine and gemcitabine/cisplatin in patients with locally advanced or metastatic urothelial cancer without prior systemic therapy: EORTC Intergroup Study 30987. J Clin Oncol. 2012;30(10):1107–13.

206. De Santis M, Bellmunt J, Mead G, Kerst JM, Leahy M, Maroto P, Skoneczna I, Marreaud S, de Wit R, Sylvester R. Randomized phase II/III trial assessing gemcitabine/ carboplatin and methotrexate/carboplatin/vinblastine in patients with advanced urothelial cancer "unfit" for cisplatin-based chemotherapy: phase II—results of EORTC study 3098. J Clin Oncol. 2009;27(33):5634–9.

207. Apolo AB, Ostrovnaya I, Halabi S, Iasonos A, Philips GK, Rosenberg JE, Riches J, Small EJ, Milowsky MI, Bajorin DF. Prognostic model for predicting survival of patients with metastatic urothelial cancer treated with cisplatin-based chemotherapy. J Natl Cancer Inst. 2013;105(7):499–503.

208. Bellmunt J, Choueiri TK, Fougeray R, Schutz FA, Salhi Y, Winquist E, Culine S, von der Maase H, Vaughn DJ, Rosenberg JE. Prognostic factors in patients with advanced transitional cell carcinoma of the urothelial tract experiencing treatment failure with platinum-containing regimens. J Clin Oncol. 2010;28(11):1850–5.

209. Niegisch G, Fimmers R, Siener R, Park SI, Albers P. Prognostic factors in second-line treatment of urothelial cancers with gemcitabine and paclitaxel (German Association of Urological Oncology trial AB20/99). Eur Urol. 2011;60(5):1087–96.

210. Galsky MD, Moshier E, Krege S, Lin CC, Hahn N, Ecke T, Sonpavde G, Godbold J, Oh WK, Bamias A. Nomogram for predicting survival in patients with unresectable and/or metastatic urothelial cancer who are treated with cisplatin-based chemotherapy. Cancer. 2013;119(16):3012–9.

211. Kluth LA, et al. Gender-specific differences in clinicopathologic outcomes following radical cystectomy: an international multi-institutional study of more than 8000 patients. Eur Urol. 2013. doi:10.1016/j.eururo.2013.11.040

212. Sonpavde G, Khan MM, Svatek RS, Lee R, Novara G, Tilki D, Lerner SP, Amiel GE, Skinner E, Karakiewicz PI, Bastian PJ, Kassouf W, Fritsche HM, Izawa JI, Ficarra V, Dinney CP, Lotan Y, Fradet Y, Shariat SF. Prognostic risk stratification of pathological stage T2N0 bladder cancer after radical cystectomy. BJU Int. 2010;108(5):687–92. doi: 10.1111/j.1464-410X.2010.09902.x. Epub 2010 Nov 19. PMID: 21087453

213. Sonpavde G, Khan MM, Svatek RS, Lee R, Novara G, Tilki D, Lerner SP, Amiel GE, Skinner E, Karakiewicz PI, Bastian PJ, Kassouf W, Fritsche HM, Izawa JI, Scherr DS, Ficarra V, Dinney CP, Lotan Y, Fradet Y, Shariat SF. Prognostic risk stratification of pathological stage T3N0 bladder cancer after radical cystectomy. J Urol. 2011;185(4):1216–21. doi: 10.1016/j.juro.2010.11.082. Epub 2011 Feb 22. PMID: 21334687.

214. Takata, et al. Clin Cancer Res. 2005;11:2625–36.

215. Smith, et al. Lancet Oncol. 2011;12: 137–43.

Richard M. Bambury, Robert B. Sims,
and Jonathan E. Rosenberg

10.1 Clinical Trial Design Concepts in Bladder Cancer

The development of new and improved therapeutic strategies is a key goal of the oncology community and such efforts are ongoing in the field of bladder cancer. New treatments are tested for safety and efficacy in humans using a prospective, phased clinical trial structure.

Phase I oncology trials are typically performed when a new drug or compound has some evidence of anticancer activity in the preclinical setting. While it is hoped that patients will derive clinical benefit from participation, the primary objective of these trials is to find a safe dose and schedule of the compound for further testing in phase II and III trials. Pharmacokinetic studies are also performed to assess how the drug is distributed and excreted by the human body and patients are monitored for any toxicity that may arise. These trials often start by using 10 % of the lethal dose of drug in animal species (measured as milligrams per square meter of body surface area) [1]. Three patients are treated and observed for toxicity and if no dose-limiting toxicity (DLT) occurs then the dose is escalated for the next three patients. What constitutes a DLT is defined separately for each individual trial but is typically defined as clinically significant grade ≥ 3 toxicity or a toxicity requiring dose reduction or treatment discontinuation. If no more than one patient in a cohort of three experiences a DLT then three additional patients are treated at that level, and the dose is further escalated if these three experience no DLT. In summary, dose levels are escalated as long as no more than one in six patients experience a DLT at which point dose escalation stops. Doses are often escalated in proportion to a modified Fibonacci series of numbers [2]. Such a phase I trial design is commonly termed the "3+3" design. Newer phase I designs aimed at speeding up this process include methods for intrapatient dose escalation and greater dose escalation between cohorts [2]. For some classes of therapeutics, DLTs may not occur. In such instances (e.g. tumor vaccines), a phase I study is performed to find the minimum dose and schedule of drug with maximum biologic activity. Pharmacokinetic and pharmacodynamic endpoints such as plasma drug concentration and measurement of tumor targeted T cells may be used in such cases [3]. Patients considered for enrollment in phase I trials generally have exhausted standard therapies and have few good therapeutic options.

R.M. Bambury, M.B., M.R.C.P.I. (✉) • R.B. Sims
J.E. Rosenberg
Department of Genitourinary Medical Oncology,
Sidney Kimmel Center for Prostate and Urologic
Cancers, Memorial Sloan Kettering Cancer Center/
Weill Cornell Medical College, 353 East 68th Street,
New York, NY 10065, USA
e-mail: bamburyr@mskcc.org;
richardbambury@me.com

B.R. Konety and S.S. Chang (eds.), *Management of Bladder Cancer:
A Comprehensive Text With Clinical Scenarios*, DOI 10.1007/978-1-4939-1881-2_10,
© Springer Science+Business Media New York 2015

Historically, phase II trials were performed to assess whether a new drug or combination of drugs has evidence of efficacy in a given tumor type [2]. Increasingly investigators are designing these trials to enroll only patients whose tumors contain a relevant molecular target, in addition to or instead of a specific anatomic or histopathologic subtype. RECIST response rate or progression-free survival are the most commonly used primary endpoints, and results are typically compared to previously reported efficacy rates for current standard of care regimens [4, 5]. To minimize the number of patients exposed to a futile drug, a commonly used statistical approach is the optimal two-stage design whereby the trial is terminated early if the drug does not show sufficient levels of activity [6]. Given the limitations associated with comparing the effects of a new drug on treated patients by comparing with historic controls, randomized phase II designs are increasingly used. These trials use endpoints such as response rate or progression-free survival rather than more robust endpoints such as overall survival that are needed for registrational phase III trials. Furthermore the statistical design does not need to be as stringent as that used for phase III trials as the goal of the trial is to detect a signal of activity, rather than to definitively prove clinical benefit (e.g. alpha level of 0.10 rather 0.05 may be used). Both of the above differences allow these trials to be smaller and provide quicker results than their phase III counterparts although results should not be used to alter practice or for regulatory approval [3].

Phase III trials are intended to provide data which is sufficiently robust to provide guidance to practicing physicians when making decisions about how to manage their patients [2]. Overall survival and quality of life in a cohort of patients treated with an investigational compound compared with a cohort treated with current standard of care are the most relevant measures. Quality of life is more difficult to assess than overall survival due its subjective nature, although efforts are ongoing to incorporate such data collection into newer phase III trials. To maximize the applicability of phase III trial results to the real world setting, they often enroll patients in numerous treatment locations and sometimes involve international collaboration. Treatment assignment should be randomized to eliminate known and unknown selection biases. Analysis of results should be performed by "intention to treat" meaning all patients assigned to a treatment arm are analyzed when computing results regardless of whether or not they received the assigned treatment [2].

Molecular markers predictive of response are increasingly important in cancer medicine. Theoretically, such "predictive biomarkers" are used to ensure those patients who will benefit from a given compound receive it and to eliminate futile therapy with the associated toxicity and cost for others. Biomarker discovery should now be integrated in all phases of clinical trials by attempting to find associations between response to therapy and molecular characteristics of the tumor. Although a full discussion of the methodologies which can be used are outside the scope of this chapter, two successful examples in cancer medicine include human epidermal growth factor receptor 2 (HER2) immunohistochemistry to select patients for trastuzumab treatment in breast cancer and epidermal growth factor receptor (*EGFR*) gene mutations to select for erlotinib treatment in lung cancer [7, 8].

Historically, it has been difficult to perform clinical trials of novel agents in bladder cancer for a number of reasons. Accruing sufficient numbers of patients has been a problem because locally advanced or metastatic bladder cancer is not as common as some of the other major cancer types. Overall, bladder cancer has an annual incidence rate in the USA of 23/100,000 persons compared with 49/100,000 for colorectal cancer and 70/100,000 for lung cancer [9]. Of these only about 50 % develop muscle-invasive or metastatic disease during their disease course, and it is only these patients who are considered for systemic therapy using current treatment paradigms. The patient population is comprised mainly of elderly patients (median age at diagnosis is 73) with a current or former smoking history, (with all of the associated toxicities) making many patients ineligible for clinical trials of novel agents with uncertain toxicity profiles.

For example, approximately 50 % of patients are ineligible for standard cisplatin-based chemotherapy due to co-morbidities (renal dysfunction, neuropathy, hearing loss) or performance status. Systemic cisplatin-based chemotherapy in the neoadjuvant setting was eventually shown to improve survival for muscle invasive bladder cancer, but accrual to these trials was fraught with difficulty due to issues highlighted above as well as the need for co-operation from urologists in referring patients for treatment prior to cystectomy. One example of such difficulty was a neoadjuvant chemotherapy trial that took 11 years to enroll 317 patients at 126 institutions between 1987 and 1998 [10]. A more recent example was a Spanish adjuvant chemotherapy trial which terminated early in 2007 due to poor accrual after only 142 of a planned 340 patients were enrolled [11].

The optimal trial design for an investigational agent in bladder cancer is dependent on the disease state under investigation as well as the properties of the compound. In non-muscle invasive bladder cancer, novel therapies can be screened for activity by using a "marker lesion" study. In this design, a small solitary tumor is left in place after resection of other disease, and treatment with a novel systemic or intravesical agent is initiated [12, 13]. Cystoscopic follow up and tumor size measurement are used to assess response to therapy and if lesions are progressing then resection is performed. Development of a novel systemic treatment active against non-muscle invasive disease could reduce the significant morbidity and cost of lifelong surveillance, multiple endoscopic resections and intravesical treatment with which these patients are currently managed [14]. BCG refractory non-muscle invasive bladder cancer is often treated with cystectomy because prognosis is guarded with continuation of conservative management (one study in patients with recurrent T1 disease treated with bladder sparing approaches described a 71 % rate of progression to muscle invasive disease and a 48 % rate of cancer-related death at 5 years follow-up) [15]. In muscle invasive bladder cancer, the current standard of care involves neoadjuvant cisplatin-based chemotherapy followed by radical cystectomy [16]. This

treatment paradigm provides an ideal research setting for the addition of novel agents to conventional chemotherapy regimens because a detailed assessment of the molecular characteristics of the tumor pre- and post-treatment is possible. An objective measurement of the compounds' anticancer activity based on pathologic response is also possible. The molecular information gleaned can be used to discover biomarkers predictive of treatment response as well as confirming that the target of interest is in fact inhibited. Once phase I and II trials have demonstrated evidence of efficacy and safety for a novel compound, a randomized phase III study is performed to investigate for superiority over the current standard of care. In the era of precision medicine, with compounds directed at specific molecular targets, the investigation of potential predictive biomarkers either in the initial inclusion criteria and/or in the subsequent results analysis should be strongly considered.

Potential bladder cancer randomized clinical trial designs and endpoints for different disease states are outlined in Table 10.1. The specifics of design for any given clinical trial will be dependent on the particular agent under investigation so the designs outlined are intended only as a general guide.

10.2 Novel Treatment Strategies Under Investigation for Bladder Cancer

10.2.1 Signaling Pathway Blockade

Cancer cells typically bear thousands of genetic alterations but only a small number are thought to be "driver" events leading to transformation of a normal cell to the malignant state [18]. Cells that have activating alterations in growth-promoting oncogenes are reliant on continued activity of these protein products for sustained proliferation and survival in a state termed "oncogene addiction" [19]. Therapeutic manipulation of this phenomenon by blockade of the overactive signaling molecule or its downstream effectors has lead to successful development of

Table 10.1 Endpoint options for randomized phase II and III clinical trials in bladder cancer

Disease state	Current standard of care [17]	Randomized trial design for experimental arm	Primary endpoint Randomized phase II	Primary endpoint Phase III	Secondary endpoints Phase III
NMIBC—newly diagnosed high grade or Tis/T1	TURBT+ I.V. BCG	Novel agent added to or replacing I.V. BCG	Recurrence-free survival or Complete response rate if marker lesion study	Recurrence-free survival	Progression-free survival Bladder intact survival Overall survival Toxicity
NMIBC—BCG refractory	Cystectomy	TURBT+novel systemic or I.V. agent with immediate cystectomy if failure	Progression-free survival or Complete response rate if marker lesion study	Overall survival	Progression-free survival Distant metastasis free survival Bladder intact survival Toxicity
MIBC—pre-cystectomy and cisplatin eligible	Neoadjuvant cisplatin-based chemotherapy followed by cystectomy	Novel systemic agent added to or replacing systemic chemotherapy	pT0 rate	Overall survival	pT0 rate Distant metastasis-free survival Toxicity
MIBC—pre-cystectomy and cisplatin ineligible	Cystectomy	Neoadjuvant systemic treatment	pT0 rate	Overall survival	pT0 rate Distant metastasis-free survival Toxicity
MIBC—post-cystectomy	Observation or adjuvant chemotherapy	Adjuvant systemic treatment regimen	Recurrence-free survival	Overall survival	Recurrence-free survival Distant metastasis-free survival Toxicity
Advanced bladder cancer[a] 1st line	Cisplatin-based chemotherapy	Novel agent added to or replacing systemic chemotherapy	Progression-free survival	Overall survival	Progression-free survival Response rate Toxicity
Advanced bladder cancer[a] ≥2nd line	Second-line chemotherapy	Novel agent added to or replacing systemic chemotherapy	Progression-free survival	Overall survival	Progression-free survival Response rate Toxicity

NMIBC Non-muscle invasive bladder cancer, *BCG* Bacillus calmette-guerin, *MIBC* Muscle invasive bladder cancer, *I.V.* intravesical, *pT0* Absence of any tumor on pathologic examination of cystectomy specimen
[a]Metastatic or locally advanced disease

drugs in many cancers including chronic myeloid leukemia, lung cancer, and melanoma [20–22]. Many bladder tumors have activating genetic alterations which may render them susceptible to signaling pathway blockade using the same approach. The frequency of specific alterations can vary with grade and stage of disease. Furthermore, the specific type of alteration may have an effect in its biologic relevance and its potential as a therapeutic target. For example, emerging data in melanoma patients suggests that imatinib is effective in tumors with exon 11 or 13 point mutations of the *KIT* gene, but is unlikely to be effective in patients with *KIT* amplification [23]. An outline of the most commonly found activating alterations in potentially targetable signaling pathways based on a recently published series of muscle invasive bladder cancers is shown in Table 10.2 [24].

Activating alterations of the phosphoinositide 3-kinase(PI3K)/Akt/mTOR (mammalian target of rapamycin) pathway occur in approximately 30 % of muscle invasive bladder cancers [25]. Specifically, one study reported activation of

Table 10.2 Oncogenic alterations with a frequency of $\geq$5 % in a series of 97 localized high-grade carcinomas of bladder origin [24]

	% of patients affected	Type of mutation(s)
RB pathway		
CDKN2A	25	Deletion or point mutations
CCND1	14	Amplification
CCNE1	5	Amplification
RB	15	Point mutations or deletion
E2F3	21	Amplification
Overall	61	
RAS/RAF pathway		
FGFR3	13	Activating point mutations
ERBB2	6	Amplification
FGFR1	6	Amplification
RAF1	6	Amplification
Overall	36	
MTOR pathway		
PIK3CA	18	Activating point mutations
TSC1	7	Inactivating point mutations
Overall	30	

Note: 85 % patients had $\geq$ pT2 disease and 90 % were of predominantly urothelial carcinoma histology

PIK3CA in 18 %, inactivation of *PTEN* in 4 %, activation of *AKT* in 2 %, and inactivation of *TSC1* in 7 % [24]. Therapeutic molecules targeting PI3K and mTOR are under active development in this disease. One report highlighting the potential of this approach described the case of a patient with metastatic urothelial carcinoma who achieved a durable complete response with everolimus, a drug targeting the mTOR complex. Upon tumor genome sequencing the patient was found to have an inactivating *TSC1* point mutation and further study in other patients highlighted the potential of these mutations to be predictive of response to everolimus therapy [26]. This finding requires prospective validation in other TSC1 mutant tumors.

Activating point mutations of *FGFR3* have been reported in 13 % of muscle invasive urothelial bladder cancers [24]. These mutations are even more common in non-muscle invasive bladder cancer with reported frequencies of 66 % and 38 % in Ta and T1 disease respectively [27].

Activating translocations of *FGFR3* have also been described although their frequency is not yet clear [28]. Furthermore, FGFR3 protein is overexpressed in up to 40 % of FGFR3 wild-type tumors so that in total approximately 50 % of muscle invasive bladder cancers may have activating genetic alterations or protein overexpression of FGFR3 and suggesting this pathway as a viable therapeutic target [27]. Although one trial in metastatic disease has failed to show significant activity for the FGFR3 inhibitor dovitinib, there are ongoing efforts to target this pathway using therapeutic compounds with improved pharmacokinetic and pharmacodynamic profiles [29].

Loss of cell-cycle control through inactivation of the RB (retinoblastoma protein) pathway is observed in 60 % of muscle invasive bladder cancers [24]. This occurs through *RB* mutation or deletion in 15 %, *CDKN2A* deletion in 24 %, *CCND1* amplification in 14 %, and *E2F3* amplification in 21 % [24]. Interest in targeting this pathway in bladder cancer has risen given the successful use of the RB pathway inhibitor PD0332991 in breast cancer [30]. CDK4 (Cyclin-dependent kinase 4) inhibitors such as PD0332991 work by inhibiting CDK4/Cyclin D1 complex which is an upstream downregulator of the RB protein. Preclinical evidence suggests that these agents need intact RB protein to work effectively so patients with *RB* deletion or inactivating mutation may not benefit. [31, 32] Clinical trials testing these agents in bladder cancer will determine their efficacy in different genetic subsets of this disease.

Monoclonal antibodies and small molecule tyrosine kinase inhibitors targeting the human epidermal growth factor receptor 2 (HER2) and epidermal growth factor receptor (EGFR) proteins have led to therapeutic advances in subsets of breast, gastroesophageal, lung, and other cancers [22, 33, 34]. These strategies have been most useful in subsets of the disease bearing genetic alterations leading to over activation of the relevant protein through amplification or point mutation. The HER2 encoding *ERRB2* gene is amplified in 6 % of bladder cancers and according to one report the EGFR protein is expressed in 74 % of cases (although this is not necessarily accompanied by *EGFR* gene alteration) [24, 35].

These proteins may prove to be viable therapeutic targets in subsets of bladder cancer patients.

Aurora A kinase and polo-like kinase 1 are proteins involved in orderly cell mitosis. Overexpression of either molecule had been associated with poor prognosis in bladder cancer patients [36, 37]. These proteins are also overexpressed in other tumor types and ongoing development of therapeutic molecules targeting them may lead to effective treatment options in bladder cancer patients [38].

Heat shock proteins (HSPs) are believed to act as "molecular chaperones" by stabilizing the signaling molecules which promote cell survival [39]. Members of this family including HSP 27, HSP70-2, and HSP 90 are upregulated in cells during times of stress [39]. They may also play a role in carcinogenesis and chemoresistance in many tumor types including bladder cancer [40, 41]. OGX427 is an antisense oligonucleotide which suppresses cellular expression of HSP 27 [42]. It is under active investigation in bladder cancer patients as a single agent and in combination with cytotoxic chemotherapy (NCT01780545, NCT01454089, and NCT00959868).

10.2.2 Immunotherapy Strategies

Intravesical bacillus Calmette-Guerin (BCG), a live attenuated form of mycobacterium bovis, is an effective treatment for non-muscle invasive bladder cancer. When used in the adjuvant setting after cystoscopic resection of non-muscle invasive bladder cancer it decreases recurrence rates by 70 % [43]. Although the precise mechanism of action is unclear, BCG triggers both acquired and innate local immune responses which correlate well with its antitumor efficacy [44]. The efficacy of this immunotherapy in early bladder cancer management provides proof of principle that it is an immunogenic disease with opportunity for benefit from newer immunotherapy approaches.

DN24-02 is an autologous active cellular immunotherapy currently undergoing clinical investigation in the adjuvant setting for resected muscle invasive bladder cancer (NCT01353222). A patient's own peripheral blood mononuclear cells are collected via standard leukapheresis and activated ex-vivo against a recombinant HER2-derived fusion protein to stimulate an immune response against HER2. Only patients expressing HER2 protein (accounting for approximately 80 % of bladder cancer patients) are eligible for inclusion in the study [45]. Early laboratory data provide encouraging evidence that treated patients are mounting an appropriate immune response to HER2 expressing cells but data on clinical outcomes are awaited [46]. This approach has proven efficacy in prostate cancer where, using the same manufacturing platform, sipuleucel T, improved median overall survival from 22 to 26 months (HR=0.78, $p=0.032$) in asymptomatic or minimally symptomatic metastatic castrate-resistant patients [47].

Other emerging immunotherapy strategies which may have a role in the future treatment of bladder cancer include immune checkpoint blockade with antibodies targeting CTLA-4, PD-1, or PD-L1. Indeed, PD-L1 expression is associated with higher stage and grade bladder cancers [48]. The PD-L1 monoclonal antibody MPDL3280A is under active investigation and promising preliminary data from a phase I trial reported objective responses in 16 of 30 (52 %) UC patients with PD-L1 positive tumors [49]. Furthermore, the emerging field of chimeric antigen receptor-modified T cells may lead to wide ranging treatment breakthroughs in the management of hematologic as well as solid tumor malignances [50].

10.2.3 Anti-Angiogenic Strategies

As in other solid tumors, angiogenesis plays a key role in bladder cancer development and progression [51, 52]. Despite this, trials investigating the use of tyrosine kinase inhibitors sunitinib and pazopanib [both of which inhibit signaling from the pro-angiogenic vascular endothelial growth factor receptor (VEGFR) and platelet-derived growth factor receptor (PDGFR)] produced little evidence of efficacy [53–55]. Bevacizumab is a monoclonal antibody targeting the VEGF protein and has known efficacy in metastatic lung, colon, cervical, and other cancers. Two single-arm phase II trials have evaluated its efficacy and toxicity in urothelial cancer when added to platinum-based chemotherapy with encouraging response rates (49 and 72 %) and median overall survival (13.9 and 20.4 months) was reported [56, 57]. An ongoing randomized phase III clinical trial is evaluating its efficacy in advanced bladder cancer when added to the cisplatin/gemcitabine regimen (NCT00942331). Trebananib is an angiopoietin inhibitor which also has anti-angiogenic properties and will be investigated in combination with docetaxel for advanced urothelial cancer in the near future (NCT01907308).

References

1. Leventhal B, Wittes R. Research methods in clinical oncology. New York, NY: Raven; 1988.
2. DeVita V, Lawrence T, Rosenberg S. DeVita, Hellman, and Rosenberg's Cancer: principles & practice of oncology. 9th ed. Philadelphia, PA: Wolters Kluwer Health/Lippincott Williams & Wilkins; 2011.
3. Simon RM et al. Clinical trial designs for the early clinical development of therapeutic cancer vaccines. J Clin Oncol. 2001;19(6):1848–54.
4. Eisenhauer EA et al. New response evaluation criteria in solid tumours: revised RECIST guideline (version 1.1). Eur J Cancer. 2009;45(2):228–47.
5. Seymour L et al. The design of phase II clinical trials testing cancer therapeutics: consensus recommendations from the clinical trial design task force of the national cancer institute investigational drug steering committee. Clin Cancer Res. 2010;16(6):1764–9.
6. Simon R. Optimal two-stage designs for phase II clinical trials. Control Clin Trials. 1989;10(1):1–10.
7. Simon R, Maitournam A. Evaluating the efficiency of targeted designs for randomized clinical trials. Clin Cancer Res. 2004;10(20):6759–63.
8. Lindeman NI et al. Molecular testing guideline for selection of lung cancer patients for EGFR and ALK tyrosine kinase inhibitors: guideline from the College of American Pathologists, International Association for the Study of Lung Cancer, and Association for Molecular Pathology. J Thorac Oncol. 2013;8(7):823–59.
9. Siegel R, Naishadham D, Jemal A. Cancer statistics, 2012. CA Cancer J Clin. 2012;62(1):10–29.
10. Grossman HB et al. Neoadjuvant chemotherapy plus cystectomy compared with cystectomy alone for locally advanced bladder cancer. N Engl J Med. 2003; 349(9):859–66.
11. Paz-Ares LG, et al. Randomized phase III trial comparing adjuvant paclitaxel/gemcitabine/cisplatin (PGC) to observation in patients with resected invasive bladder cancer: results of the Spanish Oncology Genitourinary Group (SOGUG) 99/01 study. ASCO meeting abstracts, 2010;28 (18_suppl):LBA4518.
12. Dalbagni G et al. Phase II trial of intravesical gemcitabine in bacille Calmette-Guerin-refractory transitional cell carcinoma of the bladder. J Clin Oncol. 2006;24(18):2729–34.
13. Brausi MA et al. Can gemcitabine instillation ablate solitary low-risk non-muscle-invasive bladder cancer? Results of a phase II marker lesion study. Urol Int. 2011;87(4):470–4.
14. James AC, Gore JL. The costs of non-muscle invasive bladder cancer. Urol Clin North Am. 2013;40(2): 261–9.
15. Raj GV et al. Treatment paradigm shift may improve survival of patients with high risk superficial bladder cancer. J Urol. 2007;177(4):1283–6. discussion 1286.
16. Hussain MH et al. Bladder cancer: narrowing the gap between evidence and practice. J Clin Oncol. 2009; 27(34):5680–4.
17. Network NCC. Bladder cancer, Version 1.2013. NCCN guidelines for bladder cancer management. www.nccn.org. Accessed July 3, 2013.
18. Torti D et al. A preclinical algorithm of soluble surrogate biomarkers that correlate with therapeutic inhibition of the MET oncogene in gastric tumors. Int J Cancer. 2012;130(6):1357–66.
19. Weinstein IB. Cancer. Addiction to oncogenes – the Achilles heal of cancer. Science. 2002;297(5578):63–4.
20. O'Brien SG et al. Imatinib compared with interferon and low-dose cytarabine for newly diagnosed chronic-phase chronic myeloid leukemia. N Engl J Med. 2003;348(11):994–1004.
21. Chapman PB et al. Improved survival with vemurafenib in melanoma with BRAF V600E mutation. N Engl J Med. 2011;364(26):2507–16.
22. Rosell R et al. Erlotinib versus standard chemotherapy as first-line treatment for European patients with advanced EGFR mutation-positive non-small-cell lung cancer (EURTAC): a multicentre, open-label, randomised phase 3 trial. Lancet Oncol. 2012;13(3): 239–46.
23. Carvajal RD. Another option in our kit of effective therapies for advanced melanoma. J Clin Oncol. 2013;31(26):3173–5.
24. Iyer G et al. Prevalence and co-occurrence of actionable genomic alterations in high-grade bladder cancer. J Clin Oncol. 2013;31(25):3133–40.
25. Balar AV, et al. Alterations in the PI3K/Akt signaling pathway and association with outcome in invasive high-grade urothelial cancer in American Society of Clinical Oncology 2012 Genitourinary Cancers Symposium, San Francisco, CL; 2012.
26. Iyer G et al. Genome sequencing identifies a basis for everolimus sensitivity. Science. 2012;338(6104):221.
27. Tomlinson DC et al. FGFR3 protein expression and its relationship to mutation status and prognostic variables in bladder cancer. J Pathol. 2007;213(1):91–8.
28. Williams SV, Hurst CD, Knowles MA. Oncogenic FGFR3 gene fusions in bladder cancer. Hum Mol Genet. 2013;22(4):795–803.
29. Milowsky MI, et al. Final results of a multicenter, open-label phase II trial of dovitinib (TKI258) in patients with advanced urothelial carcinoma with either mutated or nonmutated FGFR3. In: ASCO 2013 Genitourinary Cancers Symposium, Orlando, FL; 2013.

30. Finn RS, et al. Results of a randomized phase 2 study of PD 0332991, a cyclin dependent kinase (CDK) 4/6 inhibitor, in combination with letrozole vs letrozole alone for first-line treatment of ER+/HER2– advanced breast cancer (BC). In: San Antonio breast Cancer Symposium 2012. San Antonio, TX; 2012.

31. Dean JL et al. Therapeutic response to CDK4/6 inhibition in breast cancer defined by ex vivo analyses of human tumors. Cell Cycle. 2012;11(14):2756–61.

32. McClendon AK et al. CDK4/6 inhibition antagonizes the cytotoxic response to anthracycline therapy. Cell Cycle. 2012;11(14):2747–55.

33. Moja L et al. Trastuzumab containing regimens for early breast cancer. Cochrane Database Syst Rev. 2012;4, CD006243.

34. Bang YJ et al. Trastuzumab in combination with chemotherapy versus chemotherapy alone for treatment of HER2-positive advanced gastric or gastro-oesophageal junction cancer (ToGA): a phase 3, open-label, randomised controlled trial. Lancet. 2010;376(9742): 687–97.

35. Chaux A et al. High epidermal growth factor receptor immunohistochemical expression in urothelial carcinoma of the bladder is not associated with EGFR mutations in exons 19 and 21: a study using formalin-fixed, paraffin-embedded archival tissues. Hum Pathol. 2012;43(10):1590–5.

36. Comperat E et al. Gene expression study of Aurora-A reveals implication during bladder carcinogenesis and increasing values in invasive urothelial cancer. Urology. 2008;72(4):873–7.

37. Lei Y et al. Prognostic significance of Aurora-A expression in human bladder cancer. Acta Histochem. 2011;113(5):514–8.

38. Matulonis UA et al. Phase II study of MLN8237 (alisertib), an investigational Aurora A kinase inhibitor, in patients with platinum-resistant or -refractory epithelial ovarian, fallopian tube, or primary peritoneal carcinoma. Gynecol Oncol. 2012;127(1):63–9.

39. Richardson PG et al. Inhibition of heat shock protein 90 (HSP90) as a therapeutic strategy for the treatment of myeloma and other cancers. Br J Haematol. 2011;152(4):367–79.

40. Garg M et al. Heat-shock protein 70–2 (HSP70-2) expression in bladder urothelial carcinoma is associated with tumour progression and promotes migration and invasion. Eur J Cancer. 2010;46(1):207–15.

41. Kamada M et al. Hsp27 knockdown using nucleotide-based therapies inhibit tumor growth and enhance chemotherapy in human bladder cancer cells. Mol Cancer Ther. 2007;6(1):299–308.

42. Hadaschik BA et al. Intravesically administered antisense oligonucleotides targeting heat-shock protein-27 inhibit the growth of non-muscle-invasive bladder cancer. BJU Int. 2008;102(5):610–6.

43. Shelley MD et al. Intravesical bacillus calmette-guerin in Ta and T1 bladder cancer. Cochrane Database Syst Rev. 2000;4, CD001986.

44. Kawai K et al. Bacillus Calmette-Guerin (BCG) immunotherapy for bladder cancer: current understanding and perspectives on engineered BCG vaccine. Cancer Sci. 2013;104(1):22–7.

45. Press MF, et al. HER2 expression in patients with surgically resected urothelial cancer at high risk of recurrence screened for the phase II randomized, open-label trial of DN24-02, an autologous cellular immunotherapy targeting HER2. In: ASCO Genitourinary Cancers Symposium, 2013. Orlando, FL; 2013.

46. Bajorin DF, et al. Preliminary safety, product parameters, and immune response assessments from a phase II randomized, open-label trial of DN24-02, an autologous cellular immunotherapy (ACI), in patients (pts) with surgically resected HER2+ urothelial cancer (UC) at high risk for recurrence. ASCO meeting abstracts, 2013;31(15_suppl):4547.

47. Kantoff PW et al. Sipuleucel-T immunotherapy for castration-resistant prostate cancer. N Engl J Med. 2010;363(5):411–22.

48. Inman BA et al. PD-L1 (B7-H1) expression by urothelial carcinoma of the bladder and BCG-induced granulomata: associations with localized stage progression. Cancer. 2007;109(8):1499–505.

49. Thomas Powles, N.J.V., Gregg Daniel Fine, Joseph Paul Eder, Fadi S. Braiteh, Yohann Loriot, Cristina Cruz Zambrano, Joaquim Bellmunt, Howard A. Burris, Siew-leng Melinda Teng, Xiaodong Shen, Hartmut Koeppen, Priti S. Hegde, Daniel S. Chen, Daniel Peter Petrylak. Inhibition of PD-L1 by MPDL3280A and clinical activity in pts with metastatic urothelial bladder cancer in ASCO annual meeting. 2014. Chicago, USA.

50. Grupp SA et al. Chimeric antigen receptor-modified T cells for acute lymphoid leukemia. N Engl J Med. 2013;368(16):1509–18.

51. Bochner BH et al. Angiogenesis in bladder cancer: relationship between microvessel density and tumor prognosis. J Natl Cancer Inst. 1995;87(21):1603–12.

52. Bernardini S et al. Serum levels of vascular endothelial growth factor as a prognostic factor in bladder cancer. J Urol. 2001;166(4):1275–9.

53. Bellmunt J et al. Phase II study of sunitinib as first-line treatment of urothelial cancer patients ineligible to receive cisplatin-based chemotherapy: baseline interleukin-8 and tumor contrast enhancement as potential predictive factors of activity. Ann Oncol. 2011;22(12):2646–53.

54. Gallagher DJ et al. Sunitinib in urothelial cancer: clinical, pharmacokinetic, and immunohistochemical study of predictors of response. Eur Urol. 2011;60(2): 344–9.

55. Necchi A et al. Pazopanib in advanced and platinum-resistant urothelial cancer: an open-label, single group, phase 2 trial. Lancet Oncol. 2012;13(8):810–6.

56. Balar AV et al. Phase II study of gemcitabine, carboplatin, and bevacizumab in patients with advanced unresectable or metastatic urothelial cancer. J Clin Oncol. 2013;31(6):724–30.

57. Hahn NM et al. Phase II trial of cisplatin, gemcitabine, and bevacizumab as first-line therapy for metastatic urothelial carcinoma: Hoosier Oncology Group GU 04–75. J Clin Oncol. 2011;29(12):1525–30.

Part II

Non Muscle Invasive Bladder Cancer

Seth P. Lerner and Alvin C. Goh

11.1 Introduction

Bladder cancer is considered one of the costliest malignancies treated in the United States (US) from diagnosis to death [1, 2]. A significant socioeconomic burden arises from the need for frequent follow-up exams, regular endoscopic treatments, and requisite surveillance imaging. With over 72,000 new diagnoses of bladder cancer expected in 2013, this disease continues to pose a substantial economic challenge [3].

Eighty percent of all newly diagnosed bladder cancers are non-muscle invasive urothelial carcinomas confined to the mucosa or lamina propria. Given its propensity for recurrence, bladder cancer frequently follows a prolonged course of follow-up and treatment [4]. While the majority of low-grade tumors do not progress, up to 20 % of non-muscle invasive lesions can proceed to muscle invasion or metastasis [5]. Additionally, patients with Ta or T1 urothelial cancer associated with carcinoma in-situ (CIS) are frequently understaged and are at higher risk for progression despite intravesical therapy.

The detection of urothelial carcinoma has traditionally relied on cystoscopy, cytologic analysis, and imaging of the upper tract. To evaluate the bladder, white light cystoscopy is used to visually inspect for abnormal lesions. Cytologic examination of voided or bladder wash specimens can be utilized in conjunction with cystoscopy to screen, diagnose, and monitor patients with bladder cancer. Several commercially available bladder cancer tumor markers are available to assist with bladder cancer detection. While putatively useful for screening and surveillance, experience with these markers has been mixed. Their specific role in the diagnosis and management of urothelial cancer remains to be defined.

Once a lesion is identified, transurethral resection is performed to assess histopathologic grade and stage. Although some factors that influence the rate of recurrence, such as tumor size, multifocality, and tumor genetics, are unchangeable, one way to reduce tumor recurrence may be more complete resection of all visible lesions and a more complete assessment of the normal appearing mucosa. What appears to be tumor "recurrence" may be residual tumor left behind or lesions missed during diagnostic and therapeutic cystoscopy [6]. Variability in the quality of tumor resection may account for differences in recurrence rates when bladder tumors of similar characteristics are compared across multiple centers.

S.P. Lerner, M.D., F.A.C.S. (✉)
Scott Department of Urology, Beth and Dave Swalm chair in Urologic Oncology, Multidisciplinary Bladder Cancer Program, Baylor College of Medicine, 7200 Cambridge, Suite A10.107, MC BCM380, Houston, TX 77030, USA
e-mail: slerner@bcm.edu

A.C. Goh, M.D.
Department of Urology, Houston Methodist Hospital, Houston, TX, USA

B.R. Konety and S.S. Chang (eds.), *Management of Bladder Cancer:*
A Comprehensive Text With Clinical Scenarios, DOI 10.1007/978-1-4939-1881-2_11,
© Springer Science+Business Media New York 2015

Improved visualization of bladder lesions might facilitate more complete resection and detection of occult lesions, thereby reducing tumor burden. Moreover, since most bladder lesions are found prior to muscle invasion and metastasis, early diagnosis, accurate staging, and aggressive intervention offer the opportunity to intervene prior to progression to a life-threatening disease.

While the goals of diagnosis and treatment of bladder cancer remain focused on reducing disease recurrence, progression, and mortality, in light of ever-rising healthcare costs, judicious application of new diagnostic strategies must be pursued. Herein, we discuss the current tools in use for bladder cancer diagnosis. We provide an overview of non-invasive diagnostic techniques, including urine cytology and FDA-approved urine markers. We review several emerging imaging technologies and data supporting their application to improve bladder cancer diagnosis, including fluorescence cystoscopy, optical coherence tomography, narrow-band imaging, confocal microscopy, and spectroscopy.

11.2 Non-Invasive Diagnostic Techniques

11.2.1 Urine Cytology

Cytologic analysis of voided urine or washed bladder specimens remains the gold standard for non-invasive bladder cancer detection and monitoring. This microscopic evaluation of stained urothelial cells relies on a histopathologic interpretation of abnormal cytologic features, including prominent nucleoli, increased nuclear-to-cytoplasmic ratio, mitotic figures, and hyperchromasia. Owing to decreased cellular adhesion, high-grade tumors are more easily detected than low-grade tumors with urine cytology. In a combined analysis of contemporary studies by the Mayo clinic, overall sensitivity is low, ranging from 19 % for low-grade tumors to 60 % for high-grade tumors [7]. A recent study of more than 800 patients comparing urine cytology to other urinary markers showed 89 % sensitivity for high-grade tumors and carcinoma in situ [8].

Variability in the sensitivity of cytology reported in the literature may be due to user-dependence and heterogeneity of experience among interpreting pathologists. A strength of cytology remains its high specificity, which ranges from 88 to 98 % [8, 9].

11.2.2 Urinary Biomarkers

A plethora of urinary tumor markers have been investigated in an effort to improve upon the diagnostic characteristics of urine cytology. Many studies have evaluated the diagnostic performance of individual and combination markers as compared to results with urine cytology. These urinary markers depend on elevations in bladder cancer-specific proteins in the urine or chromosomal aberrations present in the urothelial cells. A potential advantage of urinary markers is the ability to provide diagnostic information regarding cancer risk in a non-invasive fashion. To satisfy the characteristics of an ideal test, any proposed biomarker test should be reliable, inexpensive, non-invasive, and highly sensitive and specific. We have chosen to focus on four FDA-approved, commercially available urinary markers designed for the detection and diagnosis of bladder cancer. The diagnostic characteristics of these urinary markers are summarized in Table 11.1.

Nuclear matrix protein 22 (NMP22) is a protein related to mitosis and the distribution of chromatids to dividing cells. This class of proteins is responsible for DNA replication and gene regulation in the nucleus of the cell. The test for the marker is available both as a quantitative ELISA assay and as a point-of-care (POC) assay known as BladderChek (Stellar Pharmaceutics, Inc., London, ON). It is FDA-approved for use as an aid to cystoscopy in the diagnosis and management of bladder cancer. NMP22 is expressed in much higher concentrations in urothelial carcinoma than in normal urothelium. However, several benign conditions, including inflammation, recent instrumentation, bowel interposition, urinary tract infection, hematuria, and stones can lead to false-positive results [16]. Several studies

Table 11.1 Urine tumor markers for bladder cancer

	Target	Sensitivity	Specificity	Confounder	FDA-approved
NMP22 [10, 11]	Nuclear matrix protein	Low grade 54–63 % High grade 70–100 %	55–90 %	Hematuria, inflammation, instrumentation, urinary tract infection	Yes
BTA [12, 13]	Complement factor H-related protein	NMIBC 45–75 % MIBC 67–100 %	64–81 %	Hematuria, inflammation, instrumentation, urolithiasis	Yes
ImmunoCyt [14]	3 glycoprotein antigens (19A211, LDQ10, M344)	NMIBC 60–66 % MIBC 68–80 %	78 %	Intravesical therapy	Yes
FISH (UroVysion) [15]	Aneuploidy chr 3, 7, 17, deletion 9p21	NMIBC 64–76 % MIBC 83–100 %	89–97 %	Barbotage	Yes

have examined the diagnostic characteristics of this protein assay. The mean sensitivity and specificity for NMP22 is 75 % [17]. In a multicenter study of 1331 patients, Grossman et al. showed that NMP22 had greater ability to detect bladder cancer in high-risk patients undergoing cystoscopy and bladder biopsy than did voided cytology (sensitivity 55.7 % (95 % CI, 44.1–66.7 %) vs. 15.8 % (95 % CI, 7.6–24.0 %) [18]. However, NMP22 was less specific for bladder cancer than voided cytology (85.7 vs. 99.2 %). In addition to its improved cancer detection in combination with cystoscopy, a positive NMP22 result has been shown to be associated with a higher risk of bladder cancer recurrence [19, 20].

Bladder tumor antigen (BTA) tests detect complement factor H-related protein in the urine. This protein inhibits initiation of the complement cascade. The assay comes in a point of care solution, known as BTA stat®, which may be conducted in the office with a qualitative result. Alternatively, a quantitative enzyme-linked immunoabsorbent serologic assay (ELISA), BTA TRAK®, requires a reference laboratory for processing. The BTA tests are approved by the FDA for surveillance of bladder cancer, but not for initial diagnosis. Systematic reviews of studies using BTA stat® have shown overall sensitivity and specificity of 70 and 75 %, respectively [21]. The Finnbladder group showed in a prospective multicenter trial of 501 patients with a history of bladder cancer that BTA stat® was better at

detecting bladder cancer recurrence than was voided cytology (53.4 vs. 17.8 %, $p<0.001$). In this study, the overall specificities of BTA stat® and cytology were 85.7 % (95 % CI 81.1–89.5) and 98.3 % (95 % CI 96.0–99.4), respectively. False-positive results for the BTA tests are known to occur in the presence of urinary tract infections, stones, benign prostatic hyperplasia, intravesical therapy, hematuria, and inflammation. These confounding factors have limited the widespread applicability of these tests.

ImmunoCyt® is an immunofluorescence assay that detects several cell surface antigens, high-molecular weight form of carcinoembryonic antigen (19A211), and two mucin glycoproteins (LDQ10 and M344), which are specific for urothelial carcinoma. This test is FDA-approved for the surveillance of bladder cancer. The sensitivity of ImmunoCyt is particularly high for carcinoma in situ (85 %) and T1 tumors (80 %). In a meta-analysis of over 2,800 patients, Mowatt et al. showed an overall sensitivity and specificity of 84 % (95 % CI, 77–91 %) and 75 % (95 % CI, 78–92 %), respectively [22]. Given its performance characteristics, ImmunoCyt® has been studied in combination with urine cytology. In an Italian study of 2,217 patients undergoing evaluation and surveillance for bladder cancer, the addition of ImmunoCyt® to cytology increased sensitivity to 72.8 % while maintaining an overall specificity of 71.9 % [14]. The combination of these tests has been proposed to identify low-risk patients and reduce the frequency of cystoscopic evaluation. Intravesical therapy may increase the false-positive rate of ImmunoCyt® [23]. However, some authors have suggested that this may be an anticipatory positive, as nearly 50 % of the so-called false positives had converted to recurrences at 1 year follow-up [24]. Various technical challenges also limit the accessibility and application of this test, including labor-intensive evaluation of at least 500 cells per slide, a steep learning curve, technical expertise, and interobserver variability.

The UroVysion® test utilizes fluorescence in situ hybridization (FISH) to detect aneuploidy of chromosomes 3, 7, and 17, and deletions of 9p21. The threshold for a positive test includes five or more urothelial cells with gains of two or more chromosomes, or 12 or more cells with gain of 1 chromosome, or 12 or more cells with loss of 9p21 with a minimum examination of 25 cells [7, 25]. The performance of UroVysion® improves with increasing grade and stage. The overall sensitivity of UroVysion® has been shown to be superior to voided cytology (74 vs. 48 %), especially in high-grade disease such as carcinoma in situ (CIS) (100 vs. 67 %) [26]. In this meta-analysis of 12 studies, the overall specificity for UroVysion® was 83 % and for cytology was 96 %. By detecting chromosomal aberrations, UroVysion® may have the ability to identify occult disease prior to visible abnormalities on cystoscopy. In patients with negative cystoscopy and cytology, a positive FISH test may precede the development of a visible tumor by up to 1–2 years in 40–60 % of cases [27]. UroVysion® does not appear to be affected by hematuria or inflammation, although false positives may result with the use of barbotage or the presence of polyoma virus. The FISH assay has also been shown to be useful in monitoring patients for recurrence following BCG therapy. A positive test has been associated with a higher risk for the development of muscle invasive disease following BCG treatment and increased risk for recurrent tumors. In a study of 126 patients receiving BCG, Kamat and colleagues found that a positive FISH result in patients at any time during therapy increased the risk of recurrence by 3 to 5 times and of disease progression by 5–13 times over that in patients

with a negative FISH [28]. The authors proposed that FISH might be a useful marker to monitor BCG response and help identify potentially high-risk patients for alternative therapies. UroVysion® has also been found to have utility as an adjunct to aid in risk stratification of patients with equivocal cytology results. In a study of 120 patients with atypical cytology and a reflex FISH test, the negative predictive value of UroVysion® in patients with equivocal or negative cystoscopy was 100 % [29]. In such patients, further diagnostic work-up and biopsy may be avoided. While initially developed to detect bladder cancer, some data suggest UroVysion® on urine washings may also be useful for the detection of upper tract urothelial carcinoma. In a group of 55 patients suspected of upper tract tumors, FISH was able to detect all upper tract cancers and had a 100 % negative predictive value [30]. Compared to washing urine cytology, FISH was more sensitive (100 vs. 20.8 %), but less specific (89.5 vs. 97.4 %). The role of FISH in upper tract urothelial carcinoma remains to be defined.

A host of other biomarkers are being actively investigated for use in bladder cancer detection and surveillance. These areas of study include antigens (hyaluronic acid, survivin, NMP52), proteomic markers (CXCL1, tumor-associated trypsin inhibitor, matrix metalloproteinases), genetic markers (FGFR3 mutations), epigenetic markers (hypermethylation of E-cadherin and p16), and microRNA. As laboratory analytic techniques, including high-throughput genomic and proteomic technologies, become increasingly complex, our methods for analyzing and understanding such high-dimensional data will need to evolve. It is unlikely that one single marker will provide complete insight, but rather a group or network of factors analyzed in combination will aid in the diagnosis, risk stratification, and treatment of bladder cancer.

11.3 Current Imaging Tools

White light (WL) cystoscopy remains the gold standard for the diagnosis of bladder cancer. Ultrasound and cross-sectional imaging lack sufficient resolution to detect subtle, microstructural changes in the bladder wall. Direct visual inspection via WL and subsequent histopathologic examination through tumor biopsy are thus the primary mode of diagnosis and subsequent surveillance in bladder cancer management. As noted previously in this chapter, urine biomarkers play an important adjunctive role, particularly for detection and monitoring for high-grade disease. They are discussed in detail later in this chapter.

Flexible cystoscopy is the workhorse in the outpatient clinic. Current state-of-the-art technology employs digital systems that incorporate charged couple device (CCD) distal chip sensors. Complementary metal oxide sensors (CMOS) obviate the need for fragile fiber optics, improving durability while simultaneously providing superior optical resolution [31]. Rigid instruments and state-of-the-art cameras in the operating room also incorporate high definition (HD) with significant improvements in resolution.

11.3.1 Rationale for Add On Imaging Technology

For the majority of bladder lesions, notably papillary tumors, WL performs quite well. Experienced urologists have excellent ability to discriminate benign from malignant lesions. Cina et al. illustrated that practitioners were able to reliably distinguish cancerous from non-cancerous lesions by WL alone with 100 % sensitivity and specificity [32]. Despite these considerable advances, WL has persistent limitations with false-positive findings leading to excessive intervention with bladder biopsies, incomplete TURBT leading to residual untreated microscopic cancer, and missed diagnosis of carcinoma in situ (CIS) that is not visible by WL in up to 50 % of patients [33].

While useful in identification of malignancy, visual appearance has been shown to be unreliable in determining tumor grade or level of invasion [32]. Carcinoma in situ may not be visible by WL and easily overlooked in up to 50 % of lesions [34]. Missing such a lesion could significantly impact a patient's management and outcome [35].

Further limitations in the use of WL can be seen in endoscopic-guided tumor resection where residual tumor and inadequate staging, especially in high-grade T1 disease, occur. A second TUR shortly after initial diagnosis of T1 tumors demonstrates residual tumor in 43–62 % of cases [36–38]. The significant recurrence rate of bladder cancer can be attributed in part to non-visualized residual tumor left behind after incomplete resection [6]. Understaging of T1HG cancers at the time of cystectomy occurs in up to 40 % of patients, suggesting that inadequate tumor sampling is a contributing factor [39]. While WL remains the current standard of practice in bladder cancer diagnosis and management, better tools for detection, staging, and guidelines for treatment clearly are needed.

Newer diagnostic imaging modalities offer the hope of more precise characterization of dysplastic and malignant lesions in the bladder. These include fluorescence cystoscopy (also referred to as photodynamic diagnosis [PDD]), optical coherence tomography (OCT), narrow band imaging (NBI), Raman spectroscopy, virtual cystoscopy, and confocal microscopy (reviewed by Cauberg et al. [40], Goh et al. [41], and Liu et al. [42]).

11.4 Photodynamic Diagnosis (PDD)/Fluorescence Cystoscopy

PDD requires preoperative intravesical instillation of a fluorophore that is taken up by the urothelium and preferentially metabolized by dysplastic cells. When exposed to blue light (380–480 nm) dysplastic cells emit a characteristic red fluorescence. In the 1990s, 5-aminolevulinic acid (5-ALA) was described with the advantages of intravesical application and better fluorescence [43]. ALA is a substrate involved in heme biosynthesis and induces accumulation of excessive intracellular levels of the fluorescent substrate protoporphyrin IX (PpIX). Since neoplastic or rapidly proliferating cells tend to accumulate excess PpIX in contrast to normal tissue, 5-ALA can be used to induce red fluorescence under exposure to blue light in order to identify cancerous

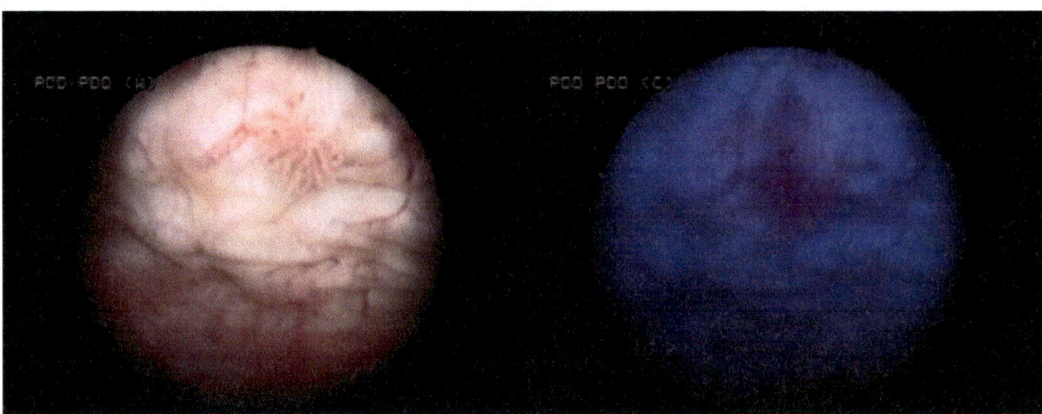

Fig. 11.1 WL shows a papillary bladder tumor (*left*). Fluorescence cystoscopy following intravesical HAL instillation shows the papillary lesion fluorescing red (*right*)

and pre-cancerous lesions [44] (Fig. 11.1). One of the limitations of 5-ALA is its relative tissue insolubility. This limited tissue penetrance has been addressed with the development of the hexyl ester derivative, hexaminolevulinate (HAL), with increased lipophilic properties.

PDD has been in use in Europe for two decades using the 5-ALA and, more recently, the hexyl ester derivative of ALA (HAL) (Hexvix, Photocure, Oslo Norway) following European Union regulatory approval in 2005. Updated EAU guidelines include PDD as an option for use when a high-grade cancer is suspected either when there is a positive cytology or history of high-grade cancer [45]. HAL in combination with the Storz D-Light system was approved by the US Food and Drug Administration in 2010 on the basis of a phase III trial conducted in Europe and North America, which demonstrated a 16 % relative reduction in recurrence at 9 months for HAL compared to WL [46].

Multiple studies have validated the ability of PDD to identify a greater number of papillary and CIS lesions and two recent meta-analyses of clinical trials using HAL provide further confirmatory evidence. Burger and colleagues reported that at least one additional Ta or T1 tumor was identified in 25 % of patients [47]. In a pooled analysis of three phase III multicenter trials investigating HAL [48–50], Liu et al. showed a fluorescence detection rate of CIS of 87 versus 75 % for WL ($p=0.006$) [51]. Several studies also suggest that use of PDD is associated with a more complete tumor resection [52–54]. With more accurate diagnosis, Jocham and co-workers demonstrated that better postoperative treatment was possible in over 20 % of patients with bladder tumors [48].

False positives are a concern as this may lead to overuse of bladder biopsies and this occurs in up to 40 % of lesions and ranges from 10 to 12 % on a per patient basis in contemporary clinical trials. [46] Surgeon experience plays a role and other causes of false-positive florescence include autofluorescence (AF), which results from activation of the tissue's endogenous fluorophores in response to blue light, tangential imaging and inflammation, including that associated with post-intravesical therapy mucosal changes and post-transurethral resection. Both ALA and HAL exhibit limited depth of penetration, restricting the evaluation of more invasive lesions. Photobleaching, or loss of fluorescence, is also a factor limiting the amount of time for examination to about 30 min [55].

11.4.1 Level I Evidence Assessing Reduction in Recurrence Probability

Several phase III trials have been reported recently evaluated the potential for ALA and HAL to reduce the risk of recurrence and the data

Table 11.2 Phase III trials using fluorescence cystoscopy vs. no treatment/placebo control

Author	Year	N	Agent	Timepoint	Recurrence-free survival (%) PDD	WLC	p value
Grossman et al. [59]	2012	516	HAL	54 months[a]	38	32	0.04
Geavlete et al. [58]	2012	362	HAL	24 months	69	54	0.001
Hermann et al. [60]	2011	145	HAL	24 months	70	53	0.02
Stenzl et al. [62]	2011	359	5-ALA	12 months	64	73	NS
Stenzl, et al. [46]	2010	551	HAL	9 months	53	44	0.026
Schumacher et al. [61]	2010	300	5-ALA	12 months	55	56	NS
Denzinger et al. [54]	2007	301	5-ALA	8 years	71[b]	45	0.0003
Daniltchenko et al. [53]	2005	102	5-ALA	5 years	41	25	0.02
Babjuk et al. [56]	2005	122	5-ALA	24 months	40	28	0.008
Filbeck et al. [57][c]	2002	191	5-ALA	24 months	90	66	0.004

[a]Median HAL 55 months vs. median WL 53 months; Long-term follow up of Stenzl, et al. (2010)
[b]Long-term follow up of Filbeck et al (2002); Median ALA 86 months vs. median WL 83 months
[c]Residual tumor and planned re-TRUBT at 5–6 weeks 25.2 % vs. 4.5 % for WL vs. ALA, respectively

are summarized in Table 11.2 [46, 53, 54, 56–62]. An excellent review of the literature regarding HAL was recently published and the authors concluded that the improved tumor detection and reduction of residual disease after TURBT is associated with a modest but significant reduction in recurrence post TURBT. No data to date suggest that PDD is associated with a reduction in progression. These trials have shown no significant differences in adverse events between patients undergoing fluorescence cystoscopy and those undergoing WL [18, 46, 48]. Burger and colleagues analyzed 600 patients comparing HAL and 5-ALA and found both superior to WL with reduced residual tumor post TURBT and recurrence probability with no significant difference between the two protoporphyrins [52]. The FDA approval does not include patients within 90 days post-BCG treatment, nor does it cover multiple uses in the same patient. A recent study of 25 patients suggested a benefit with PDD in 19 % of patients but with a higher false-positive biopsy rate. Registry studies have been proposed to address both of these opportunities.

11.4.2 Cost-Effectiveness

Several studies have documented that bladder cancer is the most expensive cancer from diagnosis until death. Patients diagnosed at localized stage experience higher lifetime costs compared to patients diagnosed at regional stage in part due to longer survival from diagnosis to death [63]. Konety and colleagues reported in 2007 that the average cost of TURBTs in the US was $26,653 and that monitoring and treatment of recurrence consumes an estimated 60 % of total bladder cancer-related costs [64].

Cost analyses of the use of the hexylester derivative of ALA (hexylaminolevulinic acid) suggest that its use can reduce the overall cost of care at least in part due to a lower overall cancer burden. Sievert et al. reported that the cost of a TURBT would be reduced by $187 representing a 9.2 % benefit by eliminating the need for site-directed biopsies of normal appearing mucosa and a 20 % reduction in the need for a second resection within 6 months [65]. Utilizing data from a randomized trial of ALA conducted in Germany, Burger and colleagues estimated annual savings of $224 per year with use of fluorescence cystoscopy [66]. It is not clear that the studies by Sievert and Burger accounted for the fully capitalized cost of purchasing a blue light system in the US. More recently, Garfield developed a decision tree model to evaluate the cost-effectiveness of using fluorescence cystoscopy at the time of initial TURBT and found that with 4.5 years of follow-up the total cost burden was $25,921 compared to $30,581 in patients who were managed with white light cystoscopy alone [67].

11.4.3 Novel Fluorophores

Hypericin is a derivative of St. John's wart that is less susceptible to photobleaching, with improved specificity and can be used in the same imaging system as for the porphyrin-related substrates. D'Hallewin and colleagues reported 94 % sensitivity for hypericin-induced fluorescent detection of CIS and 95 % specificity, which was superior to 5-ALA and HAL [68]. The drug showed excellent tolerability and fluorescence lasted up to 16 h following instillation. A potential limitation of hypericin is low water solubility, which may be overcome with use of solvents, such as polyvinylpyrrolidone (PVP) and albumin [69, 70]. In preclinical animal models, PVP-hypericin accumulated 3.5-fold preferentially in malignant vs. benign urothelium [71]. Examination of these new aqueous formulations of hypericin demonstrated overall tumor detection sensitivity and specificity ranging from 81–95 % and 53–91 %, respectively. Using image analysis of fluorescence images in 23 patients, Kah and colleagues were able to distinguish low- and high-grade lesions and suggest that this technique may help identify CIS lesions [72].

11.5 Optical Coherence Tomography (OCT)

OCT is a real-time high-resolution imaging technology that utilizes near infrared light (890–1300 nm). It measures the unique backscatter properties of different tissue characteristics to provide a cross-sectional image of biologic tissues. It permits detection of microarchitectural features to a resolution of 10–20 μm in a fashion similar to B-mode ultrasound [73]. Compared to high frequency ultrasound, OCT is able to distinguish structures up to 10–25 times smaller [74]. OCT can be applied to any surface structure and was initially developed for imaging the retina and since has been applied in a variety of gastrointestinal lesions, cervical dysplasia, and skin disorders. The feasibility of in vivo detection of human bladder pathology by OCT was demonstrated by Zagaynova and colleagues [75]. Current endoscopic implementations of this technology utilizes a 2.7-mm diameter probe that can be passed

through a standard cystoscope facilitating real-time examination with a relatively short learning curve for interpretation of surface microarchitecture to a depth of 1–2 mm.

OCT is able to resolve layers of the bladder and distinguish benign from malignant characteristics (Fig. 11.2). Manyak et al. reported 100 % sensitivity and 89 % specificity for classifying lesions as benign or malignant in 24 patients [76]. In a series of 32 patients, Goh and colleagues showed 100 % sensitivity, 90 % specificity, and 100 % negative predictive value for detection of muscle invasion [77]. False positives do occur in the setting of disruptions of the bladder wall from erosion, scarring, or granuloma. Integration of fluorescence cystoscopy (FC) with OCT may improve the diagnostic characteristics of both imaging modalities [78]. Schmidbauer and colleagues evaluated this in 68 patients and found on a per patient basis FC plus OCT improved specificity of FC from 62.5 to 87.5 % [79]. The utility of OCT in the diagnosis of CIS and its role in bladder cancer management has yet to be elucidated in large controlled studies. We have completed a multicenter trial in the US with the primary aim to assess the accuracy and positive predictive value of OCT for determining tumor stage correlated by histopathology (NCT00831558). Preliminary findings indicate that OCT is very accurate in distinguishing non-invasive tumors (Ta) from invasive (T1–T3). This may help with intra-operative determination of the need for deep resection into muscularis propria to optimize pathologic staging.

There is a wealth of data produced with each digitized OCT image. Computer-aided texture analysis reduces the subjectivity of image interpretation and provides an objective method to distinguish cancer from benign tissue [80]. Optical brightness has been used to classify cervical intraepithelial neoplasia [81]. Cauberg et al. have evaluated the utility of this for optical grading of bladder cancer [82]. We have observed a continuum of lower to higher degrees of brightness with increased depth of invasion (unpublished).

Recent technical innovations in OCT involve thinner profile probes that may be used with flexible instruments and to access the upper urinary tract and a portable laptop computer that

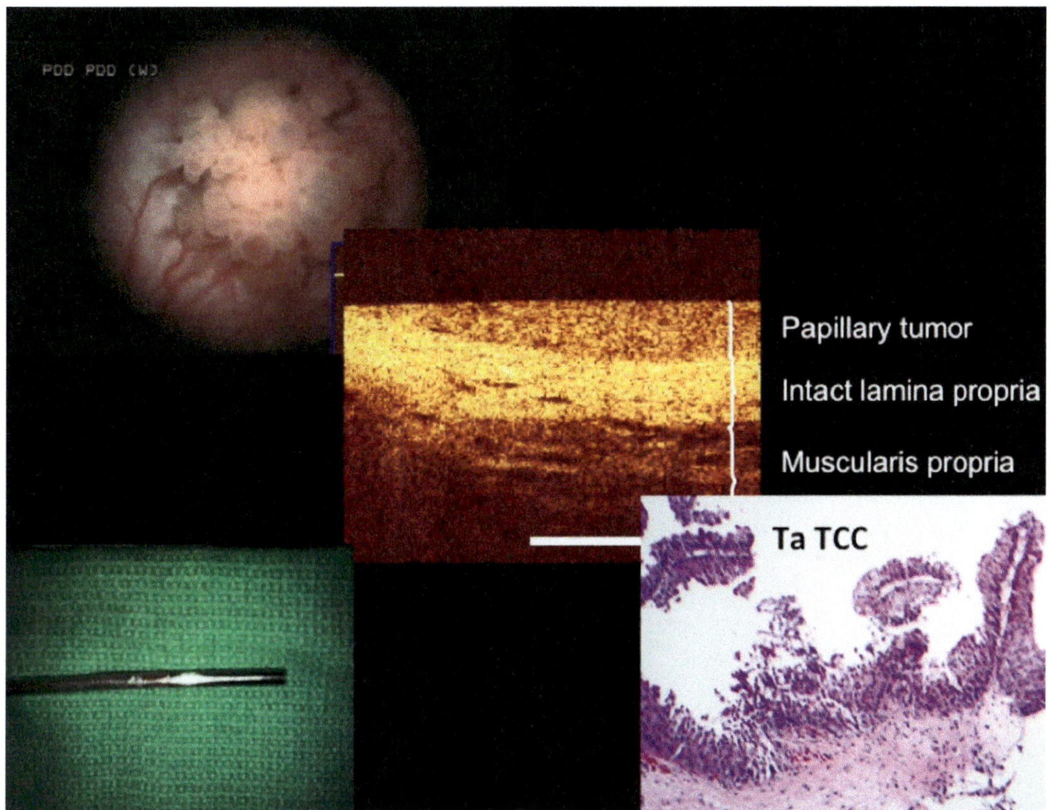

Fig. 11.2 White light cystoscopic view of a papillary bladder tumor (*top left*); OCT (*middle*) demonstrates the mucosal layer is expanded, but intact, without evidence of invasion. The lamina propria is intact and appears bright and clearly defined, while the muscularis propria layer appears dark below. Histologic analysis shows a TaG1 urothelial carcinoma (*bottom right*). OCT 2.7 mm probe *bottom left*

may facilitate use in the outpatient clinic. CIS can be particularly challenging to identify as up to 50 % of lesions appear normal by WL. Ren and colleagues at Stony Brook have developed an experimental OCT system that produces three-dimensional (3-D) images and have used this system to describe the variable morphologies of CIS [83]. Their in vivo preclinical work suggests that 3-D OCT enhanced the sensitivity of WL and FC and improved the specificity of NBI for detection of CIS [84].

11.6   Narrow-Band Imaging (NBI)

NBI enhances the contrast between abnormal lesions and normal urothelium by restricting the optical spectrum used for visualization. A narrowed bandwidth is accomplished with filters, which permit transmission of light at wavelengths of 415 and 540 nm [85]. Hypervascularity is highlighted because hemoglobin strongly absorbs light at these wavelengths. Since this technique simply filters the light, it is easily integrated into a standard endoscopic platform. Another advantage is that no additional dyes or markers are necessary.

NBI cystoscopy relies on the inherent hypervascularity of urothelial carcinomas to enhance visual contrast, and thereby detection of lesions. Given identical optics, NBI provides the same resolution of macroscopic lesions as WL. Areas with increased angiogenesis have a blue tint and appear darker than normal mucosa (Fig. 11.3). Several studies have shown that NBI endoscopy offers better detection of bladder cancer than

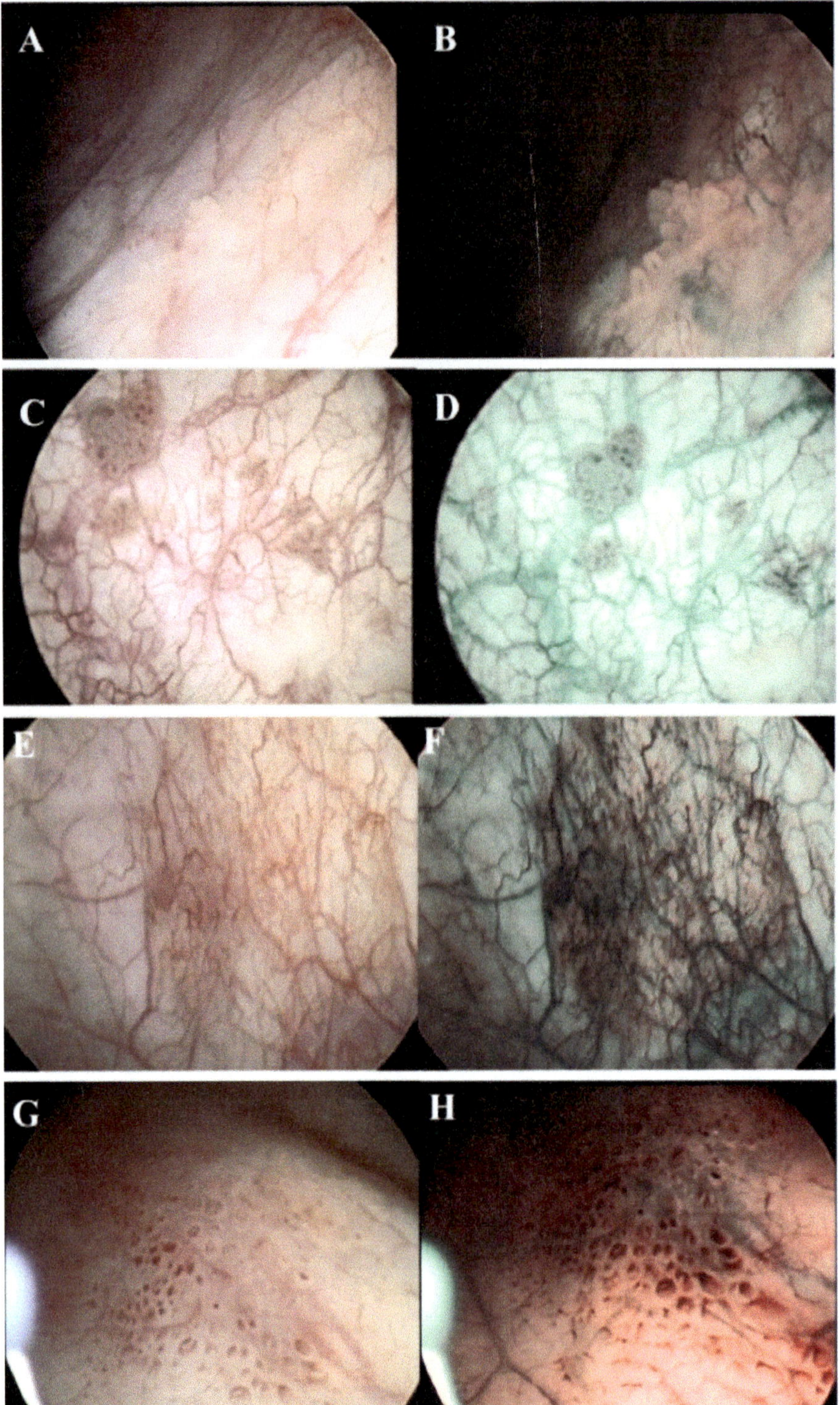

Fig. 11.3 WL and NBI images. (**a**) A small papillary tumor. (**b**) Improved detection by NBI. (**c**) WL image of multiple pTaG1 tumors. (**d**) Enhanced contrast of same tumors with NBI. (**e**) WL image of CIS. (**f**) Enhanced visualization of CIS with NBI. (**g**) False-positive lesion near the right orifice identified by WL (**h**) Same lesion identified by NBI (reactive tissue). Cauberg et al. Elsevier 2010 (with Permission)

WL. A recent meta-analysis of 8 studies and 1,022 patients showed the sensitivity and specificity of NBI and WL were 94 % (95 % CI 91–96) vs. 85 % (95 % CI 80–89) and 85 % (95 % CI 81–88) vs. 87 % (95 % CI 83–90), respectively [86]. In the largest reported single-center series ($n=427$), Herr et al. demonstrated that NBI identified CIS better than WL (100 % versus 83 % sensitivity, $p=0.01$) [87]. A recent subset analysis of patients in this cohort with recurrent tumors showed an apparent reduction in the recurrence rate of tumors detected and treated with NBI cystoscopy [88]. The authors reported an absolute improvement of 7 months recurrence-free survival after adoption of NBI technology. BCG therapy and inflammatory conditions have been shown to increase the false-positive rate of this technology. Two studies have shown similar overall false-positive rates of 32–36 % for NBI [87, 89]. The false-detection rates raise concerns regarding the cost and potential morbidity of unnecessary biopsies, although these results appear to be similar to those associated with WL and PDD. Further controlled multicenter studies are needed to confirm the diagnostic and therapeutic benefit of NBI for bladder cancer.

11.7 Confocal Laser Endomicroscopy (CLE)

CLE is an emerging imaging technology that can provide microscopic, real-time, histopathologic information on live tissue. This technique employs a fiber optic bundle carrying laser light tuned to 488 nm and fluorescent dyes for contrast. Until recently, technical challenges have limited the use of this technology in an endoscopic solution. Currently, 1.4 mm and 2.6 mm-diameter flexible microendoscopy probes are commercially available and can pass through standard cystoscopic equipment. Of the imaging modalities discussed thus far, CLE has the highest resolution (up to 2–5 μm and to a depth to 240 μm).

CLE is capable of resolving micron-scale detail of tissue microarchitecture down to the cellular level, making it well suited for the detection of epithelial carcinomas, such as bladder cancer. Current clinical data derive largely from the gastrointestinal literature, where CLE has been shown to be useful in the identification of esophageal, gastric, and colorectal neoplasias [90, 91]. Recently, the feasibility of using CLE to detect, characterize, and differentiate bladder cancer from normal urothelium in vivo and ex vivo has been demonstrated [92, 93]. Some limitations of CLE include the need for intravenous or intravesical fluorescein dye as a contrast agent, a finite window for imaging, en face contact required for image acquisition, limited depth of penetration, and a small field of view. As an adjunct to conventional cystoscopy, CLE may be used to focus on areas of suspicion, confirm microscopic abnormalities, and potentially reduce unnecessary biopsies. The diagnostic characteristics and therapeutic utility of this technology in the genitourinary system appear promising and is the subject of active investigation.

11.8 Emerging Technology

With each imaging modality offering different resolution, depth of penetration, and field of view, it is likely that a combination of techniques, macroscopic (WL, PDD, NBI) and microscopic (OCT, CLE), may be integrated to provide enhanced endoscopic characterization of bladder tumors. In an ex vivo study, one group has shown the feasibility of utilizing PDD to target suspicious bladder tumors and then following immediately with CLE [94]. A future application may be to use real-time, intraoperative microscopic imaging techniques to guide and assess the adequacy of tumor resection.

On the horizon are several advanced imaging techniques currently in development that may assist in diagnosis and treatment of bladder cancer (Table 11.3). Virtual cystoscopy utilizes multi-detector computed tomographic 3-D volume-rendered reconstructions to detect bladder lesions as small as 5 mm in size [41]. Limitations include the inability to detect flat lesions and radiation exposure from cross-sectional imaging. Endoluminal high-frequency

Table 11.3 Imaging modalities

	Cystoscopy (WLC, PDD NBI)	OCT	CLE	VC	HFUS	CARS
Contrast media	None or HAL	None	Fluorescein	Air or Iodinated	None	None
Resolution	mm–cm	10–20 µm	2–5 µm	5 mm	100 µm	0.07–0.1 µm
Depth of penetration	Surface	1–2 mm	240 µm	Surface	10–20 mm	300 µm
Acquisition	Real-time	Real-time	Real-time	Post-processing	Real-time	Real-time

WLC White light cystoscopy, *PDD* Photodynamic diagnosis, *BI* Narrow band imaging, *OCT* Optical coherence tomography, *CLE* Confocal laser endomicroscopy, *VC* Virtual cystoscopy, *HFUS* Endoluminal High frequency ultrasound, *CARS* Coherent anti-stokes Raman scattering

ultrasound (HFUS) allows greater depth of penetration (up to 20 mm), but less spatial resolution than OCT. It has been shown to be useful for identifying muscle invasion in larger bladder tumors [95]. Two-photon laser microscopy takes advantage of the autofluorescence of cells and of extracellular matrix components using light in the ultraviolet spectrum. An ex vivo examination of normal urothelium and of carcinoma in situ demonstrated the discriminatory capability with this technique to resolution at the sub-micron level [96]. Coherent anti-stokes Raman scattering (CARS) microscopy is a novel, label-free imaging modality which utilizes a combination of lasers to excite intrinsic chemical bonds (C–H) to generate optical contrast [97]. This nonlinear technique offers the potential of high-resolution (0.07–0.1 µm), real-time image acquisition without the need for dyes or stains. CARS microscopy has been shown to be capable of characterizing prostatic glandular structure and cavernosal nerves in fresh tissue specimens from patients undergoing radical prostatectomy [98]. Investigation is currently underway to assess its suitability for bladder cancer detection.

11.9 Conclusion

Bladder cancer remains a challenging disease to diagnosis and to manage. The application of new technology from biomarker analysis to novel imaging techniques offers the opportunity to improve detection and treatment. Accumulating data support the use of fluorescence cystoscopy to enhance bladder cancer detection and reduce tumor recurrence following treatment. Continued prospective study is necessary to evaluate the feasibility and efficacy of emerging imaging methods for bladder cancer.

References

1. Riley GF, Potosky AL, Lubitz JD, Kessler LG. Medicare payments from diagnosis to death for elderly cancer patients by stage at diagnosis. Med Care. 1995;33(8):828–41.
2. Botteman MF, Pashos CL, Redaelli A, Laskin B, Hauser R. The health economics of bladder cancer: a comprehensive review of the published literature. Pharmacoeconomics. 2003;21(18):1315–30.
3. Siegel R, Naishadham D, Jemal A. Cancer statistics, 2013. CA Cancer J Clin. 2013;63(1):11–30.
4. Herr HW. Natural history of superficial bladder tumors: 10- to 20-year follow-up of treated patients. World J Urol. 1997;15(2):84–8.
5. Holmang S, Hedelin H, Anderstrom C, Holmberg E, Busch C, Johansson SL. Recurrence and progression in low grade papillary urothelial tumors. J Urol. 1999;162(3 Pt 1):702–7.
6. Brausi M, Collette L, Kurth K, van der Meijden AP, Oosterlinck W, Witjes JA, et al. Variability in the recurrence rate at first follow-up cystoscopy after TUR in stage Ta T1 transitional cell carcinoma of the bladder: a combined analysis of seven EORTC studies. Eur Urol. 2002;41(5):523–31.
7. Halling KC, King W, Sokolova IA, Meyer RG, Burkhardt HM, Halling AC, et al. A comparison of cytology and fluorescence in situ hybridization for the detection of urothelial carcinoma. J Urol. 2000;164(5):1768–75.
8. Todenhofer T, Hennenlotter J, Esser M, Mohrhardt S, Tews V, Aufderklamm S, et al. Combined application of cytology and molecular urine markers to improve the detection of urothelial carcinoma. Cancer Cytopathol. 2013;121(5):252–60.
9. Lokeshwar VB, Habuchi T, Grossman HB, Murphy WM, Hautmann SH, Hemstreet 3rd GP, et al. Bladder

tumor markers beyond cytology: International Consensus Panel on bladder tumor markers. Urology. 2005;66(6 Suppl 1):35–63.

10. Zippe C, Pandrangi L, Agarwal A. NMP22 is a sensitive, cost-effective test in patients at risk for bladder cancer. J Urol. 1999;161(1):62–5. Epub. 1999/02/26.

11. Grossman HB, Messing E, Soloway M, Tomera K, Katz G, Berger Y, et al. Detection of bladder cancer using a point-of-care proteomic assay. JAMA. 2005;293(7):810–6. Epub 2005/02/17.

12. Giannopoulos A, Manousakas T, Gounari A, Constantinides C, Choremi-Papadopoulou H, Dimopoulos C. Comparative evaluation of the diagnostic performance of the BTA stat test, NMP22 and urinary bladder cancer antigen for primary and recurrent bladder tumors. J Urol. 2001;166(2):470–5. Epub 2001/07/18.

13. Toma MI, Friedrich MG, Hautmann SH, Jakel KT, Erbersdobler A, Hellstern A, et al. Comparison of the ImmunoCyt test and urinary cytology with other urine tests in the detection and surveillance of bladder cancer. World J Urol. 2004;22(2):145–9. Epub 2004/03/03.

14. Comploj E, Mian C, Ambrosini-Spaltro A, Dechet C, Palermo S, Trenti E, et al. uCyt+/ImmunoCyt and cytology in the detection of urothelial carcinoma: an update on 7422 analyses. Cancer Cytopathol. 2013;121(7):392–7. Epub. 2013/03/16.

15. Bonberg N, Taeger D, Gawrych K, Johnen G, Banek S, Schwentner C, et al. Chromosomal instability and bladder cancer: the UroVysion(TM) test in the UroScreen study. BJU Int. 2013;112(4):E372–82. Epub 2013/01/29.

16. Ponsky LE, Sharma S, Pandrangi L, Kedia S, Nelson D, Agarwal A, et al. Screening and monitoring for bladder cancer: refining the use of NMP22. J Urol. 2001;166(1):75–8.

17. Liou LS. Urothelial cancer biomarkers for detection and surveillance. Urology. 2006;67(3 Suppl 1):25–33. discussion –4.

18. Grossman HB, Gomella L, Fradet Y, Morales A, Presti J, Ritenour C, et al. A phase III, multicenter comparison of hexaminolevulinate fluorescence cystoscopy and white light cystoscopy for the detection of superficial papillary lesions in patients with bladder cancer. J Urol. 2007;178(1):62–7.

19. Lau P, Chin JL, Pautler S, Razvi H, Izawa JI. NMP22 is predictive of recurrence in high-risk superficial bladder cancer patients. Can Urol Assoc J. 2009;3(6):454–8.

20. Shariat SF, Savage C, Chromecki TF, Sun M, Scherr DS, Lee RK, et al. Assessing the clinical benefit of nuclear matrix protein 22 in the surveillance of patients with nonmuscle-invasive bladder cancer and negative cytology: a decision-curve analysis. Cancer. 2011;117(13):2892–7.

21. Glas AS, Roos D, Deutekom M, Zwinderman AH, Bossuyt PM, Kurth KH. Tumor markers in the diagnosis of primary bladder cancer. A systematic review. J Urol. 2003;169(6):1975–82.

22. Mowatt G, Zhu S, Kilonzo M, Boachie C, Fraser C, Griffiths TR, et al. Systematic review of the clinical effectiveness and cost-effectiveness of photodynamic diagnosis and urine biomarkers (FISH, ImmunoCyt, NMP22) and cytology for the detection and follow-up of bladder cancer. Health Technol Assess. 2010;14(4):1–331. iii–iv.

23. Lodde M, Mian C, Negri G, Vittadello F, Comploj E, Palermo S, et al. Effect of intravesical instillation on performance of uCYT+test. Urology. 2004;63(5):878–81.

24. Piaton E, Daniel L, Verriele V, Dalifard I, Zimmermann U, Renaudin K, et al. Improved detection of urothelial carcinomas with fluorescence immunocytochemistry (uCyt+assay) and urinary cytology: results of a French Prospective Multicenter Study. Lab Invest. 2003;83(6):845–52.

25. Huysentruyt CJ, Baldewijns MM, Ruland AM, Tonk RJ, Vervoort PS, Smits KM, et al. Modified UroVysion scoring criteria increase the urothelial carcinoma detection rate in cases of equivocal urinary cytology. Histopathology. 2011;58(7):1048–53.

26. Hajdinjak T. UroVysion FISH test for detecting urothelial cancers: meta-analysis of diagnostic accuracy and comparison with urinary cytology testing. Urol Oncol. 2008;26(6):646–51.

27. Yoder BJ, Skacel M, Hedgepeth R, Babineau D, Ulchaker JC, Liou LS, et al. Reflex UroVysion testing of bladder cancer surveillance patients with equivocal or negative urine cytology: a prospective study with focus on the natural history of anticipatory positive findings. Am J Clin Pathol. 2007;127(2):295–301.

28. Kamat AM, Dickstein RJ, Messetti F, Anderson R, Pretzsch SM, Gonzalez GN, et al. Use of fluorescence in situ hybridization to predict response to bacillus Calmette-Guerin therapy for bladder cancer: results of a prospective trial. J Urol. 2012;187(3):862–7.

29. Schlomer BJ, Ho R, Sagalowsky A, Ashfaq R, Lotan Y. Prospective validation of the clinical usefulness of reflex fluorescence in situ hybridization assay in patients with atypical cytology for the detection of urothelial carcinoma of the bladder. J Urol. 2010;183(1):62–7.

30. Mian C, Mazzoleni G, Vikoler S, Martini T, Knuchel-Clark R, Zaak D, et al. Fluorescence in situ hybridisation in the diagnosis of upper urinary tract tumours. Eur Urol. 2010;58(2):288–92.

31. Quayle SS, Ames CD, Lieber D, Yan Y, Landman J. Comparison of optical resolution with digital and standard fiberoptic cystoscopes in an in vitro model. Urology. 2005;66(3):489–93.

32. Cina SJ, Epstein JI, Endrizzi JM, Harmon WJ, Seay TM, Schoenberg MP. Correlation of cystoscopic impression with histologic diagnosis of biopsy specimens of the bladder. Hum Pathol. 2001;32(6):630–7.

33. Rink M, Babjuk M, Catto JW, Jichlinski P, Shariat SF, Stenzl A, et al. Hexyl aminolevulinate-guided fluorescence cystoscopy in the diagnosis and follow-up of patients with non-muscle-invasive bladder cancer: a critical review of the current literature. Eur Urol. 2013;64(4):624–38.

34. Soloway MS, Murphy W, Rao MK, Cox C. Serial multiple-site biopsies in patients with bladder cancer. J Urol. 1978;120(1):57–9.
35. Millan-Rodriguez F, Chechile-Toniolo G, Salvador-Bayarri J, Palou J, Vicente-Rodriguez J. Multivariate analysis of the prognostic factors of primary superficial bladder cancer. J Urol. 2000;163(1):73–8.
36. Klan R, Loy V, Huland H. Residual tumor discovered in routine second transurethral resection in patients with stage T1 transitional cell carcinoma of the bladder. J Urol. 1991;146(2):316–8.
37. Schwaibold HE, Sivalingam S, May F, Hartung R. The value of a second transurethral resection for T1 bladder cancer. BJU Int. 2006;97(6):1199–201.
38. Brauers A, Buettner R, Jakse G. Second resection and prognosis of primary high risk superficial bladder cancer: is cystectomy often too early? J Urol. 2001;165(3):808–10.
39. Shariat SF, Palapattu GS, Karakiewicz PI, Rogers CG, Vazina A, Bastian PJ, et al. Discrepancy between clinical and pathologic stage: impact on prognosis after radical cystectomy. Eur Urol. 2007;51(1):137–49. discussion 49–51.
40. Cauberg Evelyne CC, de la Rosette JJ, de Reijke TM. Emerging optical techniques in advanced cystoscopy for bladder cancer diagnosis: a review of the current literature. Indian J Urol. 2011;27(2):245–51.
41. Goh AC, Lerner SP. Application of new technology in bladder cancer diagnosis and treatment. World J Urol. 2009;27(3):301–7.
42. Liu JJ, Droller MJ, Liao JC. New optical imaging technologies for bladder cancer: considerations and perspectives. J Urol. 2012;188(2):361–8.
43. Kennedy JC, Pottier RH, Pross DC. Photodynamic therapy with endogenous protoporphyrin IX: basic principles and present clinical experience. J Photochem Photobiol B. 1990;6(1–2):143–8.
44. Batlle AM. Porphyrins, porphyrias, cancer and photo-dynamic therapy–a model for carcinogenesis. J Photochem Photobiol B. 1993;20(1):5–22.
45. Babjuk M, Burger M, Zigeuner R, Shariat SF, van Rhijn BW, Comperat E, et al. EAU guidelines on non-muscle-invasive urothelial carcinoma of the bladder: update 2013. Eur Urol. 2013;64(4):639–53.
46. Stenzl A, Burger M, Fradet Y, Mynderse LA, Soloway MS, Witjes JA, et al. Hexaminolevulinate guided fluorescence cystoscopy reduces recurrence in patients with nonmuscle invasive bladder cancer. J Urol. 2010;184(5):1907–13.
47. Burger M, Grossman HB, Droller M, Schmidbauer J, Hermann G, Dragoescu O, et al. Photodynamic diagnosis of non-muscle-invasive bladder cancer with hexaminolevulinate cystoscopy: a meta-analysis of detection and recurrence based on raw data. Eur Urol. 2013;64(5):846–54.
48. Jocham D, Witjes F, Wagner S, Zeylemaker B, van Moorselaar J, Grimm MO, et al. Improved detection and treatment of bladder cancer using hexaminolevu-linate imaging: a prospective, phase III multicenter study. J Urol. 2005;174(3):862–6. discussion 6.
49. Schmidbauer J, Witjes F, Schmeller N, Donat R, Susani M, Marberger M. Improved detection of uro-thelial carcinoma in situ with hexaminolevulinate fluorescence cystoscopy. J Urol. 2004;171(1):135–8.
50. Fradet Y, Grossman HB, Gomella L, Lerner S, Cookson M, Albala D, et al. A comparison of hexami-nolevulinate fluorescence cystoscopy and white light cystoscopy for the detection of carcinoma in situ in patients with bladder cancer: a phase III, multicenter study. J Urol. 2007;178(1):68–73. Discussion.
51. Liu H, Wu M, Thomas YK, Lerner SP. Fluorescence and white light cystoscopy for detecting carcinoma in situ of the bladder. J Urol. 2008;179(4):326.
52. Burger M, Stief CG, Zaak D, Stenzl A, Wieland WF, Jocham D, et al. Hexaminolevulinate is equal to 5-aminolevulinic acid concerning residual tumor and recurrence rate following photodynamic diagnostic assisted transurethral resection of bladder tumors. Urology. 2009;74(6):1282–6.
53. Daniltchenko DI, Riedl CR, Sachs MD, Koenig F, Daha KL, Pflueger H, et al. Long-term benefit of 5-aminolevulinic acid fluorescence assisted transure-thral resection of superficial bladder cancer: 5-year results of a prospective randomized study. J Urol. 2005;174(6):2129–33. discussion 33.
54. Denzinger S, Burger M, Walter B, Knuechel R, Roessler W, Wieland WF, et al. Clinically relevant reduction in risk of recurrence of superficial bladder cancer using 5-aminolevulinic acid-induced fluores-cence diagnosis: 8-year results of prospective ran-domized study. Urology. 2007;69(4):675–9.
55. Steinbach P, Weingandt H, Baumgartner R, Kriegmair M, Hofstadter F, Knuchel R. Cellular fluorescence of the endogenous photosensitizer protoporphyrin IX following exposure to 5-aminolevulinic acid. Photochem Photobiol. 1995;62(5):887–95.
56. Babjuk M, Soukup V, Petrik R, Jirsa M, Dvoracek J. 5-aminolaevulinic acid-induced fluorescence cys-toscopy during transurethral resection reduces the risk of recurrence in stage Ta/T1 bladder cancer. BJU Int. 2005;96(6):798–802.
57. Filbeck T, Pichlmeier U, Knuechel R, Wieland WF, Roessler W. Clinically relevant improvement of recurrence-free survival with 5-aminolevulinic acid induced fluorescence diagnosis in patients with super-ficial bladder tumors. J Urol. 2002;168(1):67–71.
58. Geavlete B, Multescu R, Georgescu D, Jecu M, Stanescu F, Geavlete P. Treatment changes and long-term recurrence rates after hexaminolevulinate (HAL) fluorescence cystoscopy: does it really make a differ-ence in patients with non-muscle-invasive bladder cancer (NMIBC)? BJU Int. 2012;109(4):549–56.
59. Grossman HB, Stenzl A, Fradet Y, Mynderse LA, Kriegmair M, Witjes JA, et al. Long-term decrease in bladder cancer recurrence with hexaminolevulinate enabled fluorescence cystoscopy. J Urol. 2012;188(1):58–62.
60. Hermann GG, Mogensen K, Carlsson S, Marcussen N, Duun S. Fluorescence-guided transurethral resec-tion of bladder tumours reduces bladder tumour

recurrence due to less residual tumour tissue in Ta/T1 patients: a randomized two-centre study. BJU Int. 2011;108(8 Pt 2):E297–303.

61. Schumacher MC, Holmang S, Davidsson T, Friedrich B, Pedersen J, Wiklund NP. Transurethral resection of non-muscle-invasive bladder transitional cell cancers with or without 5-aminolevulinic Acid under visible and fluorescent light: results of a prospective, randomised, multicentre study. Eur Urol. 2010;57(2): 293–9.

62. Stenzl A, Penkoff H, Dajc-Sommerer E, Zumbraegel A, Hoeltl L, Scholz M, et al. Detection and clinical outcome of urinary bladder cancer with 5-aminolevulinic acid-induced fluorescence cystoscopy: a multicenter randomized, double-blind, placebo-controlled trial. Cancer. 2011;117(5):938–47.

63. Avritscher EB, Cooksley CD, Grossman HB, Sabichi AL, Hamblin L, Dinney CP, et al. Clinical model of lifetime cost of treating bladder cancer and associated complications. Urology. 2006;68(3):549–53.

64. Konety BR, Joyce GF, Wise M. Bladder and upper tract urothelial cancer. J Urol. 2007;177(5):1636–45.

65. Sievert KD, Amend B, Nagele U, Schilling D, Bedke J, Horstmann M, et al. Economic aspects of bladder cancer: what are the benefits and costs? World J Urol. 2009;27(3):295–300.

66. Burger M, Zaak D, Stief CG, Filbeck T, Wieland WF, Roessler W, et al. Photodynamic diagnostics and non-invasive bladder cancer: is it cost-effective in long-term application? A Germany-based cost analysis. Eur Urol. 2007;52(1):142–7.

67. Garfield SS, Gavaghan MB, Armstrong SO, Jones JS. The cost-effectiveness of blue light cystoscopy in bladder cancer detection: United States projections based on clinical data showing 4.5 years of follow up after a single hexaminolevulinate hydrochloride instillation. Can J Urol. 2013;20(2):6682–9.

68. D'Hallewin MA, Kamuhabwa AR, Roskams T, De Witte PA, Baert L. Hypericin-based fluorescence diagnosis of bladder carcinoma. BJU Int. 2002;89(7):760–3.

69. Kubin A, Meissner P, Wierrani F, Burner U, Bodenteich A, Pytel A, et al. Fluorescence diagnosis of bladder cancer with new water soluble hypericin bound to polyvinylpyrrolidone: PVP-hypericin. Photochem Photobiol. 2008;84(6):1560–3.

70. Sim HG, Lau WK, Olivo M, Tan PH, Cheng CW. Is photodynamic diagnosis using hypericin better than white-light cystoscopy for detecting superficial bladder carcinoma? BJU Int. 2005;95(9):1215–8.

71. Vandepitte J, Van Cleynenbreugel B, Hettinger K, Van Poppel H, de Witte PA. Biodistribution of PVP-hypericin and hexaminolevulinate-induced PpIX in normal and orthotopic tumor-bearing rat urinary bladder. Cancer Chemother Pharmacol. 2011;67(4):775–81.

72. Kah JC, Lau WK, Tan PH, Sheppard CJ, Olivo M. Endoscopic image analysis of photosensitizer fluorescence as a promising noninvasive approach for pathological grading of bladder cancer in situ. J Biomed Opt. 2008;13(5):054022.

73. Pan Y, Xie H, Fedder GK. Endoscopic optical coherence tomography based on a microelectromechanical mirror. Opt Lett. 2001;26(24):1966–8.

74. Fujimoto JG, Pitris C, Boppart SA, Brezinski ME. Optical coherence tomography: an emerging technology for biomedical imaging and optical biopsy. Neoplasia. 2000;2(1–2):9–25.

75. Zagaynova EV, Shirmanova MV, Kirillin MY, Khlebtsov BN, Orlova AG, Balalaeva IV, et al. Contrasting properties of gold nanoparticles for optical coherence tomography: phantom, in vivo studies and Monte Carlo simulation. Phys Med Biol. 2008;53(18):4995–5009.

76. Manyak MJ, Gladkova ND, Makari JH, Schwartz AM, Zagaynova EV, Zolfaghari L, et al. Evaluation of superficial bladder transitional-cell carcinoma by optical coherence tomography. J Endourol. 2005;19(5):570–4.

77. Goh AC, Tresser NJ, Shen SS, Lerner SP. Optical coherence tomography as an adjunct to white light cystoscopy for intravesical real-time imaging and staging of bladder cancer. Urology. 2008;72(1):133–7.

78. Wang ZG, Durand DB, Schoenberg M, Pan YT. Fluorescence guided optical coherence tomography for the diagnosis of early bladder cancer in a rat model. J Urol. 2005;174(6):2376–81.

79. Schmidbauer J, Remzi M, Klatte T, Waldert M, Mauermann J, Susani M, et al. Fluorescence cystoscopy with high-resolution optical coherence tomography imaging as an adjunct reduces false-positive findings in the diagnosis of urothelial carcinoma of the bladder. Eur Urol. 2009;56(6):914–9.

80. Lingley-Papadopoulos CA, Loew MH, Zara JM. Wavelet analysis enables system-independent texture analysis of optical coherence tomography images. J Biomed Opt. 2009;14(4):044010.

81. Belinson SE, Ledford K, Rasool N, Rollins A, Wilan N, Wang C, et al. Cervical epithelial brightness by optical coherence tomography can determine histological grades of cervical neoplasia. J Low Genit Tract Dis. 2013;17(2):160–6.

82. Cauberg EC, de Bruin DM, Faber DJ, de Reijke TM, Visser M, de la Rosette JJ, et al. Quantitative measurement of attenuation coefficients of bladder biopsies using optical coherence tomography for grading urothelial carcinoma of the bladder. J Biomed Opt. 2010;15(6):066013.

83. Ren H, Yuan Z, Waltzer W, Shroyer K, Pan Y. Enhancing detection of bladder carcinoma in situ by 3-dimensional optical coherence tomography. J Urol. 2010;184(4):1499–506.

84. Ren H, Park KC, Pan R, Waltzer WC, Shroyer KR, Pan Y. Early detection of carcinoma in situ of the bladder: a comparative study of white light cystoscopy, narrow band imaging, 5-ALA fluorescence cystoscopy and 3-dimensional optical coherence tomography. J Urol. 2012;187(3):1063–70.

85. Gono K, Obi T, Yamaguchi M, Ohyama N, Machida H, Sano Y, et al. Appearance of enhanced tissue

features in narrow-band endoscopic imaging. J Biomed Opt. 2004;9(3):568–77.

86. Zheng C, Lv Y, Zhong Q, Wang R, Jiang Q. Narrow band imaging diagnosis of bladder cancer: systematic review and meta-analysis. BJU Int. 2012;110(11 Pt B):E680–7.

87. Herr HW, Donat SM. A comparison of white-light cystoscopy and narrow-band imaging cystoscopy to detect bladder tumour recurrences. BJU Int. 2008;102(9):1111–4.

88. Herr HW, Donat SM. Reduced bladder tumour recurrence rate associated with narrow-band imaging surveillance cystoscopy. BJU Int. 2011;107(3):396–8.

89. Cauberg EC, Kloen S, Visser M, de la Rosette JJ, Babjuk M, Soukup V, et al. Narrow band imaging cystoscopy improves the detection of non-muscle-invasive bladder cancer. Urology. 2010;76(3):658–63.

90. Goetz M. Endomicroscopy and targeted imaging of gastric neoplasia. Gastrointest Endosc Clin N Am. 2013;23(3):597–606.

91. Dong YY, Li YQ, Yu YB, Liu J, Li M, Luan XR. Meta-analysis of confocal laser endomicroscopy for the detection of colorectal neoplasia. Colorectal Dis. 2013;15(9):e488–95.

92. Sonn GA, Jones SN, Tarin TV, Du CB, Mach KE, Jensen KC, et al. Optical biopsy of human bladder neoplasia with in vivo confocal laser endomicroscopy. J Urol. 2009;182(4):1299–305.

93. Wiesner C, Jager W, Salzer A, Biesterfeld S, Kiesslich R, Hampel C, et al. Confocal laser endomicroscopy for the diagnosis of urothelial bladder neoplasia: a technology of the future? BJU Int. 2011;107(3): 399–403.

94. Bonnal JL, Rock Jr A, Gagnat A, Papadopoulos S, Filoche B, Mauroy B. Confocal laser endomicroscopy of bladder tumors associated with photodynamic diagnosis: an ex vivo pilot study. Urology. 2012;80(5):1162. e1-5.

95. Yuan Z, Wang Z, Pan R, Liu J, Cohen H, Pan Y. High-resolution imaging diagnosis and staging of bladder cancer: comparison between optical coherence tomography and high-frequency ultrasound. J Biomed Opt. 2008;13(5):054007.

96. Cicchi R, Crisci A, Cosci A, Nesi G, Kapsokalyvas D, Giancane S, et al. Time- and Spectral-resolved two-photon imaging of healthy bladder mucosa and carcinoma in situ. Opt Express. 2010;18(4):3840–9.

97. Evans CL, Xie XS. Coherent anti-stokes Raman scattering microscopy: chemical imaging for biology and medicine. Annu Rev Anal Chem (Palo Alto, Calif). 2008;1:883–909.

98. Gao L, Zhou H, Thrall MJ, Li F, Yang Y, Wang Z, et al. Label-free high-resolution imaging of prostate glands and cavernous nerves using coherent anti-Stokes Raman scattering microscopy. Biomed Opt Express. 2011;2(4):915–26.

68-Year-old man with asymptomatic
microscopic hematuria, significant tobacco
history, negative upper tract imaging, and
persistently atypical and suspicious cytology

Christopher S. Gomez, Mark S. Soloway,
Jorge Raul Caso, Claudia P. Rojas, and Merce Jorda

12.1 Diagnosis and Risk Factors

The evaluation of patients with asymptomatic microscopic hematuria is an important aspect of the practice of urologists. There is a lack of consensus on the ideal evaluation and follow-up of these patients. The need for quality studies and lack of evidence for the proper evaluation was recognized by the AUA in their most recent guideline.

Our patient is one of the 23 % of men over the age of 60 that is found to have microscopic hematuria. His age and gender place him into a high-risk category for urothelial cancer of the bladder (UC). Regardless of additional risk factors, up to 5 % of men over the age of 60 with microscopic hematuria will be found to have bladder cancer on subsequent investigations [1].

Younger men and women of any age are less likely to be found to have a serious condition as the cause of microscopic hematuria (0–7 %) [2]. The low probability of urinary tract malignancy in patients younger than 35 led the AUA to recommend that cystoscopy is not mandatory in the evaluation of asymptomatic microscopic hematuria in this age group and may be performed at the physician's discretion. A more recent study by Loo et al. suggests that this age could be extended to 50 years old if there are not other risk factors, e.g. cigarette or cigar smoking, radiation exposure, occupational exposure to carcinogens [3]. Men have a higher incidence of bladder cancer with a ratio of 3 to 5:1. This ratio exceeds 6:1 in several Mediterranean countries, which is likely accounted for by environmental exposure and cigarette smoking [4].

Tobacco smoking continues to be the most important risk factor for the development of bladder cancer with risks up to sixfold higher than that of non-smokers. The risk of bladder cancer increases with increasing duration and intensity

C.S. Gomez, M.D. • M.S. Soloway, M.D. (✉)
J.R. Caso, M.D., M.P.H.
Department of Urology, University of Miami Miller
School of Medicine, 9601 Collins Ave, Apt 1410,
Miami, FL 33154, USA
e-mail: gomezurology@gmail.com;
MSoloway@med.miami.edu; JCaso@med.miami.edu

C.P. Rojas, M.D. • M. Jorda, M.D., Ph.D., M.B.A.
Department of Pathology, University of Miami Miller
School of Medicine, 1400 NW 12th Ave, Miami,
FL 33136, USA
e-mail: Crojas@med.miami.edu;
mjorda@med.miami.edu

B.R. Konety and S.S. Chang (eds.), *Management of Bladder Cancer:*
A Comprehensive Text With Clinical Scenarios, DOI 10.1007/978-1-4939-1881-2_12,
© Springer Science+Business Media New York 2015

of smoking. The intensity and duration of smoking poses an equal risk to both sexes. The risk associated with smoking is modifiable and after 15 years of cessation, the risk of developing bladder cancer approaches that of a non-smoker [4]. There is a lack of public knowledge on the association of smoking and bladder cancer [5]. Many physicians are also not aware of this association. This is a problem as there is often a several month delay from the onset of hematuria to the referral for an investigation of the cause of hematuria. If the hematuria is related to a malignancy in the urinary tract this delay may alter the prognosis. Macroscopic hematuria in a person with a history of smoking should necessitate a prompt referral to an urologist for cystoscopy and upper urinary tract imaging. Of note, cigar smoking is also associated with urothelial cancer of the urinary tract particularly if the smoke is inhaled.

12.2 Imaging

Our patient has had normal "upper tract imaging." According to the most recent AUA guideline [6], upper tract imaging for this patient should be a multiphasic CT urography without and with IV contrast. The consensus was that multiphasic CT urography has the highest sensitivity and specificity for detecting lesions of the renal parenchyma and upper urinary tract.

If the patient has an allergy to iodinated contrast or is pregnant, magnetic resonance urography is an alternative. MRI is becoming more familiar and common practice to urologists in diagnosing renal lesions with sensitivities >90 %. MRU is capable of detecting upper tract malignancies with sensitivity of 80 % and specificity of 97 % [7]. If our patient has normal imaging with either of these studies, one could be confident that no further radiographic imaging is necessary.

If a patient with microscopic hematuria presents with a "normal" renal ultrasound, is this sufficient to rule out a lesion in the upper tract? Ultrasound has poor sensitivity for detecting upper tract urothelial malignancies with rates of 50–77 % [8, 9]. Given this poor sensitivity for detection of upper tract lesions in our patient with

risk factors for urothelial carcinoma and an atypical cytology, one should evaluate the entire urothelium to ensure the absence of a urothelial or renal neoplasm. Evaluation of the upper tract should be performed with either CTU or MRU.

The use of intravenous urography has a poor sensitivity when compared to CTU with a sensitivity of 50–60 % for detecting upper tract UC [10]. Retrograde pyelography (RPG) is a reasonable alternative to evaluate the entire upper tract. However, this is an invasive test and has no advantages when compared to CTU or MRU. If our patient had a relative or absolute contraindication for a multiphasic CT with iodinated contrast, MRI or RPG provides an alternative.

12.3 Cystoscopy

Adequate evaluation of the lower urinary tract by an experienced urologist should identify most papillary or sessile urothelial tumors. Carcinoma in situ as a primary bladder cancer is unusual but in most instances can be identified as an erythematous patch of abnormal appearing urothelium. In any event any abnormal appearing lesion in the bladder or prostatic urothelium should be biopsied and a diagnosis of bladder cancer established. In the scenario as presented we will assume this has been performed and no evident cancer was observed.

If the cytology report was reported as "consistent with cancer" random mucosal biopsies would be obtained even in the absence of a visible lesion. A false-positive cytology particularly if indicated as showing high-grade cells is rarely a false positive and the clinician must search the entire urothelium for the source of the cancer cells. In this case we have only atypical/suspicious cells in the urine.

12.4 Urine Cytology

The next important aspect of our case is the report indicating that the cytology contained atypical cells.

Urine cytology or the examination of the urine for cancer cells is an important laboratory study useful in the initial detection of UC and for surveillance of patients once they have been treated. Several systems of classification have been proposed since Papanicolaou laid the groundwork for the study of urine cytology in 1947; in broad terms samples are categorized as unsatisfactory, normal, atypical, suspicious, or malignant [11–13]. There is variability between institutions with regards to the criteria and expected prognostic implications within each grouping, particularly in the middle ground between clearly normal or malignant samples [12]. This has lead to some authors referring to the original "class III" classification described by Papanicolaou—consisting of abnormal cells which are not sufficiently pathognomonic—as a "wastebasket" that includes specimens with little chance of malignancy as well as those with nearly certain high-grade malignancy [12, 14, 15].

Although it has been a standard diagnostic test for many years, the most recent AUA guideline on the evaluation of asymptomatic microhematuria states that the use of urine cytology and urine-based markers are not recommended as a part of the routine evaluation for an individual with asymptomatic microhematuria [6]. The committee felt that false positives lead to unnecessary biopsies and emotional stress to the patient. High-grade urothelial cancer is more easily and accurately diagnosed than low-grade cancer with urine cytology [15–17]. False negatives can occur when the urothelium is instrumented or otherwise irritated such as with stones or an inflammatory process [16–18].

To help standardize reporting of these samples, Renshaw suggested classifying specimens using five features: cell clusters, vacuolated cytoplasm, degree of atypia, quantity of atypia, and quality of atypia[14]. Characteristics of high-grade cancer include increased size, pleomorphism, and high nuclear to cytoplasmic ratio (N:C) (Fig. 12.1a). Focal pseudo-degenerated atypia with diffuse, dark chromatin in cells with intact nuclear membranes is associated with a significant risk of a high-grade tumor. Necrosis and anisonucleosis, if found consistently, is a highly specific (but with low sensitivity) marker of neoplasia [14]. Low-grade tumors are charac-

terized by papillary or loosely cohesive clusters of cells, an increased N:C, eccentric nuclei, finely granular chromatin, and irregular nuclear membranes [14, 17] (Fig. 12.1b). However, the presence of papillary clusters in voided urine should also raise the differential diagnosis of lithiasis, strictures, and instrumentations effect. Vacuolated or bubbly cytoplasm is common in reactive cells and should be called negative [14, 15].

Since the specificity of urinary cytology is very high for high-grade UC, these unnecessary biopsies are likely related to atypical or suspicious readings by the cytopathologist. A cytology report that states "malignant cells are present" raises an alarm and requires additional imaging and testing. Depending on the clinician a report stating "suspicious for malignancy" might initiate a similarly extensive evaluation [19, 20]. Patients who have malignant cells identified on cytology and have normal upper tract imaging and cystoscopy require random bladder biopsies and possibly a biopsy from the prostatic urethra if there is no abnormality seen in the bladder. This more invasive approach is warranted due to the high specificity of urine cytology that approaches 100 % when malignant cells are identified by the trained cytopathologist [21]. Whereas atypical samples will likely be treated as negative and receive little or no additional workup [13–15]. Adding to the confusion, "atypical" and "suspicious" may be applied interchangeably between different cytopathologists to indicate class III samples. This diagnosis occurs with a variable frequency that can range from rare 2 to 25 % of samples [13, 15].

When cytology results do not have a clear "malignant" or "no malignant cells identified" diagnosis, communication with the pathologist and a good understanding of cytology reporting is imperative.

Proper sample acquisition is an important aspect of obtaining reliable urine cytology. The accuracy of urinary cytology increases when more samples are investigated. It is important to ensure centrifugation of the entire specimen to allow for more representative urothelial cell recruitment. This is true for both voided and bladder washing samples [22]. Bladder washings will increase the cell yield and thus improve the sensitivity, however samples obtained via lower or upper tract instrumentation have a higher probability of atypia being reported when compared to voided samples [13, 23]. Cytology obtained from a urinary diversion has a higher rate of atypia.

Reporting of atypical cytology can vary and there have been attempts to subdivide atypical urine samples, indicating the degree to which the cytopathologist feels a carcinoma may be present. In 2004, the Papanicolaou society recommended that an atypical cytology with changes suggestive but not definitive for carcinoma provide additional information. Findings were to be subclassified as reactive changes versus low-grade urothelial carcinoma, reactive changes versus high-grade urothelial carcinoma, favor papillary urothelial neoplasm of low malignant potential, or suspicious for high-grade urothelial carcinoma [16]. Subclassification of atypia is not universally used or recognized. In practice, some institutions may group these cytologies as atypical but subcategorize them as more or less suspicious for carcinoma using terms such as "cells of uncertain significance" versus "cannot exclude high-grade urothelial cancer" [12] and "favor a reactive process" versus "unclear if reactive or neoplastic" [15] (Fig. 12.1c, d). Furthermore, the malignant potential of this diagnosis is not well understood so we have adopted a pattern of close surveillance rather than more invasive testing when a report states atypical cells are identified.

Retrospective reviews have provided some information on the outcome of individuals who have had such a report and have been monitored. The chance of identifying UC has varied from 17 to 66 % and most studies have significant selection bias by including only patients who have had a bladder biopsy. Ubago et al. retrospectively reviewed 1,320 atypical urine cytology diagnoses over a 10-year period. They found that 21 % of the atypical specimens "progressed" to a malignant diagnosis with either positive cytology or cancer on a subsequent biopsy. Upper urinary tract specimens had the highest rate of progression (38 %): urinary diversion specimens had the lowest (12 %). This report included 57 cases in which a positive biopsy was obtained within 2 days after the atypical cytology. Piaton et al. found that there were significant differences if they divided atypia into either "atypical of undetermined significance" (AUC-US) or "atypical cannot exclude high grade" (AUC-H). Fifty-four percent of the patients with AUC-H had a subsequent diagnosis of a high-grade tumor and only 17 % of patient with AUC-US developed a high-grade lesion [24].

To augment the diagnostic accuracy of urinary cytology, in particular a relatively low sensitivity, fluorescence in situ hybridization (FISH) has been proposed [25, 26]. Probes to detect aneuploidy of chromosomes 3, 7, and 17, as well as a locus-specific probe to detect loss of 9p21 are used and collectively known as the UroVysion™ assay [25, 26] (Fig. 12.1e, f). Although it has shown usefulness in clarifying which patients with atypical urine cytology later have a UC, there are more false-positive results. In an early study, 7 out of 11 patients who had a negative biopsy but a positive FISH later developed a carcinoma; significantly, 4 out of 7 had undergone progression when they recurred [26]. However, most so-called "anticipatory positive" results have been reported in low-grade tumors [27]. Among patients undergoing evaluation for hematuria, although researchers found the sensitivity improved by nearly 2× over cytology, the improvement was in part due to better detection of low-grade tumors. A positive FISH without subsequent diagnosis of cancer was detected in 89 out of 473 patients, with a benign cause for the hematuria found in just over half. The remaining patients had no identifiable cause [25]. Another study examining the use of FISH in the surveillance of patients with bladder cancer found that 18 out of 21 patients with a recurrence had a positive FISH, as did 22 out of 43 patients who did not [28].

The authors disagree on the relative importance of the chromosomal abnormalities. The 9p21 deletion was found to predict 75 % of the patients undergoing bladder cancer surveillance who had a recurrence [28]. Others studies suggest, however, that aneuploidy of chromosomes 7 and 17 is more commonly associated with tumor

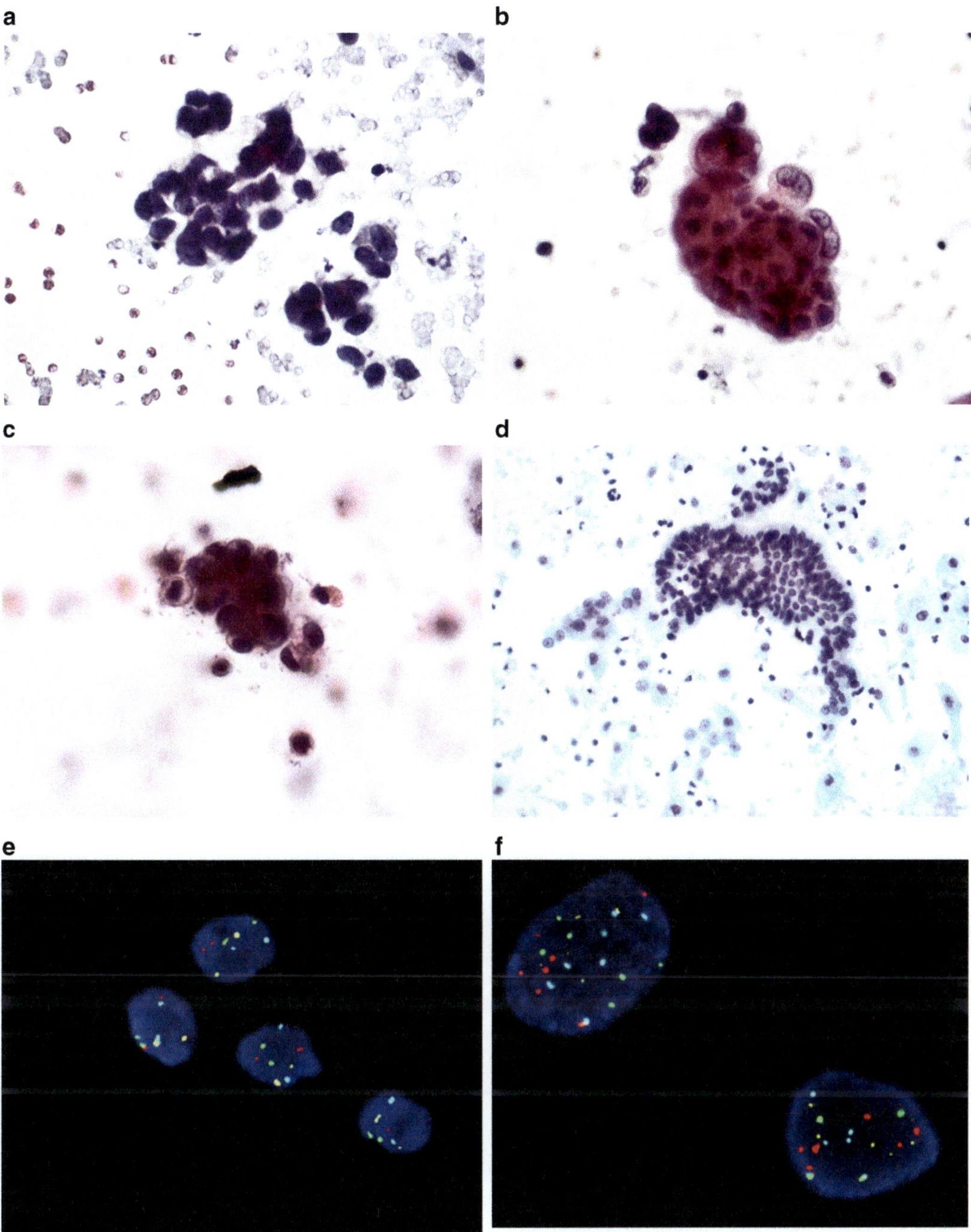

Fig. 12.1 (**a**) Loose cohesive cluster of highly atypical cell with markedly increased N/C ratio, unevenly distributed coarse chromatin, marked hyperchromasia, and irregular nuclear membranes consistent with high-grade urothelial carcinoma. (**b**) Papillary-like aggregate of cells, high N/C ratio, and nuclei eccentrically located with finely granular chromatin consistent with low-grade urothelial carcinoma. (**c**) Loose cohesive cluster of cells with relative hyperchromasia and irregularity of nuclear membrane consistent with atypia cannot exclude high grade. (**d**) Papillary-like aggregate with indistinct cell borders, dense and homogenous cytoplasm, inconspicuous irregular nuclear membrane, and fine and evenly distributed chromatin; consistent with atypia of undetermined significance. (**e**) Negative fluorescent in situ hybridization (FISH) urovision assay. (**f**) Positive FISH detecting aneuploidy of chromosome 3, 7, and 17

than aneuploidy of chromosome 3 or loss of 9pq21 [29]. In trying to improve on the rate of false-positive results, in particular limiting the effect of reactive urothelium, a tetraploid pattern has been suggested to be a generally benign finding, although not exclusive of neoplasia. Using these criteria, the authors have been able to decrease false-positive results in reactive cases 2/3 to 1/3 of samples [30]. Other cited causes of false positives—besides inflammatory conditions such as prostatic hypertrophy, stones, strictures, and polyps—include barbotage collection of the urine specimen, human polyoma virus infection, and seminal vesicle cells [18, 25, 29].

12.5 Conclusion and Recommendations

The patient in this scenario has some high-risk features for a urothelial malignancy because of his age, sex, and smoking history. The presence of microscopic hematuria suggests that he should be followed with a repeat urinalysis and one can consider a repeat evaluation should the hematuria persist [6]. The likelihood that he will have cancer on a subsequent investigation is quite low, however, in the absence of gross hematuria or a frankly positive cytology. Our case is unique and focuses on the fact that this gentleman has an atypical cytology. While a review of the literature shows that this is not synonymous with a positive cytology or malignancy, there is an increased risk of future urothelial carcinoma.

This increased risk deserves close surveillance while minimizing morbidity. Random bladder biopsies for an atypical cytology are not recommended and would represent over treatment and morbidity exposure to the ~80 % of these patients who will never develop a urothelial malignancy. The use of selective upper tract ureteral washings is of low value and again not recommended for this individual. Sadek et al. have shown that upper tract cytology is often contaminated from the bladder causing false-positive readings and a low specificity [31]. Introducing upper tract washings with poor reliability would likely lead to further investigations and morbidity. Rather,

repeat upper tract imaging can be performed if the urine cytology remains atypical or microscopic hematuria persists. The use of additional urine tumor markers (i.e. FISH) is not indicated at this time. The lower specificity of FISH will subject patients to unnecessary invasive procedures and increase the cost of surveillance.

Repeat voided urine cytology and flexible cystoscopy at 6 months is a reasonable approach with a high sensitivity for detecting both high-grade and low-grade malignant lesions while minimizing morbidity and anxiety for the patient. Bladder wash cytology might be considered at the time of the flexible endoscopy to provide more and better preserved cells. If repeat urine cytology shows malignant cells while the cystoscopy remains normal, then further investigations with bladder and prostatic urethral biopsies as well as a RPG if the lower tract is normal would be indicated.

References

1. Britton JP. Effectiveness of haematuria clinics. Br J Urol. 1993;71(3):247–52.
2. Benbassat J, Gergawi M, Offringa M, Drukker A. Symptomless microhaematuria in schoolchildren: causes for variable management strategies. QJM. 1996;89:845–54.
3. Loo RK, Lieberman SF, Slezak JM, et al. Stratifying risk of urinary tract malignant tumors in patients with asymptomatic microscopic hematuria. Mayo Clin Proc. 2013;88:129–38.
4. Parkin DM. The global burden of urinary bladder cancer. Scand J Urol Nephrol. 2008;42:12–20.
5. Nieder AM, John S, Messina CR, et al. Are patients aware of the association between smoking and bladder cancer? J Urol. 2006;176:2405–8.
6. Diagnosis, evaluation and follow-up of asymptomatic microhematuria (AMH) in adults: AUA Guideline. 2012.
7. Takahashi N, Glockner JF, Hartman RP, et al. Gadolinium enhanced magnetic resonance urography for upper urinary tract malignancy. J Urol. 2010;183:1330–6.
8. Datta SN, Allen GM, Evans R, et al. Urinary tract ultrasonography in the evaluation of hematuria-areort of over 1000 cases. Ann R Coll Surg Engl. 2002;84:203–5.
9. Edwards TJ, Dickinson AJ, Natale S, et al. A prospective analysis of the diagnostic yield resulting from the attendance of 4020 patients at a protocol-driven haematuria clinic. BJU. 2006;97:301–5.
10. Chlapoutakis K, Theocharopoulos N, Yarmentitis S, et al. Performance of computed tomographic urography

in diagnosis of upper urinary tract urothelial carcinoma, in patients presenting with hematuria: systematic review and meta-analysis. Eur J Radiol. 2010;73:334–8.

11. Papanicolaou GN. Cytology of the urine sediment in neoplasms of the urinary tract. J Urol. 1947;57: 375–9.

12. Owens CL, Vandenbussche CJ, Burroughs FH, Rosenthal DL. A review of reporting systems and terminology for urine cytology. Cancer Cytopathol. 2013;121:9–14.

13. Muus Ubago J, Mehta V, Wojcik EM, Barkan GA. Evaluation of atypical urine cytology progression to malignancy. Cancer Cytopathol. 2013;121:387–91.

14. Renshaw AA. Subclassifying atypical urinary cytology specimens. Cancer. 2000;90:222–9.

15. Brimo F, Vollmer RT, Case B, Aprikian A, Kassouf W, Auger M. Accuracy of urine cytology and the significance of an atypical category. Am J Clin Pathol. 2009;132:785–93.

16. Layfield LJ, Elsheikh TM, Fili A, Nayar R, Shidham V. Papanicolaou Society of Cytopathology. Review of the state of the art and recommendations of the Papanicolaou Society of Cytopathology for urinary cytology procedures and reporting : the Papanicolaou Society of Cytopathology Practice Guidelines Task Force. Diagn Cytopathol. 2004;30:24–30.

17. Murphy WM, Soloway MS, Jukkola AF, Crabtree WN, Ford KS. Urinary cytology and bladder cancer. The cellular features of transitional cell neoplasms. Cancer. 1984;53:1555–65.

18. Kapur U, Venkataraman G, Wojcik EM. Diagnostic significance of "atypia" in instrumented versus voided urine specimens. Cancer. 2008;114:270–4.

19. Nabi G, Greene D, Donnel MO. Suspicious urinary cytology with negative evaluation for malignancy in the diagnostic investigation of haematuria: how to follow up? J Clin Pathol. 2004;57:365–8.

20. Stenberg I, Rona R, Olsfanger S, Lew S, Leibovitch I. The clinical significance of class III (suspicious) urine cytology. Cytopathol Off J Br Soc Clin Cytol. 2011;329–33.

21. Lokeshwar VB, Habuchi T, Grossman HB, et al. Bladder tumor markers beyond cytology: International consensus panel on bladder tumor markers. Urology. 2005;66:35–63.

22. Planz B, Jochims E, Deix T, et al. The role of urinary cytology for detection of bladder cancer. EJSO. 2005;31:304–8.

23. Raab SS, Grzybicki DM, Brbin CM, et al. Urine cytology discrepancies—frequency, causes and outcomes. Am J Clin Pathol. 2007;127:946–53.

24. Piaton E, Advenier AS, Benaïm G, et al. A typical urothelial cells (AUC): a Bethesda-derived wording applicable to urinary cytopathology. Ann Pathol. 2011;31(1):11–7.

25. Sarosdy MF, Kahn PR, Ziffer MD, Love WR, Barkin J, Abara EO, et al. Use of a multitarget fluorescence in situ hybridization assay to diagnose bladder cancer in patients with hematuria. J Urol. 2006;176:44–7.

26. Halling KC, King W, Sokolova IA, Meyer RG, Burkhardt HM, Halling AC, et al. A comparison of cytology and fluorescence in situ hybridization for the detection of urothelial carcinoma. J Urol. 2000;164:1768–75.

27. Nieder AM, Soloway MS, Herr HW. Should we abandon the FISH test? Eur Urol. 2007;51:1469–71.

28. Tomasini JM, Konety BR. Urinary markers/cytology: what and when should a urologist use. Urol Clin North Am. 2013;40:165–73.

29. Tapia C, Glatz K, Obermann EC, Grilli B, Barascud A, Herzog M, et al. Evaluation of chromosomal aberrations in patients with benign conditions and reactive changes in urinary cytology. Cancer Cytopathol. 2011;119:404–10.

30. Dimashkieh H, Wolff DJ, Smith TM, Houser PM, Nietert PJ, Yang J. Evaluation of urovysion and cytology for bladder cancer detection: a study of 1835 paired urine samples with clinical and histologic correlation. Cancer Cytopathol. 2013;121:591–7.

31. Sadek S, Soloway MS, Hook S, Civantos F. The value of upper tract cytology after transurethral resection of bladder tumor in patients with bladder transitional cell cancer. J Urol. 1999;161:77–9. discussion 79–80.

Localized Surgical Therapy and Surveillance

13

Manish I. Patel and Paul D. Sved

Abbreviations

NMIBC	Non-muscle-invasive bladder cancer
TURBT	Transurethral resection of bladder tumor
UTI	Urinary tract infection
EORTC	European organization for the research and treatment of cancer
CIS	Carcinoma in situ
BMAP	Bladder mapping
EAU	European association of urology
PUNLMP	Papillary neoplasm of low malignant potential
FC	Fluorescent cystoscopy
WL	White light
UTT	Upper tract tumor

M.I. Patel, M.B.B.S., Ph.D., F.R.A.C.S. (✉)
Westmead Hospital, University of Sydney,
Suite 10, 16-18 Mons Rd, Westmead, NSW 2145,
Australia
e-mail: mpatel@med.usyd.edu.au

P.D. Sved, M.B.B.S., M.S., F.R.A.C.S.
Royal Prince Alfred Hospital, University of Sydney,
Suite 312, 100 Carillon Avenue, Newtown,
NSW 2042, Australia
e-mail: psved@sydney.edu.au

13.1 Introduction

The significance of the initial surgical management of NMIBC by TURBT cannot be overstated. This technically demanding procedure will set the foundation for the management of the patient. A competently performed TURBT will optimize patient outcome. Similarly, follow-up must be systematic and vigilant in order to minimize the risk and consequences of tumor recurrence or progression.

13.2 Preoperative Assessment

13.2.1 Imaging Studies

CT urography is the imaging modality of choice in the evaluation of patients scheduled to undergo TURBT [1]. It has greater sensitivity and specificity than either standard intravenous urography or ultrasound. CT urography provides information on tumor stage and also enables the simultaneous evaluation of the renal parenchyma and upper tract urothelium.

13.2.2 Laboratory Investigations

Prior to a TURBT, the urine should be cultured and any infection treated. In addition, a full blood count, coagulation studies, and measurement of electrolytes and creatinine should be obtained.

B.R. Konety and S.S. Chang (eds.), *Management of Bladder Cancer:*   179
A Comprehensive Text With Clinical Scenarios, DOI 10.1007/978-1-4939-1881-2_13,
© Springer Science+Business Media New York 2015

13.2.3 Medical Clearance

Patients diagnosed with bladder cancer are often elderly and may have a history of smoking. Therefore, a preoperative medical and anesthesia review is beneficial and may reduce the rate of procedure cancellation at the time of surgery [2]. Medical conditions which must be diagnosed or optimized prior to urological surgery in this patient population commonly include chronic airways disease, ischemic heart disease and peripheral vascular disease, diabetes mellitus and chronic renal impairment. Antiplatelet agents such as clopidogrel should be stopped 7–10 days and warfarin discontinued 3–5 days prior to surgery, respectively. The INR should be checked on the day of surgery. For patients who require continuous thromboprophylaxis, low molecular-weight heparin may be required but discontinued 24 h before surgery.

13.2.4 Antibiotic Prophylaxis

As stated earlier, all patients should have a negative urine culture prior to TURBT. This may require specific antibiotics to eliminate organisms found on an initial culture. The question of routine antibiotic prophylaxis at the time of surgery has been controversial. In a recent review of 42 randomized controlled trials involving 7,496 patients undergoing transurethral surgery, it was found that antibiotic prophylaxis significantly reduced the incidence of bacteriuria, symptomatic UTI, bacteremia, and fever ≥ 38.5 °C [3]. These findings also pertained to low-risk patients, including those without catheters and negative urine cultures and were most apparent in those who underwent TURBT and TURP. The AUA recommends antibiotic prophylaxis for all patients undergoing TURBT [4]. The antibiotics of choice are either a fluoroquinolone or trimethoprim-sulfamethoxazole. A proposed alternative is intravenous aminoglycoside $\pm$ ampicillin or a first/second-generation cephalosporin.

13.3 Transurethral Resection of Bladder Tumors

Transurethral resection of bladder tumors (TURBT) is a key initial step in the management of bladder cancer. It serves both diagnostic and therapeutic purposes. An increasing body of evidence also now links the quality of the initial TURBT to prognosis. The aims of the TURBT are to obtain a specimen of sufficient size and quality to enable accurate histological characterization, to determine the depth of invasion and the presence or absence of both lymphovascular involvement and abnormal urothelium adjacent to the primary lesion.

TURBT may be performed under either general or regional anesthesia according to patient factors and preferences of the surgeon and anesthesiologist. Neuromuscular blockade may be necessary for tumors on the lateral bladder wall to avoid an obturator nerve reflex [5].

After induction of anesthesia, the patient is placed in the dorsal lithotomy position with care taken to ensure all pressure areas are padded and protected. Patients with a history of a joint replacement or spinal abnormality may be positioned whilst awake to minimize the risk of unintended joint dislocation or spinal nerve irritation. A bimanual examination of the pelvis is undertaken before (and after) resection. A complete endoscopic evaluation of the urethra and bladder is performed using both a 30° and 70° lens. Evaluation of the anterior bladder wall may be aided by gentle suprapubic pressure. Either water or 1.5 % glycine may be used as an irrigant for monopolar resection and 0.9 % saline if bipolar electrocautery is used.

After the entire bladder is examined, the tumor(s) are resected using the cutting current on the loop resectoscope. Whilst electrocautery settings are at the discretion of the operating surgeon, cutting currents of 140–150 W and coagulation of 40–50 W are commonly used [6]. The principles of TURBT are (1) resection of all visible tumor, (2) sampling of urothelium adjacent

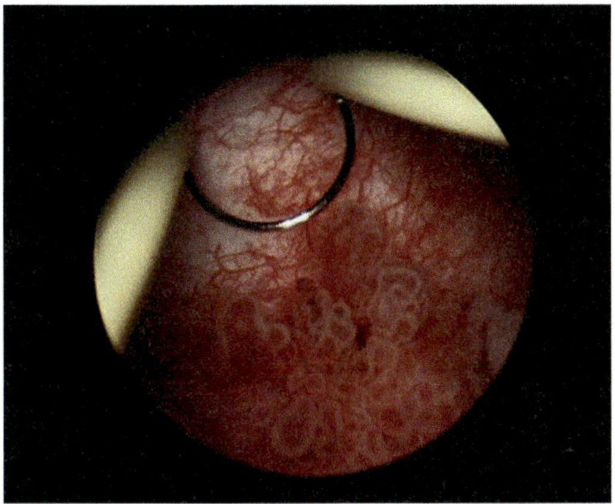

Fig. 13.1 Papillary TCC with resectoscope in position to resect lesion

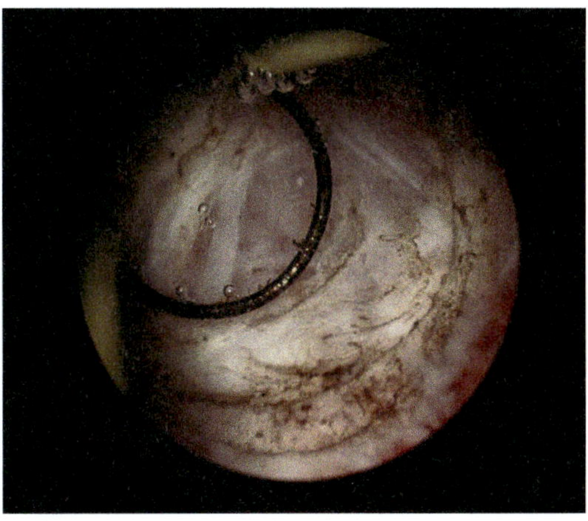

Fig. 13.2 Lesion resected to deep muscle without perforation

to the tumor, and (3) resection of tissue at the tumor base until normal muscle fibers are visible [7]. Before contact is made with the tissue, the loop is electrified. Delicate movements of the loop and sheath are made to adjust the depth and width of resection. Resection may be either en bloc or performed in staged phases. En bloc resection involves simultaneous resection of the tumor and its base. This is best suited to smaller lesions (<2 cm diameter) and has the advantage of reduced diathermy artifact [7, 8]. Staged resection involves resection of the tumor sequentially, commencing at its luminal surface until its base is reached and normal detrusor is identified as seen in Figs. 13.1 and 13.2. The base and muscle may be sent for separate analysis to optimize the analysis of tumor depth [9]. During resection the bladder is emptied with meticulous care taken to ensure all tissues are retrieved by straining irrigant that is drained from the bladder. Small, low-grade appearing papillary tumors may be removed by cold-cup biopsy forceps [6]. Following resection, hemostasis is achieved by selective cauterization of bleeding vessels with care taken to avoid the ureteric orifices. For extensive resections, a roller electrode may be used for hemostasis. Depending on the extent of resection the urologist will decide whether a Foley catheter

or continuous bladder irrigation is necessary. If irrigation is commenced it is important to ensure free efflux of irrigant and urine before the patient leaves the operating room to avoid bladder distension and delayed perforation.

13.4 TURBT in Specific Circumstances

13.4.1 Tumors at the Ureteral Orifices

Cautery close to the ureteral orifice may cause scarring and lead to ureteric obstruction [10]. Resection of the orifice may lead to reflux and, rarely, disruption of the vesicoureteric junction. Following resection here, a ureteric stent may be required. The ICUD has recommended a CT urogram or DTPA renal scan 3–6 weeks after resection.

13.4.2 Tumors on the Lateral and Anterior Walls

Resection of lateral wall tumors may result in obturator nerve stimulation, sudden leg adduction, and perforation [11]. Strategies to prevent or minimize this include: (1) avoid overfilling the bladder during resection, (2) reduce cutting current, (3) "tapping" or "staccato" activation of the cutting current, (4) using bipolar cautery, and (5) neuromuscular blockade. Resection of tumors on the anterior wall may be facilitated by an application of suprapubic pressure by an assistant [5]. This may also be helpful when performing TURBT in obese patients.

13.4.3 Tumors in Bladder Diverticulae

Resection of tumors in diverticulae provides a unique challenge due to the lack of a muscularis propria and the inherent limitations in assessment of the depth of invasion. In addition, the risk of perforation is increased. The ICUD has recommended diverticulectomy, partial or total cystectomy to deal with large or high-grade tumors arising in a diverticulum. Small, papillary, low-grade-appearing tumors may be dealt with by careful fulguration to avoid perforation [10].

13.5 Reresection

Repeat TURBT is now a standard of care in selected cases of high-grade non-muscle-invasive urothelial carcinoma and forms part of the key recommendations of treatment guidelines published by the EAU, AUA, and ICUD [10, 12]. Tumors requiring reresection include all those invading the lamina propria (T1) and high-grade Ta tumors where detrusor muscle has not been sampled [13]. Reresection serves three main purposes: (1) to ensure complete clearance of the primary tumor, (2) to minimize the risk of understaging, and (3) to provide prognostic information to aid decision-making. In addition, there is some evidence that reresection may improve response to intravesical treatment.

The rate of early recurrence after TURBT varies widely and is often attributed to an incomplete primary resection [14]. This was shown in an EORTC analysis of seven phase 3 trials. The rate of recurrence at 3 months varied from 0 to 46 %, with multivariate analysis demonstrating

that the quality of initial resection was the only explanation for the wide variation [15]. Others have shown that surgeon experience is an important factor in the quality and completeness of the initial resection [16, 17]. Reresection is important to ensure complete clearance of the primary lesion, especially where less experienced surgeons are involved.

Several studies have indicated that the depth of tumor invasion is often underestimated on an initial TURBT. The absence of muscularis propria in the initial resection has proven to be an important predictor of clinical understaging. In a study by Herr et al. [18], of 23 patients with T1 lesions without muscle in the initial TURBT specimen, 49 % had their disease reclassified as T2 on repeat resection. In comparison, only 14 % of T1 lesions containing muscle in the initial resection were subsequently upstaged. Similarly, Dutta et al. [19] reported a 64 % rate of understaging in T1 tumors if muscle was absent in the TURBT specimen when compared to final analysis of the cystectomy specimen. Understaging has also been reported in Ta disease when muscle is absent [20]. For these reasons, a reresection has been recommended to ensure accurate staging in all high-grade non-muscle-invasive (Ta and T1) bladder cancers.

The results of a reresection also have prognostic implications. Herr et al. [21] first reported that of 260 patients with T1 tumors on initial resection, those with residual T1 disease at repeat resection had a 5-year progression rate to muscle-invasive disease of 82 %. In comparison, only 19 % of those with no residual T1 disease progressed. Similar findings were reported in a later study from the same group [22]. Based on these findings, the authors suggested that patients with residual invasive disease at reresection may be better served with immediate cystectomy rather than a trial of intravesical BCG.

Finally, a randomized trial of adjuvant mitomycin C with or without reresection in T1 disease found higher rates of both recurrence and progression in the group that did not undergo reresection [23]. These results suggest that repeat resection may also provide a direct therapeutic advantage when combined with intravesical treatment.

13.6 Cold-Cup Biopsy

Random bladder biopsies distant to the site of the primary tumor are commonly performed to detect the presence of CIS, which is often difficult to identify but if present may alter management. Cold-cup biopsies are taken from normal- and suspicious-looking urothelium including the sidewalls, trigone, posterior wall, and dome using an angled biopsy forceps mounted on a 30-degree lens. This process is often referred to as BMAP [24]. The current EAU guidelines recommend biopsies from normal bladder mucosa when cytology is positive or when an exophytic tumor has a non-papillary appearance [25]. The EAU and ICUD also stipulate that biopsies of the prostatic urethra should be considered when a tumor is located at the bladder neck or trigone, when there are multiple tumors and when consideration is being given to orthotopic bladder substitution [25, 26].

Despite the recommendations, the accuracy of cold-cup BMAP remains questionable. Gudjonsson et al. recently reported a sensitivity of just over 50 % in detecting CIS by cold-cup BMAP in 162 patients who underwent cystectomy [24]. Others have raised concerns regarding the potential for tumor implantation at the biopsy site in the presence of CIS [27]. The ICUD have concluded that random bladder biopsies do not alter management in most cases and should be limited to cases where discordance exists between urine cytology and cystoscopic findings and in bladder mapping prior to consideration of a partial cystectomy [10].

13.7 Fulguration

Patients with recurrent low-grade, non-invasive bladder cancer may not require repeated visits to the operating room and general anesthesia in order to monitor and control their disease. Several investigators have proposed alternative strategies including flexible cystoscopy with fulguration of small lesions in an office or clinic setting under local anesthesia to reduce cost and morbidity [28]. The success and safety of this approach depends on the ability of the surgeon to correctly identify low grade disease and is based on our understanding of the risk of progression of low-grade disease, which is less than 10 % [29].

Herr et al. [30] found that experienced urologists could correctly identify 93 % of lesions that had recurred after initial diagnosis of non-invasive disease as low grade. When combined with urine cytology, the accuracy increased to 99 %.

O'Neill and Lowrance [28] have described their technique as follows: Prior to the procedure, a voided urine specimen is checked with a dipstick to exclude infection and is also sent for formal cytology. A single dose of oral antibiotic is administered. Men are positioned supine and women in low lithotomy. Lidocaine gel (2 %) is administered per urethra. A 17-French flexible cystoscope with 5-French working port is inserted with sterile water irrigation. A monopolar Bugbee electrode with coagulation setting at 25 W is used. Firstly the papillary fronds are cauterized, then the central portion of the lesion and, finally, the base. The patient is warned that the cauterization may feel like a fine pin-prick. After the procedure, the patient is educated about the possibility of bladder spasms, hematuria, and urinary retention. Simple analgesia is prescribed and discharged from the clinic after voiding.

The respective roles of TURBT and office fulguration in the management of low-grade non-muscle-invasive bladder cancer is described in Fig. 13.3 [31].

13.8 Follow-Up of NMIBC: Introduction

Correct follow-up schedules used in the management of bladder cancer are important as a large number of tumors are destined to recur; some with progressive disease. Optimal follow-up should enable early identification of recurrences and more critically progression. At the same time, those at low risk of recurrence or progression should be spared onerous and frequent follow-up which not only decreases quality of life but can be expensive and stretch current health

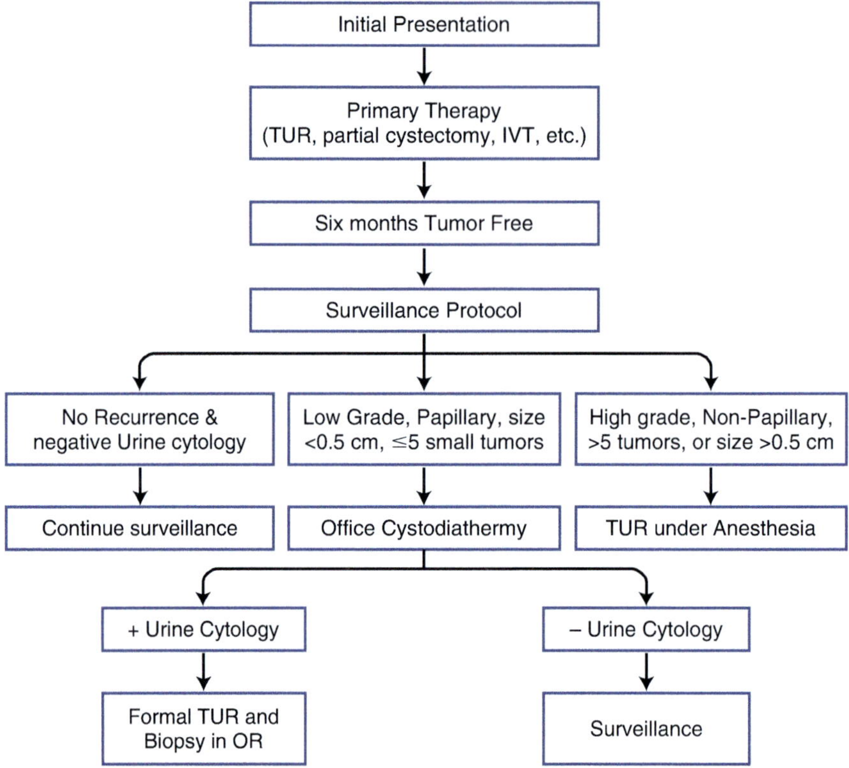

Fig. 13.3 Treatment algorithm for low-grade NMIBC. IVT, intravesical therapy; OR, operating room 31

resources. Unfortunately, the quality of evidence upon which to base follow-up schedules are of low quality so many recommendations are based on common practice.

13.9 Risk Stratification

Proper follow-up strategies can only be applied to a patient with NMIBC once the risk of recurrence and progression has been assessed. A simple way to stratify patient's risk of recurrence is by stage (T1 vs Ta) or grade (high grade vs low grade). The AUA has defined two risk groups: low risk (pTa, low grade) and high risk (pT1, high grade, and/or CIS) using these criteria [12].

Clinical prognostic factors may also be used, in addition to pathological factors to stratify patients. The EORTC have developed a prognostic model for recurrence and progression [29]. The risk table groups patients into four risk categories for both the probability of recurrence and progression according to their total score (Table 13.1).

The data from 2,596 individual patients from seven EORTC trials were used to develop these tables but unfortunately these patients were from an era where reresection of T1 tumors was not routine. On multivariate analysis, the most important factors influencing time to progression were T category, CIS, and grade. These tables will be updated by the EORTC for patients treated with BCG and maintenance. The NMIBC guidelines panel for the EAU has classified patients into low, intermediate, and high risk based on the tables (Table 13.2) [25].

One of the criticisms of the EORTC tables is that many of the patients, particularly the high-risk patients would have been undertreated by today's standard and so are closer to the untreated natural history of disease. External validation of the risk tables in a high-risk population of NMIBC population treated with BCG and maintenance

Table 13.1 EORTC tables for calculating risk of recurrence and progression [29]

Factor	Recurrence	Progression
Number of tumors		
Single	0	0
2–7	3	3
≥8	6	3
Tumor size		
<3 cm	0	0
≥3 cm	3	3
Prior recurrence rate		
Primary	0	0
<1 rec/year	2	2
>1 rec/year	4	2
T category		
Ta	0	0
T1	1	4
CIS		
No	0	0
Yes	1	6
Grade		
G1	0	0
G2	1	0
G3	2	5
Total score	0–17	0–23

Table 13.2 Probability of recurrence and progression according to score and classification system by the NMIBC guidelines panel of the EAU [25]

Recurrence score	Probability of recurrence at 5 years		Recurrence risk group
	(%)	(95 % CI)	
0	31	24–37	Low risk
1–4	46	42–49	Intermediate risk
5–9	62	58–65	Intermediate risk
10–17	78	73–84	High risk

Progression score	Probability of progression at 5 years		Progression risk group
	(%)	(95 % CI)	
0	0.8	0–1.7	Low risk
2–6	6	5–8	Intermediate risk
7–13	17	14–20	High risk
14–23	45	35–55	High risk

have revealed a progression sensitivity of 88 % and NPV of 95 % but PPV of only 17 % suggesting adequate discrimination between patients with different prognosis but poor calibration in patients treated with BCG [32].

An alternative to the EORTC risk tables is the scoring model from CUETO [33]. In this model based on 1,062 patients from four BCG trials, the prognostic factors of age, gender, tumor status, T stage, and grade were used. The risk of recurrence and progression was similar in CUETO and EORTC categorized low- and intermediate-risk patients. High-risk patients however had lower probabilities of recurrence and progression in the CUETO model, presumably because of the use of BCG with maintenance.

The EORTC risk tables or CUETO scores are an important method of risk stratification which will subsequently determine future treatment and surveillance.

13.10 Cystoscopy Schedule

The follow-up surveillance of NMIBC depends primarily on cystoscopic inspection of the bladder. This is an invasive, time-consuming and costly procedure, so optimization of this strategy is important.

13.10.1 First Cystoscopy

The first cystoscopy after a complete TURBT is of great importance due to its prognostic value. Although recurrence at 3 months depends on the quality and completeness of the initial TURBT and whether intravesical therapy has been administered, it has been shown that early tumor recurrence at 3 m is clearly prognostic for recurrence [34–36] and progression [29, 37, 38].

13.10.2 Further Cystoscopies

Traditionally when the first 3-month cystoscopy is normal, further cystoscopies have been scheduled 3 monthly for 2 years, followed by 6 monthly until the end of the fifth year. This approach has

Table 13.3 Protocol for surveillance

Risk category	Schedule of CE after 3 months and to 2 years	Schedule of CE 2–5 years	Schedule after 5 years	Upper tract imaging	Other tools
Low	9 months then yearly	Yearly	Cease follow-up	Not required	Nil
Intermediate	6 monthly	Yearly	Yearly for 10 years	CT urogram second yearly	Plus cytology
High	3 monthly	6 monthly	Yearly life-long	CT urogram yearly	Plus cytology

Authors' suggestion based on guidelines and data

more recently been tailored based on the EORTC/ EAU risk categorization (grade C recommendation) [39]. The intensive schedule described is now only recommended for high-risk patients. Low-risk patients who have a negative 3-month cystoscopy should have their next one 9 months later, and then yearly for 5 years. This is supported by a randomized study that shows time between cystoscopies can be safely doubled for low-risk patients [40]. A recommended schedule of follow-up cystoscopy is given in Table 13.3.

13.10.3 When to Stop Cystoscopy

There are no clear data defining when cystoscopic examination can be safely stopped in patients with bladder cancer, however in patients with high-risk tumors, long-term and possibly lifelong surveillance is required as even after more than a 5-year tumor free period after BCG, greater than 20 % will have a recurrence at 15 years [41].

There are conflicting data for low-risk patients. In one study, of 115 patients who were recurrence free at 5 years, 98 % remained so at 20 years [42]. Another similar study found 92 % were recurrence free long term [43]. Long-term recurrence does however occur even for low-risk tumors. Leblanc reported 14 % of recurrences were detected after 5 years from first diagnosis for TaG1 tumors [44]. Patients with PUNLMP were identified to have greater than 15 % recurrence rates after 5 years. Thus in low-risk patients while recurrence after 5 years is possible it is low, and most would recommend discontinuation of cystoscopy after this time [39]. There are no data to guide cessation of cystoscopy for intermediate-

risk patients, but logically this should be in somewhere between low and high risk and tailored to the patients' biology and personal factors [39].

13.10.4 Improving Surveillance Cystoscopy

An improvement in the sensitivity and specificity of cystoscopy could allow for decreased cystoscopies performed. FC and NBI have reported improved sensitivities but lower specificities compared to WL cystoscopy in the detection of bladder cancers. Most studies have evaluated these modalities as part of a TURBT, with very few employing it as a surveillance tool [45, 46]. The use of FC with flexible cystoscopy can improve the detection of bladder cancer by up to 28 % [47]. Similarly a study of surveillance has shown that NBI will decrease recurrences from 92 to 62 % compared to WL cystoscopy [48]. Other cystoscopic diagnostic tools such as Raman spectroscopy and optical coherence have yet to be tested in surveillance studies.

13.10.5 Bladder Biopsies

Bladder biopsies are required when suspicious lesions are identified at cystoscopy or the patient has positive cytology with no obvious disease. After BCG treatment however, the bladder is often inflamed and some will perform routine random biopsies of the bladder in this situation. Dalbagni et al. have however shown that at 3 m, the absence of positive cytology can safely negate the need for biopsy of erythematous lesions [49].

13.11 Place of Urinary Markers

A thorough evaluation of urinary markers is outside the scope of this chapter; a detailed discussion is however provided in Chap. XX. Urinary markers for surveying patients during follow-up offer the allure of being less invasive at possibly lower costs. These markers may be used as (1) an adjunct to cystoscopy to reduce the false-negative rate or (2) a substitute to cystoscopy and ideally these markers would have high sensitivity and specificity. Interestingly, in a study of patient preference on the use of urinary markers, if a test has less than 90–95 % sensitivity in comparison to cystoscopy, patients would still prefer flexible cystoscopy as their method of follow-up [50]. Currently no urinary marker fulfils these criteria and cannot replace cystoscopy follow-up [39].

Urine cytology is a standard test routinely used in conjunction with cystoscopic follow-up to detect disease which may be missed, such as CIS, upper tract disease and prostatic urethral involvement. In a study of 15,161 participants, urine cytology demonstrated an overall sensitivity and specificity of 44 % and 96 % respectively [45]. For low-risk, high–risk, and CIS tumors the sensitivity increased from 27 to 69 % and 78 % respectively. The results of sensitivity and specificity of urinary markers in the detection of NMIBC recurrence are given in Table 13.4.

Table 13.4 Sensitivity and Specificity of Urinary Markers used for bladder cancer surveillance [51]

Marker	Sensitivity (%)	Specificity (%)
Cytology	12–47	83–97
FISH	64 (median)	73 (median)
Immunocyte	81 (median)	75 (median)
Telomerase	29–66	NA
BTA-Trak	60–83	60–79
BTA-stat	29–74	56–86
NMP-22	50–85	46–93
MSA	72–97	80–100
CYFRA	75–88	73–95
Ubiquitin	21–80	72–95

13.12 Imaging

Ultrasound for the detections of small bladder tumors has low sensitivity particularly for small tumors and cannot be recommended to replace cystoscopy.

CT scan has reported sensitivities if 79–90 % and specificities of 91–95 % in comparison to cystoscopy for the detection of bladder tumors [52]. The accuracy of CT however does decrease in patients with recurrence as scar from TURBT and tumors in the bladder base can make identification difficult. Virtual CT cystoscopy has a reported sensitivity similar to multi-detector CT, but higher than virtual MRI cystoscopy or virtual ultrasound cystoscopy [52]. Unfortunately, none of the imaging methods available are sensitive enough to replace cystoscopy.

13.13 Upper Tract Evaluation

The risk of development of upper tract UTT in patients with NMIBC is dependent on tumor multiplicity, tumor presence in the trigone, bladder CIS, tumor grade and stage [53]. In a study of 1,529 patients with NMIBC, the risk of UTT recurrence over a median time of 4.2 years was 0.6 %, 1.8 % and 4.1 % for low-, intermediate- and high-risk patients respectively [53]. The time to recurrence of UUT from initial TURBT ranges from a median of 43 to 88 months.

Upper tract tumors are routinely diagnosed by CT urography but an alternative is MRI urography in patients with contrast allergy. Yearly upper-tract imaging is recommended in high-risk patients and second yearly for intermediate risk. Low-risk patients do not require it.

13.14 Conclusion

The lack of evidence makes clear guidelines in the follow-up evaluation of NMIBC difficult. All bladder tumors ought to have a cystoscopy at 3 m following TURBT. Further cystoscopies should be performed based on risk category. Low-risk patients can be discharged after 5 years of surveillance however high-risk patients need lifelong surveillance as well as yearly UTT surveillance. Urine cytology can be used as an adjunct to cystoscopy but other urinary markers do not have a clear role in follow-up at this time.

References

1. Kamat AM, Hegarty PK, Gee JR, Clark PE, Svatek RS, Hegarty N, et al. ICUD-EAU International Consultation on Bladder Cancer 2012: screening, diagnosis, and molecular markers. Eur Urol. 2013;63(1):4–15. PubMed PMID: 23083902.
2. Cousins J, Howard J, Borra P. Principles of anaesthesia in urological surgery. BJU Int. 2005;96(2):223–9. PubMed PMID: 16001964.
3. Alsaywid BS, Smith GH. Antibiotic prophylaxis for transurethral urological surgeries: systematic review. Urol Ann. 2013;5(2):61–74. PubMed PMID: 23798859. Pubmed Central PMCID: 3685747.
4. Wolf Jr JS, Bennett CJ, Dmochowski RR, Hollenbeck BK, Pearle MS, Schaeffer AJ, et al. Best practice policy statement on urologic surgery antimicrobial prophylaxis. J Urol. 2008;179(4):1379–90. PubMed PMID: 18280509.
5. Kirkali Z, Chan T, Manoharan M, Algaba F, Busch C, Cheng L, et al. Bladder cancer: epidemiology, staging and grading, and diagnosis. Urology. 2005;66(6 Suppl 1):4–34. PubMed PMID: 16399414.
6. Pan D, Soloway MS. The importance of transurethral resection in managing patients with urothelial cancer in the bladder: proposal for a transurethral resection of bladder tumor checklist. Eur Urol. 2012;61(6):1199–203. PubMed PMID: 22464897.
7. Furuse H, Ozono S. Transurethral resection of the bladder tumour (TURBT) for non-muscle invasive bladder cancer: basic skills. Int J Urol. 2010;17(8):698–9. PubMed PMID: 20649827.
8. Solsona E, Iborra I, Ricos JV, Monros JL, Dumont R, Casanova J, et al. Recurrence of superficial bladder tumors in prostatic urethra. Eur Urol. 1991;19(2):89–92. PubMed PMID: 1902417.
9. Soloway MS, Patel J. Surgical techniques for endoscopic resection of bladder cancer. Urol Clin North Am. 1992;19(3):467–71. PubMed PMID: 1636231.
10. Burger M, Oosterlinck W, Konety B, Chang S, Gudjonsson S, Pruthi R, et al. ICUD-EAU International Consultation on Bladder Cancer 2012: non-muscle-invasive urothelial carcinoma of the bladder. Eur Urol. 2013;63(1):36–44. PubMed PMID: 22981672.
11. Nieder AM, Meinbach DS, Kim SS, Soloway MS. Transurethral bladder tumor resection: intraoperative and postoperative complications in a residency setting. J Urol. 2005;174(6):2307–9. PubMed PMID: 16280830.
12. Hall MC, Chang SS, Dalbagni G, Pruthi RS, Seigne JD, Skinner EC, et al. Guideline for the management of nonmuscle invasive bladder cancer (stages Ta, T1, and Tis): 2007 update. J Urol. 2007;178(6):2314–30. PubMed PMID: 17993339.
13. Ramirez-Backhaus M, Dominguez-Escrig J, Collado A, Rubio-Briones J, Solsona E. Restaging transurethral resection of bladder tumor for high-risk stage Ta and T1 bladder cancer. Curr Urol Rep. 2012;13(2):109–14. PubMed PMID: 22367558.
14. Mariappan P, Smith G, Lamb AD, Grigor KM, Tolley DA. Pattern of recurrence changes in noninvasive bladder tumors observed during 2 decades. J Urol. 2007;177(3):867–75. PubMed PMID: 17296362. Discussion 75.
15. Brausi M, Collette L, Kurth K, van der Meijden AP, Oosterlinck W, Witjes JA, et al. Variability in the recurrence rate at first follow-up cystoscopy after TUR in stage Ta T1 transitional cell carcinoma of the bladder: a combined analysis of seven EORTC studies. Eur Urol. 2002;41(5):523–31. PubMed PMID: 12074794.
16. Han KS, Joung JY, Cho KS, Seo HK, Chung J, Park WS, et al. Results of repeated transurethral resection for a second opinion in patients referred for nonmuscle invasive bladder cancer: the referral cancer center experience and review of the literature. J Endourol. 2008;22(12):2699–704. PubMed PMID: 19025393.
17. Mariappan P, Zachou A, Grigor KM, Edinburgh Uro-Oncology Group. Detrusor muscle in the first, apparently complete transurethral resection of bladder tumour specimen is a surrogate marker of resection quality, predicts risk of early recurrence, and is dependent on operator experience. Eur Urol. 2010;57(5):843–9. PubMed PMID: 19524354.
18. Herr HW. The value of a second transurethral resection in evaluating patients with bladder tumors. J Urol. 1999;162(1):74–6. PubMed PMID: 10379743.
19. Dutta SC, Smith Jr JA, Shappell SB, Coffey CS, Chang SS, Cookson MS. Clinical under staging of high risk nonmuscle invasive urothelial carcinoma treated with radical cystectomy. J Urol. 2001;166(2):490–3. PubMed PMID: 11458053.
20. Vasdev N, Dominguez-Escrig J, Paez E, Johnson MI, Durkan GC, Thorpe AC. The impact of early re-resection in patients with pT1 high-grade non-muscle invasive bladder cancer. Ecancermedicalscience. 2012;6:269. PubMed PMID: 22988482. Pubmed Central PMCID: 3436501.
21. Herr HW, Donat SM, Dalbagni G. Can restaging transurethral resection of T1 bladder cancer select patients for immediate cystectomy? J Urol. 2007;177(1):75–9. PubMed PMID: 17162005. Discussion 9.
22. Herr HW, Donat SM. Quality control in transurethral resection of bladder tumours. BJU Int. 2008;102(9 Pt B):1242–6. PubMed PMID: 19035888.
23. Divrik RT, Yildirim U, Zorlu F, Ozen H. The effect of repeat transurethral resection on recurrence and progression rates in patients with T1 tumors of the blad-

der who received intravesical mitomycin: a prospective, randomized clinical trial. J Urol. 2006;175(5):1641–4. PubMed PMID: 16600720.

24. Gudjonsson S, Blackberg M, Chebil G, Jahnson S, Olsson H, Bendahl PO, et al. The value of bladder mapping and prostatic urethra biopsies for detection of carcinoma in situ (CIS). BJU Int. 2012;110(2 Pt 2):E41–5. PubMed PMID: 22035276.

25. Babjuk M, Oosterlinck W, Sylvester R, Kaasinen E, Bohle A, Palou-Redorta J, et al. EAU guidelines on non-muscle-invasive urothelial carcinoma of the bladder, the 2011 update. Eur Urol. 2011;59(6):997–1008. PubMed PMID: 21458150.

26. Hautmann RE, Abol-Enein H, Davidsson T, Gudjonsson S, Hautmann SH, Holm HV, et al. ICUD-EAU International Consultation on Bladder Cancer 2012: urinary diversion. Eur Urol. 2013;63(1):67–80. PubMed PMID: 22995974.

27. Levi AW, Potter SR, Schoenberg MP, Epstein JI. Clinical significance of denuded urothelium in bladder biopsy. J Urol. 2001;166(2):457–60. PubMed PMID: 11458047.

28. O'Neil BB, Lowrance WT. Office-based bladder tumor fulguration and surveillance: indications and techniques. Urol Clin North Am. 2013;40(2):175–82. PubMed PMID: 23540776.

29. Sylvester RJ, van der Meijden AP, Oosterlinck W, Witjes JA, Bouffioux C, Denis L, et al. Predicting recurrence and progression in individual patients with stage Ta T1 bladder cancer using EORTC risk tables: a combined analysis of 2596 patients from seven EORTC trials. Eur Urol. 2006;49(3):466–5. PubMed PMID: 16442208. Discussion 75–7.

30. Herr HW, Donat SM, Dalbagni G. Correlation of cystoscopy with histology of recurrent papillary tumors of the bladder. J Urol. 2002;168(3):978–80. PubMed PMID: 12187203.

31. Donat SM, North A, Dalbagni G, Herr HW. Efficacy of office fulguration for recurrent low grade papillary bladder tumors less than 0.5 cm. J Urol. 2004;171(2 Pt 1):636–9.

32. Fernandez-Gomez J, Madero R, Solsona E, Unda M, Martinez-Pineiro L, Ojea A, et al. The EORTC tables overestimate the risk of recurrence and progression in patients with non-muscle-invasive bladder cancer treated with bacillus Calmette-Guerin: external validation of the EORTC risk tables. Eur Urol. 2011;60(3):423–30. PubMed PMID: 21621906.

33. Fernandez-Gomez J, Madero R, Solsona E, Unda M, Martinez-Pineiro L, Gonzalez M, et al. Predicting nonmuscle invasive bladder cancer recurrence and progression in patients treated with bacillus Calmette-Guerin: the CUETO scoring model. J Urol. 2009;182(5):2195–203. PubMed PMID: 19758621.

34. Holmang S, Johansson SL. Stage Ta-T1 bladder cancer: the relationship between findings at first followup cystoscopy and subsequent recurrence and progression. J Urol. 2002;167(4):1634–7. PubMed PMID: 11912378.

35. Kurth KH, Denis L, Bouffioux C, Sylvester R, Debruyne FM, Pavone-Macaluso M, et al. Factors affecting recurrence and progression in superficial bladder tumours. Eur J Cancer. 1995;31A(11):1840–6. PubMed PMID: 8541110.

36. Parmar MK, Freedman LS, Hargreave TB, Tolley DA. Prognostic factors for recurrence and followup policies in the treatment of superficial bladder cancer: report from the British Medical Research Council Subgroup on Superficial Bladder Cancer (Urological Cancer Working Party). J Urol. 1989;142(2 Pt 1):284–8. PubMed PMID: 2501516.

37. Herr HW. Progression of stage T1 bladder tumors after intravesical bacillus Calmette-Guerin. J Urol. 1991;145(1):40–3. PubMed PMID: 1984096. Discussion 3–4.

38. Solsona E, Iborra I, Dumont R, Rubio-Briones J, Casanova J, Almenar S. The 3-month clinical response to intravesical therapy as a predictive factor for progression in patients with high risk superficial bladder cancer. J Urol. 2000;164(3 Pt 1):685–9. PubMed PMID: 10953125.

39. Babjuk M, Burger M, Zigeuner R, Shariat SF, van Rhijn BW, Comperat E, et al. EAU guidelines on non-muscle-invasive urothelial carcinoma of the bladder. Eur Urol. 20131;64(4):639--53. PubMed PMID: 23827737.

40. Olsen LH, Genster HG. Prolonging follow-up intervals for non-invasive bladder tumors: a randomized controlled trial. Scand J Urol Nephrol Suppl. 1995;172:33–6. PubMed PMID: 8578253.

41. Holmang S, Strock V. Should follow-up cystoscopy in bacillus Calmette-Guerin-treated patients continue after five tumour-free years? Eur Urol. 2012;61(3):503–7. PubMed PMID: 22119022.

42. Mariappan P, Smith G. A surveillance schedule for G1Ta bladder cancer allowing efficient use of check cystoscopy and safe discharge at 5 years based on a 25-year prospective database. J Urol. 2005;173(4):1108–11. PubMed PMID: 15758711.

43. Fitzpatrick JM, West AB, Butler MR, Lane V, O'Flynn JD. Superficial bladder tumors (stage pTa, grades 1 and 2): the importance of recurrence pattern following initial resection. J Urol. 1986;135(5):920–2. PubMed PMID: 3959241.

44. Leblanc B, Duclos AJ, Benard F, Cote J, Valiquette L, Paquin JM, et al. Long-term followup of initial Ta grade 1 transitional cell carcinoma of the bladder. J Urol. 1999;162(6):1946–50. PubMed PMID: 10569544.

45. Mowatt G, Zhu S, Kilonzo M, Boachie C, Fraser C, Griffiths TR, et al. Systematic review of the clinical effectiveness and cost-effectiveness of photodynamic diagnosis and urine biomarkers (FISH, ImmunoCyt, NMP22) and cytology for the detection and follow-up of bladder cancer. Health Technol Assess. 2010;14(4):1–331. iii–iv. PubMed PMID: 20082749.

46. Cauberg EC, Kloen S, Visser M, de la Rosette JJ, Babjuk M, Soukup V, et al. Narrow band imaging cystoscopy improves the detection of non-muscle-invasive bladder cancer. Urology. 2010;76(3):658–63. PubMed PMID: 20223505.

47. Loidl W, Schmidbauer J, Susani M, Marberger M. Flexible cystoscopy assisted by hexaminolevulinate induced fluorescence: a new approach for bladder cancer detection and surveillance? Eur Urol. 2005;47(3):323–6. PubMed PMID: 15716195.

48. Herr HW, Donat SM. Reduced bladder tumour recurrence rate associated with narrow-band imaging surveillance cystoscopy. BJU Int. 2011;107(3):396–8. PubMed PMID: 20707789.

49. Dalbagni G, Rechtschaffen T, Herr HW. Is transurethral biopsy of the bladder necessary after 3 months to evaluate response to bacillus Calmette-Guerin therapy? J Urol. 1999;162(3 Pt 1):708–9. PubMed PMID: 10458348.

50. Yossepowitch O, Herr HW, Donat SM. Use of urinary biomarkers for bladder cancer surveillance: patient perspectives. J Urol. 2007;177(4):1277–82. PubMed PMID: 17382711. Discussion 82.

51. Soukup V, Babjuk M, Bellmunt J, Dalbagni G, Giannarini G, Hakenberg OW, et al. Follow-up after surgical treatment of bladder cancer: a critical analysis of the literature. Eur Urol. 2012;62(2):290–302. PubMed PMID: 22609313.

52. Cohan RH, Caoili EM, Cowan NC, Weizer AZ, Ellis JH. MDCT Urography: Exploring a new paradigm for imaging of bladder cancer. AJR Am J Roentgenol. 2009;192(6):1501–8. PubMed PMID: 19457811.

53. Millan-Rodriguez F, Chechile-Toniolo G, Salvador-Bayarri J, Huguet-Perez J, Vicente-Rodriguez J. Upper urinary tract tumors after primary superficial bladder tumors: prognostic factors and risk groups. J Urol. 2000;164(4):1183–7. PubMed PMID: 10992362.

45-Year-old healthy man with his first large,
high-grade ta cancer

José L. Domínguez-Escrig
and Eduardo Solsona Narbón

Abbreviations

5-ALA	5-Aminolevulinic acid
AUA	American Urology Association
BCG	Bacillus Calmette-Guerin
Cis	Carcinoma in situ
CUETO	Club Urológico Español de Tratamiento Oncológico
EAU	European Association of Urology
HAL	Hexaminolevulinic acid
IBCG	International Bladder Cancer Group
MMC	Mytomicin C
NBI	Narrow band imaging
NICE	National Institute of Clinical Excellence
PDD	Photodynamic diagnosis
PFS	Progression-free survival
RFS	Recurrence-free survival
RE-TUR	Re trans-urethral resection
TUR	Trans-urethral resection
WLC	White light cystoscopy

J.L. Domínguez-Escrig, L.M.S., M.D., F.R.C.S. (Urol) (✉)
E.S. Narbón
Servicio de Urología, Fundacion Instituto Valenciano
de Oncologia, C. Profesor Beltrán Báguena N. 8.,
46009, Valencia, Spain
e-mail: jldominguezescrig@hotmail.com;
solsona@pulso.com; http://www.ivo.es

With a worldwide age-standardized incidence rate of 9 per 100,000 for men and 2 per 100,000 for women, bladder cancer is the most common malignancy of the urinary tract, representing the 7th and 17th most frequent malignancy in men and women, respectively. The worldwide age-standardized mortality rates are 3 and 1 per 100,000 for men and women, respectively. With a higher incidence in the developed world, the EU age standardized mortality rate are 8 and 3 per 100,000 for men and women, respectively [1].

Approximately 75–85 % of cases present with a disease that is confined to the mucosa (Ta, CIS) or sub-mucosa (T1), being grouped as non-muscle-invasive bladder tumors (NMIBC). However, this is a very lose heading as evidenced at a molecular level and by the very different clinical behavior of these tumors. Regarding pTa G3 urothelial carcinoma of the bladder, the evidence for clinical management, often extrapolated from pT1 high-grade disease remains limited.

In this chapter, we present and discuss the clinical management of a 45-year-old healthy man with his first large, high-grade Ta cancer.

While low-grade pTa disease carries a very low (<5 %) risk of progression [2], contemporary series have demonstrated a significant risk in terms of both recurrence and progression of pTa G3 disease, with rates in the order of 50 % and 25 %, respectively, recently reported by Lebret et al. [3].

Current international guidelines recommend cystoscopic surveillance, re-resection (Re-TUR),

B.R. Konety and S.S. Chang (eds.), *Management of Bladder Cancer:
A Comprehensive Text With Clinical Scenarios*, DOI 10.1007/978-1-4939-1881-2_14,
© Springer Science+Business Media New York 2015

and intravesical adjuvant therapy with Bacillus Calmette-Guerin (BCG).

Firstly, we shall review the case, with particular attention to the pathology at our multidisciplinary meeting. Formal review of the slides by a dedicated uro-pathologist is paramount when evaluating the tumor, defining stage and grade, as well as, giving surrogate information of the quality of the resection performed.

Equally important, we routinely perform imaging of the upper tract in all high-risk tumors, in the presence of positive cytology, as well as, following recommendations of the EAU guidelines, in all cases when the tumor is located at the trigone. As most units, we conventionally performed intravenous urography (IVU), used to detect filling defects and hydronephrosis. Recently, we have updated our local guidelines and moved to CT-urography to assess the upper urinary tract.

In a recent review of 935 patients by Stenberg et al., evaluating the usefulness of routine upper tract imaging in patients followed for pTa and pT1 NMIBC, only 51 were found to develop tumors. The 5- and 10-year upper tract disease-free probabilities were 98 % and 94 % versus 93 % and 88 %, for patients with pTa and pT1 tumors, respectively. In this series, only 29 % of patients were diagnosed on routine imaging, with an overall efficacy of only 0.49 % [4].

While the involvement of upper urinary tract is low in NMIBC, with reported incidences ranging from 0.3 to 2.4 % [4–7], it increases significantly when the tumor is located in the trigone, as evidenced by Palou et al. In this retrospective study of 1,529 cases with primary NMIBC, synchronous upper tract involvement was found in 7.5 % of patients with tumors located in the trigone. In this series, if trigonal location and multiplicity had been considered, 66.7 % of tumors would have been diagnosed [8].

Furthermore, the risk of recurrence in the upper urinary tract increases in multifocal and high-risk tumors [9]. This is particularly important in the case of carcinoma in situ, with an incidence as high as 24.6 % observed in our series [6, 10].

Accurate tumor staging and grading is necessary in order to plan the optimal treatment for each patient as they are among the most important predictors of recurrence and disease progression in non-muscle-invasive bladder cancer (NMIBC).

Prediction is now facilitated by risk calculator software readily available to all professionals from different sources. The most widely implemented nomogram is the European Organization for Research and Treatment of Cancer (EORTC) Risk Tables for Ta T1 Bladder Cancer Version 1.0, http://www.eortc.be/tools/bladdercalculator (programmed by Richard Sylvester, EORTC Data Center, Brussels, Belgium). Combining data from 2,596 patients with NMIBC from seven EORTC trials, it is a simple scoring system based on six variables: Number of tumors, tumor size, prior recurrence rate, stage (T), grade, and presence or absence of carcinoma in situ [11]. Applying these tables to our particular case and considering a solitary, primary tumor, > 3 cm in diameter, stage pTa, high-grade (G3) without associated pTcis, we shall obtain that the estimated rates for disease recurrence and progression are 38 % (35–41) and 5 % (4–7) at 1 year, respectively, while rates of 62 % (58–65) and 17 % (14–20), respectively, are obtained at 5 years.

However, this scoring system may be less useful in our particular case, as we are dealing with a high-grade G3 tumor and a candidate for BCG adjuvant therapy. Certainly, the main limitation of the EORTC risk tables is the fact that it is based on older series, with little exposure to adjuvant therapy and without maintenance protocols, thus, resulting in overall worse predicted outcomes [12]. A more contemporary scoring model, proposed by the CUETO group, may better predict recurrence and progression rates in our scenario [13]. Applying this model, that also takes into account age at diagnosis (45 years) and gender (male), the predicted rates for disease recurrence and progression are 8.24 % (5.91–10.57) and 3 % (0.82–5.18) at 1 year, respectively, while rates of 20.98 % (17.32–24.63) and 11.69 % (7.57–15.81), respectively, are expected at 5 years.

Ultimately, the mainstay of the initial management of NMIBC should be the correct staging, thus, requiring an optimal sampling of the tumor.

The response to this challenge comes in a two-fold approach: implementation of a policy of routine re-resection, the so-called second look TUR or Re-TUR, as well as, continue to develop novel techniques of imaging and endoscopy aimed to optimize tumor identification at the time of cystoscopy, as well as, non-invasive diagnostic markers.

14.1 Re-resection

The overall rate of recurrence following TUR in patients with NMIBC can be as high as 70 %, with the greatest risk being at the first follow-up cystoscopy [14]. This can be attributed, at least in part, to incomplete resection of the initial tumor or to overlooked multifocal disease. The analysis of seven phase III trials by the European Organization for Research and Treatment of Cancer EORTC confirmed substantial variations in early recurrence rates among institutions, with recurrence rates at 3 months ranging from 0 to 46 %, only explained, after multivariate analysis, by the variable quality of the resections [15]. Herr and Donat explained that the quality of TURBT can be measured with three variables: the macroscopic resection of the tumor, the presence of muscle in the sample, and the recurrence rate in the first follow-up [16].

Presence of Detrusor muscle in the TURBT specimen is a surrogate marker of resection quality. In Mariappan's series [17], reporting the presence of muscle in 67 % of all the first TUR specimens, the presence of muscle was associated in the multivariate analysis to the recurrence rate at first cystoscopy, with a 2.9 times higher probability of recurrence in the absence of muscle. Furthermore, Herr et al. identified the absence of muscle in the initial TUR specimen as a predictor of clinical under-staging. In this study, 14 % of patients with clinical stage T1 disease and muscle in the specimen were upstaged to T2 versus 49 % if no muscle was present [18]. Similarly, Dutta et al. reported a 64 % rate of under-staging in T1 tumors if muscle was absent in the specimen versus only a 30 % if muscle was present [19].

For Ta disease, when muscle was not clearly stated to be present in the TUR specimens, upstaging has been reported in up to 14.3 % [20]; contrary to the 6.4 % reported by Han when muscle was sampled [21].

The published rates of residual tumor detected by Re-TUR range from 20 to 81.5 % [17, 22]. If we stratify the data based on tumor stage, residual disease was detected in 22–74 % of Ta [22, 23] and in 26.5–81.5 % of T1 tumors [17]. Updated series on routine Re-TUR from MSKCC, including 1,312 patients with NMIBC, have been recently published by Herr and Donat, reporting residual disease in 51–78 % of patients, depending on T stage and being highest for pT1 disease at initial TUR. In this study, while re-TUR demonstrated upstaging in 15 % of patients with a pTa disease, muscle invasive disease was discovered in 30 % of those with initial pT1 tumors [16].

Divrik et al. [24] randomized 210 patients with newly diagnosed pT1, to Re-TUR or standard follow-up. In this study, 25.7 % had residual pT1 disease and 7.6 % were upstaged (pT2 or pT1 + Cis). Reported RFS rates at 1, 2 and 3 years were 86.35 %, 77.67 % and 68.72 % in the re-TUR group and 47.08 %, 42.31 % and 37.01 % in the TUR alone group, respectively. The authors also observed a reduced risk of progression compared with those in whom a Re-TUR was not performed. In the multivariate analysis, Re-TUR was found to be an independent predictor of progression, as also demonstrated following analysis of the Memorial Sloan-Kettering Cancer Center initial [16] and updated [25] series.

Following recommendations of the AUA and EAU guidelines, we routinely perform re-resection, within 6 weeks, in all high-grade tumors, pT1 disease, in cases of incomplete first resection or when muscle is absent in the pathology specimen.

Together with the routine implementation of a policy of Re-TUR, we have recently added new devices and optimized optical and software systems that are now part of our daily endoscopic armamentarium and may potentially improve our outcomes. Such systems include photodynamic diagnosis (PDD) and narrow band imaging (NBI).

Photodynamic diagnosis (PDD) uses blue light (375–440 nm) after intravesical instillation of the photosensitizers 5-aminolaevulinic acid

(ALA) or hexaminolaevulinic acid (HAL), highlighting the areas of accumulation. PDD is superior to white light cystoscopy (WLC) for the detection of tumors at cystoscopy and biopsy, being even more relevant in the case of Cis [26]. For pTa disease, relevant to our clinical scenario, the reported detection rates for PDD are still superior to WLC, 94–97 % versus 83–88 %, respectively [27, 28].

A recently published meta-analysis by Mowatt et al. reported that PDD showed higher sensitivity than WLC in the pooled estimates for both patient (92 % vs. 71 %) and biopsy (93 % vs. 65 %) level analyses, while PDD had a lower specificity (63 % vs. 81 %) [29]. False positive rates of upto 30% have been reported with fluoresence cystoscopy mainly due to false fluorescence inerpretation during the learning curve, inflammation and the previous use of BCG [30, 31]. Therefore, we believe that the timing of the RE-RTU is ideal, before starting treatment with BCG.

The 2013 EAU 2013 guidelines on non-muscle-invasive bladder cancer recommend the use of PDD in patients with a history of high-grade tumor or those with positive cytology. Although, there is no clear long-term impact on progression, neither on recurrence in the case of 5-ALA [32, 33], contemporary studies have demonstrated a benefit in terms of RFS with the use of HAL PDD-guided TUR, including pTa disease [34–38].

Narrow band imaging (NBI) filters light into two wavelengths of 540 nm (green) and 415 nm (blue) absorbed by hemoglobin, thus, enhancing the vessel-urothelium delineation and highlighting the more vascular malignant tissue [39]. NBI has demonstrated superiority to WLC on the detection of bladder tumors pTa, pT1, as well as, in bladder Cis [39–45]. Systematic review and meta-analysis of pooled data from eight studies, including 1,022 patients, recently published by Zheng et al. has concluded that NBI is an effective method for the identification of bladder tumors, including Cis and superior to WLC [46]. Furthermore, the available data indicate a significant reduction on residual tumor rates following NBI-TUR [41, 47].

Despite long follow-up studies assessing the impact on disease recurrence and progression still lacking, a study by Herr and Donat, evaluating the role of routine surveillance with NBI versus WLC on a cohort of 126 patients with low-grade NMIBC, has demonstrated a reduction on the recurrence rate (65 % vs. 94 %), number of recurrent tumors (2.8 vs. 2.8) and a longer RFS (29 months vs. 13 months), favorable to NBI [48]. Moreover, a recently published prospective randomized trial has demonstrated that compared to white light TUR, NBI-RTU translated into a 10 % reduction of the risk or recurrence (51.4 % vs. 32.9 %), at 1 year [49].

14.2 Urine Markers

In parallel to the rapid embracing of novel endoscopic aids, the focus of practicing urologists and researchers has turned to the development of non-invasive urine markers aimed to refine the diagnosis and follow-up of urothelial tumors. Among those, NMP22 ELISSA and NMP22 BladderCheck, InmunoCyt, BTA Stat and BTA-TRAK and Urovysion-FISH are currently commercially available, while others are still at different stages of clinical evaluation.

Nuclear Matrix Protein 22 tests include the laboratory-based, quantitative, immunoassay NMP22 bladder cancer test kit and the point-of-check, qualitative NMP22 BladderCheck (Matritech Inc.) with a sensitivities ranging from 47 to 100 % and 5–90 %, respectively. However, reported specificities of up to 90 % and 86 %, respectively, remain overall inferior to that of urine cytology [50]. Although it is not altered by BCG and therefore potentially useful in high-grade disease such as our clinical scenario, NMP22 performs better in low-grade disease [51]. Moreover, false positives are reported with infection, inflammation, calculi, stents, instrumentation and bowel interposition, as well as, other genitourinary malignancies [52].

InmunoCyt (Scimedx Corp.) is a novel test combining immunofluorescence and cytology to target the bladder cancer-specific M344, LDQ10, and 19A211 antigens [53]. With an improved sensitivity of up to a 100 %, particularly when compared to cytology alone in low-grade tumors, the specificity remains low, with reported rates of 69–81.6 % [53–57] and it is also affected by cystitis and BPH [50].

The qualitative, point-of-care *BTA Stat* and the quantitative, ELISA *BTA-TRAK* detect human complement factor H-related protein, a bladder tumor-associated antigen, in voided urine [58, 59]. Sensitivity and specificity rates of 57–83 % and 60–92 %, respectively, are reported for BTA Stat test, with rates of 62–91 % and 29–65 %, respectively, for BTA-TRAK [50, 60]. Importantly for our case, while it is affected by several benign conditions, similar to NMP22, false positives can be caused by BCG treatment [61].

Urovysion® FISH (Vysis-Abbott Laboratories) is a multi-target assay designed to detect aneuploidy of chromosomes 3, 7, 17 and the loss of the 9p21 locus in malignant cells [62], with sensitivity and specificity rates of 84.2 % and 91.8 %, respectively, reported by Sokolova et al., in the original. Contemporary series have reported specificity rates of 78–92 % and sensitivity rates of 69–85 % [61]. A recent meta-analysis by Hajdinjak et al. [63], involving 2,477 FISH tests from 14 studies, has reported a pooled sensitivity and specificity of 72 % (69–75 %) and 83 % (82–85 %), respectively; with sensitivity increased to 86 % (82–89 %) when pTa disease was excluded.

Relevant to our clinical scenario, FISH may potentially be useful in assessing BCG response as supported by several recently published studies demonstrating correlation of post-BCG positive FISH and tumor recurrence [64–66], as well as, progression to invasive disease. In this study, published by Kipp et al. [64], patients with a positive post-therapy FISH were found to develop recurrence earlier and to be 9.4 times as likely to develop pT2 disease.

Up to this date and based on the available evidence, regarding the routine implementation of urine markers, the 2013 EAU guidelines conclude that "A urinary marker other than cytology is not recommended for high-risk NMIBC surveillance."

14.3 Treatment

Once the case has clearly been defined as high-grade non-muscle-invasive urothelial carcinoma stage pTa G3, we would start adjuvant therapy with an induction course of 6-weekly instillations of Bacillus Calmette-Guerin [67], initiated at least 2 weeks after the Re-TUR and routinely followed by maintenance BCG therapy [68], aimed to reduce the risk of recurrence, as well as, disease progression.

Meta-analyses demonstrated that BCG after TUR is superior to TUR alone or TUR and chemotherapy for prevention of recurrence of non-muscle-invasive tumors [69–73] and highlighted the role of maintenance BCG [71]. In intermediate- and high-risk NMIBC, BCG has been shown to be superior to MMC [74], epirubicin alone [2], or in combination with interferon [75] in the reduction of disease recurrence.

Furthermore, meta-analyses have demonstrated that BCG therapy prevents, or at least delays disease progression. A meta-analysis by the EORTC-GUCG including 4,863 patients from 24 RCTs, employing five different BCG strains and in 20 of the trials, some form of BCG maintenance, has been recently published. With a median follow-up of 2.5 years, progression was seen in 9.8 % of patients treated with BCG versus 13.8 % in the control groups (TUR alone, TUR plus intravesical chemotherapy, or TUR plus other immunotherapy), representing 27 % reduction in the odds of progression with BCG maintenance treatment ($P = 0.0001$) [76]. Although, the long-term superiority of BCG regarding progression is still under debate [71], a recently published RCT with long-term follow up has demonstrated a significant reduction of metastases and improved overall- and disease-specific survival in patients treated with BCG compared to adjuvant chemotherapy [2].

Taking into account the findings of the CUETO group regarding recurrence and progression prognostic value of sex, age and tumor focality, one can conclude that our clinical scenario represents an ideal case. Being a primary single tumor, male gender and younger age

(45 years), one can expect the best possible response to BCG therapy [12, 13]. While the optimal instillation frequency and duration of maintenance remain unknown [68, 77], we normally continue BCG with 3-monthly instillations, for up to 3 years. A recent EORTC RCT including 1,355 patients has demonstrated that when BCG is given at full dose, maintenance for 3 years, but not for 1 year, reduces recurrence rate in high-risk disease. However, there were no differences in progression or overall survival [78].

Far from a potentially deleterious effect of delaying BCG therapy to after the Re-RTU, this may have a beneficial effect, as evidenced by Herr et al., in a series of 347 patients with high-risk NMIBCs, reporting a recurrence rate of 45 % in the cohort of patients undergoing restaging/second TUR before BCG treatment versus an 80 % in those who received BCG treatment after initial TUR. Multivariate analysis showed that the lack of response to BCG at first follow-up cystoscopy and a single TUR (rather than restaging TUR) before BCG therapy were significant independent factors associated with subsequent tumor recurrence and stage progression [79].

In our department, the routine long-term follow-up this patient will be by means of regular cystoscopy and urinary cytology, the first one being always performed in the operating theatre and under anesthesia, thus, allowing for biopsies or further resection should this be considered appropriate. For long-term checks, we now perform flexible cystoscopy and cytology, easily performed in the office. At present, we do not implement urinary markers for the routine surveillance of these patients.

The patient is always counseled regarding the benefits, as well as the side-effects of the adjuvant treatment, particularly about the potential for serious complications of the BCG therapy and a direct telephone contact is given to the patient. Information is paramount in order to reassure the patient and to improve compliance. More importantly, it is essential for the early recognition by the patient of potentially serious complications that develop in less than 5 % of cases and are, if managed promptly, curable [80].

Recommendations for individual situations have been provided by the International Bladder Cancer Group (IBCG) and colleagues from Fundación Puigvert [81] and have been summarized in the updated 2013 EAU Bladder Cancer Guidelines, with a systematic review of the local (cystitis, hematuria, granulomatous prostatitis, and epididymo-orchitis), as well as, systemic (fever, arthralgia, arthritis, and BCG sepsis) adverse events, with clear recommendations regarding their treatment, in particular, guidance regarding discontinuation, temporal or definitive, of BCG instillations and general rules regarding the adequate initiation of tuberculostatic drugs and/or corticoids. These are guidelines to which we adhere in our daily clinical practice.

References

1. Ferlay, Shin H, Bray F, Forman D, Mathers C, Parkin D. Globocan 2008: cancer incidence and mortality worldwide 2010. International Agency for Research on Cancer: Lyon, France. IARC CancerBase No. 10.
2. Sylvester RJ, Brausi MA, Kirkels WJ, Hoeltl W, Da Calais SF, Powell PH, Prescott S, Kirkali Z, van de Beek C, Gorlia T, de Reijke TM. Long-term efficacy results of EORTC genito-urinary group randomized phase 3 study 30911 comparing intravesical instillations of epirubicin, bacillus Calmette-Guerin, and bacillus Calmette-Guerin plus isoniazid in patients with intermediate- and high-risk stage Ta T1 urothelial carcinoma of the bladder. Eur Urol. 2010;57(5):766–73.
3. Lebret T, Bohin D, Kassardjian Z, Herve JM, Molinie V, Barre P, Lugagne PM, Botto H. Recurrence, progression and success in stage Ta grade 3 bladder tumors treated with low dose bacillus Calmette-Guerin instillations. J Urol. 2000;163(1):63–7.
4. Sternberg IA, Keren Paz GE, Chen LY, Herr HW, Donat SM, Bochner BH, Dalbagni G. Upper tract imaging surveillance is not effective in diagnosing upper tract recurrence in patients followed for non-muscle invasive bladder cancer. J Urol. 2013;190(4):1187–91.
5. Goessl C, Knispel HH, Miller K, Klan R. Is routine excretory urography necessary at first diagnosis of bladder cancer? J Urol. 1997;157(2):480–1.
6. Solsona E, Iborra I, Ricos JV, Dumont R, Casanova JL, Calabuig C. Upper urinary tract involvement in patients with bladder carcinoma in situ (Tis): its impact on management. Urology. 1997;49(3):347–52.
7. Holmang S, Hedelin H, Anderstrom C, Holmberg E, Johansson SL. Long-term followup of a bladder

carcinoma cohort: routine followup urography is not necessary. J Urol. 1998;160(1):45–8.

8. Palou J, Rodriguez-Rubio F, Huguet J, Segarra J, Ribal MJ, Alcaraz A, Villavicencio H. Multivariate analysis of clinical parameters of synchronous primary superficial bladder cancer and upper urinary tract tumor. J Urol. 2005;174(3):859–61.

9. Millan-Rodriguez F, Chechile-Toniolo G, Salvador-Bayarri J, Huguet-Perez J, Vicente-Rodriguez J. Upper urinary tract tumors after primary superficial bladder tumors: prognostic factors and risk groups. J Urol. 2000;164(4):1183–7.

10. Solsona E, Iborra I, Ricos JV, Monros JL, Dumont R, Almenar S. Extravesical involvement in patients with bladder carcinoma in situ: biological and therapy implications. J Urol. 1996;155(3):895–9.

11. Sylvester RJ, van der MEIJDEN AP, Oosterlinck W, Witjes JA, Bouffioux C, Denis L, Newling DW, Kurth K. Predicting recurrence and progression in individual patients with stage Ta T1 bladder cancer using EORTC risk tables: a combined analysis of 2596 patients from seven EORTC trials. Eur Urol. 2006;49(3):466–5.

12. Fernandez-Gomez J, Madero R, Solsona E, Unda M, Martinez-Pineiro L, Ojea A, Portillo J, Montesinos M, Gonzalez M, Pertusa C, Rodriguez-Molina J, Camacho JE, Rabadan M, Astobieta A, Isorna S, Muntanola P, Gimeno A, Blas M, Martinez-Pineiro JA. The EORTC tables overestimate the risk of recurrence and progression in patients with non-muscle-invasive bladder cancer treated with bacillus Calmette-Guerin: external validation of the EORTC risk tables. Eur Urol. 2011;60(3):423–30.

13. Fernandez-Gomez J, Madero R, Solsona E, Unda M, Martinez-Pineiro L, Gonzalez M, Portillo J, Ojea A, Pertusa C, Rodriguez-Molina J, Camacho JE, Rabadan M, Astobieta A, Montesinos M, Isorna S, Muntanola P, Gimeno A, Blas M, Martinez-Pineiro JA. Predicting nonmuscle invasive bladder cancer recurrence and progression in patients treated with bacillus Calmette-Guerin: the CUETO scoring model. J Urol. 2009;182(5):2195–203.

14. Mariappan P, Smith G, Lamb AD, Grigor KM, Tolley DA. Pattern of recurrence changes in noninvasive bladder tumors observed during 2 decades. J Urol. 2007;177(3):867–75.

15. Brausi M, Collette L, Kurth K, van der MEIJDEN AP, Oosterlinck W, Witjes JA, Newling D, Bouffioux C, Sylvester RJ. Variability in the recurrence rate at first follow-up cystoscopy after TUR in stage Ta T1 transitional cell carcinoma of the bladder: a combined analysis of seven EORTC studies. Eur Urol. 2002;41(5):523–31.

16. Herr HW, Donat SM. Quality control in transurethral resection of bladder tumours. BJU Int. 2008;102(9 Pt B):1242–6.

17. Mariappan P, Zachou A, Grigor KM. Detrusor muscle in the first, apparently complete transurethral resection of bladder tumour specimen is a surrogate marker of resection quality, predicts risk of early recurrence, and is dependent on operator experience. Eur Urol. 2010;57(5):843–9.

18. Herr HW. The value of a second transurethral resection in evaluating patients with bladder tumors. J Urol. 1999;162(1):74–6.

19. Dutta SC, Smith Jr JA, Shappell SB, Coffey CS, Chang SS, Cookson MS. Clinical under staging of high risk nonmuscle invasive urothelial carcinoma treated with radical cystectomy. J Urol. 2001;166(2):490–3.

20. Vasdev N, McKie C, Dominguez-Escrig J, El-Sherif A, Johnson M, Durkan G, Rix D, Thorpe A. The role of early re-resection in pTaG3 transitional cell carcinoma of the urinary bladder. BJMSU. 2013;4(4):158–65. Elsevier.

Ref Type: Generic

21. Schips L, Augustin H, Zigeuner RE, Galle G, Habermann H, Trummer H, Pummer K, Hubmer G. Is repeated transurethral resection justified in patients with newly diagnosed superficial bladder cancer? Urology. 2002;59(2):220–3.

22. Ali MH, Ismail IY, Eltobgy A, Gobeish A. Evaluation of second-look transurethral resection in restaging of patients with nonmuscle-invasive bladder cancer. J Endourol. 2010;24(12):2047–50.

23. Han KS, Joung JY, Cho KS, Seo HK, Chung J, Park WS, Lee KH. Results of repeated transurethral resection for a second opinion in patients referred for nonmuscle invasive bladder cancer: the referral cancer center experience and review of the literature. J Endourol. 2008;22(12):2699–704.

24. Divrik RT, Sahin AF, Yildirim U, Altok M, Zorlu F. Impact of routine second transurethral resection on the long-term outcome of patients with newly diagnosed pT1 urothelial carcinoma with respect to recurrence, progression rate, and disease-specific survival: a prospective randomised clinical trial. Eur Urol. 2010;58(2):185–90.

25. Herr HW, Donat SM, Dalbagni G. Can restaging transurethral resection of T1 bladder cancer select patients for immediate cystectomy? J Urol. 2007;177(1):75–9.

26. Liu JJ, Droller MJ, Liao JC. New optical imaging technologies for bladder cancer: considerations and perspectives. J Urol. 2012;188(2):361–8.

27. Geavlete B, Jecu M, Multescu R, Georgescu D, Geavlete P. HAL blue-light cystoscopy in high-risk nonmuscle-invasive bladder cancer–re-TURBT recurrence rates in a prospective, randomized study. Urology. 2010;76(3):664–9.

28. Schmidbauer J, Witjes F, Schmeller N, Donat R, Susani M, Marberger M. Improved detection of urothelial carcinoma in situ with hexaminolevulinate fluorescence cystoscopy. J Urol. 2004;171(1):135–8.

29. Mowatt G, N'Dow J, Vale L, Nabi G, Boachie C, Cook JA, Fraser C, Griffiths TR. Photodynamic diagnosis of bladder cancer compared with white light cystoscopy: Systematic review and meta-analysis. Int J Technol Assess Health Care. 2011;27(1):3–10.

30. Draga RO, Grimbergen MC, Kok ET, Jonges TN, van Swol CF, Bosch JL. Photodynamic diagnosis (5-aminolevulinic acid) of transitional cell carcinoma after bacillus Calmette-Guerin immunotherapy and mitomycin C intravesical therapy. Eur Urol. 2010;57(4):655–60.

31. Ray ER, Chatterton K, Khan MS, Chandra A, Thomas K, Dasgupta P, O'Brien TS. Hexylaminolaevulinate fluorescence cystoscopy in patients previously treated with intravesical bacille Calmette-Guerin. BJU Int. 2010;105(6):789–94.

32. Schumacher MC, Holmang S, Davidsson T, Friedrich B, Pedersen J, Wiklund NP. Transurethral resection of non-muscle-invasive bladder transitional cell cancers with or without 5-aminolevulinic Acid under visible and fluorescent light: results of a prospective, randomised, multicentre study. Eur Urol. 2010;57(2):293–9.

33. Stenzl A, Penkoff H, Dajc-Sommerer E, Zumbraegel A, Hoeltl L, Scholz M, Riedl C, Bugelnig J, Hobisch A, Burger M, Mikuz G, Pichlmeier U. Detection and clinical outcome of urinary bladder cancer with 5-aminolevulinic acid-induced fluorescence cystoscopy: a multicenter randomized, double-blind, placebo-controlled trial. Cancer. 2011;117(5):938–47.

34. Hermann GG, Mogensen K, Carlsson S, Marcussen N, Duun S. Fluorescence-guided transurethral resection of bladder tumours reduces bladder tumour recurrence due to less residual tumour tissue in Ta/T1 patients: a randomized two-centre study. BJU Int. 2011;108(8 Pt 2):E297–303.

35. Stenzl A, Burger M, Fradet Y, Mynderse LA, Soloway MS, Witjes JA, Kriegmair M, Karl A, Shen Y, Grossman HB. Hexaminolevulinate guided fluorescence cystoscopy reduces recurrence in patients with nonmuscle invasive bladder cancer. J Urol. 2010;184(5):1907–13.

36. Grossman HB, Stenzl A, Fradet Y, Mynderse LA, Kriegmair M, Witjes JA, Soloway MS, Karl A, Burger M. Long-term decrease in bladder cancer recurrence with hexaminolevulinate enabled fluorescence cystoscopy. J Urol. 2012;188(1):58–62.

37. Geavlete B, Multescu R, Georgescu D, Jecu M, Stanescu F, Geavlete P. Treatment changes and long-term recurrence rates after hexaminolevulinate (HAL) fluorescence cystoscopy: does it really make a difference in patients with non-muscle-invasive bladder cancer (NMIBC)? BJU Int. 2012;109(4):549–56.

38. Malmstrom PU, Grabe M, Haug ES, Hellstrom P, Hermann GG, Mogensen K, Raitanen M, Wahlqvist R. Role of hexaminolevulinate-guided fluorescence cystoscopy in bladder cancer: critical analysis of the latest data and European guidance. Scand J Urol Nephrol. 2012;46(2):108–16.

39. Cauberg EC, Kloen S, Visser M, de la Rosette JJ, Babjuk M, Soukup V, Pesl M, Duskova J, de Reijke TM. Narrow band imaging cystoscopy improves the detection of non-muscle-invasive bladder cancer. Urology. 2010;76(3):658–63.

40. Bryan RT, Billingham LJ, Wallace DM. Narrow-band imaging flexible cystoscopy in the detection of recurrent urothelial cancer of the bladder. BJU Int. 2008;101(6):702–5.

41. Geavlete B, Jecu M, Multescu R, Geavlete P. Narrow-band imaging cystoscopy in non-muscle-invasive bladder cancer: a prospective comparison to the standard approach. Ther Adv Urol. 2012;4(5):211–7.

42. Geavlete B, Multescu R, Georgescu D, Stanescu F, Jecu M, Geavlete P. Narrow band imaging cystoscopy and bipolar plasma vaporization for large nonmuscle-invasive bladder tumors—results of a prospective, randomized comparison to the standard approach. Urology. 2012;79(4):846–51.

43. Herr HW, Donat SM. A comparison of white-light cystoscopy and narrow-band imaging cystoscopy to detect bladder tumour recurrences. BJU Int. 2008;102(9):1111–4.

44. Tatsugami K, Kuroiwa K, Kamoto T, Nishiyama H, Watanabe J, Ishikawa S, Shinohara N, Sazawa A, Fukushima S, Naito S. Evaluation of narrow-band imaging as a complementary method for the detection of bladder cancer. J Endourol. 2010;24(11):1807–11.

45. Zhu YP, Shen YJ, Ye DW, Wang CF, Yao XD, Zhang SL, Dai B, Zhang HL, Shi GH. Narrow-band imaging flexible cystoscopy in the detection of clinically unconfirmed positive urine cytology. Urol Int. 2012;88(1):84–7.

46. Zheng C, Lv Y, Zhong Q, Wang R, Jiang Q. Narrow band imaging diagnosis of bladder cancer: systematic review and meta-analysis. BJU Int. 2012;110(11 Pt B):E680–7.

47. Cauberg EC, Mamoulakis C, de la Rosette JJ, de Reijke TM. Narrow band imaging-assisted transurethral resection for non-muscle invasive bladder cancer significantly reduces residual tumour rate. World J Urol. 2011;29(4):503–9.

48. Herr HW, Donat SM. Reduced bladder tumour recurrence rate associated with narrow-band imaging surveillance cystoscopy. BJU Int. 2011;107(3):396–8.

49. Naselli A, Introini C, Timossi L, Spina B, Fontana V, Pezzi R, Germinale F, Bertolotto F, Puppo P. A randomized prospective trial to assess the impact of transurethral resection in narrow band imaging modality on non-muscle-invasive bladder cancer recurrence. Eur Urol. 2012;61(5):908–13.

50. Tilki D, Burger M, Dalbagni G, Grossman HB, Hakenberg OW, Palou J, Reich O, Roupret M, Shariat SF, Zlotta AR. Urine markers for detection and surveillance of non-muscle-invasive bladder cancer. Eur Urol. 2011;60(3):484–92.

51. Mansoor I, Calam RR, Al-Khafaji B. Role of urinary NMP-22 combined with urine cytology in follow-up surveillance of recurring superficial bladder urothelial carcinoma. Anal Quant Cytol Histol. 2008;30(1):25–32.

52. Sharma S, Zippe CD, Pandrangi L, Nelson D, Agarwal A. Exclusion criteria enhance the specificity and positive predictive value of NMP22 and BTA stat. J Urol. 1999;162(1):53–7.

53. Fradet Y, Lockhard C. Performance characteristics of a new monoclonal antibody test for bladder cancer: ImmunoCyt trade mark. Can J Urol. 1997;4(3):400–5.

54. Feil G, Zumbragel A, Paulgen-Nelde HJ, Hennenlotter J, Maurer S, Krause S, Bichler KH, Stenzl A. Accuracy of the ImmunoCyt assay in the diagnosis of transitional cell carcinoma of the urinary bladder. Anticancer Res. 2003;23(2A):963–7.

55. Mian C, Pycha A, Wiener H, Haitel A, Lodde M, Marberger M. Immunocyt: a new tool for detecting transitional cell cancer of the urinary tract. J Urol. 1999;161(5):1486–9.

56. Olsson H, Zackrisson B. ImmunoCyt a useful method in the follow-up protocol for patients with urinary bladder carcinoma. Scand J Urol Nephrol. 2001;35(4):280–2.

57. Pfister C, Chautard D, Devonec M, Perrin P, Chopin D, Rischmann P, Bouchot O, Beurton D, Coulange C, Rambeaud JJ. Immunocyt test improves the diagnostic accuracy of urinary cytology: results of a French multicenter study. J Urol. 2003;169(3):921–4.

58. Kinders R, Jones T, Root R, Bruce C, Murchison H, Corey M, Williams L, Enfield D, Hass GM. Complement factor H or a related protein is a marker for transitional cell cancer of the bladder. Clin Cancer Res. 1998;4(10):2511–20.

59. Villicana P, Whiting B, Goodison S, Rosser CJ. Urine-based assays for the detection of bladder cancer. Biomark Med. 2009;3(3):265.

60. Quek ML, Sanderson K, Daneshmand S, Stein JP. New molecular markers for bladder cancer detection. Curr Opin Urol. 2004;14(5):259–64.

61. Parker J, Spiess PE. Current and emerging bladder cancer urinary biomarkers. ScientificWorldJournal. 2011;11:1103–12.

62. Sokolova IA, Halling KC, Jenkins RB, Burkhardt HM, Meyer RG, Seelig SA, King W. The development of a multitarget, multicolor fluorescence in situ hybridization assay for the detection of urothelial carcinoma in urine. J Mol Diagn. 2000;2(3):116–23.

63. Hajdinjak T. UroVysion FISH test for detecting urothelial cancers: meta-analysis of diagnostic accuracy and comparison with urinary cytology testing. Urol Oncol. 2008;26(6):646–51.

64. Kipp BR, Karnes RJ, Brankley SM, Harwood AR, Pankratz VS, Sebo TJ, Blute MM, Lieber MM, Zincke H, Halling KC. Monitoring intravesical therapy for superficial bladder cancer using fluorescence in situ hybridization. J Urol. 2005;173(2):401–4.

65. Savic S, Zlobec I, Thalmann GN, Engeler D, Schmauss M, Lehmann K, Mattarelli G, Eichenberger T, Dalquen P, Spieler P, Schoenegg R, Gasser TC, Sulser T, Forster T, Zellweger T, Casella R, Bubendorf L. The prognostic value of cytology and fluorescence in situ hybridization in the follow-up of nonmuscle-invasive bladder cancer after intravesical Bacillus Calmette-Guerin therapy. Int J Cancer. 2009;124(12):2899–904.

66. Whitson J, Berry A, Carroll P, Konety B. A multicolour fluorescence in situ hybridization test predicts recurrence in patients with high-risk superficial bladder tumours undergoing intravesical therapy. BJU Int. 2009;104(3):336–9.

67. Morales A, Eidinger D, Bruce AW. Intracavitary Bacillus Calmette-Guerin in the treatment of superficial bladder tumors. J Urol. 1976;116(2):180–3.

68. Lamm DL, Blumenstein BA, Crissman JD, Montie JE, Gottesman JE, Lowe BA, Sarosdy MF, Bohl RD, Grossman HB, Beck TM, Leimert JT, Crawford ED. Maintenance bacillus Calmette-Guerin immunotherapy for recurrent TA, T1 and carcinoma in situ transitional cell carcinoma of the bladder: a randomized Southwest Oncology Group Study. J Urol. 2000;163(4):1124–9.

69. Bohle A, Jocham D, Bock PR. Intravesical bacillus Calmette-Guerin versus mitomycin C for superficial bladder cancer: a formal meta-analysis of comparative studies on recurrence and toxicity. J Urol. 2003;169(1): 90–5.

70. Han RF, Pan JG. Can intravesical bacillus Calmette-Guerin reduce recurrence in patients with superficial bladder cancer? A meta-analysis of randomized trials. Urology. 2006;67(6):1216–23.

71. Malmstrom PU, Sylvester RJ, Crawford DE, Friedrich M, Krege S, Rintala E, Solsona E, Di Stasi SM, Witjes JA. An individual patient data meta-analysis of the long-term outcome of randomised studies comparing intravesical mitomycin C versus bacillus Calmette-Guerin for non-muscle-invasive bladder cancer. Eur Urol. 2009;56(2):247–56.

72. Shelley MD, Kynaston H, Court J, Wilt TJ, Coles B, Burgon K, Mason MD. A systematic review of intravesical bacillus Calmette-Guerin plus transurethral resection vs transurethral resection alone in Ta and T1 bladder cancer. BJU Int. 2001;88(3):209–16.

73. Shelley MD, Wilt TJ, Court J, Coles B, Kynaston H, Mason MD. Intravesical bacillus Calmette-Guerin is superior to mitomycin C in reducing tumour recurrence in high-risk superficial bladder cancer: a meta-analysis of randomized trials. BJU Int. 2004;93(4): 485–90.

74. Jarvinen R, Kaasinen E, Sankila A, Rintala E. Long-term efficacy of maintenance bacillus Calmette-Guerin versus maintenance mitomycin C instillation therapy in frequently recurrent TaT1 tumours without carcinoma in situ: a subgroup analysis of the prospective, randomised FinnBladder I study with a 20-year follow-up. Eur Urol. 2009;56(2):260–5.

75. Duchek M, Johansson R, Jahnson S, Mestad O, Hellstrom P, Hellsten S, Malmstrom PU. Bacillus Calmette-Guerin is superior to a combination of epirubicin and interferon-alpha2b in the intravesical treatment of patients with stage T1 urinary bladder cancer. A prospective, randomized, Nordic study. Eur Urol. 2010;57(1):25–31.

76. Sylvester RJ, van der MEIJDEN AP, Lamm DL. Intravesical bacillus Calmette-Guerin reduces the

risk of progression in patients with superficial bladder cancer: a meta-analysis of the published results of randomized clinical trials. J Urol. 2002;168(5):1964–70.

77. Zlotta AR, van Vooren JP, Huygen K, Drowart A, Decock M, Pirson M, Jurion F, Palfliet K, Denis O, Simon J, Schulman CC. What is the optimal regimen for BCG intravesical therapy? Are six weekly instillations necessary? Eur Urol. 2000;37(4):470–7.

78. Oddens J, Brausi M, Sylvester R, Bono A, van de Beek C, van AG, Gontero P, Hoeltl W, Turkeri L, Marreaud S, Collette S, Oosterlinck W. Final results of an EORTC-GU cancers group randomized study of maintenance bacillus Calmette-Guerin in intermediate- and high-risk Ta, T1 papillary carcinoma of the urinary bladder: one-third dose versus full dose and 1 year versus 3 years of maintenance. Eur Urol. 2013;63(3):462–72.

79. Herr HW. Restaging transurethral resection of high risk superficial bladder cancer improves the initial response to bacillus Calmette-Guerin therapy. J Urol. 2005;174(6):2134–7.

80. van der MEIJDEN AP, Sylvester RJ, Oosterlinck W, Hoeltl W, Bono AV. Maintenance Bacillus Calmette-Guerin for Ta T1 bladder tumors is not associated with increased toxicity: results from a European Organisation for Research and Treatment of Cancer Genito-Urinary Group Phase III Trial. Eur Urol. 2003;44(4):429–34.

81. Rodriguez F, Palou J, Martinez R, Rodriguez O, Rosales A, Huguet J, Villavicencio H. Practical guideline for the management of adverse events associated with BCG installations. Arch Esp Urol. 2008;61(5): 591–6.

73-year-old woman with multiple, recurrent
high-grade Ta tumors who has received
perioperative mitomycin chemotherapy and
has significant lower urinary tract symptoms

Joseph A. Gillespie and Michael A. O'Donnell

15.1 Clinical Scenario

A 73-year-old woman referred by an outside urologist has multiple, recurrent high-grade Ta tumors and lower urinary tract symptoms (LUTS). Perioperatively, the patient received a single course of mitomycin, but has not received any other intravesical treatments. In the course of this chapter, we will discuss the unique aspects of this patient's disease burden and the clinical options available to the practicing urologist. There are numerous issues that apply broadly to any patient at high risk for recurrence and progression and specifically to this patient, given her age, sex, and concomitant LUTS that could impact care and course. We have divided her care into two distinct phases for conceptual ease.

15.1.1 Phase 1: Diagnosis

The importance of accurate staging and grading are imperative for the proper implementation of treatment. The prototypal transurethral resection

J.A. Gillespie, M.D. • M.A. O'Donnell, M.D. (✉)
Department of Urology, University of Iowa,
200 Hawkins Dr., 3 RCP, Iowa City,
IA 52242-1089, USA
e-mail: joseph-gillespie@uiowa.edu;
michael-odonnell@uiowa.edu

(TUR) assiduously examines the lower urinary tract—including the entirety of the bladder mucosae, as well as the urothelium lining the urethra—and resects all tumors that are detected. A complete resection of a single papillary tumor involves the removal of it in its entirety, the inclusion of the muscle from the tumor bed, and the ablation of a circumference of uninvolved mucosa surrounding the tumor bed. As evidenced by the persistence of tumor as well as significant chance for upstaging during re-resection, the prototypal TUR is not always initially possible. Even in the most facile hands and discerning eye, the technical limitations of the resectoscope and physical limitations inherent to both patient and physician limit the ability of a single TUR to reproducibly grade and stage and to simultaneously identify and eradicate all tumor extent. The need for a re-resection is well established for all patients except those whose diagnosis poses scant risk for progression, such as those with low-grade Ta and small tumor burden, or for those whose diagnosis precludes further endoscopic treatment, as in cases of muscle invasive disease. In all other patients, we recommend a second-look TUR within 4–6 weeks of the initial procedure.

Germane to the patient in this clinical scenario is the multiplicity of her tumors, the possibility that this represents an early recurrence, and the presence of lower urinary tract symptoms

B.R. Konety and S.S. Chang (eds.), *Management of Bladder Cancer:*
A Comprehensive Text With Clinical Scenarios, DOI 10.1007/978-1-4939-1881-2_15,
© Springer Science+Business Media New York 2015

(LUTS). Tumor multiplicity and early recurrence may indicate an inadequate initial TUR and the presence of LUTS may indicate concomitancy of carcinoma in situ. Whether an early recurrence of disease represents disease recurrence or failure of surgical technique is often unknowable. Tumor size and multiplicity are risk factors for early recurrence at re-resection and the presence of residual tumor at re-resection has a high likelihood to be the result of insufficient detection or resection during the initial TUR [1].

There is also concern that this patient has been understaged. This can be the result of failure to include muscle in the biopsy specimens, failure of the pathologist to select a biopsy specimen that has muscle present, or the vagaries of pathological interpretation. Ta disease, disease that is confined to the mucosae and does not penetrate the lamina propria, is the most common form of non-muscle invasive bladder cancer (NMIBC) and represents between half and two-thirds of all cases of NMIBC [2–4]. High-grade Ta disease is, however, a relatively uncommon entity and represents only 6.9 % of all Ta confined disease [4]. Delineating invasion of the lamina propria is difficult and can be further confounded by the vestiges of the TUR. Numerous studies have shown a high degree of inter-pathologist variability with regard to specimen characterization of grade and stage. The likelihood of diagnostic concordance between the local pathologist and a central, specialty trained uropathologist is only 23 % for Ta high-grade disease [5]. A false sense of security should not be imparted by a diagnosis of "superficial" or Ta disease. This patient with high-grade disease, regardless of the stage, is at a higher risk for recurrence and progression compared to a patient with low-grade disease.

Cellular discohesion is a property of both high-grade papillary tumors and carcinoma in situ (CIS). Therefore, urine cytology is insufficient to the task of excluding the presence of CIS until all high-grade papillary tumors have been eradicated. The simultaneous presence of high-grade cells on urine cytology and LUTS should prompt an exhaustive search for CIS. It has been our experience and that of others that the presence of LUTS increases the likelihood of concomitant CIS [6]. It is of particular prognostic significance in this patient as the presence of CIS confers a substantial increase in the risk for progression and cancer-specific death. Utilizing the EORTC risk assessment tables for a patient with multiple, small, high-grade, Ta tumors that received a single instillation of chemotherapy after initial TUR, her risk of progression without CIS is 5 % at 1 year and 17 % at 5 years [7]. The presence of CIS will increase her risk of progression to 17 % at 1 year and 45 % at 5 years. While it is not possible to definitively exclude the presence of CIS in this patient with absolute certainty, a good faith investigation is imperative, given the impact it could have on the future course of her disease and any informed discussion regarding further treatment. To this end, the authors advocate the adjunctive use of fluorescence cystoscopy (FC) and random bladder biopsies for this restaging procedure.

A visual inspection of the bladder may detect the telltale red velvety lesion of CIS at TUR, but the majority of CIS lesions are missed by white light cystoscopy (WLC) [8]. Currently, it is our practice to maximize the detection of CIS by the selective inclusion of random biopsies and FC. The European Association of Urology (EAU) does not routinely recommend random or prostatic biopsies during TUR [9]. Nonetheless, it is our current practice to perform random bladder biopsies in all high-risk patients and, additionally, in male patients we take two biopsies proximal to the verumontanum at the 5 and 7 o'clock positions. Thorstenson et al., in a recent prospective study, showed substantial benefit to patients with high-risk disease with respect to a decrease in recurrence rates, increase in CIS detection and 5-year cancer-specific survival (CSS) [10]. Further studies are needed to validate their findings, but, in general, random bladder biopsies had a tendency to increase the level of treatment in patients with positive findings due to an increased detection of CIS.

FC can further increase the detection of CIS to ~90 % (as opposed to 40 % for WLC) [8]. Currently, no other endoscopic modality has surpassed this, though narrow band imaging appears to be similarly efficacious [11]. In this patient, a second look procedure is crucial before any treatment can be considered. As stated earlier, there is a substantial risk of the patient being understaged. Furthermore, not only is there known persistent disease in this patient, but a reasonable likelihood tumors went undetected during the initial resection. Furthermore, there is a need to re-resect the tumor bed of the lesions that were previously identified and extirpated as this is thought to be a common source of eventual recurrence [12]. A second-look TUR that utilizes FC will increase the capacity of the surgeon to stratify the patient according to the EORTC risk tables by enhancing the detection of CIS, increasing the number of tumors detected, and enhancing the resection of identified tumors. Accurate assessment of the risk of recurrence and progression are imperative for any further discussion of treatment.

15.1.2 Phase 2: Treatment

The natural history of high-grade NMIBC is that of unrelenting progression. Superficial disease (pTa) becomes invasive by transversing the lamina propria (pT1). Metastasis can occur prior to muscle invasion through lymphovascular spread without invasion of the detrusor muscle (pT2) and localized spread (pT3). The tools at the disposal of the urologist are few with regard to bladder preservation. Visible tumor can be extirpated surgically and disease that cannot be seen with the endoscope is treated with intravesical therapy.

In the prior section we have emphasized the TUR as a diagnostic tool and its primacy in obtaining the correct histopathological diagnosis. A transurethral resection of a bladder tumor (TURBT) is, of course, therapeutic as well as diagnostic. A TURBT is an underappreciated art and the importance of a well-performed TURBT cannot be overemphasized. The procedure needs to be systematic and, above all, complete. The surgeon must be diligent and willing to perform numerous staged resections until the bladder is absolutely free of tumor. The eradication of all identifiable tumors is imperative prior to the initiation of intravesical therapy. A hastily performed TURBT cannot be salvaged by chemotherapy or immunotherapy. Conceptually, a TURBT manages endoscopically visible (macroscopic) disease and chemotherapy or immunotherapy microscopic disease. For a patient with high-grade papillary tumors, the effect of perioperative chemotherapy and subsequent immunotherapy is modest relative to a well-performed TUR.

Multiple studies have validated the perioperative use of immediate intravesical therapy chemotherapy [13, 14]. In this patient, the only role for chemotherapy is perioperative. Instillation should occur after every TURBT in which tumor was resected and the suspicion of bladder perforation is low. The use of perioperative chemotherapy bears mentioning for several reasons, in spite of this practice being well established in the literature. In the United States, the rate of perioperative administration rates of chemotherapy after TURBT are abysmally and inexcusably poor [15]. The reason for this is multifaceted and not limited to surgeon negligence. In recent years national shortages of various chemotherapeutics have led to the sporadic unavailability of one and subsequent shortage of another. More often, however, the reasons are more mundane and are usually related to poor communication between support staff and surgeon and the unavailability is one of immediacy rather than actuality. Regardless, it is the surgeon's responsibility to ensure that a chemotherapeutic agent is judiciously and promptly administered after a TURBT, especially in patients that have the greatest potential to benefit from intravesical chemotherapy. And while overall administration rates are low, a recent study calls into question the notion that this is due to indolence or ignorance on the part of the practicing urologist. Rather, they found that in cases where a chemotherapeutic had the greatest potential to positively affect recurrence rates—i.e., the tumor was Ta or T1 and this was the initial resection or a first recurrence—and there was no contraindication for chemotherapeutic administration—i.e., a deep resection—compliance rates were very high (83 %) [15]. We prefer mitomycin C (MMC), given its costs and well established side-effect profile. If this is unavailable, we then proceed to doxorubicin and then epirubicin.

The impact of perioperative chemotherapy upon recurrence and progression in a patient with multiple high-grade Ta tumors is currently unknown. Sylvester et al. performed a meta-analysis and found an absolute decrease in recurrence rates of 11.7 % for NMIBC, including low- and high-grade disease (48.4 % vs. 37.7 %) [16]. Recent studies that have attempted to assess efficacy based upon EAU risk stratification have been underwhelming in demonstrating an effect, but also underpowered for subgroup analysis [17, 18]. It is likely that benefit of perioperative chemotherapy is very modest with respect to recurrence in high-grade disease. As the number of prognostic risk factors for recurrence increase, i.e., tumor size, multiplicity, early recurrence, tumor stage, concomitant CIS, the benefit is likely to asymptotically approach zero. Progression is not affected by the instillation of perioperative chemotherapy. Currently, both the EAU and American Urological Association (AUA) guidelines give tepid support to immediate perioperative chemotherapy for high-risk patients [9, 19]. We advocate the use of perioperative chemotherapy after TURBT for the following reasons. Most intravesical therapies have an absolute benefit that is measured in the single digits. The labor and time required for instillation at the completion of a TURBT is nominal if the drug is ordered in advance. A 1–2 % absolute benefit in reducing recurrence would justify the cost of MMC and doxorubicin relative to a TURBT (doxorubicin is ~$35/dose and MMC is ~$130/dose). Furthermore, at the time of initial resection, tumor grade is often not known. In some forms of low-grade NMIBC, the postoperative instillation of a chemotherapeutic agent may be sufficient for treatment if it is instilled at that time [9].

If a well-performed TURBT is the foundation of bladder conserving therapy for patients with NMIBC, then bacillus Calmette-Guerin (BCG) is the cornerstone for patients with high-grade disease. Both the AUA and EAU recommend BCG for the treatment of patients with a high risk for recurrence and progression [9, 19]. Several recent meta-analyses have attempted to codify the role that BCG can play in the prevention of recurrence and progression in high-grade disease. Han et al. reviewed 25 trials of patients treated with TUR or TUR and BCG for NMIBC and found tumor recurrence in 49.7 % and 40.5 %, respectively [20]. Similar findings have been replicated by multiple other meta-analyses with similar results [21, 22]. With respect to progression, Sylvester et al. reviewed 24 trials involving TUR or TUR and BCG for information on tumor progression [23]. Those treated with TUR alone progressed in 13.8 % of all cases, whereas only 9.8 % progressed when treated with TUR and BCG. Of note, induction alone appears to be insufficient for the prevention of progression. Only studies with maintenance therapy demonstrated an impact upon progression [23, 24].

BCG therapy is the therapy of choice for CIS. Due to the overwhelmingly microscopic nature of the disease—notwithstanding the occasional red velvety lesion—TURBT is insufficient to the task of eradicating CIS. The complete response rate after BCG induction and maintenance therapy is approximately 85 % [17, 25]. BCG has also been shown to decrease the risk of progression relative to other intravesical therapies (12 % progression rate vs. 16 % for chemotherapy) [16].

For BCG therapy to be successful, a substantial commitment is required of both the urologist and patient. The discomfort of intravesical therapy should not be downplayed and the need for a long-term treatment emphasized. Patients should be instructed to expect minor complications and the possibility of significant complications. In our practice, induction begins 2–3 weeks after the second-look TUR and consists of 6 weekly instillations of BCG. Six weeks after completing induction we perform a restaging procedure. In the absence of tumor, the upper tracts are assessed by upper tract washings and bilateral retrograde pyelograms. The lower urinary tract is assessed with bladder washings, random biopsies, and cystoscopy. The visualization of a tumor is considered an early recurrence and BCG treatment failure. A positive urine cytology without apparent tumor is prognostically significant, but it is not an absolute indication of BCG failure. Approximately 50 % of patients with persistence of positive cytology will become complete responders to BCG after maintenance [26].

The ideal maintenance regimen has yet to be defined in the literature. Recent studies have tended to show that for high-grade disease "more is more," i.e., full dose is better than 1/3 dose, 3 years of maintenance results in a more durable response than 1 year [27]. We perform 3 weekly instillations of BCG at 3 and 6 months after the completion of induction. Maintenance instillations continue every 6 months after that, as per SWOG protocol, for a total of 3 years [27]. In conjunction with this demanding treatment protocol, quarterly cystoscopic surveillance is additionally necessary for the direct examination of the bladder for recurrence for a minimum of 2 years [9, 19].

The persistence of tumor or positive urine cytology after the first round of maintenance is always concerning and should prompt a formal evaluation under anesthesia. Any evidence of treatment failure after maintenance results in a restaging procedure with FC as previously described, replete with upper tract (bilateral washing and retrogrades) as well as lower tract (random biopsies and washings) evaluations. Any tumor that is present should be resected. Tumor stage progression while receiving BCG therapy is an indication for cystectomy.

Any initial informed discussion of treatment options in a patient with high-grade NMIBC should include cystectomy. Patients with Ta high-grade disease should not be excluded from this discussion simply because they have been designated to have a more "superficial" disease. As stated earlier, there is significant risk for misdiagnosis in the form of understaging. The timing and stridency with which cystectomy should be counseled is in proportion to the risk of progression and death.

Cystectomy can be performed at three therapeutic intervals: immediate, early, or deferred. Deferred cystectomy—intravesical therapy followed by cystectomy upon progression to muscle invasive disease—should be avoided as it places the patient at undue risk for metastasis and death from disease. Denzinger et al. compared cancer-specific survival (CSS) in 185 consecutive patients at high risk for progression that were offered early cystectomy [28]. All patients had T1G3 disease and at least two of three characteristics that confer an increased risk of progression: multiplicity, tumor greater than 3 cm, or CIS. In total 54 elected for early cystectomy. These were subsequently cross-matched with patients that underwent a delayed cystectomy for recurrence (48 %), CIS (38 %), or progression to muscle invasive disease (34 %). The median time from initial TUR to deferred cystectomy was 11.2 months. The delayed cystectomy patients had a significant decrease in CSS at 10 years relative to the early cystectomy group (78 % vs. 51 %). Notwithstanding the substantial risk of a selection bias in this trial—the deferred cohort all failed bladder conserving therapy—this illustrates the potential risk of delaying treatment.

Immediate cystectomy—cystectomy performed without an inductive course of BCG—represents therapeutic overkill in this patient with one exception: the presence of diffuse CIS that is concomitant with high-grade papillary tumors. Extensive, diffuse CIS has a natural history this is different than focal CIS. Moreover, it represents further advanced and aggressive manifestation of the disease [29]. It is not, however, possible to quantify the risks of secondary diffuse CIS at this time with any accuracy as data in the literature are lacking. What is known is that patients with diffuse CIS are at risk for extravesical extension into the urethra and distal ureters and metastatic disease. The former is important as it complicates future intravesical treatment. The latter, while it is not a standard of care to proceed with immediate cystectomy in this case, a surgeon cannot be faulted for counseling a patient toward this end. Immediate cystectomy should otherwise be reserved for a patient with a strong preference toward cystectomy and an aversion for the rigors of BCG therapy, or in a patient that is a functional bladder cripple.

BCG therapy failure is a harbinger of eventual progression and an indication for early cystectomy. The EAU considers the following BCG treatment failures:

- Progression to muscle invasive disease at any time
- The persistence of high-grade disease after induction
- The persistence, or after initially resolving, reappearance of disease after maintenance therapy
- Stage progression while receiving BCG therapy
- Spontaneous appearance of CIS during BCG therapy

With the exception of progression to muscle invasive disease, none of these are, however, an absolute indication for cystectomy. In our practice we counsel toward early cystectomy in all of these with one exception: the persistence of high-grade disease after induction. As long as the persistence does not represent a worsening of the original diagnosis, i.e., the observed tumor is sub-centimeter and few in number, this patient still has a 50 % chance of achieving a complete response after re-induction or maintenance [26]. Further courses of BCG are not recommended because of the reduced chance of success (<20 %) coupled with the increased likelihood of tumor progression and death [30, 31].

References

1. Jakse G, Algaba F, Malmström PU, Oosterlinck W. A second-look TUR in T1 transitional cell carcinoma: why? Eur Urol. 2004;45:539–46.
2. Larsson P, Wijkström H, Thorstenson A, Adolfsson J, Norming U, Wiklund P, Onelöv E, Steineck G. A population-based study of 538 patients with newly detected urinary bladder neoplasms followed during 5 years. Scand J Urol Nephrol. 2003;37:195–201.
3. Haukaas S, Daehlin L, Maartmann-Moe H, Ulvik NM. The long-term outcome in patients with superficial transitional cell carcinoma of the bladder: a single-institutional experience. BJU Int. 1999;83:957–63.
4. Kikuchi E, Fujimoto H, Mizutani Y, Okajima E, Koga H, Hinotsu S, Shinohara N, Oya M, Miki T, Cancer Registration Committee of the Japanese Urological Association. Clinical outcome of tumor recurrence for Ta, T1 non-muscle invasive bladder cancer from the data on registered bladder cancer patients in Japan: 1999-2001 report from the Japanese Urological Association. Int J Urol. 2009;16:279–86.
5. Sylvester RJ, van der Meijden A, Witjes JA, Jakse G, Nonomura N, Cheng C, Torres A, Watson R, Kurth KH. High-grade Ta urothelial carcinoma and carcinoma in situ of the bladder. Urology. 2005;66:90–107.
6. Ranasinghe W, Persad R. The changing incidence of carcinoma in-situ of the bladder worldwide, advances in the scientific evaluation of bladder cancer and molecular basis for diagnosis and treatment. ISBN: 978-953-51-1142-9, InTech. doi:10.5772/53929. Available from http://www.intechopen.com/books/advances-in-the-scientific-evaluation-of-bladder-cancer-and-molecular-basis-for-diagnosis-and-treatment/the-changing-incidence-of-carcinoma-in-situ-of-the-bladder-worldwide
7. Sylvester RJ, van der Meijden AP, Oosterlinck W, Witjes JA, Bouffioux C, Denis L, Newling DW, Kurth K. Predicting recurrence and progression in individual patients with stage Ta T1 bladder cancer using EORTC risk tables: a combined analysis of 2596 patients from seven EORTC trials. Eur Urol. 2006;49:466–7.
8. Fradet Y, Grossman HB, Gomella L, Lerner S, Cookson M, Albala D, Droller MJ, PC B302/01 Study Group. A comparison of hexaminolevulinate fluorescence cystoscopy and white light cystoscopy for the detection of carcinoma in situ in patients with bladder cancer: a phase III, multicenter study. J Urol. 2007;178:68–73.
9. Babjuk M, Oosterlinck W, Sylvester R, Kaasinen E, Bohle A, Redorta-Palou J, Roupret M. EAU guidelines on nonmuscle-invasive urothelial carcinoma of the bladder, the 2011 update. Eur Urol. 2011;59:997–1008.
10. Thorstenson A, Schumacher M, Wiklund N, Jonsson M, Larsson P, Wijkström H, Onelöv E, Steineck G, De Verdier P. Diagnostic random bladder biopsies: reflections from a population-based cohort of 538 patients. Scand J Urol Nephrol. 2010;44:11–9.
11. Naselli A, Introini C, Timossi L, Spina B, Fontana V, Pezzi R, Germinale F, Bertolotto F, Puppo P. A randomized prospective trial to assess the impact of transurethral resection in narrow band imaging modality on non-muscle-invasive bladder cancer recurrence. Eur Urol. 2012;61:908–13.
12. Koloszy Z. Histopathological "self control" in transurethral resection of bladder tumors. Br J Urol. 1991;67:162–4.
13. Sylvester RJ, Oosterlinck W, van der Meijden AP. A single immediate postoperative instillation of chemotherapy decreases the risk of recurrence in patients with stage Ta T1 bladder cancer: a meta-analysis of published results of randomized clinical trials. J Urol. 2004;171:2186–90.
14. Sylvester RJ, Oosterlinck W, Witjes JA. The schedule and duration of intravesical chemotherapy in patients with non-muscle-invasive bladder cancer: a systematic review of the published results of randomized clinical trials. Eur Urol. 2008;53:709–19.
15. Barocas DA, Liu A, Burks FN, Suh RS, Shuster TG, Bradford T, Moylan, DA, Knapp, PM, Murtagh DS, Morris D, Dunn RL, Montie JE, Miller DC. Practice-base collaboration to imprvoe the use of immediate intravesical therapy after resection for non-muscle-invasive bladder cancer. J Urol. 2013. pii: S0022-5347(13)04620-X. doi:10.1016/j.juro.2013.06.025. [Epub ahead of print].
16. Montgomery JS, Miller DC, Weizer AZ. Quality indicators in the management of bladder cancer. J Natl Compr Canc Netw. 2013;11:492–500.
17. Sylvester RJ, van der MA, Lamm DL. Intravesical bacillus Calmette-Guerin reduces the risk of progression in patients with superficial bladder cancer: a meta-analysis of the published results of randomized clinical trials. J Urol. 2002;168:1964–70.
18. Gudjonsson S, Adell L, Merdasa F, Olsson R, Larsson B, Davidsson T, Richthoff J, Hagberg G, Grabe M, Bendahl PO, Mansson W, Liedberg F. Should all

patients with non-muscle-invasive bladder cancer receive early intravesical chemotherapy after transurethral resection? The results of a prospective randomised multicentre study. Eur Urol. 2009;55:773–80.

19. Kaasinen E, Rintala E, Hellström P, Viitanen J, Juusela H, Rajala P, Korhonen H, Liukkonen T, FinnBladder Group. Factors explaining recurrence in patients undergoing chemoimmunotherapy regimens for frequently recurring superficial bladder carcinoma. Eur Urol. 2002;42:167–74.

20. Hall MC, Chang SS, Dalbagni G, Pruthi RS, Seigne JD, Skinner EC, Wolf Jr JS, Schellhammer PF. Guideline for the management of nonmuscle invasive bladder cancer (stages Ta, T1, and Tis): 2007 update. J Urol. 2007;178:2314–30.

21. Han RF, Pan JG. Can intravesical bacillus Calmette-Guérin reduce recurrence in patients with superficial bladder cancer? A meta-analysis of randomized trials. Urology. 2006;67:1216–23.

22. Shelley MD, Wilt TJ, Court J, Coles B, Kynaston H, Mason MD. Intravesical bacillus Calmette-Guerin is superior to mitomycin C in reducing tumour recurrence in high-risk superficial bladder cancer: a meta-analysis of randomized trials. BJU Int. 2004;93:485–90.

23. Bohle A, Jocham D, Bock PR. Intravesical bacillus Calmette-Guerin versus mitomycin C for superficial bladder cancer: a formal meta-analysis of comparative studies on recurrence and toxicity. J Urol. 2003;169:90–5.

24. Shelley MD, Kynaston H, Court J, Wilt TJ, Coles B, Burgon K, Mason MD. A systematic review of intravesical bacillus lmette-Guerin plus transurethral resection vs transurethral resection alone in Ta and T1 bladder cancer. BJU Int. 2001;88:209–16.

25. Jakse G, Hall R, Bono A, Höltl W, Carpentier P, Spaander JP, van der Meijden AP, Sylvester R. Intravesical BCG in patients with carcinoma in situ of the urinary bladder: long-term results of EORTC GU Group phase II protocol 30861. Eur Urol. 2001;40:144–50.

26. Takenaka A, Yamada Y, Miyake H, Hara I, Fujisawa M. Clinical outcomes of bacillus Calmette-Guerin instillation therapy for carcinoma in situ of urinary bladder. Int J Urol. 2008;15:309–13.

27. Lamm D, Herr H, Jakse G, Kuroda M, Mostofi FK, Okajima E, Sakamoto A, Sesterhenn I, da Silva FC. Updated concepts and treatment of carcinoma in situ. Urol Oncol. 1998;4:130–8.

28. Denzinger S, Fritsche H, Otto W, Blana A, Wieland W, Burger M. Early versus deferred cystectomy for initial high-risk pT1G3 urothelial carcinoma of the bladder: do risk factors define feasibility of bladder-sparing approach? Eur Urol. 2008;53:146–52.

29. Oddens J, Brausi M, Sylvester R, Bono A, Beek C, Ande GL, Gontero P, Hoeltl W, Turkeri L, Marreaud S, Collette S, Oosterlinck W. Final results of an EORTC-GU cancers group randomized study of maintenance bacillus Calmette-Guérin in intermediate- and high-risk Ta, T1 papillary carcinoma of the urinary bladder: one-third dose versus full dose and 1 year versus 3 years of maintenance. Eur Urol. 2013;63:462–72.

30. Lamm DL, Blumenstein BA, Crissman JD, Montie JE, Gottesman JE, Lowe BA, Sarosdy MF, Bohl RD, Grossman HB, Beck TM, Leimert JT, Crawford ED. Maintenance bacillus Calmette-Guérin immunotherapy for recurrent TA, T1 and carcinoma in situ transitional cell carcinoma of the bladder: a randomized Southwest Oncology Group Study. J Urol. 2000;163:1124–9.

31. Catalona WJ, Hudson MA, Gillen DP, Andriole GL, Ratliff TL. Risks and benefits of repeated courses of intravesical bacillus Calmette-Guerin therapy for superficial bladder cancer. J Urol. 1987;137:220–4.

A 68-Year-old man with rapidly recurring multiple, low-grade, papillary Ta tumors despite perioperative mitomycin and one induction course of BCG

James S. Rosoff and Thomas E. Keane

16.1 Introduction

An estimated 72,570 cases of bladder cancer will be diagnosed in the US in 2013 [1]. Although the vast majority of the 15,210 bladder cancer deaths will be attributed to advanced cases, non-muscle-invasive bladder cancer (NMIBC) and its management can result in significant morbidity and cost to the healthcare system [2].

Approximately 70 % of newly diagnosed cases of bladder cancer are non-muscle-invasive disease, and approximately 70 % of these are classified as Ta disease (confined to the urothelium) [3]. The majority of Ta tumors are low-grade (82–97 % with an average of 93 %) [4], while low-grade Ta lesions represent approximately 20 % of all non-muscle-invasive bladder cancers. Low-grade Ta tumors recur in 50–70 % of cases and carry a 5–10 % risk of progression to invasive disease and a 1–5 % risk of death [5].

Transurethral resection (TUR) is the standard treatment for clinical Ta, low-grade tumors. Although TUR alone can completely remove these lesions, they have a high risk for recurrence. The patient in this clinical scenario is at very high risk for recurrence based on the following factors: presence of multiple tumors, large tumor volume, and a short time to recurrence (with an assumed recurrence at 3-month cystoscopy).

16.2 Intravesical Therapy

It has been shown that the risk of recurrence for NMIBC is reduced from 48 % without chemotherapy to 37 % when intravesical chemotherapy is given within 24 h of TUR [6]. This technique was initially described in the 1970s using thiotepa in the immediate postoperative period [7, 8]. Although a randomized trial of 247 patients published by the British Medical Research Council [9] showed no advantage to intravesical thiotepa, other small trials [10, 11] showed a benefit to thiotepa (possibly because a higher dose was used in those trials).

In 1981, Abrams et al. demonstrated a decrease in the number of recurrences following TUR for patients treated with intravesical doxorubicin compared to placebo [12]. Other agents, such as epirubicin [13, 14] and ethoglucid [15, 16], were also shown to reduce the recurrence rate.

J.S. Rosoff, M.D. (✉)
Department of Urology, Yale School of Medicine,
789 Howard Avenue, FMP 312, New Haven,
CT 06519, USA
e-mail: james.rosoff@yale.edu

T.E. Keane, M.B., Ch.B., F.R.C.S.I., F.A.C.S.
Department of Urology, Medical University
of South Carolina, 96 Jonathan Lucas Street,
MSC 620 – HE644CSB, Charleston, SC 29424, USA

B.R. Konety and S.S. Chang (eds.), *Management of Bladder Cancer:*
A Comprehensive Text With Clinical Scenarios, DOI 10.1007/978-1-4939-1881-2_16,
© Springer Science+Business Media New York 2015

In 1996, Lamm and Torti reviewed the existing randomized prospective trials comparing intravesical chemotherapy to TUR alone. These studies included over 1,000 patients each for thiotepa, doxorubicin, and mitomycin. The net benefit on the short-term recurrence rate was 12, 13, and 15 %, respectively [17].

A 2004 meta-analysis comprising 1,476 patients in seven randomized trials (including the negative thiotepa study above) demonstrated a reduction in the recurrence rate from 48.4 to 36.7 % with the administration of a single immediate dose of intravesical chemotherapy. This analysis also included studies investigating epirubicin (44 % of the patient total), mitomycin C (29 %), and pirarubicin (11 %). The authors also found that although patients with multiple tumors benefited from a single dose of intravesical therapy, they also eventually recurred at a much higher rate than those with a single tumor (65 % vs. 36 %) [6]. However, in a multicenter randomized trial involving 502 patients, Tolley et al. demonstrated a benefit for intravesical mitomycin C irrespective of the recurrence risk category (low, intermediate or high risk for recurrence) [18]. In an earlier analysis of the same data, this group also demonstrated a benefit to mitomycin C maintenance therapy, with a significantly decreased 2-year recurrence rate in the group receiving multiple instillations as compared to those receiving a single post-resection dose [19].

The issue of improved efficacy with longer intravesical chemotherapy treatment schedules is addressed by a meta-analysis published in 2000 by Huncharek et al. [20]. This study encompassed over 3,700 patients from 11 randomized trials and produced several important findings. First, the authors showed a much larger reduction in the overall 1-year recurrence rate (44 %) than had been shown in the single-dose studies above. Using sensitivity analyses, the authors determined that this difference was at least partially attributed to dosing schedule and treatment duration. For example, in a subset analysis of 575 patients treated on 2-year protocols, the reduction in recurrence was 73 %. A subsequent meta-analysis by the same group showed a similar decrease in the recurrence rate for patients treated with post-resection intravesical chemotherapy as compared to those treated with TUR alone [21]. However, the sensitivity analysis in this study demonstrated that the differences in treatment efficacy were due to choice of intravesical agent, with doxorubicin being less effective than the other agents. Another meta-analysis published in 2008 by Sylvester et al. attempted to determine the optimal schedule and duration of intravesical chemotherapy. The authors concluded that these parameters could not be determined based on the available data [22]. In a randomized trial investigating methods to improve the efficacy of intravesical mitomycin, Au et al. showed that strategies to alkalinize the urine and increase the concentration of the drug in the bladder resulted in a significant increase in the time to recurrence and a higher recurrence-free percentage at 5 years [23].

16.3 BCG Versus Mitomycin C

BCG is generally not used for the primary treatment of low-grade Ta bladder cancer. However, it has been investigated as second-line therapy and in patients at high recurrence risk. A multicenter randomized trial comparing short-term BCG, short-term mitomycin, and long-term mitomycin did not demonstrate an advantage of BCG over mitomycin in the short-term arms. However, the authors showed a significantly decreased 3-year recurrence rate for the long term-mitomycin arm (13.9 %) as compared to the short-term BCG arm (34.5 %) and the short-term mitomycin arm (31.4 %) [24]. In a 2003 meta-analysis, BCG was shown to be superior to mitomycin for those patients at high risk of recurrence [25]. Another meta-analysis published by Bohle et al. found similar results. The authors demonstrated a significantly reduced recurrence rate for the BCG group compared to the mitomycin group (38.6 % vs. 46.4 %) [26]. Both studies, however, showed a higher rate of local and systemic toxicity in the BCG-treated arms. Furthermore, it has been shown that the apparent advantage of BCG over mitomycin becomes negligible in the subset of patients with only papillary tumors [27]. Nevertheless, it would be reasonable to attempt treatment with BCG as a second-line agent after failure of intravesical chemotherapy.

16.4 Other Intravesical Agents

Several other intravesical chemotherapeutic agents have been investigated. Gemcitabine demonstrated increased efficacy and decreased toxicity when compared to mitomycin in a phase III randomized trial [28]. Other studies demonstrated the efficacy of gemcitabine in BCG-refractory disease, with a 47 % complete response rate at 3 months [29]. However, the durability at 1 and 2 years was limited (28 and 21 %, respectively). Docetaxel has also shown promise in the setting of BCG-refractory NMIBC [30]. In a study of 54 patients treated with intravesical docetaxel, Barlow et al. demonstrated a complete initial response in 59 % of patients. Adding maintenance therapy increased the median time to recurrence from 19 to 39 months [31]. A phase I study of 18 patients with BCG-refractory NMIBC treated with intravesical nanoparticle albumin-bound paclitaxel demonstrated a complete initial response in 28 % of patients [32]. Further studies with this and other agents are ongoing.

16.5 Active Surveillance

Since these low-grade noninvasive tumors are less likely to undergo progression of stage or grade, some urologists have advocated an active surveillance protocol with regular office cystoscopy and fulguration of tumors as needed [33]. Our patient is not an ideal candidate for this as he has a high volume of disease, but if we could clear his bladder of all visible tumors, it might be reasonable to treat any small recurrences in the office. This would avoid exposing him to the risks of repeated TURs while diminishing the overall cost to the healthcare system [34].

16.6 Radical Cystectomy

There is very limited published information on the role of cystectomy in this clinical situation. Nevertheless, cystectomy is warranted if low-grade disease progresses to refractory high-grade NMIBC or in the rare case of progression to muscle-invasive disease. Less clear, however, is the role of cystectomy in the case of rapidly recurrent disease or inability to completely resect all tumors. Amling et al. reported on a single-institution series of 531 patients who underwent radical cystectomy for urothelial carcinoma [35]. A total of 31 patients (5.8 %) underwent radical cystectomy for Ta disease that was high-grade, recalcitrant to TUR, and/or resistant to chemotherapy. Although we do not have numbers on the specific indication for cystectomy in this group, the 5- and 10-year cancer-specific survival rates were 88 and 75 %, demonstrating that death from bladder cancer does indeed occur in this subset of patients. Therefore, this suggests that cystectomy is a reasonable option for patients with Ta disease that falls into one of the above categories. In a study of 699 patients with low-grade Ta disease, 17 (2.4 %) died of bladder cancer, including 13 of 14 with progression to muscle invasion and 4 of 19 with progression to high-grade NMIBC [36]. The authors found that resected tumor weight (a surrogate for tumor volume) was associated with tumor recurrence and disease-specific mortality. Ultimately, six patients in the entire cohort underwent cystectomy (<1 %), but five of those six died of metastatic urothelial carcinoma and only one was disease-free at follow-up. Although it was only five patients, it is concerning that those individuals died of what was initially diagnosed as low-grade Ta disease. The authors conclude that current surveillance regimens are inadequate for detecting disease progression in a manner that will alter the natural history of the disease.

Low-grade invasive disease has been described though it is a rare entity. In a series of 41 cases of invasive low-grade T1 urothelial carcinoma described by Toll and Epstein, 10 of 29 evaluable patients (34 %) developed a recurrence [37]. Of those ten patients, three underwent cystectomy and two were alive without evidence disease at the time of last follow-up. Due to the small sample size and limited follow-up, the authors were unable to draw any conclusions about the prognosis of this entity. Still, it is important to consider this lesion in the setting of our clinical scenario.

In our experience, we have performed radical cystectomy due to inability to resect all tumors after three or four attempts at complete TUR. As for disease that has failed intravesical therapy, we have generally performed cystectomy after failure of a total of three cycles of induction intravesical therapy (often with two different agents). Nevertheless, the decision to proceed to cystectomy is largely dependent on other clinical variables. Although there are limited data on the role of radical surgery for unresectable low-grade Ta bladder cancer or low-grade Ta disease that does not respond to intravesical therapy, we must still consider cystectomy in these scenarios.

16.7   Conclusions

Thus, for this patient we would recommend TUR with complete resection of all visible lesions, followed by immediate intravesical treatment with mitomycin C and then an induction course of mitomycin C (6 weekly instillations) beginning 4 weeks after the initial resection. We would then follow this with office surveillance (and fulguration of any small recurrences) beginning at 3 months post-TUR. As for surveillance of the upper tracts, we would not recommend any imaging after the initial upper tract evaluation, as long as the grade and stage of the tumors remained the same. If the patient responded to the induction course of intravesical chemotherapy, we would recommend an extended course of intravesical therapy (monthly instillations for up to 3 years). If unable to obtain a durable response (> 3 months), we would then give a different intravesical agent—in this case BCG. If that were to fail and the patient was unwilling or unable to undergo continued resections, we would then consider radical cystectomy.

References

1. Siegel R, Naishadham D, Jemal A. Cancer statistics, 2013. CA Cancer J Clin. 2013;63(1):11–30. PubMed PMID: 23335087.
2. Avritscher EB, Cooksley CD, Grossman HB, Sabichi AL, Hamblin L, Dinney CP, et al. Clinical model of lifetime cost of treating bladder cancer and associated complications. Urology. 2006;68(3):549–53. PubMed PMID: 16979735.
3. Ro JY, Staerkel GA, Ayala AG. Cytologic and histologic features of superficial bladder cancer. Urol Clin North Am. 1992;19(3):435–53. PubMed PMID: 1636229.
4. Sylvester RJ, van der Meijden A, Witjes JA, Jakse G, Nonomura N, Cheng C, et al. High-grade Ta urothelial carcinoma and carcinoma in situ of the bladder. Urology. 2005;66(6 Suppl 1):90–107. PubMed PMID: 16399418.
5. Donat SM. Evaluation and follow-up strategies for superficial bladder cancer. Urol Clin North Am. 2003;30(4):765–76. PubMed PMID: 14680313.
6. Sylvester RJ, Oosterlinck W, van der Meijden AP. A single immediate postoperative instillation of chemotherapy decreases the risk of recurrence in patients with stage Ta T1 bladder cancer: a meta-analysis of published results of randomized clinical trials. J Urol. 2004;171(6 Pt 1):2186–90. quiz 435, PubMed PMID: 15126782.
7. Burnand KG, Boyd PJ, Mayo ME, Shuttleworth KE, Lloyd-Davies RW. Single dose intravesical thiotepa as an adjuvant to cystodiathermy in the treatment of transitional cell bladder carcinoma. Br J Urol. 1976;48(1):55–9. PubMed PMID: 817761.
8. Gavrell GJ, Lewis RW, Meehan WL, Leblanc GA. Intravesical thio-tepa in the immediate postoperative period in patients with recurrent transitional cell carcinoma of the bladder. J Urol. 1978;120(4):410–1. PubMed PMID: 100615.
9. The effect of intravesical thiotepa on the recurrence rate of newly diagnosed superficial bladder cancer. An MRC Study. MRC Working Party on Urological Cancer. Br J Urol. 1985;57(6):680–5. PubMed PMID: 2867800.
10. Zincke H, Benson Jr RC, Hilton JF, Taylor WF. Intravesical thiotepa and mitomycin C treatment immediately after transurethral resection and later for superficial (stages Ta and Tis) bladder cancer: a prospective, randomized, stratified study with crossover design. J Urol. 1985;134(6):1110–4. PubMed PMID: 3932685.
11. Zincke H, Utz DC, Taylor WF, Myers RP, Leary FJ. Influence of thiotepa and doxorubicin instillation at time of transurethral surgical treatment of bladder cancer on tumor recurrence: a prospective, randomized, double-blind, controlled trial. J Urol. 1983;129(3):505–9. PubMed PMID: 6403716.
12. Abrams PH, Choa RG, Gaches CG, Ashken MH, Green NA. A controlled trial of single dose intravesical adriamycin in superficial bladder tumours. Br J Urol. 1981;53(6):585–7. PubMed PMID: 7032640.
13. van der Meijden AP, Kurth KH, Oosterlinck W, Debruyne FM. Intravesical therapy with adriamycin and 4-epirubicin for superficial bladder cancer: the experience of the EORTC GU Group. Cancer Chemother Pharmacol. 1992;30(Suppl):S95–8. PubMed PMID: 1394828.
14. Oosterlinck W, Kurth KH, Schroder F, Sylvester R, Hammond B. A plea for cold biopsy, fulguration and immediate bladder instillation with Epirubicin in small superficial bladder tumors. Data from the EORTC GU Group Study 30863. Eur Urol. 1993;23(4):457–9.

15. Kurth KH, Debruyne FJ, Senge T, Carpentier PJ, Riedl H, Sylvester R, et al. Adjuvant chemotherapy of superficial transitional cell carcinoma: an E.O.R.T.C. randomized trail comparing doxorubicin hydrochloride, ethoglucid and TUR-alone. Progr Clin Biol. 1985;185B:135–42. PubMed PMID: 3898138.

16. Kurth KH, Schroder FH, Tunn U, Ay R, Pavone-Macaluso M, Debruyne F, et al. Adjuvant chemotherapy of superficial transitional cell bladder carcinoma: preliminary results of a European organization for research on treatment of cancer. Randomized trial comparing doxorubicin hydrochloride, ethoglucid and transurethral resection alone. J Urol. 1984;132(2):258–62.

17. Lamm DL, Torti FM. Bladder cancer, 1996. CA Cancer J Clin. 1996;46(2):93–112. PubMed PMID: 8624800.

18. Tolley DA, Parmar MK, Grigor KM, Lallemand G, Benyon LL, Fellows J, et al. The effect of intravesical mitomycin C on recurrence of newly diagnosed superficial bladder cancer: a further report with 7 years of follow up. J Urol. 1996;155(4):1233–8. PubMed PMID: 8632538.

19. Tolley DA, Hargreave TB, Smith PH, Williams JL, Grigor KM, Parmar MK, et al. Effect of intravesical mitomycin C on recurrence of newly diagnosed superficial bladder cancer: interim report from the Medical Research Council Subgroup on Superficial Bladder Cancer (Urological Cancer Working Party). Br Med J. 1988;296(6639):1759–61. PubMed PMID: 3136828, Pubmed Central PMCID: 2546235.

20. Huncharek M, Geschwind JF, Witherspoon B, McGarry R, Adcock D. Intravesical chemotherapy prophylaxis in primary superficial bladder cancer: a meta-analysis of 3703 patients from 11 randomized trials. J Clin Epidemiol. 2000;53(7):676–80. PubMed PMID: 10941943.

21. Huncharek M, McGarry R, Kupelnick B. Impact of intravesical chemotherapy on recurrence rate of recurrent superficial transitional cell carcinoma of the bladder: results of a meta-analysis. Anticancer Res. 2001;21(1B):765–9. PubMed PMID: 11299841.

22. Sylvester RJ, Oosterlinck W, Witjes JA. The schedule and duration of intravesical chemotherapy in patients with non-muscle-invasive bladder cancer: a systematic review of the published results of randomized clinical trials. Eur Urol. 2008;53(4):709–19. PubMed PMID: 18207317, Pubmed Central PMCID: 2587437.

23. Au JL, Badalament RA, Wientjes MG, Young DC, Warner JA, Venema PL, et al. Methods to improve efficacy of intravesical mitomycin C: results of a randomized phase III trial. J Natl Cancer Inst. 2001;93(8):597–604. PubMed PMID: 11309436.

24. Friedrich MG, Pichlmeier U, Schwaibold H, Conrad S, Huland H. Long-term intravesical adjuvant chemotherapy further reduces recurrence rate compared with short-term intravesical chemotherapy and short-term therapy with Bacillus Calmette-Guerin (BCG) in patients with non-muscle-invasive bladder carcinoma. Eur Urol. 2007;52(4):1123–9. PubMed PMID: 17383080.

25. Shelley MD, Court JB, Kynaston H, Wilt TJ, Coles B, Mason M. Intravesical bacillus Calmette-Guerin versus mitomycin C for Ta and T1 bladder cancer. Cochrane Database Syst Rev. 2003;3, CD003231. PubMed PMID: 12917955.

26. Bohle A, Jocham D, Bock PR. Intravesical bacillus Calmette-Guerin versus mitomycin C for superficial bladder cancer: a formal meta-analysis of comparative studies on recurrence and toxicity. J Urol. 2003;169(1):90–5. PubMed PMID: 12478111.

27. Malmstrom PU, Wijkstrom H, Lundholm C, Wester K, Busch C, Norlen BJ. 5-Year followup of a randomized prospective study comparing mitomycin C and bacillus Calmette-Guerin in patients with superficial bladder carcinoma. Swedish-Norwegian Bladder Cancer Study Group. J Urol. 1999;161(4):1124–7. PubMed PMID: 10081852.

28. Addeo R, Caraglia M, Bellini S, Abbruzzese A, Vincenzi B, Montella L, et al. Randomized phase III trial on gemcitabine versus mytomicin in recurrent superficial bladder cancer: evaluation of efficacy and tolerance. J Clin Oncol. 2010;28(4):543–8. PubMed PMID: 19841330.

29. Skinner EC, Goldman B, Sakr WA, Petrylak DP, Lenz HJ, Lee CT, et al. SWOG S0353: phase II trial of intravesical gemcitabine in patients with nonmuscle invasive bladder cancer who had recurrence after at least 2 prior courses of intravesical bacillus Calmette-Guerin. J Urol. 2013;15. PubMed PMID: 23597452.

30. Barlow L, McKiernan J, Sawczuk I, Benson M. A single-institution experience with induction and maintenance intravesical docetaxel in the management of non-muscle-invasive bladder cancer refractory to bacille Calmette-Guerin therapy. BJU Int. 2009;104(8):1098–102. PubMed PMID: 19389012.

31. Barlow L, McKiernan JM, Benson MC. Long-term survival outcomes with intravesical docetaxel for recurrent nonmuscle invasive bladder cancer after previous bacillus Calmette-Guerin therapy. J Urol. 2013;189(3):834–9. PubMed PMID: 23123371.

32. McKiernan JM, Barlow LJ, Laudano MA, Mann MJ, Petrylak DP, Benson MC. A phase I trial of intravesical nanoparticle albumin-bound paclitaxel in the treatment of bacillus Calmette-Guerin refractory non-muscle invasive bladder cancer. J Urol. 2011;186(2):448–51. PubMed PMID: 21680003.

33. Hernandez V, Alvarez M, de la Pena E, Amaruch N, Martin MD, de la Morena JM, et al. Safety of active surveillance program for recurrent nonmuscle-invasive bladder carcinoma. Urology. 2009;73(6):1306–10. PubMed PMID: 19375783.

34. Tiu A, Jenkins LC, Soloway MS. Active surveillance for low-risk bladder cancer. Urol Oncol. 2013;18. PubMed PMID: 23518309.

35. Amling CL, Thrasher JB, Frazier HA, Dodge RK, Robertson JE, Paulson DF. Radical cystectomy for

stages Ta, Tis and T1 transitional cell carcinoma of the bladder. J Urol. 1994;151(1):31–5. discussion 5–6, PubMed PMID: 8254828.

36. Linton KD, Rosario DJ, Thomas F, Rubin N, Goepel JR, Abbod MF, et al. Disease specific mortality in patients with low risk bladder cancer and the impact of cystoscopic surveillance. J Urol. 2013;189(3):828–33. PubMed PMID: 23017513.

37. Toll AD, Epstein JI. Invasive low-grade papillary urothelial carcinoma: a clinicopathologic analysis of 41 cases. Am J Surg Pathol. 2012;36(7):1081–6. PubMed PMID: 22510761.

A 72-Year-old woman with a 3 cm low-grade
T1 tumor located in the bladder dome and
without muscle present in the resected
specimen

J. Alfred Witjes and Florine W.M. Schlatmann

Abbreviations

5-ALA	5-Aminolevulinic acid
AUA	American Association of Urology
BCG	Bacillus Calmette-Guérin
CIS	Carcinoma in situ
EAU	European Association of Urology
EORTC	European Organization for Research and Treatment of Cancer
FC	Fluorescence cystoscopy
HG	High grade
MMC	Mitomycin C
NMIBC	Non-muscle-invasive bladder cancer
SPI	Single postoperative instillation

17.1 Confirming the Diagnosis and Identifying Prognostic Factors

The initial diagnosis is puzzling. Some aspects suggest a good prognosis; some aspects suggest trouble.

J.A. Witjes, M.D., Ph.D. (✉)
F.W.M. Schlatmann, M.D.
Department of Urology, Radboud University
Nijmegen Medical Centre, P.O. Box 9101,
Nijmegen 6500 HB, The Netherlands
e-mail: fred.witjes@radboudumc.nl

Age has not been studied frequently as risk factor for outcome in non-muscle-invasive bladder cancer (NMIBC). Two relatively recent studies specifically looked at outcome after bacillus Calmette-Guérin (BCG) instillation therapy and examined the impact of age. Joudi et al. found a significant difference in response to BCG between patients 61–70 years old versus those older than 80, 61 % versus 39 % cancer-free survival after a median follow-up of 24 months ($p=0.0002$) [1]. On a multivariate analysis, age was an independent risk factor for response to BCG.

Herr reported on 805 patients treated with BCG with multiple or recurrent high-grade NMIBC including carcinoma in situ (CIS) [2]. The first response to BCG and 2-year cancer-free survival were similar between age groups, but after 5 years 27 % of patients older than 70 years were cancer-free compared to 37 % younger than 70 years ($p=0.005$). A possible explanation for this impaired tumor response at older age is that BCG requires a competent immune system that may be less at an older age.

A recent study also found age to be a prognostic factor for recurrence after transurethral resection of a bladder tumor (TURBT) with BCG but also without BCG therapy [3]. For recurrence, age was found to be a continuous variable, with a significant worse outcome above the age of 80 (adjusted hazard ratio of 2.25, $p<0.001$). The

B.R. Konety and S.S. Chang (eds.), *Management of Bladder Cancer:*
A Comprehensive Text With Clinical Scenarios, DOI 10.1007/978-1-4939-1881-2_17,
© Springer Science+Business Media New York 2015

same study also reported more significant chance for progression, but this was restricted to patients treated with BCG and older than 80 years of age (adjusted hazard ratio of 2.8, $p=0.02$). In all, on multivariate analyses, age was an independent risk factor for recurrence and progression. Shariat et al. came to a similar conclusion in a recent review of studies published between 1966 and 2009 [4]. They hypothesized, however, that older patients face several barriers to receive appropriate treatment, resulting in less and less aggressive treatment and subtherapeutic dosing that obviously might be an additional factor for a worse outcome [4]. In summary, the age of 72 in this patient has a negative impact on her treatment outcome, although this impact would appear to be limited.

Gender, on the other hand, is a clear prognostic factor. Especially in invasive bladder cancer, women appear to present with higher stage disease, but even when corrected for initial stage and grade, their prognosis appears to be worse [5, 6]. Noon et al. reported recently on a group of more than 3,200 bladder cancer patients, and found an increased cancer-specific mortality at 5 years for women as compared to men (32 % vs. 22 %, $p<0.01$) in the high-risk NMIBC group, which they defined as high grade and/or T1 and/or CIS [6]. There was no difference in low-risk NMIBC. There are potential explanations for these differences. Women might be exposed to carcinogens differently than men (smoking, chemicals). In some countries women might have less access to health care. Since women more than men are oftentimes accustomed to bladder symptoms due to urinary tract infections they might seek help later in case of, for example, hematuria. Women do not have to strain with voiding, so from an anatomical point of view they usually have a thinner bladder wall as compared to men, with subsequent earlier muscle invasion and metastasis. Finally, hormones (estrogens) might play a role in tumor development and progression. Apart from a later presentation and worse prognosis, women also seem to be undertreated as compared to men with similar stage and grade [6].

Size as criterion would appear to be objective and simple: the bigger the tumor the worse the prognosis. Indeed several studies have found size to be of prognostic value. The European Organization for Research and Treatment of Cancer (EORTC) published their prognostic model for recurrence and progression in 2006 [7]. Size was described as <1 cm, between 1 and 3 cm and >3 cm. In the multivariate model the cutoff of 3 cm appeared of prognostic value for recurrence (hazard ratio 1.34, $p<0.0001$) and progression (hazard ratio 1.94, $p<0.0001$). This size cut off has since been used in the European Association of Urology (EAU) guideline as prognostic factor. The American Association of Urology (AUA) guideline discriminates between low volume (their index patient 2, a low-risk patient) and large volume (their index patient 3, intermediate-risk) tumors [8]. Unfortunately, the volume criteria are not further specified. Finally, a recent large multicenter retrospective study by Gontero et al. looking at prognostic factors in >2,500 T1G3 patients, also confirmed size (cut off 3 cm) as an independent prognostic factor for recurrence, progression, and even overall survival [9]. Gontero et al. used size together with age and the presence of CIS to predict tumor progression.

However, size estimation is not always easy. In small tumors usually the size of the resection loop is used as comparator, as it is typically done in marker lesion studies in NMIBC [10]. Multiple tumors, or, as in this clinical scenario, larger tumors might pose a problem. In those cases estimation of size during cystoscopy is difficult. Measurement with ultrasound or CT scan might be an alternative, but the majority of patients presenting with presumably non-invasive tumors will not undergo imaging before their TURBT. An alternative might be to take the resected tumor weight as surrogate for size. This has recently been described by Kwon et al. [11]. For recurrence, neither tumor size (cut off 3 cm) nor tumor weight (cut off 2 g, measured without the tumor base) were significant factors in a multivariate analysis. However, for progression of NMIBC, weight (hazard ratio 4.0, $p=0.018$) and grade (hazard ratio 2.6, $p=0.001$) were the two only significant prognostic factors in their multivariate analysis. In spite of the limitations of weight in case of an incomplete resection or resection of a large tumor base, this appears more objective and reproducible than size. In summary, the size of the described tumor, with the limitations of size measurement, suggests a negative impact on the disease outcome of the patient in this clinical scenario.

The major problem in our view is the combination of low grade and T1. In the first place both grading and staging are subject to substantial variability [12]. Several studies addressing review pathology have shown that the reproducibility of grade is between 42 and 70 %, and of stage between 60 and 91 % for Ta and 38 and 77 % for T1. The overall conformity of stage and grade ranges between 51 and 62 %, which actually is not that much better than a flip of a coin.

What can be the reasons for this disconcordance? Usually a local pathologist and a reviewing pathologist are looking at different slides that might reflect different parts of the tumor ("review" pathology typically is done on "three unstained slides"). Furthermore, the reviewing pathologist might not be the gold standard, since even expert urologic pathologists have a high inter- and intra-individual variation. Van Rhijn et al. for example, had 173 NMIBC tumor slides reviewed twice by four uro-pathologists [13]. For the 2004 and 1973 WHO grading, the agreement between the four pathologists was 39–74 and 39–64 %, respectively. The intra-observer agreement was better and varied from 71 to 88 %. Although the 2004 grading system has improved reproducibility of grading to a certain extent, the reproducibility still is far from 100 %.

Another recent study by May et al. confirmed that the 2004 grading system has less inter-observer variability, although the 1973 classification might be better to identify aggressive (grade 3) tumors. They also confirmed that even when separating indolent from aggressive urothelial cancers, striking pathologist-dependent differences are apparent [14]. Their explanation was that the criteria used to grade are complex and subjective, and they highlight the need for more objective (molecular) markers, since otherwise histo-morphology remains to have significant limitations.

A second concern with the diagnosis of a low-grade T1 bladder cancer is that many doubt whether this exists. Examining pathology review series in NMIBC, the number of grade 1, T1 tumors appears to be minimal to zero. In a review, for example, of three phase III fluorescence cystoscopy studies, 631 tumors and biopsies were reviewed by a local and a review pathologist, none of the 11 pT1G1 tumors as judged by a local pathologist was confirmed to be pT1G1 by the review pathologist. The review pathologist, in its turn, did not reclassify any tumor as pT1G1 [12]. This clinical scenario, however, deals with a low-grade T1 tumor, not a grade 1 T1 tumor. Since more than half of old grade 2 tumors are now classified as low-grade tumors [14], obviously low-grade pT1 tumors will be diagnosed and will exist, but its frequency, for example in our practice, is low. Apart from all these study data, the concept of a low-grade tumor that has the ability to invade seems contradictory.

Proceeding with our 72-year-old female patient, the next aspect to consider is the tumor location. The prognostic value of location of a tumor in the bladder has been addressed, but most series do not consider this an important factor. If there are any locations with worse prognostic importance it might be the bladder neck or the lateral and posterior bladder walls [15].

What could be important for this particular location of the bladder tumor is the technical aspect of the TURBT. Complete resection of tumors in the dome may be more difficult, and the risk of a bladder perforation seems increased. However, larger studies in literature have reported that tumor location is not a predisposing factor for perforation [16]. Still, we are not surprised that the resection was not deep enough in the sense that detrusor muscle was not present. The location may contribute to this, and in addition, as most urologists will know from daily practice the bladder wall thickness is less in females than in males. This has been described for young healthy adults between 15 and 40 years of age [17]. Also taking into consideration an increasing detrusor wall thickness in males with increasing age and outflow obstruction, the difference in bladder wall thickness between men and women at older age is not only significant but also relevant for a resection. As a consequence, a bladder wall perforation during TURBT is more frequently seen in females. Herkommer et al. confirmed this in their study on 1,284 patients undergoing a TURBT [18]. They found 49 bladder perforations, which were seen more frequently in females (7.2 % vs. 2.6 %, $p<0.001$) and with increasing tumor size/weight (2.4 % when the size was <2.5 cm, versus 9.2 % when the tumor was >2.5 cm, $p=0.003$). Perforations were less frequent in obese patients (5.5 % when the BMI was <25 vs. 0.6 % when the BMI was >35, $p=0.016$), and this finding is also most probably a result of a thicker bladder wall in obese patients. The final prognostic factor was tumor stage (non-invasive vs. invasive). In conclusion, it is not totally surprising that the initial resection in this 72-year-old woman was not complete.

However, does this automatically mean that we should recommend a re-resection? Considering the controversial diagnosis of a low-grade T1 tumor, we recommend a second opinion in regards to pathology evaluation be performed. In case the stage is Ta, and the overall diagnosis is low-grade Ta, a re-TURBT is not necessary. In that case, additional therapy could and should have been a single postoperative instillation (SPI) with chemotherapy according to guidelines [8, 19]. We assume that this has not been done in this case scenario. The alternative would now be to treat this patient with a course of chemotherapy or even BCG. Although this is done, especially in the US [20], this would seem to be overtreatment. We would advise, instead counseled observation with surveillance cystoscopy after 3 months.

If, however, the reviewed pathology is read as a high-grade Ta tumor, re-TURBT can be considered. The European guideline indeed advocates re-TURBT in all high-grade tumors, whereas the American guideline currently advises re-TURBT in patients with lamina propria invasion (pT1) but without muscle in the specimen [8, 19]. It is obvious that a review confirmation of any T1 tumor without detrusor muscle necessitates a re-TURBT. Although there is no consensus about strategy and timing of a re-TURBT, most authors recommend an interval of 2–6 weeks after the initial TURBT, and the re-TURBT should include resection of the primary tumor site [19].

Are there any means of improving the yield of this re-TURBT? The combination of re-TURBT with random biopsies has been reported in several studies. In an EORTC analysis, the chance of finding abnormalities with random biopsies in patients with low-risk tumors was 4.4 % (1.5 % for CIS) and with intermediate- and high-risk tumors was 11.6 % (3.5 % for CIS) [21]. This study and other studies came to the conclusion that random biopsies of normal looking mucosa do not impact on the prognosis or treatment of the patient [21, 22]. Based on these studies the European guideline indeed states that in patients with papillary non-muscle-invasive bladder tumors, mapping or random biopsies are not routinely recommended [19]. In the American guideline this is not explicitly discussed [8].

A second way to improve the accuracy of staging may be the use of one of the different methods to improve cystoscopic evaluation during TURBT. It is well recognized that the use of fluorescence cystoscopy (FC) helps to improve the detection of bladder tumors, a more complete resection of those tumors and a subsequent lower short- and long-term recurrence rate [23]. However, this is during initial resection of tumors. The value of FC on subsequent resections, especially after bladder manipulation like intravesical BCG of a recent TURBT, is less well documented. Inflammatory reactive changes in the bladder (e.g. infection, tissue repair) also cause photosensitizers to accumulate in these regions that in turn produce false-positive fluorescence. A recent expert panel meeting recognized this limitation, but still considered that the better tumor identification and subsequent better diagnosis and treatment outweighed the (minimally) increased false-positive rate [24]. More specifically the interval after BCG has been studied. Draga et al. reported on 552 procedures and 1,874 biopsies from the bladder with 5-aminolevulinic acid (5-ALA) after BCG or mitomycin C (MMC) [25]. As expected, inflammation (OR 1.53), leukocyturia (OR 1.84), and false-positive FC (OR 1.49) were more common after intravesical BCG. They advised to wait 3 months after BCG, at which time point the bladder situation has returned to normal. Of note, intavesical MMC had no effect on the performance of FC. Our personal experience suggests that the period of an increased FP rate after a resection seems shorter than after BCG intravesical therapy, thus suggesting that a period of around 6 weeks, our normal period to wait for a re-TURBT, might be a good tradeoff between a potentially higher false-positive rate with FC, the added value of FC, and a not too long period for a re-TURBT.

17.2 Additional Therapy

As mentioned above, in case of a low-grade solitary Ta tumor after pathology review, we would not do a re-TURBT and observe this patient. Ideally she would have received a SPI. A course of additional intravesical chemotherapy or BCG would seem overtreatment to us, and a cystoscopy in 3 months would be planned. For further decision making the outcome of this 3 months cystoscopy is important, since a recurrence at 3 months implies a higher risk of future recurrences and obviously a new resection and additional intravesical therapy is warranted.

All other results of the review pathology automatically results in at least a T1 tumor and/or a high-grade tumor. This implies a high-risk situation, and one might consider this a case for BCG treatment anyway.

However, a re-TURBT would certainly be helpful to identify residual tumor, to ensure the resection is complete, to identify associated CIS, and/or even to detect muscle invasive disease. In our institution, the re-TURBT would be performed approximately 6 weeks after the initial operation. We would also use FC to have optimal information about the bladder situation, since this was not used initially, in spite of a higher chance of a false-positive biopsy result. The "worst" pathology result of the initial TURBT and the re-TURBT should be used to decide the therapy choice. For example, if the pathology review of the initial sample reveals a high-grade (HG) T1 tumor, and the re-resection comes out negative including a negative deep biopsy con-

taining detrusor muscle, therapy should be based on the diagnosis of a pT1HG bladder tumor.

In the scenario of identified and resected residual tumor, but no CIS or invasive disease on additional pathology, the final classification remains a high-risk NMIBC in this patient. In such a case, both the European and American guidelines advise induction and maintenance BCG [8, 19]. The most recent EORTC study has demonstrated that in high-risk patients full-dose BCG given for a period of 3 years produces the best cancer outcomes [26]. Results with lower BCG doses or shorter treatment regimens are worse, although only the 1 year schedule with 1/3 dose regimen resulted in a significantly lower recurrence-free survival after 5 years of 54.5 % as compared to 64.2 % with 3 years and full-dose BCG. Side-effect profile in all arms was similar. This last observation is surprising. In our experience dose reduction from full dose to 1/3 dose certainly decreases side effects in some patients. Therefore, this would be our first step in patients with side effects that potentially limit optimal intravesical BCG treatment.

In the second scenario, confirming high-risk papillary non-muscle-invasive disease, but with associated CIS, the prognosis becomes worse. Clearly, this is the highest risk category in NMIBC, as is also recognized and classified for the first time in the latest 2013 EAU guideline [27]. As this 2013 EAU guideline recommends, in these patients cystectomy should be considered. Considering here additional negative risk factors as described above, namely gender and tumor size, we would indeed certainly discuss radical treatment with this patient. As is reported recently, delay of adequate therapy and tumor progression means a significant worsening of the prognosis, with a 3-year cancer-specific mortality after progression of 65 % [28]. In case the decision would be to stay conservative initially, BCG induction and maintenance therapy as described in the previous scenario is the treatment of choice, but follow-up should be very strict.

In the last scenario, muscle invasive disease, obviously further staging should be done and cystectomy should be advised as is clearly recommended in both the European and American guidelines [8, 19].

In summary, this clinical scenario of a 72-year-old woman with a 3 cm low-grade T1 bladder tumor located in the dome, in which the resection revealed no detrusor muscle, is an interesting one. We would certainly advise review of the pathology result, since a low-grade T1 tumor seldom occurs. If the review of the pathology reveals a low-grade Ta tumor, we would advise further follow-up and not an immediate course of chemotherapy or BCG. However, if a T1 and/or a high-grade tumor is found, a re-resection is mandatory, which we would do with fluorescence cystoscopy. The result of the re-resection, together with the other negative prognostic factors (gender and tumor size) will dictate further therapy that ranges from induction and planned maintenance BCG to radical cystectomy.

References

1. Joudi FN, Smith BJ, O'Donnell MA, Konety BR. The impact of age on the response of patients with superficial bladder cancer to intravesical immunotherapy. J Urol. 2006;175(5):1634–9.
2. Herr HW. Age and outcome of superficial bladder cancer treated with bacille CalmetteGuérin therapy. Urology. 2007;70(1):65–8.
3. Kohjimoto Y, Iba A, Shintani Y, Inagaki T, Uekado Y, Hara I. Impact of patient age on outcome following bladder-preserving treatment for non-muscle-invasive bladder cancer. World J Urol. 2010;28(4):425–30.
4. Shariat SF, Sfakianos JP, Droller MJ, Karakiewicz PI, Meryn S, Bochner BH. The effect of age and gender on bladder cancer: a critical review of the literature. BJU Int. 2009;105(3):300–8.
5. Mungan NA, Aben KKH, Schoenberg MP, Visser O, Coebergh JWW, Witjes JA, Kiemeney LALM. Gender differences in stage-adjusted bladder cancer survival. Urology. 2000;55(6):876–80.
6. Noon AP, Albertsen PC, Thoams F, Rosario DJ, Catto JWF. Competing mortality in patients diagnosed with bladder cancer: evidence of undertreatment in the elderly and female patients. Br J Cancer. 2013;108(7): 1534–40.
7. Sylvester RJ, van der Meijden APM, Oosterlinck W, Witjes JA, Bouffioux C, Denis L, Newling DWW, Kurth KH. Predicting recurrence and progression in individual patients with stage Ta T1 bladder cancer using EORTC risk tables: a combined analysis of 2596 patients from 7 EORTC trials. Eur Urol. 2006;49(3):466–77.
8. Hall MC, Chang SS, Dalbagni G, Pruthi RS, Seigne JD, Skinner EC, Wolf Jr JS, Schellhammer PF. Guideline for the management of nonmuscle invasive bladder cancer (stages Ta, T1, and Tis): 2007 update. J Urol. 2007;178(6):2314–30.
9. Gontero P, Sylvester R, Pisano F, Joniau S, Van der Eeckt K, Serretta V, Larrè S, di Stasi S, Van Rhijn B, Witjes JA, Grotenhuis A, Colombo R, Briganti A, Babjuk M, Soukup V, Malmstrom PU, Irani J, Malats N, Baniel J, Cai T, Cha E, Ardelt P, Varkarakis J, Bartoletti R, Spahn M, Palou J, Dalbagni G, Shariat S, Karnes J. Prognostic factors and risk groups in T1G3 patients initially treated with BCG: results of a multicenter retrospective series. AUA 2013 abstract 1697.
10. Hendricksen K, van der Heijden AG, Cornel EB, Vergunst H, de Reijke TM, van Boven E, Smits GA, Puri R, Gruijs S, Witjes JA. Two-year follow-up of the phase II marker lesion study of intravesical apaziquone for patients with non-muscle invasive bladder cancer. World J Urol. 2009;27(3):337–42.
11. Kwon DH, Song PH, Kim HT. Multivariate analysis of the prognostic significance of resection weight after transurethral resection of bladder tumor for NMIBC. Korean J Urol. 2012;53(7):457–62.
12. Witjes JA, Moonen PMJ, van der Heijden AG. Review pathology in superficial bladder cancer trial: the impact of patient risk category. Urology. 2006;67(4):751–5.
13. van Rhijn BWG, van Leenders GJLH, Ooms BCM, Kirkels WJ, Zlotta AR, Boevé ER, Jöbsis AC, van der Kwast TH. The pathologist's mean grade is constant and individualizes the prognostic value of bladder cancer grading. Eur Urol. 2010;57(6):1052–7.
14. May M, Brookman-Amissah S, Roigas J, Hartmann A, Störkel S, Kristiansen G, Gilfrich C, Borchardt R, Hoschke B, Kaufmann O, Gunia S. Prognostic accuracy of individual uropathologists in noninvasive urinary bladder carcinoma: a multicentre study comparing the 1973 and 2004 World Health Organisation Classifications. Eur Urol. 2010;57(5):850–8.
15. Vukomanovic I, Colovic V, Soldatovic I, Hadzi-Djokic J. Prognostic significance of tumor location in high-grade non-muscle-invasive bladder cancer. Med Oncol. 2012;29(3):1916–20.
16. Collado A, Chéchile GE, Salvador J, Vicente J. Early complications of endoscopic treatment for superficial bladder cancer. J Urol. 2000;164(5):1529–32.
17. Oelke M, Höfner K, Jonas U, Ubbink D, de la Rosette J, Wijkstra H. Ultrasound measurement of the detrusor wall thickness in healthy adults. Neurourol Urodyn. 2006;25(4):308–17.
18. Herkommer K, Hofer C, Gschwend JE, Kron M, Treiber U. Gender and body mass index as risk factors for bladder perforation during primary transurethral resection of bladder tumors. J Urol. 2012;187(5):1566–70.
19. Babjuk M, Oosterlinck W, Sylvester R, Kaasinen E, Böhle A, Palou-Redorta J, Rouprêt M. EAU guidelines on non-muscle-invasive urothelial carcinoma of the bladder, the 2011 update. Eur Urol. 2011;59(6): 997–1008.
20. Witjes JA, Palou J, Soloway M, Lamm D, Kamat AM, Brausi M, Persad R, Buckley R, Colombel M, Böhle A. Current clinical practice gaps in the treatment of

intermediate- and high-risk non-muscle-invasive bladder cancer (NMIBC) with emphasis on the use of bacillus Calmette-Guérin (BCG): results of an international individual patient data survey (IPDS). BJU Int. Forthcoming 2013.

21. van der Meijden A, Oosterlinck W, Brausi M, Kurth KH, Sylvester R, de Balincourt C. Significance of bladder biopsies in Ta, T1 bladder tumors: a report from the EORTC Genito-Urinary Tract Cancer Cooperative Group EORTC-GU Group Superficial Bladder Committee. Eur Urol. 1999;35(4):267–71.

22. Kiemeney LA, Witjes JA, Heijbroek RP, Koper NP, Verbeek AL, Debruyne FM. Should random urothelial biopsies be taken from patients with primary superficial bladder cancer? A decision analysis. Members of the Dutch South-East Co-Operative Urological Group. Br J Urol. 1994;73(2):164–71.

23. Burger M, Grossman HB, Droller M, Schmidbauer J, Hermann G, Drăgoescu O, Ray E, Fradet Y, Karl A, Burgués JP, Witjes JA, Stenzl A, Jichlinski P, Jocham D. Photodynamic diagnosis of non-muscle-invasive bladder cancer with hexaminolevulinate cystoscopy: a meta-analysis of detection and recurrence based on raw data. Eur Urol. Forthcoming 2013.

24. Witjes JA, Redorta JP, Jacqmin D, Sofras F, Malmström PU, Riedl C, Jocham D, Conti G, Montorsi F, Arentsen HC, Zaak D, Mostafid AH, Babjuk M. Hexaminolevulinate-guided fluorescence cystoscopy in the diagnosis and follow-up of patients with non-muscle-invasive bladder cancer: review of the evidence and recommendations. Eur Urol. 2010;57(4):607–14.

25. Draga RO, Grimbergen MC, Kok ET, Jonges TN, van Swol CF, Bosch JL. Photodynamic diagnosis (5-aminolevulinic acid) of transitional cell carcinoma after bacillus Calmette-Guérin immunotherapy and mitomycin C intravesical therapy. Eur Urol. 2010;57(4):655–60.

26. Oddens J, Brausi M, Sylvester R, Bono A, van de Beek C, van Andel G, Gontero P, Hoeltl W, Turkeri L, Marreaud S, Collette S, Oosterlinck W. Final results of an EORTC-GU cancers group randomized study of maintenance bacillus Calmette-Guérin in intermediate- and high-risk Ta, T1 papillary carcinoma of the urinary bladder: one-third dose versus full dose and 1 year versus 3 years of maintenance. Eur Urol. 2013;63(3):462–72.

27. Babjuk M, Burger M, Zigeuner R, Shariat S, van Rhijn B, Comperat E, Sylvester R, Kaasinen E, Böhle A, Palou J, Roupret M. Guidelines on Non-muscle-invasive bladder cancer (TaT1 and CIS). EAU Guidelines 2013, presented at the EAU Annual Congress 2013. Arnhem, The Netherlands: European Association of Urology; 2013. Available from http://www.uroweb.org/gls/pdf/05_TaT1_Bladder_Cancer_LR.pdf.

28. van den Bosch S, Witjes JA. Long-term cancer specific survival in patients with high-risk non muscle-invasive bladder cancer and tumour progression: a systematic review. Eur Urol. 2011;60(3):493–500.

Jennifer J. Ahn and James M. McKiernan

18.1 Introduction

Bladder cancer is the fourth most commonly diagnosed cancer in the United States (US), with an estimated 72,570 new cases and 15,210 deaths in 2013 [1]. Roughly 70–80 % of patients will first present with non-muscle invasive bladder cancer (NMIBC), and undergo local removal, or transurethral resection of bladder tumor (TURBT) as initial therapy. TURBT can be curative, however tumors recur up to 70 % of the time, and can progress in up to 40 % of patients, necessitating radical treatment [2]. Intravesical therapy serves as an adjunct to TURBT, providing local therapy while minimizing systemic toxicity, ultimately reducing disease recurrence and progression rates. Chemotherapy and immunotherapy are the two primary forms of intravesical therapy, and

J.J. Ahn, M.D.
Department of Urology, New York-Presbyterian Hospital, Columbia University, New York, NY, USA

Department of Urology, Columbia University Medical Center, Herbert Irving Pavilion, 11th Floor, 161 Fort Washington Avenue, New York, NY 10032, USA
e-mail: jja2130@columbia.edu

J.M. McKiernan, M.D. (✉)
Department of Urology, Columbia University Medical Center, Herbert Irving Pavilion, 11th Floor, 161 Fort Washington Avenue, New York, NY 10032, USA
e-mail: jmm23@columbia.edu

each has its own risks and benefits. The European Association of Urology (EAU) and American Urological Association (AUA) guidelines for NMIBC treatment are similar (Table 18.1), yet they do not provide specific details of agents, dosage, and schedules, as existing evidence regarding efficacy is variable. In this review, general principles, current agents, indications for use, and future directions will be discussed.

18.2 General Principles of Intravesical Therapy

The bladder has unique properties that lend itself to local drug administration. First, access to the bladder is easily obtained via the urethra. In addition, the urothelium serves as a barrier between the urine and the bloodstream, minimizing systemic absorption and potential toxicity. The urothelial umbrella cells are an essential component of this barrier, as they maintain their tight junctions while the bladder fills and empties. The overlying hydrophilic glycosaminoglycan (GAG) layer and plaques also serve as an additional level of protection [3]. While these unique characteristics make the bladder ideal for local therapy, ensuring drug delivery at therapeutic levels is more complex.

Factors inherent to medications that influence absorption into the urothelium include pKa, molecular weight, and lipophilicity. The urothelial

B.R. Konety and S.S. Chang (eds.), *Management of Bladder Cancer:*
A Comprehensive Text With Clinical Scenarios, DOI 10.1007/978-1-4939-1881-2_18,
© Springer Science+Business Media New York 2015

Table 18.1 AUA and EAU Guidelines on intravesical therapy [9, 10]

Risk category	AUA guidelines (2010)	EAU guidelines (2012)
Low	• TURBT • One immediate postoperative chemotherapy instillation	• TURBT • One immediate postoperative chemotherapy instillation

Intermediate	• TURBT
	• Induction BCG or MMC
	• Maintenance BCG or MMC
		• TURBT
		• One immediate postoperative chemotherapy instillation PLUS:
		  – Chemotherapy, or
		  – BCG for minimum of 1 year

High	• TURBT
	• Induction BCG + maintenance, or
	• Cystectomy
		• TURBT
		• One immediate postoperative chemotherapy instillation PLUS:
		  – Chemotherapy, or
		  – BCG for minimum of 1 year, or
		• Cystectomy

Table 18.2 Bladder properties affecting intravesical drug absorption

	Property of urothelium	Parameters for intravesical drugs
Ionization Constant (pKa)	• Ionized molecules cannot pass through lipid bilayer or protein channels	• Drugs should be highly ionized at pH of 6–7
Molecular Weight (MW)	• Protein channels are ~10 Å which is comparable to MW of 200	• Drugs should have a molecular weight >200 kDa
Partition Coefficient (p)	• Urothelium has higher water content than typical cell membrane	• Drugs should have $\log P$ from: • −0.4 to −1.2 or • −7.5 to −8.0

lipid bilayer prevents diffusion of ionized molecules, while protein channels of ~10 Å allow for transport of smaller molecules. Thus, the ionization constant (pKa), partition coefficient (measure of lipophilicity), and molecular size are important characteristics of potential intravesical drugs (Table 18.2).

Mishina and colleagues established that intravesical drugs should (1) have a $\log P$ (partition coefficient) between −0.4 and −1.2 or −7.5 and −8.0, 2) have a molecular weight >200 kDa, and (3) be highly non-ionized at a pH of 6–7 [4]. This maximizes uptake into the urothelium, while avoiding systemic absorption. Additionally, they concluded that mitomycin c (MMC) was the best medication available at that time, based upon the above criteria, but was still not the optimal anticancer drug.

Patient characteristics also impact intravesical drug delivery, including urine volume and hydration status, urine pH, and the integrity of the bladder wall [5]. Au and colleagues have developed models assessing multiple parameters to maximize drug delivery, and have shown that optimizing MMC delivery yields improvement in recurrence-free survival versus conventional administration [6]. Current approaches to improving drug delivery include altering membrane permeability with hyperthermia, electric current, or chemical enhancement, designing drug formulations that enhance urothelial uptake, such as liposomes or nanoparticles, and utilizing gene therapy to target molecular pathways. Each of these will be discussed in further detail in the context of the respective therapeutic agents.

While intravesical therapy is ideal for providing local treatment, it is not without adverse effects. Typical local toxicity includes dysuria, hematuria, and cystitis, but is usually well-tolerated and treatable. Systemic absorption is rare, but can cause significant toxicity such as myelosuppression [7]. General principles to minimize local and systemic toxicity are as follows: avoid treatment in the setting of an active urinary tract infection (UTI), gross hematuria, and traumatic catheterization. It is also imperative that the urothelium is intact, and thus one should allow for adequate healing after TUR, typically 2–4 weeks. Other patient factors that may delay wound healing include prior pelvic radiotherapy, diabetes mellitus, poor nutritional status, and steroid use. Specific contraindications and adverse effects will be discussed as applicable with each individual agent.

18.3 Chemotherapy

18.3.1 Postoperative Instillation

Intravesical administration of chemotherapy was first reported in 1955 [8] and despite consistent use since then, the ideal drugs and optimal conditions for efficacy are still under active investigation. Current AUA and EAU guidelines recommend administration of some form of intravesical therapy for low-, intermediate-, and high-risk NMIBC. Immediate postoperative instillation of intravesical chemotherapy has been shown to reduce tumor recurrence with a variety of agents, and is now routinely recommended by the EAU for all cases of NMIBC, and by the AUA for suspected low-risk disease [9, 10]. The proposed mechanism is that the chemotherapeutic agent destroys any residual tumor or circulating tumor cells released after TURBT, thereby preventing tumor cell implantation and reducing tumor recurrence. However, this theoretical mechanism of action has not been proven in any definitive matter. In a comprehensive meta-analysis which included 1,476 patients [11], Sylvester et al. found that a single instillation of postoperative intravesical chemotherapy reduced tumor recurrence from 48.4 % (TURBT alone) to 36.7 % (TURBT + chemotherapy) at a median follow-up of 3.4 years ($p < 0.0001$). The majority of included patients had a single tumor on primary presentation, making it less applicable to those with multiple, recurrent tumors, though the subset analysis of patients with multiple tumors

did show a trend toward reduction in recurrence, from 81.5 % (TURBT) to 65.2 % (TURBT + chemotherapy), $p = 0.06$. The analyzed trials used various agents, including thiotepa, epirubicin, MMC, and pirarubicin. Thiotepa was found to be inferior to the other three agents, while the latter three were found to be equivalent.

While immediate postoperative intravesical chemotherapy instillation is recommended, it is, in reality, given infrequently. A SEER-Medicare analysis found a perioperative MMC instillation rate of <6 % prior to 2011 [12], despite level 1 evidence supporting its role in decreasing recurrence rates. The primary contraindication to giving postoperative intravesical therapy is suspected bladder perforation. Unfortunately, single postoperative instillation of chemotherapy has not been shown to impact progression or survival. But side effects are generally transient in the absence of perforation, and the subsequent reduction in recurrence prevents future TURBTs and associated anesthesia and hospitalization costs, making it a recommended standard of care for patients with urothelial cancer.

18.3.2 Adjuvant/Maintenance Treatment

After transurethral biopsy results become available, the decision of whether or not to give adjuvant intravesical treatment arises. Current AUA and EAU guidelines recommend no further adjuvant therapy for those with low-risk disease, but advocate for intravesical bacillus Calmette-Guerin (BCG) or chemotherapy for those with intermediate-risk disease, while those at high risk for progression should also receive induction BCG with maintenance therapy. Recommendations for adjuvant chemotherapy stem from several trials showing a significant reduction in recurrence compared with TURBT alone, though progression and survival are not affected, similar to single postoperative instillations [13]. Several different chemotherapy agents have been utilized in the adjuvant setting and with maintenance, and many have been compared to BCG. Unfortunately, these studies often include heterogeneous patient populations, dosing

Table 18.3 Properties of intravesical agents

Agent	Mechanism of action	Molecular weight (kDa)	Dose
Mitomycin C	Alkylating agent—cross-links DNA, inhibits DNA synthesis	334	20–60 mg
Thiotepa	Alkylating agent—cross-links DNA, inhibits DNA synthesis	189	30–60 mg
Doxorubicin Epirubicin	Anthracyclines—inhibit nucleic acid synthesis and topoisomerase II	579	20–50 mg
Valrubicin	Semisynthetic anthracycline—inhibits nucleic acid synthesis and topoisomerase II	720	800 mg
Gemcitabine	Nucleoside analog—inhibits DNA synthesis	299	2,000 mg
Docetaxel	Microtubule stabilizer—inhibits mitosis and induces apoptosis	808	75 mg
Paclitaxel	Microtubule stabilizer—inhibits mitosis and induces apoptosis	854	500–600 mg
Apaziquone	Synthetic pro-drug of MMC (alkylating agent)	288	4 mg
BCG	Stimulates immune response via TH1 pathway	N/A	40–120 mg (depends on strain)
Interferon-α2b	Stimulates immune response via TH1 pathway	N/A	50 million units
Mycobacterial cell wall-DNA complex (MCC)	Mycobacterial cell wall stimulates immune response without live vaccine	N/A	8 mg

amounts and schedules, complicating interpretation. For the intermediate-risk group, no agent is currently recommended highly over another, as each has various potential risks and benefits, while BCG is superior for high-risk patients. Relevant evidence for each agent will be shown below (Table 18.3).

18.3.3 Mitomycin C

Mitomycin C (MMC) is the most widely studied and commonly used intravesical chemotherapy, with roles in the perioperative, adjuvant, and BCG failure settings. It is an alkylating agent which causes DNA cross-linking, strand breakage, and ultimately inhibition of synthesis. A randomized Medical Research Council (MRC) study compared TURBT with postoperative MMC to TURBT alone, administering 40 mg in 40 ml water for a dwell time of 1 h, within 24 h of TURBT. At a median follow-up of 7 years, MMC reduced recurrence by 34 % ($p=0.010$) across all risk groups, though progression and survival were not affected [14]. Further studies support early postoperative administration, as MMC given on the same day as TURBT reduced recurrence by a HR 2.2 (1.49–3.25, $p<0.001$), compared with waiting for ≥1 day after TURBT [15]. Immediate postoperative MMC typically has minimal toxicity, though if perforation is suspected, administration is contraindicated. Delayed healing of TURBT sites may also occur even after a single dose and this can lead to prolonged mitomycin-induced dystrophic calcifications. However, in most cases of NMIBC, immediate postoperative MMC is indicated as it is safe and reduces recurrence rates.

For adjuvant therapy, 20–60 mg of MMC is typically given for a course of 4–8 weeks. Randomized trials utilizing varying doses (20–60 mg), schedules (weekly to monthly), and duration of therapy (≤3 years) have yielded a wide range of recurrence rates (17–68 %), making it difficult to establish the ideal dosage and schedule for adjuvant MMC therapy [16]. With regards to efficacy, in one meta-analysis, chemotherapy reduced recurrence rates 21–82 % more than BCG, when stratified for studies that treated chemotherapy-naïve patients [17]. However, when including previously treated patients, there was no significant difference in recurrence. Further meta-analyses addressing progression rates found no significant difference between BCG and chemotherapy/MMC overall [18]. However, in studies adding BCG maintenance, progression rates were decreased compared to adjuvant MMC (OR = 0.66, 95 % CI 0.47–0.94; p = 0.02), suggesting superiority of BCG [19]. A recent report of 10-year results from a randomized study comparing BCG to MMC (both with maintenance therapy) found no difference in progression or overall survival, contradicting prior meta-analyses [20].

While BCG with maintenance may be superior to MMC in reducing recurrence and progression rates, MMC is still a reasonable adjuvant treatment option in intermediate-risk disease, as it has an improved side effect profile in certain studies. One meta-analysis showed cystitis rates of 54 % (BCG) vs. 39 % (MMC), p < 0.001, though discontinuation rates due to toxicity were not significantly different [21]. In addition, MMC (MW 334 kDa) does not carry the risk of systemic toxicity that BCG does. There are, however, potential complications of adjuvant MMC therapy including irritative voiding symptoms, bladder contraction, contact dermatitis, and dystrophic calcification at prior TURBT sites. These can occur commonly but are not life-threatening, but can be serious.

Given MMC's ability to reduce recurrence in the perioperative and adjuvant setting, efforts have been geared toward maximizing its efficacy. Au and colleagues illustrated that administering 40 mg MMC in 20 ml water (rather than 40 ml), restricting fluids, and alkalinizing urine with sodium bicarbonate provided the lowest recurrence rates in a randomized trial [6]. Another optimization strategy is that of thermochemotherapy (TCT) technology, which utilizes local microwave current to improve drug penetration, while also providing a direct cytotoxic effect. A recent meta-analysis determined that use of TCT-MMC in the adjuvant setting reduced the recurrence rate by 59 % versus standard MMC [22], while a trial of 83 patients showed a 10-year disease-free survival rate of 53 % (TCT-MMC)

versus 15 % (MMC), p < 0.001 [23]. Common adverse events of TCT therapy include bladder spasms (22 %) and bladder pain (18 %), lower urinary tract symptoms (LUTS) (26 %), and hematuria (6 %). A unique side effect is that of a posterior wall thermal reaction, a discolored area seen on cystoscopy with surrounding hyperemia, presumably from contact with the catheter device which provides the microwave current.

Electromotive drug administration (EMDA) provides electric current, thereby enhancing urothelial membrane permeability and drug transport. In a randomized trial, this technique resulted in decreased recurrence rates compared to MMC alone, and similar to those of BCG [24]. EMDA MMC has also been studied in the preoperative setting, given 30 min prior to TURBT, and showed significantly increased time to recurrence (52 months) compared to immediate postoperative instillation (16 months) and TUR alone (12 months, log-rank p < 0.0001) [25]. BCG + EMDA-MMC sequential therapy has also shown superiority over BCG alone, with improved recurrence (42 % vs. 58 %, p = 0.001), progression (9 % vs. 22 %, p = 0.005), and cancer-specific death rates (6 % vs. 16 %, p = 0.01) [26]. Toxicity was similar across all three groups (21–26 % of patients reporting local side effects). Both TCT and EMDA assistance have shown promising results, and should be evaluated further to determine the optimal timing, dosage, and ideal patient populations. In addition, further investigation is needed to determine their effects on progression or survival.

18.3.4 Thiotepa

Use of intravesical thiotepa was first reported in 1961, but is not commonly used currently due to its toxicity profile and low efficacy. It is an alkylating agent which has been used to treat different malignancies, but a randomized trial by the MRC showed no improvement in recurrence with one perioperative dose or maintenance therapy, as compared to TURBT alone [27]. In addition, thiotepa has a low molecular weight (189 kDa), allowing for systemic absorption, and unacceptable rates of toxicity such as myelosuppression, making it virtually obsolete in the current era [2].

18.3.5 Anthracyclines: Doxorubicin, Epirubicin, Valrubicin

Anthracyclines are a class of chemotherapeutic agents commonly used throughout oncology. They serve as intercalating agents, thereby blocking DNA and RNA synthesis, and as inhibitors of topoisomerase II, preventing transcription and DNA repair mechanisms. Doxorubicin, epirubicin, pirarubicin, and valrubicin have all been used intravesically with minimal systemic side effects, given their high MW (579–724 kDa). When compared to BCG, doxorubicin and epirubicin display higher rates of recurrence in most trials [16]. Long-term follow-up of EORTC 30911, comparing epirubicin, BCG, and BCG plus isoniazid for intermediate- and high-risk patients, showed that any BCG therapy decreased recurrence, distant metastases, and cancer-specific death rates, though not progression [28]. As a result, anthracyclines are not frequently used in the adjuvant setting.

Evidence is strongest for immediate postoperative instillation of anthracyclines over TURBT alone. Administration of 80 mg epirubicin in 50 ml saline within 24 h after TURBT reduced recurrence from 77 % (TURBT alone) to 62 % (TURBT + epirubicin), $p=0.016$, in a multicenter randomized study, though the effect was greater in patients with primary, low-risk tumors [29]. Valrubicin is approved by the US Food and Drug Administration (FDA) for use in BCG refractory carcinoma in situ (CIS), with reported complete response rates of ~20 % in short-term follow-up [30]. However, valrubicin has not been extensively studied for CIS prior to BCG failure and is not frequently used in this population. Side effects of anthracyclines are predominantly local, including chemical cystitis and irritative voiding symptoms which respond to local symptomatic treatment.

18.3.6 Gemcitabine

Gemcitabine is used systemically for metastatic or invasive urothelial cancer, and has garnered much interest in the intravesical setting. It functions as a nucleoside analog, and halts DNA synthesis, inducing cell death. Additionally, it inhibits ribonucleotide reductase, preventing both DNA synthesis and repair, inducing apoptosis [31]. Between its MW of 299 kDa and its lipid solubility, gemcitabine is an ideal intravesical agent, and has shown promise in the adjuvant setting [2]. A randomized trial assessed its role in the immediate postoperative setting, comparing gemcitabine to placebo instillation, but yielded no difference in recurrence, and was terminated early [32]. Several studies have compared gemcitabine to MMC in the adjuvant setting, and favored gemcitabine, displaying trends toward reduced recurrence and progression (though not reaching statistical significance), with significantly reduced toxicity profiles (39 % vs. 72 %) [33, 34]. However, most of these studies enrolled BCG failure patients, making them less applicable to the average intermediate-risk patient. In another study with a similar population, gemcitabine was found to be superior to BCG with fewer recurrences (53 % vs. 88 %, $p=0.002$), and both treatments were well-tolerated [35]. Results of the phase 2 SWOG S0353 trial were recently reported, showing an initial response rate of 47 %, and a 2-year response rate of 21 %, with maintenance therapy [36]. Again, this population was heavily pretreated, and thus its applicability in the setting of primary intermediate- and high-risk tumors is not yet known. However, gemcitabine is well-tolerated at a dose of 2,000 mg in 50–100 ml saline, and is a promising alternative to MMC, in intermediate-risk tumors and after BCG failure.

18.3.7 Taxanes

Taxanes serve as microtubule stabilizers, thereby preventing cell division, causing M-phase cell cycle arrest. Intravesical docetaxel (808 kDa) was first studied in a BCG refractory population, yielding a 22 % complete response rate without maintenance at 4-year follow-up, with 44 % of patients experiencing grade 1–2 toxicity [37]. Paclitaxel (854 kDa) has also been used in the BCG refractory setting, in enhanced drug formulations of paclitaxel-hyaluronic acid (HA) and *nab*-paclitaxel (nanoparticle albumin-bound).

The HA formulation increases solubility, and in a phase 1 trial of 16 patients with BCG-refractory CIS, 60 % experienced a short-term complete response, with 44 % (7/16) experiencing adverse events [38]. A phase 2 study is currently enrolling patients with G1–G2 Ta lesions. *Nab*-paclitaxel allows for higher drug concentrations, which was a disadvantage of docetaxel, as the maximum deliverable dose was never reached. Phase 1 studies illustrated drug safety, with no grade 2 or higher toxicities reported, at a maximum deliverable dose of 500 mg *nab*-paclitaxel in 100 mg NS [39]. While taxanes have been used mostly in the BCG refractory setting, enhancing drug delivery seems to be effective and well-tolerated, and further studies are warranted.

18.3.8 Apaziquone

Apaziquone is a synthetic pro-drug of MMC, and preclinical studies showed that much lower concentrations were required for similar cytotoxic effect. A phase 2 study enrolling 53 patients was recently published, with 51 patients completing the 6-week course of 4 mg in 40 ml water. Overall, 92 % of patients reported at least one adverse event, and at 18 months, 45 % of patients displayed recurrence [40]. While apaziquone carries theoretical advantages, including a lower MW (288 kDa) than MMC (334 kDa) for improved penetration, and lower doses to minimize toxicity, further studies are needed to determine its role in the treatment of NMIBC. Although unpublished, two phase 3 trials comparing apaziquone with placebo revealed no theoretical advantage to immediate post-TUR instillation of the medication using a primary endpoint of tumor recurrence rate at 2 years.

18.3.9 Future Therapies

Given that intravesical therapy is effective, but imperfect, other strategies are currently under investigation. Combination therapy has been utilized, including gemcitabine and MMC [41], and MMC, doxorubicin, and cisplatin [42], with the rationale that each agent has different cell cycle targets, and in combination they may yield greater efficacy, similar to systemic chemotherapy. The former study protocol entailed 1 g of gemcitabine in 50 ml of water for 90 min, followed by 40 mg of MMC in 20 ml water for 90 min. Initial 6 weeks of induction therapy were followed by monthly maintenance for 12 months, in a largely pretreated population. Overall, 14/47 (30 %) of patients were recurrence-free at a median follow-up of 26 months. Four patients did not complete induction therapy secondary to adverse effects.

CG0070 is an oncolytic adenovirus that utilizes knowledge of urothelial cancer molecular pathways. The adenovirus replicates preferentially in cells with defective retinoblastoma gene pathways, targeting cancerous cells. It also encodes granulocyte macrophage-colony stimulating factor (GM-CSF), inducing cytotoxicity, and has been shown to be safe in a recent phase 1 trial, with a phase 2 trial pending [43]. Oportuzumab monatox employs recombinant fusion technology, linking anti-EpCAM antibody to Pseudomonas exotoxin A. This allows for preferential binding to urothelial cancer cells, inducing apoptosis via the exotoxin [44]. Liposomes are another drug delivery mechanism, which capitalize on the inner aqueous core and outer phospholipid layer to improve the solubility of hydrophobic drugs [45]. They have been used to enhance interferon delivery in a human urothelial carcinoma cell line, as well as in animal models for interstitial cystitis treatment [3]. Other methods under investigation include the use of magnetic nanoparticles, mucoadhesive carriers, and polymeric hydrogels. While many of these platforms have yet to be assessed in clinical trials, they have shown promising results in animal models and warrant further examination.

18.4 Immunotherapy

18.4.1 History

Mycobacterium bovis was first discovered in the nineteenth century as the cause of bovine tuberculosis. Initial efforts to create a human vaccine with *M. bovis* were unsuccessful, as it proved too virulent. However in the early 1900s, French scientists Albert Calmette and Camille Guérin were able to generate an avirulent strain that became known as bacillus of Calmette and Guérin (BCG). BCG has subsequently been used as an anti-tuberculosis vaccine, largely outside of the United States. Its role in oncology arose from an observation that patients with tuberculosis had a lower incidence of cancer than those who died of other causes [46]. Further research demonstrated that in animal models, BCG mediated an indirect inflammatory response, inducing tumor necrosis and regression, as well as preventing and eradicating metastases [47, 48]. Successful reports of intralesional BCG treatment for human malignant melanoma [49] engendered significant interest in its applicability throughout oncology.

The first intravesical application of BCG for bladder cancer was reported in 1976 by Morales and colleagues [50]. Ten patients were given 6 weekly intravesical treatments of 120 mg BCG in 50 ml saline, along with intradermal BCG. With encouraging results, subsequent randomized controlled trials were conducted, with BCG yielding a significant reduction in recurrence, compared with TUR alone [51]. In 1990, the FDA approved intravesical BCG as a primary treatment for patients with CIS, and as prophylaxis for recurrent papillary tumors, and it remains a cornerstone of treatment for NMIBC.

18.4.2 Mechanism of Action

Upon intravesical instillation, BCG first binds fibronectin, a glycoprotein which mediates cell adhesion. Subsequent internalization of BCG into benign and malignant urothelial cells occurs, initiating a cascade of inflammatory responses. Major histocompatibility complex II (MHC II)-mediated BCG antigen presentation stimulates CD4+ T cells, inducing a T helper type 1 (T_H1) response. An increase in urinary cytokines such as interferon-γ, interleukin (IL)-2, IL-12, and tumor necrosis factor (TNF)-α is seen as early as week 1 of treatment [52], demonstrating activation of the T_H1 pathway. This activation promotes cell-mediated antitumor activity, conferred by

CD8+ T cells, natural killer (NK) cells, and macrophages [53]. Indeed, patients with higher levels of T_H1-related cytokines have shown improved clinical response to BCG, while those with increased T_H2 cytokines, such as IL-10, often fail BCG treatment [54]. Promoting the T_H1 response and inhibiting the T_H2 pathway are areas of active research towards optimizing immunotherapy.

18.4.3 Administration

After determining that intradermal BCG was unnecessary [55, 56], BCG is now routinely administered intravesically only. Treatment typically begins 2–4 weeks after tumor resection to allow for bladder re-epithelialization. Several strains exist in different strengths, but the ultimate aim is to achieve a dose of roughly 10^8 to 10^9 colony-forming units (CFU). To achieve this, the following amounts of vaccine are reconstituted in 50 ml of saline: Sanofi-Pasteur 81 mg, Tice 50 mg, Tokyo 40 mg, RIVM 120 mg [57]. Urine culture and urinalysis should be obtained prior to administration to ensure absence of active UTI or significant hematuria. After atraumatic sterile catheterization, reconstituted BCG is delivered via catheter for a dwell time of 1–2 h. Patients should minimize fluid intake in the hours prior to instillation to avoid dilution of BCG or the need to void prior to completing the dwell time. Some urologists suggest that patients rotate every 15 min to ensure even contact between BCG and the urothelium, however there is no literature to support or refute this anecdotal practice [57]. Contraindications to administration include active urinary tract infection, traumatic catheterization, complete incontinence, gross hematuria, recent TURBT (<2 weeks), and a history of BCG sepsis.

18.4.4 Side Effects and Management

Common side effects of BCG therapy include irritative voiding symptoms and low-grade fevers (<38.5 °C). These typically are self-limited, and resolve within 48 h of treatment [57]. Symptomatic treatment can be employed as the treating physi-

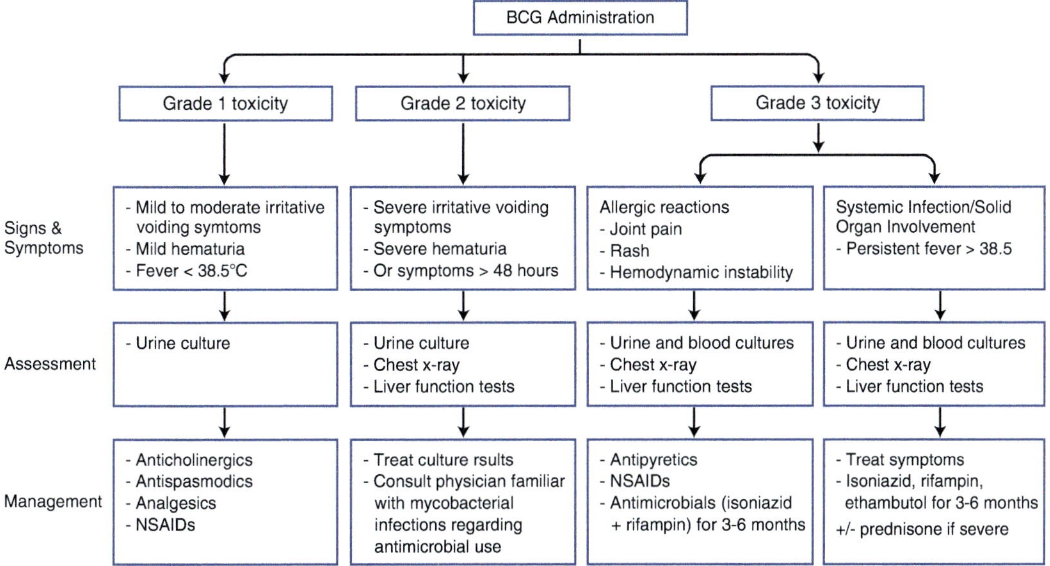

Fig. 18.1 Algorithm for management of BCG toxicity

cian sees fit, typically with anti-spasmodics and anti-pyretics (Fig. 18.1). In a recent EORTC-GU Cancer Group randomized controlled trial assessing duration of maintenance and dose reduction, only 7.8 % of all patients discontinued therapy secondary to side effects [58], a rate much lower than in previous maintenance trials [59]. While rates of discontinuation and local toxicity were acceptable at ~10–15 %, the feared complication is that of systemic absorption of BCG, leading to BCG sepsis, which requires anti-tuberculous therapy and close observation.

Another complication which requires anti-tuberculous therapy is that of solid organ involvement, e.g. prostate, epididymis, liver, kidney [60]. Some trials support the role of short-term fluoroquinolone administration prior to BCG to reduce the incidence of moderate to severe side effects [61, 62]. However, there are currently no specific recommendations or guidelines for peri-BCG antibiotic administration at this time.

18.4.5 Indications for BCG

The EAU and AUA both recommend BCG with maintenance as treatment for high-risk urothelial carcinoma of the bladder (e.g. high-grade tumors,

CIS, T1). This stems from evidence that it significantly reduces rates of recurrence compared to TURBT alone [51]. When comparing BCG to intravesical chemotherapy, recurrence rates are lower with BCG, particularly with the addition of BCG maintenance [63]. BCG is also superior in reducing rates of progression, making it the recommended agent for high-risk disease, if tolerated by the patient [60, 64, 65].

For patients with intermediate-risk disease, the overall risk of recurrence is ~50 %, but risk of progression is only ~10 %, compared to 25–50 % for patients with high-risk disease [28]. Thus, toxicity must be considered when choosing BCG. The EAU recommends BCG+≥1 year of maintenance or intravesical chemotherapy for intermediate-risk disease, while the AUA recommends induction BCG or MMC with the option of maintenance therapy. Long-term results of an EORTC phase 3 study evaluating BCG vs. epirubicin showed significant benefit of BCG to the intermediate-risk group, including a reduction in recurrence (HR 0.59, $p<0.001$), progression or distant metastases (HR 0.42, $p=0.027$), and death due to bladder cancer (HR 0.35, $p=0.02$) [28]. Thus, for patients with intermediate-risk disease, BCG is the most effective treatment, but the risk of adverse effects must be weighed against benefits. There is no role for BCG in patients with low-risk bladder cancer due to the low risk of recurrence and progression.

18.4.6 Maintenance

The efficacy of maintenance was first illustrated in SWOG 8507, in which maintenance therapy reduced time to recurrence and worsening of disease, though only 16 % of the original maintenance group completed the full 3-year schedule [59]. Subsequent meta-analyses have confirmed the utility of maintenance in reducing recurrence and progression [64], though the need for 36 months of maintenance and strength of BCG administered during maintenance remains under investigation. Dose reduction has been utilized to try to reduce toxicity while maintaining efficacy. One-third dose BCG has been shown to be as effective as full-dose BCG in reducing progression with less toxicity [66]. A recent EORTC trial addressing one-third dose vs. full-dose and 1 year vs. 3 years maintenance determined that full-dose BCG did not confer increased toxicity over one-third dose [58]. Additionally, high-risk patients displayed decreased recurrence rates with 3 years vs. 1 year of full-dose maintenance, but survival and progression were not affected. Initial induction therapy was also dose-reduced for the respective groups, making applicability somewhat complicated, as dose reduction is conventionally applied to maintenance therapy only. Though the ideal schedule has not been established, it seems that reducing the dose to one-third strength maintains efficacy and may reduce toxicity. The benefit of extending maintenance past 1 year is not entirely clear, especially when considering cost and side effects, but maintenance of at least 1 year is indeed useful and thus recommended for intermediate- and high-risk disease.

18.4.7 Optimization and Patient Factors

While there is no reliable way to predict a patient's response to BCG, there are several factors that are known to impact recurrence rates.

Advanced age has been found to correlate with increased recurrence rates in several studies. A Spanish Urological Club for Oncological Treatment (CUETO) meta-analysis found that age >70 years conferred greater risk of recurrence and progression on univariate analysis, compared with age ≤60 and 61–70. However, this significance disappeared on multivariate analysis ($p=0.052$) [67]. Herr reported on 805 patients who received BCG for NMIBC, and found that recurrence-free survival was 16 months in the group >70 years versus 20 months in those <70 years ($p=0.005$) [68]. Progression rates were not significantly different in this cohort. Joudi et al. analyzed results of a BCG-interferon multicenter trial, and found that patients >80 years had a recurrence-free survival rate of 39 % compared with 61 % for patients 61–70 years old ($p=0.0002$) [69]. Age continued to be a significant factor on multivariate analysis in both of these studies. The drivers of this observation are not entirely clear, but the hypothesis is that elderly patients tend to have depressed immune systems, preventing a robust T_H1 response, thereby decreasing efficacy. Whether elderly patients would benefit from a different dosing schedule or adjunctive therapies is not yet known.

Another factor that has been investigated is the role of high-dose vitamin supplements. Previous reports indicated that megadose vitamin therapy during BCG treatment reduced the 5-year risk of recurrence from 91 to 41 % ($p=0.0014$), when compared with recommended daily allowance (RDA) vitamins [55]. However, a larger randomized controlled trial enrolling 670 patients showed no change in recurrence rates between groups receiving megadose (Oncovite) or RDA vitamins [70]. Given these data, there are currently no AUA or EAU recommendations regarding high-dose vitamin use during BCG therapy.

Patient immune status may also play a role in predicting or monitoring BCG efficacy. Conversion of purified protein derivative (PPD) from negative to positive has been correlated with decreased recurrence in prior studies [71], while others have shown no association. Luftenegger and colleagues did find, however, that patients with a positive PPD prior to BCG treatment were more likely to develop fevers with BCG treatment. Furthermore, development of fevers >37.5 °C correlated with a lower recurrence rate of 30 %, compared with 48 % in patients who did not develop fevers ($p = 0.039$). Fevers may reflect a more robust immune response, particularly in those with prior exposure, resulting in a greater cytotoxic effect. However, other reports have examined the relationship between prior *M. tuberculosis* infection and BCG efficacy and found no correlation. Presence of leukocyturia has also been associated with decreased recurrence though it is not entirely clear why [72].

BCG has conventionally been contraindicated for immunosuppressed patients, as they are less likely to mount an effective immune response. However, Herr and Dalbagni recently reported on a series of 45 immunosuppressed patients with high-risk NMIBC who underwent induction BCG without maintenance, but with the option of repeat induction upon recurrence [73]. The cohort consisted of those on anti-rejection medications for transplants ($n = 12$), undergoing chemotherapy for other neoplasms ($n = 23$), and on high-dose prednisone for autoimmune diseases ($n = 10$). Overall, 91 % (41/45) of patients had a complete response at 6 months, but median recurrence-free and progression-free survival rates were significantly lower in the transplant group than those in the chemotherapy and autoimmune disease groups. Seventy-five percent of patients experienced local toxicity, but there were no reports of bacterial or BCG sepsis. While further studies are needed to determine the long-term efficacy of BCG in immunosuppressed patients, this experience illustrates that it is a reasonable and safe alternative, particularly in a patient population that is less likely to be fit for surgery.

Overall, BCG is the most effective intravesical therapy for reducing recurrence and progression rates, particularly with the addition of maintenance therapy. Optimal dosing and maintenance schedules are still being determined, further complicated by the fact that individual patient and tumor characteristics affect overall efficacy. A recent study described a calibrated mathematical model that takes into account existing data regarding BCG mechanism, the immune system, urothelial carcinoma, and the bladder mucosa. It proposed models of modified BCG regimens aimed at maximizing efficacy while minimizing side effects, including extended dwell times and longer intervals between treatments [74]. Such types of analyses may be more effective than undertaking new clinical trials with slight adjustments in therapy, as these can be time-consuming, expensive, and often require a significant number of patients to yield definitive results.

18.4.8 Other Immunotherapies

Mycobacterial cell wall-DNA complex (MCC) was developed as an alternative to BCG, capitalizing on the antitumor properties while obviating the risk of systemic BCG exposure. It has shown a response rate of 46 % at 26 weeks and 29 % at 18 months (at a dose of 8 mg) in a cohort of 55 patients, 85 % of whom had prior intravesical therapy [75]. Adverse events occurred in 33 % of the patients, with one patient discontinuing treatment. Interpretation of these results are complicated, as half of the patients are prior BCG failures, and MCC may be most effective in the BCG-naïve population, but this has yet to be determined. No systemic toxicity of BCG sepsis has been reported with MCC, which may be its major advantage. A phase 3 trial comparing MCC to mitomycin C has been recently suspended by the manufacturer for undisclosed reasons.

Interferons (IFN) have been investigated as another intravesical agent, as the IFN-α class stimulates the T_H1 and NK cell response as BCG does. IFN-α2b has shown efficacy as a single agent in the short term, however recurrence rates are similar to placebo with longer follow-up [76, 77]. The combination of BCG-IFN is more effective than single-agent IFN, but is comparable to BCG alone, as shown in the only randomized trial comparing the two [70]. Patients with BCG failure may benefit from combined therapy, as it produced a disease-free rate of 45 % at a median follow-up of 24 months in a phase 2 trial of 467 patients, with 6.7 % discontinuation rate due to intolerance [78, 79].

Alternative means of delivering immunotherapy are under investigation as well, including an ongoing phase 2 trial of rAd-IFN/Syn3 (Instiladrin), which utilizes a recombinant adenovirus gene delivery system to induce sustained levels of IFN expression [80]. IL-2 levels have been shown to be predictive of response to BCG, and intravesical administration of IL-2 has shown some efficacy [53]. IL-12 also works in the T_H1 pathway, but did not yield promising results in a small in vivo study, despite displaying efficacy in murine models. Another investigational approach is the inhibition of IL-10, a T_H2 pathway cytokine, which does not induce an antitumor effect. While BCG remains the cornerstone of immunotherapy, hopefully these alternative modulators of the immune response will optimize the efficacy of BCG while reducing the toxicity.

18.5 Conclusion

Intravesical therapy is an essential tool in the urologist's management of NMIBC, ranging from a single perioperative dose of chemotherapy to prolonged courses of intravesical immunotherapy followed by salvage agents. Immediate postoperative chemotherapy should be given to the majority of patients in the absence of contraindications as the benefit of reducing recurrence outweighs the low morbidity. For intermediate-risk patients, both adjuvant chemotherapy and BCG are reasonable options, with BCG plus maintenance likely providing the greatest reduction in recurrence and progression risk. However, the potential side effects of BCG are not insignificant, and one must determine if the patient is a suitable candidate. In high-risk disease, BCG is the most effective intravesical treatment, and requires maintenance therapy for maximum long-term efficacy. However, recurrence and progression rates are significant, and thus cystectomy should always be considered in the setting of BCG failure. Using new targeted therapy, optimizing drug delivery and predicting patient response are areas of research which could significantly improve the ability of intravesical therapy to reduce the high recurrence and progression rates of NMIBC, with the aim of ultimately reducing the significant morbidity and mortality of bladder cancer.

Conflict of Interest
Dr. McKiernan: none.
Dr. Ahn: none.

Disclosures *Funding sources*:
Dr. McKiernan: Celgene, Prostate Cancer Foundation.
Dr. Ahn: none.

References

1. Siegel R, Naishadham D, Jemal A. Cancer statistics, 2013. CA Cancer J Clin. 2013;63(1):11–30. Epub 2013/01/22.
2. Logan C, Brown M, Hayne D. Intravesical therapies for bladder cancer—indications and limitations. BJU Int. 2012;110 Suppl 4:12–21. Epub 2012/12/05.
3. GuhaSarkar S, Banerjee R. Intravesical drug delivery: challenges, current status, opportunities and novel strategies. J Control Release. 2010;148(2):147–59. Epub 2010/09/14.
4. Mishina T, Watanabe H, Kobayashi T, Maegawa M, Nakao M, Nakagawa S. Absorption of anticancer drugs through bladder epithelium. Urology. 1986;27(2):148–57. Epub 1986/02/01.
5. Shen Z, Shen T, Wientjes MG, O'Donnell MA, Au JL. Intravesical treatments of bladder cancer: review. Pharm Res. 2008;25(7):1500–10. Epub 2008/03/29.
6. Au JL, Badalament RA, Wientjes MG, Young DC, Warner JA, Venema PL, et al. Methods to improve efficacy of intravesical mitomycin C: results of a randomized phase III trial. J Natl Cancer Inst. 2001;93(8):597–604. Epub 2001/04/20.
7. Nargund VH, Tanabalan CK, Kabir MN. Management of non-muscle-invasive (superficial) bladder cancer. Semin Oncol. 2012;39(5):559–72. Epub 2012/10/09.
8. Bateman JC. Chemotherapy of solid tumors with triethylene thiophosphoramide. N Engl J Med. 1955;252(21):879–87. Epub 1955/05/26.
9. Babjuk M, Oosterlinck W, Sylvester R, Kaasinen E, Bohle A, Palou-Redorta J, et al. EAU guidelines on non-muscle-invasive urothelial carcinoma of the bladder, the 2011 update. Acta Urol Esp. 2012;36(7):389–402. Epub 2012/03/06.
10. Hall MC, Chang SS, Dalbagni G, Pruthi RS, Seigne JD, Skinner EC, et al. Guideline for the management of nonmuscle invasive bladder cancer (stages Ta, T1, and Tis): 2007 update. J Urol. 2007;178(6):2314–30. Epub 2007/11/13.
11. Sylvester RJ, Oosterlinck W, van der Meijden AP. A single immediate postoperative instillation of chemotherapy decreases the risk of recurrence in patients with stage Ta T1 bladder cancer: a meta-analysis of

published results of randomized clinical trials. J Urol. 2004;171(6 Pt 1):2186–90. quiz 435. Epub 2004/05/06.

12. Chamie K, Saigal CS, Lai J, Hanley JM, Setodji CM, Konety BR, et al. Compliance with guidelines for patients with bladder cancer: variation in the delivery of care. Cancer. 2011;117(23):5392–401. Epub 2011/07/23.

13. Pawinski A, Sylvester R, Kurth KH, Bouffioux C, van der Meijden A, Parmar MK, et al. A combined analysis of European Organization for Research and Treatment of Cancer, and Medical Research Council randomized clinical trials for the prophylactic treatment of stage TaT1 bladder cancer. European Organization for Research and Treatment of Cancer Genitourinary Tract Cancer Cooperative Group and the Medical Research Council Working Party on Superficial Bladder Cancer. J Urol. 1996;156(6):1934–40. Discussion 40–1. Epub 1996/12/01.

14. Tolley DA, Parmar MK, Grigor KM, Lallemand G, Benyon LL, Fellows J, et al. The effect of intravesical mitomycin C on recurrence of newly diagnosed superficial bladder cancer: a further report with 7 years of follow up. J Urol. 1996;155(4):1233–8. Epub 1996/04/01.

15. Kaasinen E, Rintala E, Hellstrom P, Viitanen J, Juusela H, Rajala P, et al. Factors explaining recurrence in patients undergoing chemoimmunotherapy regimens for frequently recurring superficial bladder carcinoma. Eur Urol. 2002;42(2):167–74. Epub 2002/08/06.

16. Shelley MD, Mason MD, Kynaston H. Intravesical therapy for superficial bladder cancer: a systematic review of randomised trials and meta-analyses. Cancer Treat Rev. 2010;36(3):195–205. Epub 2010/01/19.

17. Huncharek M, Kupelnick B. Impact of intravesical chemotherapy versus BCG immunotherapy on recurrence of superficial transitional cell carcinoma of the bladder: metaanalytic reevaluation. Am J Clin Oncol. 2003;26(4):402–7. Epub 2003/08/07.

18. Huncharek M, Kupelnick B. The influence of intravesical therapy on progression of superficial transitional cell carcinoma of the bladder: a metaanalytic comparison of chemotherapy versus bacilli Calmette-Guerin immunotherapy. Am J Clin Oncol. 2004;27(5):522–8. Epub 2004/12/15.

19. Bohle A, Bock PR. Intravesical bacille Calmette-Guerin versus mitomycin C in superficial bladder cancer: formal meta-analysis of comparative studies on tumor progression. Urology. 2004;63(4):682–6. Discussion 6–7. Epub 2004/04/10.

20. Gardmark T, Jahnson S, Wahlquist R, Wijkstrom H, Malmstrom PU. Analysis of progression and survival after 10 years of a randomized prospective study comparing mitomycin-C and bacillus Calmette-Guerin in patients with high-risk bladder cancer. BJU Int. 2007;99(4):817–20. Epub 2007/01/25.

21. Bohle A, Jocham D, Bock PR. Intravesical bacillus Calmette-Guerin versus mitomycin C for superficial bladder cancer: a formal meta-analysis of comparative studies on recurrence and toxicity. J Urol. 2003;169(1):90–5. Epub 2002/12/13.

22. Lammers RJ, Witjes JA, Inman BA, Leibovitch I, Laufer M, Nativ O, et al. The role of a combined regimen with intravesical chemotherapy and hyperthermia in the management of non-muscle-invasive bladder cancer: a systematic review. Eur Urol. 2011;60(1):81–93. Epub 2011/05/03.

23. Colombo R, Salonia A, Leib Z, Pavone-Macaluso M, Engelstein D. Long-term outcomes of a randomized controlled trial comparing thermochemotherapy with mitomycin-C alone as adjuvant treatment for non-muscle-invasive bladder cancer (NMIBC). BJU Int. 2011;107(6):912–8. Epub 2010/10/30.

24. Di Stasi SM, Giannantoni A, Stephen RL, Capelli G, Navarra P, Massoud R, et al. Intravesical electromotive mitomycin C versus passive transport mitomycin C for high risk superficial bladder cancer: a prospective randomized study. J Urol. 2003;170(3):777–82. Epub 2003/08/13.

25. Di Stasi SM, Valenti M, Verri C, Liberati E, Giurioli A, Leprini G, et al. Electromotive instillation of mitomycin immediately before transurethral resection for patients with primary urothelial non-muscle invasive bladder cancer: a randomised controlled trial. Lancet Oncol. 2011;12(9):871–9. Epub 2011/08/13.

26. Di Stasi SM, Giannantoni A, Giurioli A, Valenti M, Zampa G, Storti L, et al. Sequential BCG and electromotive mitomycin versus BCG alone for high-risk superficial bladder cancer: a randomised controlled trial. Lancet Oncol. 2006;7(1):43–51. Epub 2006/01/04.

27. The effect of intravesical thiotepa on tumour recurrence after endoscopic treatment of newly diagnosed superficial bladder cancer. A further report with long-term follow-up of a Medical Research Council randomized trial. Medical Research Council Working Party on Urological Cancer, Subgroup on Superficial Bladder Cancer. Br J Urol. 1994;73(6):632–8. Epub 1994/06/01.

28. Sylvester RJ, Brausi MA, Kirkels WJ, Hoeltl W, Calais Da Silva F, Powell PH, et al. Long-term efficacy results of EORTC genito-urinary group randomized phase 3 study 30911 comparing intravesical instillations of epirubicin, bacillus Calmette-Guerin, and bacillus Calmette-Guerin plus isoniazid in patients with intermediate- and high-risk stage Ta T1 urothelial carcinoma of the bladder. Eur Urol. 2010;57(5):766–73.

29. Gudjonsson S, Adell L, Merdasa F, Olsson R, Larsson B, Davidsson T, et al. Should all patients with non-muscle-invasive bladder cancer receive early intravesical chemotherapy after transurethral resection? The results of a prospective randomised multicentre study. Eur Urol. 2009;55(4):773–80. Epub 2009/01/21.

30. Steinberg G, Bahnson R, Brosman S, Middleton R, Wajsman Z, Wehle M. Efficacy and safety of valrubicin for the treatment of Bacillus Calmette-Guerin

refractory carcinoma in situ of the bladder. The Valrubicin Study Group. J Urol. 2000;163(3):761–7. Epub 2000/02/25.

31. Dalbagni G, Russo P, Sheinfeld J, Mazumdar M, Tong W, Rabbani F, et al. Phase I trial of intravesical gemcitabine in bacillus Calmette-Guerin-refractory transitional-cell carcinoma of the bladder. J Clin Oncol. 2002;20(15):3193–8. Epub 2002/08/01.

32. Bohle A, Leyh H, Frei C, Kuhn M, Tschada R, Pottek T, et al. Single postoperative instillation of gemcitabine in patients with non-muscle-invasive transitional cell carcinoma of the bladder: a randomised, double-blind, placebo-controlled phase III multicentre study. Eur Urol. 2009;56(3):495–503. Epub 2009/06/30.

33. Shelley MD, Jones G, Cleves A, Wilt TJ, Mason MD, Kynaston HG. Intravesical gemcitabine therapy for non-muscle invasive bladder cancer (NMIBC): a systematic review. BJU Int. 2012;109(4):496–505. Epub 2012/02/09.

34. Addeo R, Caraglia M, Bellini S, Abbruzzese A, Vincenzi B, Montella L, et al. Randomized phase III trial on gemcitabine versus mytomicin in recurrent superficial bladder cancer: evaluation of efficacy and tolerance. J Clin Oncol. 2010;28(4):543–8. Epub 2009/10/21.

35. Di Lorenzo G, Perdona S, Damiano R, Faiella A, Cantiello F, Pignata S, et al. Gemcitabine versus bacille Calmette-Guerin after initial bacille Calmette-Guerin failure in non-muscle-invasive bladder cancer: a multicenter prospective randomized trial. Cancer. 2010;116(8):1893–900. Epub 2010/02/18.

36. Skinner EC, Goldman B, Sakr WA, Petrylak DP, Lenz HJ, Lee CT, et al. SWOG S0353: phase II trial of intravesical gemcitabine in patients with non-muscle invasive bladder cancer who recurred following at least two prior courses of intravesical BCG. J Urol. 2013;190(4):1200–4. Epub 2013/04/20.

37. McKiernan JM, Masson P, Murphy AM, Goetzl M, Olsson CA, Petrylak DP, et al. Phase I trial of intravesical docetaxel in the management of superficial bladder cancer refractory to standard intravesical therapy. J Clin Oncol. 2006;24(19):3075–80. Epub 2006/07/01.

38. Bassi PF, Volpe A, D'Agostino D, Palermo G, Renier D, Franchini S, et al. Paclitaxel-hyaluronic acid for intravesical therapy of bacillus Calmette-Guerin refractory carcinoma in situ of the bladder: results of a phase I study. J Urol. 2011;185(2):445–9. Epub 2010/12/21.

39. McKiernan JM, Barlow LJ, Laudano MA, Mann MJ, Petrylak DP, Benson MC. A phase I trial of intravesical nanoparticle albumin-bound paclitaxel in the treatment of bacillus Calmette-Guerin refractory nonmuscle invasive bladder cancer. J Urol. 2011;186(2):448–51. Epub 2011/06/18.

40. Hendricksen K, Cornel EB, de Reijke TM, Arentsen HC, Chawla S, Witjes JA. Phase 2 study of adjuvant intravesical instillations of apaziquone for high risk nonmuscle invasive bladder cancer. J Urol. 2012;187(4):1195–9. Epub 2012/02/18.

41. Lightfoot AJ, Breyer BN, Rosevear HM, Erickson BA, Konety BR, O'Donnell MA. Multi-institutional analysis of sequential intravesical gemcitabine and mitomycin C chemotherapy for non-muscle invasive bladder cancer. Urol Oncol. 2013;32(1):e15–9. Epub 2013/03/21.

42. Chen CH, Yang HJ, Shun CT, Huang CY, Huang KH, Yu HJ, et al. A cocktail regimen of intravesical mitomycin-C, doxorubicin, and cisplatin (MDP) for non-muscle-invasive bladder cancer. Urol Oncol. 2012;30(4):421–7. Epub 2010/09/28.

43. Burke JM, Lamm DL, Meng MV, Nemunaitis JJ, Stephenson JJ, Arseneau JC, et al. A first in human phase 1 study of CG0070, a GM-CSF expressing oncolytic adenovirus, for the treatment of nonmuscle invasive bladder cancer. J Urol. 2012;188(6):2391–7. Epub 2012/10/24.

44. Kowalski M, Guindon J, Brazas L, Moore C, Entwistle J, Cizeau J, et al. A phase II study of oportuzumab monatox: an immunotoxin therapy for patients with noninvasive urothelial carcinoma in situ previously treated with bacillus Calmette-Guerin. J Urol. 2012;188(5):1712–8. Epub 2012/09/25.

45. Giannantoni A, Di Stasi SM, Chancellor MB, Costantini E, Porena M. New frontiers in intravesical therapies and drug delivery. Eur Urol. 2006;50(6):1183–93. Discussion 93. Epub 2006/09/12.

46. Pearl R. Cancer and tuberculosis. Am J Hygiene. 1929;9:97–159.

47. Old LJ, Clarke DA, Benacerraf B. Effect of Bacillus Calmette-Guerin infection on transplanted tumours in the mouse. Nature. 1959;184 Suppl 5:291–2. Epub 1959/07/25.

48. Zbar B, Bernstein ID, Rapp HJ. Suppression of tumor growth at the site of infection with living Bacillus Calmette-Guerin. J Natl Cancer Instit. 1971;46(4):831–9. Epub 1971/04/01.

49. deKernion JB, Golub SH, Gupta RK, Silverstein M, Morton DL. Successful transurethral intralesional BCG therapy of a bladder melanoma. Cancer. 1975;36(5):1662–7. Epub 1975/11/01.

50. Morales A, Eidinger D, Bruce AW. Intracavitary Bacillus Calmette-Guerin in the treatment of superficial bladder tumors. J Urol. 1976;116(2):180–3. Epub 1976/08/01.

51. Lamm DL, Thor DE, Harris SC, Reyna JA, Stogdill VD, Radwin HM. Bacillus Calmette-Guerin immunotherapy of superficial bladder cancer. J Urol. 1980;124(1):38–40. Epub 1980/07/01.

52. Kawai K, Miyazaki J, Joraku A, Nishiyama H, Akaza H. Bacillus Calmette-Guerin (BCG) immunotherapy for bladder cancer: current understanding and perspectives on engineered BCG vaccine. Cancer Sci. 2013;104(1):22–7. Epub 2012/11/28.

53. Askeland EJ, Newton MR, O'Donnell MA, Luo Y. Bladder cancer immunotherapy: BCG and beyond. Adv Urol. 2012;2012:181987. Epub 2012/07/11.

54. Saint F, Patard JJ, Maille P, Soyeux P, Hoznek A, Salomon L, et al. Prognostic value of a T helper 1 urinary cytokine response after intravesical bacillus Calmette-Guerin treatment for superficial bladder cancer. J Urol. 2002;167(1):364–7. Epub 2001/12/18.

55. Lamm DL, Riggs DR, Shriver JS, vanGilder PF, Rach RF, DeHaven JI. Megadose vitamins in bladder cancer: a double-blind clinical trial. J Urol. 1994;151(1):21–6. Epub 1994/01/01.

56. Luftenegger W, Ackermann DK, Futterlieb A, Kraft R, Minder CE, Nadelhaft P, et al. Intravesical versus intravesical plus intradermal bacillus Calmette-Guerin: a prospective randomized study in patients with recurrent superficial bladder tumors. J Urol. 1996;155(2):483–7. Epub 1996/02/01.

57. Shah JB, Kamat AM. Strategies for optimizing bacillus Calmette-Guerin. Urol Clin N Am. 2013;40(2):211–8. Epub 2013/04/02.

58. Oddens J, Brausi M, Sylvester R, Bono A, van de Beek C, van Andel G, et al. Final results of an EORTC-GU cancers group randomized study of maintenance bacillus Calmette-Guerin in intermediate- and high-risk Ta, T1 papillary carcinoma of the urinary bladder: one-third dose versus full dose and 1 year versus 3 years of maintenance. Eur Urol. 2013;63(3):462–72. Epub 2012/11/13.

59. Lamm DL, Blumenstein BA, Crissman JD, Montie JE, Gottesman JE, Lowe BA, et al. Maintenance bacillus Calmette-Guerin immunotherapy for recurrent TA, T1 and carcinoma in situ transitional cell carcinoma of the bladder: a randomized Southwest Oncology Group Study. J Urol. 2000;163(4):1124–9. Epub 2000/03/29.

60. Gontero P, Bohle A, Malmstrom PU, O'Donnell MA, Oderda M, Sylvester R, et al. The role of bacillus Calmette-Guerin in the treatment of non-muscle-invasive bladder cancer. Eur Urol. 2010;57(3):410–29. Epub 2009/12/09.

61. Colombel M, Saint F, Chopin D, Malavaud B, Nicolas L, Rischmann P. The effect of ofloxacin on bacillus calmette-guerin induced toxicity in patients with superficial bladder cancer: results of a randomized, prospective, double-blind, placebo controlled, multicenter study. J Urol. 2006;176(3):935–9. Epub 2006/08/08.

62. Damiano R, De Sio M, Quarto G, Di Lorenzo G, Perdona S, Palumbo IM, et al. Short-term administration of prulifloxacin in patients with nonmuscle-invasive bladder cancer: an effective option for the prevention of bacillus Calmette-Guerin-induced toxicity? BJU Int. 2009;104(5):633–9. Epub 2009/03/21.

63. Jarvinen R, Kaasinen E, Sankila A, Rintala E, FinnBladder G. Long-term efficacy of maintenance bacillus Calmette-Guerin versus maintenance mitomycin C instillation therapy in frequently recurrent TaT1 tumours without carcinoma in situ: a subgroup analysis of the prospective, randomised FinnBladder I study with a 20-year follow-up. Eur Urol. 2009;56(2):260–5. Epub 2009/04/28.

64. Sylvester RJ, van der MA, Lamm DL. Intravesical bacillus Calmette-Guerin reduces the risk of progression in patients with superficial bladder cancer: a meta-analysis of the published results of randomized clinical trials. J Urol. 2002;168(5):1964–70. Epub 2002/10/24.

65. Sylvester RJ, van der Meijden AP, Witjes JA, Kurth K. Bacillus calmette-guerin versus chemotherapy for the intravesical treatment of patients with carcinoma in situ of the bladder: a meta-analysis of the published results of randomized clinical trials. J Urol. 2005;174(1):86–91. Discussion-2. Epub 2005/06/11.

66. Martinez-Pineiro JA, Martinez-Pineiro L, Solsona E, Rodriguez RH, Gomez JM, Martin MG, et al. Has a 3-fold decreased dose of bacillus Calmette-Guerin the same efficacy against recurrences and progression of T1G3 and Tis bladder tumors than the standard dose? Results of a prospective randomized trial. J Urol. 2005;174(4 Pt 1):1242–7. Epub 2005/09/08.

67. Fernandez-Gomez J, Solsona E, Unda M, Martinez-Pineiro L, Gonzalez M, Hernandez R, et al. Prognostic factors in patients with non-muscle-invasive bladder cancer treated with bacillus Calmette-Guerin: multivariate analysis of data from four randomized CUETO trials. Eur Urol. 2008;53(5):992–1001. Epub 2007/10/24.

68. Herr HW. Age and outcome of superficial bladder cancer treated with bacille Calmette-Guerin therapy. Urology. 2007;70(1):65–8. Epub 2007/07/28.

69. Joudi FN, Smith BJ, O'Donnell MA, Konety BR. The impact of age on the response of patients with superficial bladder cancer to intravesical immunotherapy. J Urol. 2006;175(5):1634–9. Discussion 9–40. Epub 2006/04/08.

70. Nepple KG, Lightfoot AJ, Rosevear HM, O'Donnell MA, Lamm DL. Bladder Cancer Genitourinary Oncology Study G. Bacillus Calmette-Guerin with or without interferon alpha-2b and megadose versus recommended daily allowance vitamins during induction and maintenance intravesical treatment of nonmuscle invasive bladder cancer. J Urol. 2010;184(5):1915–9.

71. Saint F, Salomon L, Quintela R, Cicco A, Hoznek A, Abbou CC, et al. Do prognostic parameters of remission versus relapse after Bacillus Calmette-Guerin (BCG) immunotherapy exist? Analysis of a quarter century of literature. Eur Urol. 2003;43(4):351–60.

72. Saint F, Patard JJ, Irani J, Salomon L, Hoznek A, Legrand P, et al. Leukocyturia as a predictor of tolerance and efficacy of intravesical BCG maintenance therapy for superficial bladder cancer. Urology. 2001;57(4):617–21. Discussion 21–2. Epub 2001/04/18.

73. Herr HW, Dalbagni G. Intravesical bacille Calmette-Guerin (BCG) in immunologically compromised patients with bladder cancer. BJU Int. 2013;111(6):984–7. Epub 2013/01/29.

74. Rentsch CA, Biot C, Gsponer JR, Bachmann A, Albert ML, Breban R. BCG-mediated bladder cancer immunotherapy: identifying determinants of treatment response using a calibrated mathematical model. PloS one. 2013;8(2):e56327. Epub 2013/03/02.

75. Morales A, Phadke K, Steinhoff G. Intravesical myco-bacterial cell wall-DNA complex in the treatment of carcinoma in situ of the bladder after standard intra-vesical therapy has failed. J Urol. 2009;181(3):1040–5. Epub 2009/01/20.

76. Glashan RW. A randomized controlled study of intra-vesical alpha-2b-interferon in carcinoma in situ of the bladder. J Urol. 1990;144(3):658–61. Epub 1990/09/01.

77. Belldegrun AS, Franklin JR, O'Donnell MA, Gomella LG, Klein E, Neri R, et al. Superficial bladder cancer: the role of interferon-alpha. J Urol. 1998;159(6):1793–801. Epub 1998/05/23.

78. Joudi FN, Smith BJ, O'Donnell MA, National BCGIPIG. Final results from a national multicenter phase II trial of combination bacillus Calmette-Guerin plus interferon alpha-2B for reducing recurrence of superficial bladder cancer. Urologic oncology. 2006;24(4):344–8. Epub 2006/07/05.

79. O'Donnell MA, Lilli K, Leopold C. National Bacillus Calmette-Guerin/Interferon Phase 2 Investigator G. Interim results from a national multicenter phase II trial of combination bacillus Calmette-Guerin plus interferon alfa-2b for superficial bladder cancer. J Urol. 2004;172(3):888–93.

80. Nagabhushan TL, Maneval DC, Benedict WF, Wen SF, Ihnat PM, Engler H, et al. Enhancement of intra-vesical delivery with Syn3 potentiates interferon-alpha2b gene therapy for superficial bladder cancer. Cytokine Growth Factor Rev. 2007;18(5–6):389–94. Epub 2007/08/19.

Case: 55-year-old man with CIS and high-grade ta tumors who received a 6-week induction course of BCG

Sima P. Porten and Colin P. Dinney

Abbreviations

BCG   Bacillus Calmette-Guerin
CIS   Carcinoma in situ
EORTC   European Organization for Research and Treatment of Cancer
FDA   Food and Drug Administration
FISH   Fluorescence in situ hybridization
HAL   Hexaminolevulinate
NMIBC   Non-muscle Invasive Bladder Cancer
PDD   Photodynamic diagnosis
SWOG   Southwest Oncology Group
TUR   Transurethral resection

The majority of bladder tumors present as non-muscle invasive disease (NIMBC), with recurrence in approximately 70 % and progression in up to 20 % of patients [1, 2]. To mitigate this fate and reduce the nuisance and cost of recurrence, intravesical immunotherapy with bacillus Calmette-Guerin (BCG) is indicated for patients with higher-risk disease. Many present similarly to case described above, with high-grade tumors and concomitant carcinoma in situ (CIS), and immunotherapy with BCG is the most effective intravesical treatment proven to decrease both progression and recurrence based on evidence from high-quality meta-analyses and randomized controlled trials [3–5].

The beneficial effect of BCG is greatest in those with intermediate- and high-grade disease, as those with only low-grade, low-volume, Ta tumors (approximately 50 % of cases) have a less than 5 % probability for progression [3]. In the above case, based on the presence of CIS, high-grade disease, and more than one tumor, one could assume that this patient would be at least at intermediate risk and BCG would be beneficial. However, predicting the possibility of recurrence and progression prior to intravesical treatment may be further refined using a risk calculator such as the one created by the European Organization for Research and Treatment of Cancer (EORTC) (http://www.eortc.be/tools/bladdercalculator/) [6]. Assuming the tumor is less than 3 cm, our patient above has an intermediate probability of recurrence (38 % at 1 year, 62 % at 5 years), and a high risk of progression (17 % at 1 year, 45 % at 5 years). Alternatively, Fernandez-Gomez et al. developed a risk stratification nomogram for patients treated with BCG therapy [7]. Using this calculator, at 5 years our patient has a 36 % probability of recurrence and a 34 % chance of progression after BCG therapy.

Current evidence suggests that intravesical BCG should be administered according to the protocol described in the Southwest Oncology Group trial 8507 (SWOG) [8]. Induction consists

S.P. Porten, M.D., M.P.H. (✉) • C.P. Dinney, M.D.
Department of Urology, MD Anderson Cancer Center, The University of Texas, 1515 Holcombe Blvd, Unit 1373, Houston, TX 77030, USA
e-mail: sporten@mdanderson.org; cdinney@mdanderson.org

B.R. Konety and S.S. Chang (eds.), *Management of Bladder Cancer:*
A Comprehensive Text With Clinical Scenarios, DOI 10.1007/978-1-4939-1881-2_19,
© Springer Science+Business Media New York 2015

of 6 weekly treatments of BCG, followed by maintenance consisting of 3 weekly treatments at 3 and 6 months and then every 6 months for a total of up to 36 months. Using this regimen, it is possible for >70 % of patients who have an initial response to remain tumor free for more than 5 years and disease progression can be significantly reduced by 37 % in the setting of papillary or CIS lesions [4, 8]. As the risk for recurrence and progression is lifelong in these patients, induction is clearly not enough to produce prolonged immune stimulation [9, 10]. The optimal duration or schedule for maintenance treatment is not clear and has been debated. Recent data from a European randomized control trial reinforced the need for 3 years of maintenance BCG in high-risk patients (which we define as high-grade, T1 disease, or CIS) as recurrence was significantly decreased (hazard ratio 1.61; 95 % CI, 1.13–2.30; $p=0.009$) [11]. For those with intermediate disease (recurrent Ta disease), 1 year of treatment may be enough, as there was no difference in recurrence or progression compared to 3 years of treatment. We prefer 3 years of maintenance BCG for all patients who undergo induction regardless of assessed risk, unless side effects are truly intolerable.

Prior to beginning 6-week induction course of BCG it is mandatory to ensure both the absence of invasive disease and a "clean slate" or complete resection. A routine re-staging transurethral resection should be strongly considered in patients with high-grade tumors and is necessary in patients with T1 tumors, even if muscle is present at the time of initial resection [12, 13]. Residual disease can be found in 51–78 % of patients, with upstaging of 15 % of patients who had initial Ta disease [14]. Furthermore, in patients with high-risk NIMBC (high grade Ta/T1 tumors with concomitant CIS, such as our patient above), those who underwent a second transurethral resection (TUR) prior to BCG had a recurrence rate of 45 % compared to 80 % in those who had BCG after initial TUR after 12 months of follow-up [13]. Multivariate analysis confirmed that a single TUR prior before BCG was a significant independent factor of subsequent tumor recurrence and progression.

Photodynamic diagnosis (PDD) is a recent technologic advance that can improve tumor identification and ensure complete tumor resection either at initial resection or a re-staging procedure. Intravesical Hexaminolevulinate HCl (HAL) or Cysview (Photocure US, Princeton, NJ, USA) is administered prior to cystoscopy and drives the accumulation of protoporphyrin IX which preferentially occurs in malignant cell and fluoresces red under a blue light. [15] A recent meta-analysis pooling the results of multiple studies evaluating the addition of PDD to white light cystoscopy showed a significant increase in detection of Ta, T1, and CIS tumors and an approximately 11 % reduction in recurrence [16]. In 27 %, CIS was only detected by PDD ($p<0.001$). Currently, Cysview is approved by the Food and Drug Administration (FDA) for one-time use only in patients with known or suspected NMIBC. Additionally, approval was granted with only the Karl Storz D-Light C PDD system, which includes a rigid cystoscope necessitating an operating room procedure. PDD should be strongly considered in these patients, especially at re-staging procedures prior to induction with BCG, and possibly in the context of a clinical trial randomizing patients to white versus blue light cystoscopy to determine whether improved debulking by fluorescent cystoscopy will improve the response to intravesical BCG.

After 6-week induction course, standard protocol is to perform an office white light cystoscopy with cytology at 3 months to evaluate for response. One of four possible situations could be encountered. The first possibility is the presence of overt, visible tumor. Assuming a complete, thorough resection with reliable staging, this is a poor prognostic factor if a patient is truly refractory (representing approximately 40 % of failures). Subsequent treatment is determined after repeat risk assessment based on pathology from a repeat TUR performed in the operating room. Options include re-induction with BCG, continuation of intravesical maintenance therapy, or early radical cystectomy (within the first 24 months after diagnosis which can improve survival in 20 %) and will be discussed in subsequent chapters [17].

After intravesical treatment, it is sometimes difficult to discern if CIS (characterized by an erythematous, flat lesion) is still present, due to the inflamed appearance of the bladder mucosae. Cytology can be helpful in this second situation, where visual inspection with cystoscopy is considered negative or non-diagnostic. Cytology detects high-grade cancer cells shed in the urine and is highly specific with reported rates up to 96 % [18, 19]. For patients with a negative surveillance cystoscopy and positive cytology, cystoscopy performed in the operating room with bladder mapping (random biopsies of the bladder with TUR of the prostatic urethra at 5 and 7 o'clock) in men and evaluation of the upper tracts should be strongly considered. However, the true utility of a positive cytology at this time point is somewhat controversial. The detection rate of bladder mapping is modest with sensitivity and specificity for CIS in the bladder or the prostatic urethra of 51 and 83 % or 46 and 89 %, respectively [20]. PDD may provide additional information above and beyond random bladder mapping in surveillance of CIS after treatment with BCG, however further studies need to be conducted to support this indication [21]. Additionally, there is a possibility that complete response of CIS to BCG has not yet occurred at 3 months. In the SWOG trial, Lamm et al. reported that in patients receiving only induction BCG there was an increase in complete response from 58 % at 3 months to 68 % at 6 months [8]. Also, 64 % of patients with residual CIS at 3 months resolved at 6 months after the first cycle of maintenance therapy (started after the 3 months surveillance cystoscopy). Therefore, if positive cytology with no visible tumor would not alter the decision to continue with BCG, its utility at the 3-month surveillance visit could be considered questionable. However, we still recommend cytology at this time point as it increases the detection rate for recurrent tumor over cystoscopy alone from 52 to 60 %, and can help identify possible sites of occult or missed disease, despite increased cost [22].

Fluorescence in situ hybridization (FISH) analysis is known to detect bladder cancer recurrence at the molecular level before a lesion is seen on cystoscopy, even in the setting of intravesical immunotherapy [23, 24]. UroVysion (Abbot/Vysis, Downers Grove, IL) is a commercially available FISH system that detects aneuploidy in chromosomes 3, 7, and 17, and a loss of 9p21 locus in tumor cells shed in the urine. Compared to other urinary markers (BTA-STAT, NMP-22, or ImmunoCyt) studied in the surveillance setting, FISH has the greatest utility and accuracy. The sensitivity and specificity of this marker are 77 % (73–81 %) and 98 % (96–100 %), respectively depending on the clinical situation it is applied to. As with cytology, the increased detection rate (around 72 %) comes with increased costs, mainly due to invasive and expensive evaluation of false positives [22]. Unlike cytology which is poor predictor of therapy failure, FISH may be prognostic and predict patient response to BCG [25–28]. A recent prospective study by Kamat et al. demonstrated that patients who had a positive FISH result at 3 months after starting BCG had a higher risk of future tumor recurrence (58.3 % vs. 15.3 %, $p < 0.001$) and progression (25 % vs. 6.8 %, $p = 0.013$), even if there was no clinical evidence of recurrence of progression at that time. Based on these findings, FISH may be a useful prognostic marker and assist in patient counseling at the 3 months surveillance visit in all patients undergoing treatment with intravesical BCG, especially in those with positive cytology.

A third and more problematic possibility is a negative cystoscopy with atypical or indeterminate cytology, which happens often, especially after intravesical treatment [29, 30]. One option is observation and continuation with maintenance BCG, which leaves the possibility of missed cancer (intra- or extravesical). Alternatively, biopsy in the operating room with the associated costs and risk of surgery could be performed in every patient. FISH can be used in this setting to determine the need for further evaluation and was recently found to be a cost-effective strategy [31, 32]. Our standard practice in this situation is to continue with maintenance BCG therapy and scheduled surveillance with repeat office cystoscopy and cytology in 3 months.

Lastly, if a patient had a negative surveillance evaluation, with a normal cystoscopy and negative cytology, maintenance BCG should be administered as planned.

In conclusion, the initial management for patients with intermediate- to high-risk NIMBC consists of meticulous staging, complete resection, comprehensive BCG, and timely surveillance. The use of adjunctive tools such as PDD and urinary markers (FISH) can further help risk-stratify and treat those most likely to fail treatment.

References

1. Jemal A, Bray F, Center MM, Ferlay J, Ward E, Forman D. Global cancer statistics. CA Cancer J Clin. 2011;61(2):69–90.
2. Heney NM, Ahmed S, Flanagan MJ, et al. Superficial bladder cancer: progression and recurrence. J Urol. 1983;130(6):1083–6.
3. Sylvester RJ, Brausi MA, Kirkels WJ, et al. Long-term efficacy results of EORTC genito-urinary group randomized phase 3 study 30911 comparing intravesical instillations of epirubicin, bacillus Calmette-Guerin, and bacillus Calmette-Guerin plus isoniazid in patients with intermediate- and high-risk stage Ta T1 urothelial carcinoma of the bladder. Eur Urol. 2010;57(5):766–73.
4. Sylvester RJ, van der MA, Lamm DL. Intravesical bacillus Calmette-Guerin reduces the risk of progression in patients with superficial bladder cancer: a meta-analysis of the published results of randomized clinical trials. J Urol. 2002;168(5):1964–70.
5. Sylvester RJ, van der Meijden AP, Witjes JA, Kurth K. Bacillus calmette-guerin versus chemotherapy for the intravesical treatment of patients with carcinoma in situ of the bladder: a meta-analysis of the published results of randomized clinical trials. J Urol. 2005;174(1):86–91. discussion 91–2.
6. Sylvester RJ, van der Meijden AP, Oosterlinck W, et al. Predicting recurrence and progression in individual patients with stage Ta T1 bladder cancer using EORTC risk tables: a combined analysis of 2596 patients from seven EORTC trials. Eur Urol. 2006;49(3):466–5. discussion 466–477.
7. Fernandez-Gomez J, Madero R, Solsona E, et al. Predicting nonmuscle invasive bladder cancer recurrence and progression in patients treated with bacillus Calmette-Guerin: the CUETO scoring model. J Urol. 2009;182(5):2195–203.
8. Lamm DL, Blumenstein BA, Crissman JD, et al. Maintenance bacillus Calmette-Guerin immunotherapy for recurrent TA, T1 and carcinoma in situ transitional cell carcinoma of the bladder: a randomized Southwest Oncology Group Study. J Urol. 2000;163(4):1124–9.
9. Reichert DF, Lamm DL. Long term protection in bladder cancer following intralesional immunotherapy. J Urol. 1984;132(3):570–3.
10. Herr HW. Extravesical tumor relapse in patients with superficial bladder tumors. J Clin Oncol. 1998;16(3):1099–102.
11. Oddens J, Brausi M, Sylvester R, et al. Final results of an EORTC-GU cancers group randomized study of maintenance bacillus Calmette-Guerin in intermediate- and high-risk Ta, T1 papillary carcinoma of the urinary bladder: one-third dose versus full dose and 1 year versus 3 years of maintenance. Eur Urol. 2013;63(3):462–72.
12. Ramirez-Backhaus M, Dominguez-Escrig J, Collado A, Rubio-Briones J, Solsona E. Restaging transurethral resection of bladder tumor for high-risk stage Ta and T1 bladder cancer. Curr Urol Rep. 2012;13(2):109–14.
13. Herr HW. Restaging transurethral resection of high risk superficial bladder cancer improves the initial response to bacillus Calmette-Guerin therapy. J Urol. 2005;174(6):2134–7.
14. Herr HW, Donat SM. Quality control in transurethral resection of bladder tumours. BJU Int. 2008;102(9 Pt B):1242–6.
15. Jocham D, Stepp H, Waidelich R. Photodynamic diagnosis in urology: state-of-the-art. Eur Urol. 2008;53(6):1138–48.
16. Burger M, Grossman HB, Droller M, et al. Photodynamic diagnosis of non-muscle-invasive bladder cancer with hexaminolevulinate cystoscopy: a meta-analysis of detection and recurrence based on raw data. Eur Urol. 2013;64(5):846–54.
17. Herr HW, Sogani PC. Does early cystectomy improve the survival of patients with high risk superficial bladder tumors? J Urol. 2001;166(4):1296–9.
18. Lotan Y, Roehrborn CG. Sensitivity and specificity of commonly available bladder tumor markers versus cytology: results of a comprehensive literature review and meta-analyses. Urology. 2003;61(1):109–18. discussion 118.
19. Konety BR. Molecular markers in bladder cancer: a critical appraisal. Urol Oncol. 2006;24(4):326–37.
20. Gudjonsson S, Blackberg M, Chebil G, et al. The value of bladder mapping and prostatic urethra biopsies for detection of carcinoma in situ (CIS). BJU Int. 2012;110(2 Pt 2):E41–5.
21. Witjes JA, Redorta JP, Jacqmin D, et al. Hexaminolevulinate-guided fluorescence cystoscopy in the diagnosis and follow-up of patients with non-muscle-invasive bladder cancer: review of the evidence and recommendations. Eur Urol. 2010;57(4):607–14.
22. Kamat AM, Karam JA, Grossman HB, Kader AK, Munsell M, Dinney CP. Prospective trial to identify optimal bladder cancer surveillance protocol: reducing costs while maximizing sensitivity. BJU Int. 2011;108(7):1119–23.
23. Bubendorf L, Grilli B. UroVysion multiprobe FISH in urinary cytology. Methods Mol Med. 2004;97:117–31.
24. Sarosdy MF, Schellhammer P, Bokinsky G, et al. Clinical evaluation of a multi-target fluorescent in situ hybridization assay for detection of bladder cancer. J Urol. 2002;168(5):1950–4.

25. Whitson J, Berry A, Carroll P, Konety B. A multicolour fluorescence in situ hybridization test predicts recurrence in patients with high-risk superficial bladder tumours undergoing intravesical therapy. BJU Int. 2009;104(3):336–9.
26. Highshaw RA, Tanaka ST, Evans CP. deVere White RW. Is bladder biopsy necessary at three or six months post BCG therapy? Urol Oncol. 2003;21(3):207–9.
27. Kamat AM, Dickstein RJ, Messetti F, et al. Use of fluorescence in situ hybridization to predict response to bacillus Calmette-Guerin therapy for bladder cancer: results of a prospective trial. J Urol. 2012;187(3):862–7.
28. Mengual L, Marin-Aguilera M, Ribal MJ, et al. Clinical utility of fluorescent in situ hybridization for the surveillance of bladder cancer patients treated with bacillus Calmette-Guerin therapy. Eur Urol. 2007;52(3):752–9.
29. Raitanen MP, Aine R, Rintala E, et al. Differences between local and review urinary cytology in diagnosis of bladder cancer. An interobserver multicenter analysis. Eur Urol. 2002;41(3):284–9.
30. Hara T, Takahashi M, Gondo T, et al. Discrepancies between cytology, cystoscopy and biopsy in bladder cancer detection after Bacille Calmette-Guerin intravesical therapy. Int J Urol. 2009;16(2):192–5.
31. Gayed BA, Seideman C, Lotan Y. Cost effectiveness of fluorescence in situ hybridization in patients with atypical cytology for the detection of urothelial carcinoma. J Urol. 2013;190(4):1181–6.
32. Skacel M, Fahmy M, Brainard JA, et al. Multitarget fluorescence in situ hybridization assay detects transitional cell carcinoma in the majority of patients with bladder cancer and atypical or negative urine cytology. J Urol. 2003;169(6):2101–5.

Tracy M. Downs, Daniel J. Lee, and Douglas S. Scherr

20.1 Introduction

Urothelial carcinoma of the bladder (UCB) remains a significant health problem, accounting for more than 15,000 deaths annually [1]. Approximately 75 % of UCB patients will present with non-muscle-invasive bladder cancer (NMIBC), which includes stages Ta, T1, or carcinoma in situ (CIS). However, 50–70 % of those patients will eventually recur and approximately 10–20 % will progress to muscle-invasive disease [2].

Intravesical therapy has been increasingly utilized to help reduce the risks of recurrence and progression. The use of bacillus Calmette-Guerin (BCG) was first described in 1976, and has since become the primary first-line treatment for NMIBC [3]. Several large meta-analyses of randomized controlled trials have confirmed that the addition of BCG after transurethral resection (TUR) significantly improves recurrence rates compared to TUR alone [4–8], however up to

50 % of patients will develop recurrence within 5 years of induction therapy with BCG [9].

The management of patients who develop recurrence after BCG therapy has continued to evolve. The 2013 guidelines by the European Association of Urology [10] defined the different categories of unsuccessful treatment with intravesical BCG. The presence of a muscle-invasive bladder cancer (MIBC) on follow-up was defined as BCG failure. BCG-refractory disease was defined as: (1) the presence of a high-grade (HG) NMIBC present 3 months after BCG treatment; (2) the presence of CIS at both 3 and 6 months post-BCG treatment; or (3) the appearance of HG tumor during BCG therapy. The recurrence of HG tumor after completion of BCG therapy despite initial response can be defined as BCG relapsing. BCG intolerance indicates those who experienced severe side effects from BCG that prevented further instillation before completing induction.

T.M. Downs, M.D., F.A.C.S. (✉)
Department of Urology, University of Wisconsin
School of Medicine and Public Health,
1685 Highland Avenue, Madison, WI 53705, USA
e-mail: downs@urology.wisc.edu

D.J. Lee, M.D. • D.S. Scherr, M.D.
James Buchanan Brady Department of Urology,
Weill Cornell Medical College, New York
Presbyterian Hospital, 525 East 68th Street,
Starr 900, New York, NY 10065, USA
e-mail: djl7001@nyp.org; dss2001@med.cornell.edu

20.1.1 Rationale for Additional BCG After Recurrence

Although RC may offer the best oncologic outcomes in patients who recur and/or progress after BCG treatment, the potential benefits of RC must be weighed against the risk and impact on quality of life. Certain patients may be unable to tolerate RC because of coexisting medical conditions, or

B.R. Konety and S.S. Chang (eds.), *Management of Bladder Cancer:
A Comprehensive Text With Clinical Scenarios*, DOI 10.1007/978-1-4939-1881-2_20,
© Springer Science+Business Media New York 2015

would refuse definitive therapy in favor of a less invasive alternative with decreased treatment-related morbidities. For BCG failure, namely MIBC after BCG treatment, RC is the gold standard [10].

BCG-refractory patients can be considered a high-risk group and strongly considered for RC. In patients who have HG NMIBC recurrence within 3 months of BCG treatment, there is an associated progression rate of 82 % compared to a rate of 25 % for those who were not BCG refractory [11, 12]. A second and third course of BCG can give response rates of 30–50 % and 10–18 %, respectively [13–16]. However, among patients who developed recurrence after two treatments of BCG, up to 80 % of the patients will progress and develop MIBC or metastatic disease [16].

In patients who have CIS present at 3 months, an additional course of BCG can achieve a complete response in greater than 50 % of patients [17]. However, patients with CIS who recur after BCG have a 50 % disease progression rate with higher rates of disease-specific mortality [16, 18].

20.1.2 Side Effects

Intravesical BCG can produce moderate to severe local and systemic side effects. In the Southwest Oncology Group (SWOG) trial on maintenance BCG, only 16 % of the patients were able to complete all of the instillations of the 3-year maintenance trial [19]. The European Organization for Research and Treatment of Cancer (EORTC) trial 30911 similarly found that only 29 % of the patients were able to tolerate the full 3-year maintenance instillations of BCG [20]. In another large trial of 1,300 patients, EORTC 30962 found that there was no correlation between duration of BCG treatment and the number of instillations with the number or severity of the side effects [21]. Side effects requiring stoppage of treatment were experienced within the first year on the maintenance schedule for both the EORTC 30911 and 30962, indicating that the side effect profile is not likely dependent on the number of instillations.

20.2 Options for BCG Failures

20.2.1 BCG and Interferon

20.2.1.1 Indications
Interferons are glycoproteins that are produced in response to antigenic stimuli, and have been implicated in multiple antitumor activities including the inhibition of nucleotide synthesis, stimulation of cytokine release, enhanced natural killer cell activity, inhibition of angiogenesis, and upregulation of tumor antigens [22]. Interferon as a solitary agent is more expensive and less effective than BCG in preventing recurrence, eradicating residual disease, and treating CIS. As a single agent, the long-term efficacy rates of interferon for treating CIS is less than 15 % [23], with recurrence rates of 16–60 % that are generally higher to those of BCG alone [24, 25]. Several trials combining BCG and interferon suggest that the combination of BCG and interferon can decrease the potential dosage of BCG and reduce its side effects while maintaining similar efficacy rates, especially in those who had recurrence after BCG treatment (Table 20.1).

20.2.1.2 Side Effects
Interferon is well tolerated with few systemic symptoms that are often well-tolerated. The most common symptoms are flu-like symptoms (~20 %), and cystitis rates are usually <5 %.

20.2.1.3 Results
A recently published randomized controlled trial [28] of interferon with epirubicin compared to BCG for treatment after resection of HG T1 UCB found a significantly lower 5-year recurrence-free survival rate for those treated with the combined interferon/epirubicin compared to BCG (38 % vs. 59 %, respectively).

The progression-free survival rates (78 % vs. 77 %, respectively) and cancer-specific survival rates (90 % vs. 92 %, respectively) were not significantly different between the two arms of the trial. The treatment failure rate in each arm was 75 % (complete response rate—75 % in each study arm).

Table 20.1 Select large trials of interferon

Reference	Patient population	N	Treatment	Follow-up	Definition of "failure"	Outcome	Comment
Rajala et al. [26]	HG NMIBC	200	Epirubicin vs. IFN vs. TUR alone	72 months	Time to initial recurrence starting 3 months after TUR	Recurrence: 46 % vs. 68 % vs. 73 %	Single immediate postoperative instillation of IFN of 50 MU did not reduce risk of recurrence
Boccardo et al. [27]	HG NMIBC	287	MMC vs. IFN	NA	Recurrence starting 3 months after TUR	Median time to recurrence 36 months vs. 21 months	MMC was more effective than IFN in preventing recurrence
Hemdan et al. [28]	HG T1 UCB	250	BCG vs. epirubicin+IFN	7 years	Recurrence starting 6 months after TUR	Complete response: **25** % vs. **25** % RFS 59 % vs. 38 %	BCG was more effective than combination epirubicin+IFN in recurrence-free survival
Joudi et al. [29]	BCG refractory and BCG naïve	1,007	Low dose BCG+IFN (for refractory) vs. BCG+IFN (for BCG naïve)	24 months	Recurrence starting 3 months after TUR	Disease free: BCG refractory: 45 % BCG naïve: 59 %	BCG+IFN was effective in BCG naïve and refractory patients
Nepple et al. [30]	BCG naïve	670	BCG+RDA vitamins vs. BCG+mega Vit vs. BCG/IFN+RDA vs. BCG/IFN+mega Vit	24 months	Recurrence starting 3 months after TUR	Disease-free: 63 % vs. 59 % vs. 55 % vs. 61 %	Addition of IFN to 1/3 dose BCG provides no further benefit

More recently, interferon has been studied as a combination treatment with BCG, especially in patients who developed recurrence after BCG therapy. In a large multicenter phase II trial, 467 patients who had recurrence on BCG were then treated with a 6-week induction course of low-dose BCG plus 50 million units of interferon with three similar treatments at 3, 9, and 15 months after induction. At a median follow-up of 2 years, 45 % remained tumor free for those treated with BCG/interferon in the salvage setting, compared to a rate of 60 % in the BCG-naïve group; only 8 % of the patients experienced progression in each group [29, 31]. In a subset analysis, having two or more BCG failures, higher stage disease and shorter time to recurrence were independently predictive of a poor response to BCG/ interferon [32]. These trials indicate that BCG/ interferon can be used effectively in the salvage setting, with potentially decreased toxicity associated with the lower BCG doses used. When interpreting the results of all trials that seek to look at BCG-refractory disease, however, one must know how the definition of BCG failure was designed. For example, in those individuals that have persistent CIS 3 months after completing an induction course of BCG, by simply waiting an additional 3 months with no further therapy, approximately 20 % of patients will convert to a negative bladder biopsy [33]. As a result, in all trials that evaluate BCG-refractory therapies, it is important to understand their definition of BCG failure, as most trials will have a built-in 20 % response rate before the trial even begins. The optimal time to evaluate BCG failure is at 6 months. In addition, it is unclear if BCG alone in continued maintenance dosing is as effective as BCG + interferon.

20.2.1.4 Costs

Each treatment of interferon ranges from US$670 to US$1,340, while BCG costs around $150 per vial. The data from the trials and the difference in costs indicate that interferon is not more cost-effective and should not be used as a first-line agent.

20.2.2 Valrubicin

20.2.2.1 Indications

Valrubicin is a semisynthetic analog of doxorubicin, and is currently the only FDA-approved intravesical chemotherapeutic agent for the treatment of BCG-refractory carcinoma in-situ (CIS) in patients who are not candidates for RC. Its structure is modified from doxorubicin to allow rapid intracellular uptake with decreased cardiotoxicity. The mechanisms of action of valrubicin are to inhibit nucleoside incorporation into the nucleic acids, causing cell cycle arrest, and the inhibition of topoisomerase II that stops DNA synthesis.

20.2.2.2 Side Effects

Valrubicin is very well tolerated with low side-effects. The majority of adverse events are related to lower urinary tract symptoms with minimal systemic absorption.

20.2.2.3 Results

In a multi-institutional, nonrandomized open-label trial, 90 patients were enrolled who developed recurrence after BCG for CIS, and received 6 weekly instillations of 800 mg of valrubicin [34]. Nineteen (21 %) of the patients demonstrated a complete response initially, but only 8 % (7/90) remained disease-free at a follow-up of 2.5 years [34]. Recurrence occurred in 79 patients, and 44 eventually underwent RC, with 15 % having $\geq$pT3 disease on surgical pathology. In a complementary phase II/III trial of 80 patients with BCG-refractory disease that received valrubicin [35], the complete response rate was 18 %, with recurrence free survival rates of 10 % and 4 % at 1 and 2 years, respectively.

20.2.2.4 Costs

Each treatment of valrubicin is approximately $6,000 per treatment [36]. Future studies will be necessary to validate utility and cost-effectiveness of valrubicin and similar intravesical therapeutic agents.

20.2.3 Mitomycin C

20.2.3.1 Indications

Mitomycin C (MMC) is an alkylating agent that prevents DNA synthesis. The 2007 American Urologic Association guidelines support the use of a single instillation of MMC in the immediate postoperative period to reduce the risk of recurrence in patients with NMIBC (Table 20.2). However it has also been used as a weekly instillation for 6–8 weeks at dose ranges from 20 to 60 mg and in various maintenance schedules.

20.2.3.2 Side Effects

MMC is well tolerated, with the most common side effects including contact dermatitis (ranging from 8 to 19 %) and LUTS. In a small population of patients, a significant cystitis can occur that results in severe hematuria, dysuria, and bladder inflammation.

20.2.3.3 Results

In a meta-analysis comparing MMC with TUR compared to TUR alone [40], MMC provided a relative risk reduction of 38 % in tumor recurrence. In another meta-analysis comparing nine clinical trials of BCG compared to MMC, with a median overall follow-up time of 26 months [8], the tumor progression rates were 7.67 % for those who received BCG compared to 9.44 % for MMC. Overall, there were no significant differences in the tumor progression rates between those who received BCG compared to MMC. However, only those who received maintenance BCG had 34 % decreased odds of developing tumor progression compared to MMC ($p=0.02$).

The evidence for using MMC in BCG-refractory NMIBC is limited. In a randomized trial of 261 patients with NMIBC comparing BCG and MMC [38], only 19 % (4/21) of those who received MMC after failing BCG were disease-free at 3 years. In a randomized phase III trial of gemcitabine compared to MMC for patients with recurrent NMIBC (83.5 % of whom were BCG-refractory), the recurrence rate was 61 % for those who received MMC.

Long-term maintenance MMC may also improve recurrence rates. In a large randomized trial [39], 495 patients were treated with either short-term BCG or MMC (6-week instillations) or long-term MMC (6 weekly MMC treatments followed by monthly treatments for 3 years).

Table 20.2 Select large trials of mitomycin C

Reference	Patient population	N	Treatment	Follow-up	Outcome	Comment
Lamm et al. [37]	HG NMIBC	469	Maintenance BCG vs. Maintenance MMC	30 months	Recurrence 34.6 % vs. 46.7 % Median time to recurrence 44 months vs. 22 months	Maintenance BCG superior to MMC in prevention of recurrence, but no difference in survival
Malmstrom et al. [38]	HG NMIBC	261	Maintenance BCG vs. MMC	64 months	Disease free: 47 % vs. 34 % No difference in progression or overall survival	BCG more effective in recurrence prophylaxis, but no difference for survival or progression
Friedrich et al. [39]	NMIBC	495	BCG×6 weeks vs. MMC×6 weeks vs. MMC×3 years	2.9 years	Recurrence 25.1 % vs. 25.7 % vs. 10.4 %. 3-yr RFS: 65.5 % vs. 68.6 % vs. 86.1 %	Long-term MMC reduces the risk of recurrence without enhanced toxicity

Patients who underwent long-term MMC had higher recurrence-free survival rates (86.1 %) than short-term BCG or MMC (68.6 % and 65.5 %, respectively) without any increases in adverse events.

20.2.3.4 Costs

Each administration of immediate intravesical mitomycin C at the completion of a TURBT cost $246 per single dose of mitomycin C (MMC). Lee et al. estimated that routine utilization of postoperative chemotherapy would have prevented cancer recurrence in 46,000 patients annually, thereby leading to $3,847 of cost savings per patient [41].

20.2.4 Gemcitabine

20.2.4.1 Indications

Gemcitabine is an antimetabolite that is cytotoxic and blocks DNA synthesis and causes apoptosis. Gemcitabine has been used to treat advanced bladder cancer with effective results and a relatively safe adverse effect profile. Multiple randomized clinical trials have been published utilizing intravesical gemcitabine for NMIBC (Table 20.3).

20.2.4.2 Side Effects

Intravesical gemcitabine is generally well tolerated with trial dropout rates generally <10 %, however severe dysuria and a low rate of grade 3 adverse events were noted in two phase II trials [42, 43].

20.2.4.3 Results

As a first-line agent for NMIBC, one trial compared intravesical gemcitabine (6 weekly instillations of 2,000 mg) to BCG (6 weekly instillations) [45], and found higher recurrence rates for gemcitabine compared to BCG (53.1 % vs. 28.1 %, respectively), with a mean recurrence-free survival of 25.6 months for gemcitabine compared to 39.4 months for BCG. However, this trial only enrolled 64 patients at a single center. Three other trials focused on the use of intravesical gemcitabine for patients with recurrence after BCG therapy. In a randomized phase III trial [44] comparing intravesical gemcitabine to MMC for patients who developed recurrence after prior therapy, intravesical gemcitabine had higher disease-free rates (72 %) than MMC (61 %), and lower progression rates (40 % vs. 45.5 %, respectively). In another trial, Di Lorenzo et al. [46] randomized 92 patients who developed NMIBC recurrence after BCG therapy to receive 6 weeks

Table 20.3 Select large trials of gemcitabine

Reference	Patient population	N	Treatment	Follow-up	Outcome	Comment
Addeo et al. [44]	Recurrent NMIBC after BCG	120	Gemcitabine vs. MMC	36 months	Recurrence: 28 % vs. 39 % Progression 11 % vs. 18 % Adverse events 39 % vs. 72 %	Gemcitabine has more favorable efficacy and toxicity profile than MMC
Porena et al. [45]	NMIBC	64	Gemcitabine vs. BCG	44 months	Recurrence 53.1 % vs. 28.1 % RFS 25.6 months vs. 39.4 months No difference in toxicity	Gemcitabine inferior to BCG in preventing recurrence; but possible alternative for those who are BCG intolerant
Di Lorenzo et al. [46]	Recurrent NMIBC after BCG	92	Gemcitabine vs. BCG		Recurrence 52.5 % vs. 87.5 % RFS 3.9 months vs. 3.2 months	Gemcitabine decreases recurrence rates in BCG-refractory patients, but no difference in RFS or progression

of gemcitabine (with additional 3 weekly treatments at 3, 6, and 12 months) or BCG (at the same schedule). In this study, treatment with gemcitabine was associated with lower recurrence rates (52.5 % vs. 87.5 %), lower progression rates (33 % vs. 37.5 %), and longer recurrence-free survival rates (3.9 months vs. 3.2 months) than compared to another round of BCG. These findings were confirmed by a phase II single arm SWOG trial [42] of intravesical gemcitabine for patients who had recurrence after two prior courses of BCG, which found disease-free rates of 47 %, 28 %, and 21 % at 3 months, 1 year, and 2 years, respectively. A combination of intravesical therapies may help improve recurrence and progression rates in BCG-refractory patients. A retrospective review [47] of 47 patients who received 6 weeks of intravesical gemcitabine followed by an instillation of MMC found a complete response rate of 68 %, with 1- and 2-year recurrence-free survival rates of 48 % and 38 %, respectively. Thirty percent of the patients remained free of recurrence with a median time to follow-up of 26 months.

20.2.4.4 Costs

Although promising, these findings need to be substantiated with a prospective randomized trial. Intravesical gemcitabine appears to be safe and effective in BCG-refractory disease as a second-line agent, but has yet to show any effectiveness as a first-line agent in NMIBC. In addition, gemcitabine is one of the more expensive intravesical agents, with costs ranging from US$540 to US$1,080 per dose.

20.2.5 Intravesical Docetaxel

Docetaxel is a microtubule depolymerization inhibitor that has been effective for a wide variety of malignancies. The initial phase I clinical trials of intravesical docetaxel for BCG-refractory NMIBC found a 56 % complete response rate after a 6 weekly instillation course with minimal side effects. In the largest series of intravesical docetaxel use in patients with BCG-refractory NMIBC, 59 % had a complete response initially, with 1- and 3-year recurrence-free survival rates of 40 % and 25 %, respectively. Intravesical docetaxel is well-tolerated, with no grade 3 or 4 toxicities reported in the studies.

20.3 Novel Therapies

20.3.1 *nab*-Paclitaxel

Many of the novel agents in development aim to improve delivery of the target drug to tumor cells. Nanoparticle albumin-bound paclitaxel (*nab*-paclitaxel) is a novel agent in the taxane family that is added to albumin to improve solubility and intracellular transport, two characteristics that are essential for successful intravesical agents. In phase III trials for breast cancer, *nab*-paclitaxel was shown to have better efficacy and safety profile compared to standard paclitaxel in systemic breast cancer therapy [48]. A phase I trial using intravesical *nab*-paclitaxel was performed with 18 patients who had recurrent NMIBC after prior intravesical therapy (including MMC and/or BCG), and were given 6 weekly instillations of *nab*-paclitaxel on a dose escalation scheme. Of the 18 patients, 28 % (5/18) had a complete initial response 12 weeks after therapy, with no patients reporting grade 2 or higher local toxicities. The phase II trial of intravesical *nab*-paclitaxel is ongoing with larger cohorts and follow-up time, and will provide more information on the efficacy of this novel agent for recurrent NMIBC.

20.3.2 Improved Immunotherapy

Oportuzumab monatox (VB4-845) is a recombinant fusion protein with a humanized anti-epithelial cell adhesion molecule antibody linked to Psuedomonas exotoxin A. When the drug is internalized by the tumor cell, the exotoxin is released and causes apoptosis. In a phase II trial [49], 46 patients who were refractory to BCG were given oportuzumab monatox. Overall the complete response rates at 3 and 12 months were 40 % and 15.6 %, respectively. The treatment was well tolerated with the majority of the adverse events being mild to moderate in severity in local bladder symptoms.

Another novel delivery system uses gene therapy and recombinant adenovirus to transduce urothelium to improve delivery of interferon and maintain high levels of interferon. In a phase I trial [50] in 17 BCG-refractory patients, recombinant adenovirus-mediated interferon was combined with a novel excipient, SCH 209702, to improve transduction. There was no dose-limiting toxicity noted, and no grade 3 or higher adverse events. High and prolonged interferon levels were noted in the urine, and 43 % had a complete response at 3 months and 14.3 % were disease free at more than 2 years follow up.

20.3.3 Device-Assisted Therapy

Three main device-assisted therapy techniques are under investigation in the treatment of recurrent or refractory-BCG NMIBC: thermochemotherapy, electromotive drug administration, and photodynamic therapy.

Using a special catheter with internal thermocouples, the Synergo® system heats the bladder wall to about 41–44 °C during the installation of agents such as MMC, while simultaneously cooling the urethra to prevent damage. The heated environment can improve cellular membrane permeability and therefore penetration of MMC, and can increase the cytotoxicity of MMC itself [51]. In an early retrospective series of 52 patients comparing MMC with chemohyperthermia (C-HT) to MMC alone, the complete response rate was found to be 66 % in the C-HT group compared to 22 % in MMC alone [52]. This improvement in response to MMC with C-HT was confirmed in multiple subsequent studies. In a meta-analysis of 22 studies on C-HT, the overall risk ratio of those treated with C-HT compared to MMC alone was 41 %, indicating a recurrence risk reduction of 59 % with C-HT [53, 54]. This response appears durable, as the estimated 10-year disease-free survival rate for C-HT patients was 52.8 % compared to 14.6 % for MMC alone [54]. At a median follow-up of 90 months, recurrence rates were 40 % for C-HT

patients and 80 % for those receiving MMC alone [54]. This improvement in efficacy with C-HT can also be seen in patients with recurrent/refractory NMIBC. In two prospective trials of patients with recurrence after BCG, 1- and 2-year disease-free survival rates were 77–85 % and 56–59 %, respectively, after receiving C-HT [55, 56].

Electromotive drug administration (EMDA) creates an electrical gradient across the bladder wall to temporarily enhance cell permeability to intravesical agents such as MMC. In a prospective trial of 108 patients with NMIBC comparing MMC alone, MMC with EMDA, and BCG alone, a complete response at 6 months was seen in 31 %, 58 %, and 64 %, respectively [57]. A large multicenter prospective randomized trial compared three treatment arms in patients without prior intravesical therapy for NMIBC: TUR alone, TUR with MMC, and EDMA with MMC [58]. Compared to TUR alone or MMC, those who received EDMA with MMC had lower recurrence rates (64 % and 59 % compared to 38 %, respectively), and significantly higher disease-free intervals (12 and 16 months compared to 52 months, respectively). Although no trials have been performed with EDMA on patients who developed recurrence after BCG or prior intravesical therapy, these results appear durable and are promising for future utilization.

Photodynamic therapy (PDT) utilizes photosensitizers that can be activated by specific wavelengths of light to cause cell death by the creation of free radicals that targets the microvasculature and drives an acute inflammatory response. The first generations of photosensitizers had severe adverse effects. Photofrin® was extremely effective resulting in high tumor-free rates, but caused prolonged skin photosensitivity [59]. Another early trial was performed with oral 5-aminolevulinic acid (5-ALA), which caused notable adverse effects such as hypotension and tachycardia [60]. A single-center study of intravesical 5-ALA [61] found a recurrence-free rate of 51.6 % after a median follow-up of 23.7 months, with minimal adverse events. The recurrence-free rate in patients who had failed prior BCG therapy was 40 % (4/10). A prospective trial of a next-generation photosensitizer, Radachlorin, in 34 patients who had recurrence of NMIBC after BCG therapy found that the recurrence-free rate at 1 and 2 years was 90.9 % and 64.4 %, respectively [62], with no grade ≥3 adverse events reported. Although promising, further randomized prospective trials will be required to evaluate the use of PDT in the management of NMIBC.

20.4 Role of Radical Cystectomy in BCG-Refractory Disease

In non-muscle-invasive bladder cancer (NMIBC) approximately 70 % of patients present as pTa, 20 % as pT1, and 10 % with carcinoma in situ (CIS) lesions. Recurrence is the main problem (in ≤80 % of patients) for pTa NMIBC patients, whereas progression (in ≤45 % of patients) is the main threat in pT1 and CIS NMIBC [63]. Management of intermediate- and high-risk bladder cancer patients remains one of the most difficult problems in urologic practice. Because these tumors are potentially lethal, early identification of patients suited for BCG treatment or radical cystectomy is essential [64].

The same principles apply when giving BCG for recurrent disease as it does when considering BCG for treatment of the primary non-muscle-invasive bladder tumor. The choice between further chemotherapy or additional BCG immunotherapy depends on the risk that needs to be reduced; recurrence or progression. For example, in a multifocal low-grade papillary tumor (pTa) the 5-year risk of disease progression, based on the EORTC risk calculator [65] is very low (5–8 %), so the goal of BCG therapy in this clinical scenario is to reduce or delay disease recurrence. On the other hand, in a patient diagnosed with her first bladder tumor being a pT1G3 single tumor which is 5 cm in size, the estimated 5-year risk of disease progression, based on the EORTC risk calculator [65] is 17 %, so the goal of BCG therapy for such a patient is to reduce or prevent disease progression.

A logical and very challenging question in intermediate- and high-risk NMIBC patients whose tumors recur after treatment with intra-vesical BCG therapy is: "When is radical cystectomy indicated?" The European Association of Urology (EAU) published an update in 2013 [10], which highlights the NMIBC patients with the highest risk of disease progression. These are patients with the following characteristics [65–67]: (a) multiple and/or large (>3 cm) T1, (HG/G3) tumors, (b) T1, (HG/G3) tumors with concurrent CIS, (c) recurrent T1, (HG/G3) tumors, (d) T1, G3 and CIS in prostatic urethra, and (e) micropapillary variant of urothelial carcinoma. In these cases, discussing immediate radical cystectomy and conservative treatment with BCG instillation is recommended by the EAU. Delay of radical cystectomy in such cases might lead to decreased disease-specific survival (Level 3 evidence) [68].

To understand these recommendations, we need to review the prognostic factors for disease progression, understand the rationale for radical cystectomy in NMIBC, and analyze the published literature to ascertain if it is possible to identify patients at high risk of BCG failure who would benefit from immediate radical cystectomy or be limited to a single cycle of intravesical therapy prior to radical cystectomy.

20.5 Prognostic Factors for Progression

Fortunately, progression to muscle-invasive bladder cancer (MIBC) is much less frequent than recurrence in NMIBC. Sylvester et al. [65], in an attempt to individualize prediction of progression, calculated the probability of disease progression using data from 2,596 patients who participated in seven European Organisation for Research and Treatment of Cancer (EORTC) trials. The weight score was based on six variables (Table 20.4) and the EAU adopted this system in its guidelines and defined patients at low, intermediate and high risk for disease progression [10, 65]. Five-year probabilities of disease progression range from <1 to 45 % depending on the risk score (Table 20.5) [65]. Multiplicity and tumor size are stronger predictors of recurrence [65], while the most important variables for

Table 20.4 Weighting used to calculate recurrence and progression scores [65]

Factor	Recurrence	Progression
Number of tumors		
Single	0	0
2–7	3	3
>8	6	3
Tumor diameter		
<3 cm	0	0
>3 cm	3	3
Prior recurrence		
Primary	0	0
<1 recurrence/year	2	2
>1 recurrence/year	4	2
Stage category		
Ta	0	0
T1	1	4
Concomitant CIS		
Yes	0	0
No	1	6
Grade (WHO 1973)		
G1	0	0
G2	1	0
G3	2	5
Total score	0–17	0–23

Table 20.5 Probability of progression according to total score [10, 65]

	Probability of progression		
	1 year % (95 % CI)	5 years % (95 % CI)	Progression risk group
Progression score			
0	0.2 (0–0.7)	0.8 (0–1.7)	Low risk
2–6	1 (0.4–1.6)	6 (5–8)	Intermediate risk
7–13	5 (4–7)	17 (14–20)	High risk
14–23	17 (10–24)	45 (35–55)	High risk

CI confidence interval

prediction of progression are CIS, grade 3 and stage T1. The main limitation of the EORTC risk tables is that most patients were treated by "old" intravesical regimens and guidelines [63].

The improvements in repeat/second-look TURBT, single chemotherapeutic instillation after TUR, and increased use of induction and maintenance BCG therapy were not mainstays of clinical care in the clinical trials used to construct the EORTC risk tables. Fernando-Gomez et al.

[69] reported the data on prognostic factors from four Club Urologico Espanol de Tratamiento Oncologico (CUETO) trials, in which 1,062 patients received 5–6 months of BCG. Recurrence at first cystoscopy, stage, grade and prior tumor were each prognostic factors for progression in the multivariate analysis. Concomitant CIS was only significant in the univariate analysis [69]. Patients in the CUETO study included a higher percentage of high-risk patients than in the EORTC study and the administration of BCG in the CUETO study was more efficacious in treating CIS [65, 69]. A similar limitation exists in both the EORTC and CUETO studies. The percentage of CIS and G3 was low in both studies (i.e. 4 % and 10 % [65] and 7.5 % and 25 % [69], respectively). A separate analysis of high-risk patients was not reported in CUETO [69], but a separate analysis of 194 patients with T1G3 in the EORTC study [65] reported that the presence of CIS conferred a poor prognosis, with a 1- and 5-year progression probabilities of 29 % and 74 % respectively.

20.5.1 Substaging of T1 Non-muscle-Invasive Bladder Cancer

The varied prognosis of T1 NMIBC underscores the heterogeneous nature of this disease as the clinical outcomes vary from patient to patient. A critical challenge involves our ability to accurately stage pT1 tumors. Bol et al. [70] found an 80 % agreement, amongst three expert pathologists, when he asked them to reevaluate 130 Ta and T1 tumors. Thirty-five of the original 63 T1 tumors (35/63–56 %) were downstaged to pTa and 8/63 (13 %) were upstaged to muscle-invasive bladder cancer by the reviewers. Thus only 31 % of the original T1 tumors were reclassified similar to the original pT1 stage [70]. Several studies have demonstrated that substaging of T1 NMIBC (pT1a/pT1b/pT1c) is an important predictor of progression [71–75]. Two studies specifically addressed T1 substaging in patients treated with BCG therapy. Kondylis et al. [76] found no difference in progression for substage, and Orsola et al. [75] found a significant difference in progression-free survival (PFS) for T1a compared to T1b+T1c. One of the limitations, with pT1 substaging is that the muscularis mucosae and vascular plexus is not able to be identified in up to 35 % of cases [71–75]. Cheng et al. [77] explored alternative approaches to substaging, and measured depth of invasion by micrometer. In 100 % of the cases ($N=83$ TUR specimens) depth of invasion could be measured. Five-year PFS was 93 % for patients with <1.5 mm invasion compared to 67 % for patients with >1.5 mm subepithelial invasion. Additionally, Van der Aa et al. [78] defined microinvasive pT1 as a single spot of invasion seen only within one high-power field (under the microscope) and classified pT1 cases not meeting these two criteria as extensive invasive pT1. He could reproduce his system in 43/53 (81 %) of the tumors. While these data support pathologic substaging, the optimal system has yet to be determined and substaging is not routinely applied in routine pathologic assessment.

While a variety of molecular markers have been investigated to provide a better assessment of NMIBC prognosis [79–82], to date the value of such markers over conventional clinicopathologic variables is not clear.

20.6 Rationale for Cystectomy in NMIBC

Unfortunately, treatment options are limited for patients with recurrence after BCG therapy. Patients with BCG-refractory NMIBC have a 50 % chance of disease progression and should be considered for cystectomy [16]. Historically, the response rates to repeat BCG courses decrease significantly and each additional course is accompanied by a 7 % increase in the risk of progression [16].

Up to one-third of patients with high-grade T1 urothelial carcinoma initially treated with BCG die of bladder cancer [83, 84]. Nieder et al. [85] reported a 19 % death rate from bladder cancer, in patients who underwent radical cystectomy after failing BCG for high-grade Ta or T1 bladder

cancer. Herr and colleagues [86] reported 15-year clinical outcomes for patients with high-grade T1 showing that 52 % of patients progressed to muscle invasion and 31 % died of their disease. In the same year, Cookson et al. [83] reported 15-year results in 84 patients with high-risk NMIBC treated with TUR±BCG. Disease progression occurred in 53 % of patients, 36 % underwent cystectomy and 34 % died of bladder cancer. Soloway et al. [87] retrospectively reviewed their institutional database to compare the pathologic stage after radical cystectomy in patients who received BCG across two different time periods. Patients who underwent radical cystectomy between 1992 and 2002 (group 1) were compared to those who had radical cystectomy between 2003 and 2007 (group 2). A total of 168 of 445 (38 %) patients received BCG prior to radical cystectomy and 152 patients were in the final analysis (group 1—$N=77$; group 2—$N=75$). No significant difference in the final pathologic stage was noted between the two groups. In group 1 patients, final pathologic stage was 43 %, 26 % and 11 %, respectively, for muscle-invasive disease, extravesical disease and lymph node metastasis. In group 2 patients, final pathologic stage was 52 %, 32 % and 16 %, respectively, for muscle-invasive disease, extravesical disease and lymph node metastasis. There was no statistically significant difference between the groups for final pathologic stage ($p=0.5$), and no difference was seen in a 5-year disease-specific survival ($p=0.2$).

Herr and Sogani [88] published one of the earlier studies to analyze disease-specific survival in patients who underwent early radical cystectomy versus delayed cystectomy in patients with high-risk superficial bladder cancer. Out of 307 patients with high-risk NMIBC treated with TURBT and BCG therapy, 90 (29 %) underwent radical cystectomy for recurrent tumor during a follow-up of 15–20 years. Of the 90 patients, 44 (49 %) survived a median of 96 months. Thirty-five out of 90 patients (39 %) recurred with NMIBC and 55/90 (61 %) recurred with muscle-invasive disease. In the group of patients who recurred with NMIBC, 92 % and 56 % survived who underwent radical cystectomy less than 2 years after initial BCG therapy compared to >2 years after BCG therapy. In the group of patients who recurred with MIBC, 41 % and 18 % survived when radical cystectomy was performed within and after 2 years of receiving BCG therapy. In the early and delayed groups, the median time to cystectomy was 11 months (range 3–23 months) and 55 months (range 25–228) respectively.

Lerner et al. [89] performed a secondary data analysis of a large prospective data set from the SWOG 8507 randomized trial of maintenance BCG to better understand patterns of recurrence and the impact of timing of recurrences on survival. A total of 501 patients were evaluated who were treated with induction BCG therapy and then were randomized to maintenance BCG or observation. Recurrence patterns were defined as early (<12 months) or late (>12 months) following randomization. Disease worsening events were defined as events that included diagnosis of T2 or greater, cystectomy, systemic chemotherapy, radiation therapy or other therapy indicative of abandonment of strategies for treatment of superficial disease. Two-hundred and fifty-one patients had disease recurrence (251/501 = 50 %) and 229 (46 %) died. Fifty-nine percent of the patients who died had recurrence following randomization. Early recurrence occurred in 117 (47 %) and late recurrence in 134 (53 %) patients respectively. The hazard ratio for death for patients who had early recurrence was 2.53 (95 % CI: 1.66–3.86; $p<0.001$) compared with those who did not progress or relapse, whereas late recurrence was associated with a hazard ratio of 2.31 (95 % CI: 1.44–3.70; $p<0.001$). Early recurrence was not associated with a higher risk of death relative to late recurrence ($p=0.69$). There was no significant difference in progression to T2 or greater between early and late recurrence (38/117—32 % vs. 34/134—25 %; $p=0.21$). Cystectomy was infrequently performed in this cohort of patients; 56/251 (22 %) who had recurrence underwent radical cystectomy. Although disease recurrence was associated with a higher risk of death, the timing of the recurrence (early vs. late) was not associated with a higher risk of death. Interestingly, the early recurrence group was more likely to have T2 or greater disease

(32 % vs. 25 %) with the median time from randomization to radical cystectomy being 20 months for patients with progression to muscle-invasive cancer. The 5-year survival probability for T2 or greater was 56 % from randomization and 44 % from time of radical cystectomy. For Tis or T1 the 5-year survival probability was 95 % at randomization and 54 % from the time of radical cystectomy. While the 5-year postoperative survival probability was lower than contemporary published series, these findings in this study are very similar to the findings reported by Herr et al. [88] For example, the 5-year survival after cystectomy was very similar for recurrent NMIBC after BCG therapy (56 % delayed RC group Herr study, 54 % Lerner study). The median time to radical cystectomy for the NMIBC group in the Herr study is 55 months compared to 42 months for the Lerner study [89]. In patients who recurred following BCG with MIBC, the 5-year survival for the early cystectomy group in the Herr study is 41 % (median time—11 months; range 3–23 months) and in the Lerner study 44 %, with the median time to cystectomy 20 months. Both studies highlight the impact of delaying radical cystectomy on disease-specific survival and how crucial or imperative it is to be selective and cautious in recommending bladder-sparing strategies in this high-risk group of bladder cancer patients.

Although cystectomy with urinary diversion is the treatment most likely to prevent disease progression, this procedure is associated with considerable short- and long-term morbidity and it may not be a feasible option for patients with significant comorbidities [90, 91].

20.7 Identifying Patients at High Risk of BCG Failure

Currently, there are no prognostic variables capable of accurately predicting, on an individual patient level, response to BCG therapy. The clinicopathologic variables associated with an increased risk of BCG failure include female gender [69], older age [92], multifocality [69], recurrent tumors [69], concurrent CIS (especially in the prostatic urethra) [67], lymphovascular invasion [93], detectable disease at 3-month surveillance cystoscopy [94], depth (and multifocality) of lamina propria invasion [95], timing of failure (i.e. early vs late) [96], and two or more prior courses of BCG therapy [32].

The goal in these high-risk patients is to identify prognostic factors for the patients who will benefit from immediate radical cystectomy or limited intravesical therapy (single cycle of intravesical therapy). Masood et al. [97] reported their prognostic factors in 21 pT1G3 patients treated with early cystectomy. Multifocal disease and CIS were associated with upstaging to MIBC, while absence of these variables was associated with pT0 at radical cystectomy [97]. Denzinger et al. [98] in a cohort of 132 T1G3 patients treated with BCG found that the combination of CIS, size and multifocal disease was predictive for cancer-related death [98]. Solsona et al. [94] reported the results on 191 high-risk NMIBC patients treated with intravesical therapy (BCG in 75 cases). In a multivariate model, prognostic factors associated with disease progression were: the presence of tumor at 3-month cystoscopy, T1, CIS, G3 or prostate mucosa involvement. The authors advocated for early cystectomy in these clinical scenarios [94]. Griffiths et al. [99] reported the outcome of primary carcinoma in situ (CIS) and CIS associated with Ta or T1 transitional cell carcinoma of the bladder treated with BCG. In this cohort of 135 patients, all underwent a standard course of six BCG instillations (no maintenance BCG). Patients were divided into group 1 ($N=23$) primary CIS only, group 2 ($N=37$) primary CIS and Ta, and group 3 ($N=75$) primary CIS and T1. The overall progression rates at 5 years were 20 %, 18 % and 49 %, respectively, for groups 1, 2 and 3. Cancer-specific survival rates were 83 %, 86 % and 59 %, respectively, for groups 1, 2 and 3. Patients in group 3 (CIS and T1) treated with BCG had disease progression significantly early than patients in groups 1 and 2 (log-rank test: $p=0.013$). While a complete response to BCG in group 3 (CIS and T1) significantly delayed time to progression (Cox regression $p=0.001$), it did not reduce death from transitional cell carcinoma. The authors concluded that while a single course of BCG was remarkably effective for primary CIS and CIS associated with Ta transitional cell carcinoma, it is suboptimal in patients with primary CIS associated with T1 transitional cell carcinoma.

20.7.1 The EORTC Risk Group Stratification Tables and Patients at High Risk of BCG Failure

For the majority of intermediate- and high-risk patients, it is reasonable for patients to receive adjuvant BCG therapy following TURBT. As outlined in other aspects of this chapter, close surveillance is critical because a narrow time window exists for cystectomy to be performed for high risk or T1G3 NMIBC patients when BCG fails [94, 98–102]. Denzinger et al. [101] offered early cystectomy to 105 patients with pT1G3 disease using several of the prognostic factors in the EORTC tables that are used to risk stratify patients. Study patients with two or three additional risk factors (size >3 cm, multifocality, and CIS) were offered early cystectomy. Fifty-four (51 %) of patients opted for early cystectomy while 49 % deferred cystectomy [101]. Early cystectomy was associated with a significantly better 10-year cancer-specific survival rate compared to deferred cystectomy—78 % versus 51 % ($p<0.01$) in this nonrandomized comparison [101]. The results of the group successfully managed with BCG were not reported.

The EORTC recurrence and progression tables (see Tables 20.4 and 20.5) potentially offer the clinician a rationale way to guide which patients should receive adjuvant BCG therapy patients (0 or 1 cycle) or immediate cystectomy. Similar to other published studies [94, 98, 99] the prognostic factors with the highest risk of disease progression are multifocal disease (3 points for progression; Table 20.4), clinical T1 (4 points for progression; Table 20.4), tumor size (3 points for progression; Table 20.4), concomitant CIS (6 points for progression; Table 20.4), and high grade (5 points for progression; Table 20.4). For newly diagnosed patients (primary

Table 20.6 EORTC risk tables: progression score in TaG3 and T1G3 patients

Primary tumor—Ta G3		Primary tumor—T1 G3	
Clinical scenarios	Progression score points	Clinical scenario	Progression score points
TaG3 <3 cm	0 + 5	T1G3 <3 cm	4 + 5
Single	0	Single	0
No CIS	0	No CIS	0
	Total score = 5		Total score = 9
TaG3	0 + 5	T1G3	4 + 5
<3 cm	0	<3 cm	0
Multifocal	3	Multifocal	3
No CIS	0	No CIS	0
	Total score = 8		Total score = 12
TaG3	0 + 5	T1G3	4 + 5
>3 cm	3	>3 cm	3
Single	0	Single	0
No CIS	0	No CIS	0
	Total score = 8		Total score = 12
TaG3	0 + 5	**T1G3**	4 + 5
>3 cm	3	**>3 cm**	3
Multifocal	3	**Multifocal**	3
No CIS	0	**No CIS**	0
	Total score = 11		**Total score = 15**
TaG3	0 + 5	**T1G3**	4 + 5
<3 cm	0	**<3 cm**	0
Single	0	**Single**	0
(+) CIS	6	**(+) CIS**	6
	Total score = 11		**Total score = 15**
TaG3	0 + 5	**T1G3**	4 + 5
<3 cm	0	**<3 cm**	0
Multifocal	3	**Multifocal**	3
(+) CIS	6	**(+) CIS**	6
	Total score = 14		**Total score = 18**
TaG3	0 + 5	**T1G3**	4 + 5
>3 cm	3	**>3 cm**	3
Single	0	**Single**	0
(+) CIS	6	**(+) CIS**	6
	Total score = 14		**Total score = 18**
TaG3	0 + 5	**T1G3**	4 + 5
> 3 cm	3	**> 3 cm**	3
Multifocal	3	**Multifocal**	3
(+) CIS	6	**(+) CIS**	6
	Total score = 17		**Total score = 21**

Bold represents clinical scenarios with total progression scores ≥13 (highest risk patients)

tumor), a progression score of ≥13 could be useful to help identify the highest-risk patients for BCG failure or patients in whom early cystectomy should be considered (Table 20.6). For example, the patient with a single tumor <3 cm T1G3 and concomitant CIS (T1—4 points, Grade 3—5 points, CIS—6 points) would have a total progression risk score of 15 (1-year probability of progression of 17 % and 5-year probability of progression of 45 %). In the newly diagnosed patient with stage TaG3 and associated CIS, the patient would also need to have multiple tumors or a tumor >3 cm in order to have a progression risk score $\geq$13. The prognostic factors in the EORTC recurrence and progression tables using the total progression score might be a reasonable approach in the management of this high-risk NMIBC patient group.

20.8 Conclusion

The management of patients who develop recurrence after BCG therapy has continued to evolve. Improved definitions of BCG failure, and a better understanding of prognostic factors associated with disease progression provide valuable knowledge to both patients and urologists. While radical cystectomy offers the best oncologic outcomes in patients who recur and/or progress after BCG treatment, several intravesical therapies and novel treatments exist for appropriately selected BCG failure patients and for patients unfit for radical cystectomy. Advancements in molecular medicine may afford the promise of improved patient outcomes in these high-risk non-muscle-invasive bladder cancer patients.

References

1. Siegel R, Naishadham D, Jemal A. Cancer statistics. CA Cancer J Clin. 2013;63:11–30.
2. Rubben H, Lutzeyer W, Fischer N, Deutz F, Lagrange W, Giani G. Natural history and treatment of low and high risk superficial bladder tumors. J Urol. 1988;139:283–5.
3. Morales A, Eidinger D, Bruce AW. Intracavitary Bacillus Calmette-Guerin in the treatment of superficial bladder tumors. J Urol. 1976;116:180–3.
4. Malmstrom PU, Sylvester RJ, Crawford DE, et al. An individual patient data meta-analysis of the long-term outcome of randomised studies comparing intravesical mitomycin C versus bacillus Calmette-Guerin for non-muscle-invasive bladder cancer. Eur Urol. 2009;56:247–56.
5. Shelley MD, Kynaston H, Court J, et al. A systematic review of intravesical bacillus Calmette-Guerin plus transurethral resection vs transurethral resection alone in Ta and T1 bladder cancer. BJU Int. 2001;88:209–16.
6. Shelley MD, Wilt TJ, Court J, Coles B, Kynaston H, Mason MD. Intravesical bacillus Calmette-Guerin is superior to mitomycin C in reducing tumour recurrence in high-risk superficial bladder cancer: a meta-analysis of randomized trials. BJU Int. 2004;93:485–90.
7. Han RF, Pan JG. Can intravesical bacillus Calmette-Guerin reduce recurrence in patients with superficial bladder cancer? A meta-analysis of randomized trials. Urology. 2006;67:1216–23.
8. Bohle A, Jocham D, Bock PR. Intravesical bacillus Calmette-Guerin versus mitomycin C for superficial bladder cancer: a formal meta-analysis of comparative studies on recurrence and toxicity. J Urol. 2003;169:90–5.
9. Morales A. Long-term results and complications of intracavitary bacillus Calmette-Guerin therapy for bladder cancer. J Urol. 1984;132:457–9.
10. Babjuk M, Burger M, Zigeuner R, et al. EAU guidelines on non-muscle-invasive urothelial carcinoma of the bladder: update. Eur Urol. 2013;64:639–53.
11. Herr HW. Timing of cystectomy for superficial bladder tumors. Urol Oncol. 2000;5:162–5.
12. Herr HW. Tumor progression and survival of patients with high grade, noninvasive papillary (TaG3) bladder tumors: 15-year outcome. J Urol. 2000;163:60–1. Discussion 1–2.
13. Pansadoro V, De Paula F. Intravesical bacillus Calmette-Guerin in the treatment of superficial transitional cell carcinoma of the bladder. J Urol. 1987;138:299–301.
14. Brake M, Loertzer H, Horsch R, Keller H. Recurrence and progression of stage T1, grade 3 transitional cell carcinoma of the bladder following intravesical immunotherapy with bacillus Calmette-Guerin. J Urol. 2000;163:1697–701.
15. Brake M, Loertzer H, Horsch R, Keller H. Long-term results of intravesical bacillus Calmette-Guerin therapy for stage T1 superficial bladder cancer. Urology. 2000;55:673–8.
16. Catalona WJ, Hudson MA, Gillen DP, Andriole GL, Ratliff TL. Risks and benefits of repeated courses of intravesical bacillus Calmette-Guerin therapy for superficial bladder cancer. J Urol. 1987;137:220–4.
17. Sylvester RJ, van der Meijden A, Witjes JA, et al. High-grade Ta urothelial carcinoma and carcinoma in situ of the bladder. Urology. 2005;66:90–107.
18. Nadler RB, Catalona WJ, Hudson MA, Ratliff TL. Durability of the tumor-free response for intravesical bacillus Calmette-Guerin therapy. J Urol. 1994;152:367–73.
19. Lamm DL, Blumenstein BA, Crissman JD, et al. Maintenance bacillus Calmette-Guerin immunotherapy for recurrent TA, T1 and carcinoma in situ transitional cell carcinoma of the bladder: a randomized Southwest Oncology Group Study. J Urol. 2000;163:1124–9.
20. Sylvester RJ, Brausi MA, Kirkels WJ, et al. Long-term efficacy results of EORTC genito-urinary group randomized phase 3 study 30911 comparing intravesical instillations of epirubicin, bacillus Calmette-Guerin, and bacillus Calmette-Guerin plus isoniazid in patients with intermediate- and high-risk stage Ta T1 urothelial carcinoma of the bladder. Eur Urol. 2010;57:766–73.

21. Brausi M, Oddens J, Sylvester R, et al. Side effects of Bacillus Calmette-Guerin (BCG) in the treatment of intermediate- and high-risk Ta, T1 papillary carcinoma of the bladder: results of the EORTC genitourinary cancers group randomised phase 3 study comparing one-third dose with full dose and 1 year with 3 years of maintenance BCG. Eur Urol. 2014;65:69–76.

22. Naitoh J, Franklin J, O'Donnell MA, Belldegrun AS. Interferon alpha for the treatment of superficial bladder cancer. Adv Exp Med Biol. 1999;462:371–86. discussion 87-92.

23. Belldegrun AS, Franklin JR, O'Donnell MA, et al. Superficial bladder cancer: the role of interferon-alpha. J Urol. 1998;159:1793–801.

24. Glashan RW. A randomized controlled study of intravesical alpha-2b-interferon in carcinoma in situ of the bladder. J Urol. 1990;144:658–61.

25. Kalble T, Beer M, Mendoza E, et al. BCG vs interferon A for prevention of recurrence of superficial bladder cancer. A prospective randomized study. Urol A. 1994;33:133–7.

26. Rajala P, Kaasinen E, Raitanen M, Liukkonen T, Rintala E. Perioperative single dose instillation of epirubicin or interferon-alpha after transurethral resection for the prophylaxis of primary superficial bladder cancer recurrence: a prospective randomized multicenter study—FinnBladder III long-term result. J Urol. 2002;168:981–5.

27. Boccardo F, Cannata D, Rubagotti A, et al. Prophylaxis of superficial bladder cancer with mitomycin or interferon alfa-2b: results of a multicentric Italian study. J Clin Oncol. 1994;12:7–13.

28. Hemdan T, Johansson R, Jahnson S, Hellstrom P, Tasdemir I, Malmstrom PU. Five year outcome of a randomized prospective study comparing bacillus Calmette-Guerin with epirubicin and interferon alpha 2b in patients with T1 bladder cancer. J Urol. 2014;19(5):1244–9.

29. Joudi FN, Smith BJ, O'Donnell MA. Final results from a national multicenter phase II trial of combination bacillus Calmette-Guerin plus interferon alpha-2B for reducing recurrence of superficial bladder cancer. Urol Oncol. 2006;24:344–8.

30. Nepple KG, Lightfoot AJ, Rosevear HM, O'Donnell MA, Lamm DL. Bacillus Calmette-Guerin with or without interferon alpha-2b and megadose versus recommended daily allowance vitamins during induction and maintenance intravesical treatment of nonmuscle invasive bladder cancer. J Urol. 2010;184:1915–9.

31. O'Donnell MA, Lilli K, Leopold C. Interim results from a national multicenter phase II trial of combination bacillus Calmette-Guerin plus interferon alfa-2b for superficial bladder cancer. J Urol. 2004;172:888–93.

32. Rosevear HM, Lightfoot AJ, Birusingh KK, Maymi JL, Nepple KG, O'Donnell MA. Factors affecting response to bacillus Calmette-Guerin plus interferon

33. Herr HW, Dalbagni G. Defining bacillus Calmette-Guerin refractory superficial bladder tumors. J Urol. 2003;169:1706–8.

34. Steinberg G, Bahnson R, Brosman S, Middleton R, Wajsman Z, Wehle M. Efficacy and safety of valrubicin for the treatment of Bacillus Calmette-Guerin refractory carcinoma in situ of the bladder. The Valrubicin Study Group. J Urol. 2000;163:761–7.

35. Dinney CP, Greenberg RE, Steinberg GD. Intravesical valrubicin in patients with bladder carcinoma in situ and contraindication to or failure after bacillus Calmette-Guerin. Urol Oncol. 2013;31:1635–42.

36. Svatek RS, Hollenbeck BK, Holmang S, et al. Economics of bladder cancer: costs and considerations of caring for this disease. Eur Urol. 2014;pii: S0302-2838(14):00018–9.

37. Lamm DL, Blumenstein BA, David Crawford E, et al. Randomized intergroup comparison of bacillus calmette-guerin immunotherapy and mitomycin C chemotherapy prophylaxis in superficial transitional cell carcinoma of the bladder a southwest oncology group study. Urol Oncol. 1995;1:119–26.

38. Malmstrom PU, Wijkstrom H, Lundholm C, Wester K, Busch C, Norlen BJ. 5-year followup of a randomized prospective study comparing mitomycin C and bacillus Calmette-Guerin in patients with superficial bladder carcinoma. Swedish-Norwegian Bladder Cancer Study Group. J Urol. 1999;161:1124–7.

39. Friedrich MG, Pichlmeier U, Schwaibold H, Conrad S, Huland H. Long-term intravesical adjuvant chemotherapy further reduces recurrence rate compared with short-term intravesical chemotherapy and short-term therapy with Bacillus Calmette-Guerin (BCG) in patients with non-muscle-invasive bladder carcinoma. Eur Urol. 2007;52:1123–9.

40. Huncharek M, McGarry R, Kupelnick B. Impact of intravesical chemotherapy on recurrence rate of recurrent superficial transitional cell carcinoma of the bladder: results of a meta-analysis. Anticancer Res. 2001;21:765–9.

41. Lee CT, Barocas D, Globe DR. Economic and humanistic consequences of preventable bladder tumor recurrences in non-muscle invasive bladder cancer cases. J Urol. 2012;188:2114–9.

42. Skinner EC, Goldman B, Sakr WA, et al. SWOG S0353: phase II trial of intravesical gemcitabine in patients with nonmuscle invasive bladder cancer and recurrence after 2 prior courses of intravesical bacillus Calmette-Guerin. J Urol. 2013;190:1200–4.

43. Dalbagni G, Russo P, Bochner B, et al. Phase II trial of intravesical gemcitabine in bacille Calmette-Guerin-refractory transitional cell carcinoma of the bladder. J Clin Oncol. 2006;24:2729–34.

44. Addeo R, Caraglia M, Bellini S, et al. Randomized phase III trial on gemcitabine versus mytomicin in recurrent superficial bladder cancer: evaluation of efficacy and tolerance. J Clin Oncol. 2010;28:543–8.

45. Porena M, Del Zingaro M, Lazzeri M, et al. Bacillus Calmette-Guerin versus gemcitabine for intravesical therapy in high-risk superficial bladder cancer: a randomised prospective study. Urol Int. 2010;84:23–7.

46. Di Lorenzo G, Perdona S, Damiano R, et al. Gemcitabine versus bacille Calmette-Guerin after initial bacille Calmette-Guerin failure in non-muscle-invasive bladder cancer: a multicenter prospective randomized trial. Cancer. 2010;116:1893–900.

47. Lightfoot AJ, Breyer BN, Rosevear HM, Erickson BA, Konety BR, O'Donnell MA. Multi-institutional analysis of sequential intravesical gemcitabine and mitomycin C chemotherapy for non-muscle invasive bladder cancer. Urol Oncol. 2014;32(1):35.e15–9.

48. Gradishar WJ, Tjulandin S, Davidson N, et al. Phase III trial of nanoparticle albumin-bound paclitaxel compared with polyethylated castor oil-based paclitaxel in women with breast cancer. J Clin Oncol. 2005;23:7794–803.

49. Kowalski M, Guindon J, Brazas L, et al. A phase II study of oportuzumab monatox: an immunotoxin therapy for patients with noninvasive urothelial carcinoma in situ previously treated with bacillus Calmette-Guerin. J Urol. 2012;188:1712–8.

50. Dinney CP, Fisher MB, Navai N, et al. Phase I trial of intravesical recombinant adenovirus mediated interferon-alpha2b formulated in Syn3 for Bacillus Calmette-Guerin failures in nonmuscle invasive bladder cancer. J Urol. 2013;190:850–6.

51. van der Heijden AG, Verhaegh G, Jansen CF, Schalken JA, Witjes JA. Effect of hyperthermia on the cytotoxicity of 4 chemotherapeutic agents currently used for the treatment of transitional cell carcinoma of the bladder: an in vitro study. J Urol. 2005;173:1375–80.

52. Colombo R, Da Pozzo LF, Lev A, Freschi M, Gallus G, Rigatti P. Neoadjuvant combined microwave induced local hyperthermia and topical chemotherapy versus chemotherapy alone for superficial bladder cancer. J Urol. 1996;155:1227–32.

53. Lammers RJ, Witjes JA, Inman BA, et al. The role of a combined regimen with intravesical chemotherapy and hyperthermia in the management of non-muscle-invasive bladder cancer: a systematic review. Eur Urol. 2011;60:81–93.

54. Colombo R, Salonia A, Leib Z, Pavone-Macaluso M, Engelstein D. Long-term outcomes of a randomized controlled trial comparing thermochemotherapy with mitomycin-C alone as adjuvant treatment for non-muscle-invasive bladder cancer (NMIBC). BJU Int. 2011;107:912–8.

55. Nativ O, Witjes JA, Hendricksen K, et al. Combined thermo-chemotherapy for recurrent bladder cancer after bacillus Calmette-Guerin. J Urol. 2009;182:1313–7.

56. van der Heijden AG, Kiemeney LA, Gofrit ON, et al. Preliminary European results of local microwave hyperthermia and chemotherapy treatment in intermediate or high risk superficial transitional cell carcinoma of the bladder. Eur Urol. 2004;46:65–71. Discussion-2.

57. Di Stasi SM, Giannantoni A, Stephen RL, et al. Intravesical electromotive mitomycin C versus passive transport mitomycin C for high risk superficial bladder cancer: a prospective randomized study. J Urol. 2003;170:777–82.

58. Di Stasi SM, Valenti M, Verri C, et al. Electromotive instillation of mitomycin immediately before transurethral resection for patients with primary urothelial non-muscle invasive bladder cancer: a randomised controlled trial. Lancet Oncol. 2011;12:871–9.

59. Nseyo UO, Shumaker B, Klein EA, Sutherland K. Photodynamic therapy using porfimer sodium as an alternative to cystectomy in patients with refractory transitional cell carcinoma in situ of the bladder. Bladder Photofrin Study Group. J Urol. 1998;160:39–44.

60. Waidelich R, Stepp H, Baumgartner R, Weninger E, Hofstetter A, Kriegmair M. Clinical experience with 5-aminolevulinic acid and photodynamic therapy for refractory superficial bladder cancer. J Urol. 2001;165:1904–7.

61. Berger AP, Steiner H, Stenzl A, Akkad T, Bartsch G, Holtl L. Photodynamic therapy with intravesical instillation of 5-aminolevulinic acid for patients with recurrent superficial bladder cancer: a single-center study. Urology. 2003;61:338–41.

62. Lee JY, Diaz RR, Cho KS, et al. Efficacy and safety of photodynamic therapy for recurrent, high grade nonmuscle invasive bladder cancer refractory or intolerant to bacille Calmette-Guerin immunotherapy. J Urol. 2013;190:1192–9.

63. van Rhijn BW, Burger M, Lotan Y, et al. Recurrence and progression of disease in non-muscle-invasive bladder cancer: from epidemiology to treatment strategy. Eur Urol. 2009;56:430–42.

64. Zuiverloon TC, Nieuweboer AJ, Vekony H, Kirkels WJ, Bangma CH, Zwarthoff EC. Markers predicting response to bacillus Calmette-Guerin immunotherapy in high-risk bladder cancer patients: a systematic review. Eur Urol. 2012;61:128–45.

65. Sylvester RJ, van der Meijden A, Oosterlinck W. Predicting recurrence and progression in individual patients with stage Ta T1 bladder cancer using EORTC risk tables: a combined analysis of 2596 patients from seven EORTC trials. Eur Urol. 2006;49:466–77.

66. Fernandez-Gomez J, Madero R, Solsona E, et al. Predicting nonmuscle invasive bladder cancer recurrence and progression in patients treated with bacillus Calmette-Guerin: the CUETO scoring model. J Urol. 2009;182:2195–203.

67. Palou J, Sylvester RJ, Faba OR, et al. Female gender and carcinoma in situ in the prostatic urethra are prognostic factors for recurrence, progression, and disease-specific mortality in T1G3 bladder cancer patients treated with bacillus Calmette-Guerin. Eur Urol. 2012;62:118–25.

68. Raj GV, Herr H, Serio AM, et al. Treatment paradigm shift may improve survival of patients with high risk superficial bladder cancer. J Urol. 2007;177:1283–6. Discussion 6.

69. Fernandez-Gomez J, Solsona E, Unda M, et al. Prognostic factors in patients with non-muscle-invasive bladder cancer treated with bacillus Calmette-Guérin: multivariate analysis of data from four randomized CUETO trials. Eur Urol. 2008;53:992–1002.

70. Bol M, Baak J, Buhr-Wildhagen S. Reproducibility and prognostic variability of grade and lamina propria invasion in stages Ta, T1 urothelial carcinoma of the bladder. J Urol. 2003;169:1291–4.

71. Holmang S, Hedelin H, Anderstrom C, Holmberg E, Hohansson S. The importance of the depth of invasion in stage T1 bladder carcinoma: a prospective cohort study. J Urol. 1997;157:800–3.

72. Smits G, Schaafsma E, Klemeney L, Caris C, Debruyne F, Witjes J. Microstaging of pT1 transitional cell carcinoma of the bladder: identification of subgroups with distinct risks of progression. Urology. 1998;52:1009–13.

73. Hasui Y, Osada Y, Kitada S, Nishi S. Significance of invasion to the muscularis mucosae on the progression of superficial bladder cancer. Urology. 1994;43:782–6.

74. Angulo J, Lopez J, Grignon D, Sanchez-Chapado M. Muscularis mucosa differentiates two populations with different prognosis in stage T1 bladder cancer. Urology. 1995;45:47–53.

75. Orsola A, Trias I, Raventos C. Initial high-grade T1 urothelial cell carcinoma: feasibility and prognostic significance of lamina propria invasion microstaging (T1a/b/c) in BCG-treated and BCG-non-treated patients. Eur Urol. 2005;48:231–8.

76. Kondylis F, Demirci S, Ladaga L, Kolm P, Schellhammer P. Outcomes after intravesical bacillus Calmette-Guerin are not affected by substaging of high grade T1 transitional cell carcinoma. J Urol. 2000;163:1120–3.

77. Cheng L, Neumann R, Weaver A, Spotts B, Bostwick D. Predicting cancer progression in patient with T1 bladder carcinoma. J Clin Oncol. 1999;17:3182–7.

78. van der Aa M, van Leenders G, Steyerberg E. A new system for substaging pT1 papillary bladder cancer: a prognostic evaluation. Hum Pathol. 2005;36:981–6.

79. Stein J, Grossfeld G, Ginsberg D. Prognostic markers in bladder cancer: a contemporary review of the literature. J Urol. 1998;160:645–59.

80. Karam J, Shariat S, Hsleth J, Knowles M. Genomics: a preview of genomic medicine. BJU Int. 2006;102:1221–7.

81. van Rhijn B, Vis A, van der Kwast T. Molecular grading of urothelial cell carcinoma with fibroblast growth factor receptor 3 and MIB-1 is superior to pathologic grade for the prediction of clinical outcome. J Clin Oncol. 2003;21:1912–21.

82. Spruck III C, Ohneseit P, Gonzalez-Zulueta M. Two molecular pathways to transitional cell carcinoma of the bladder. Cancer Res. 1994;54:784–8.

83. Cookson MS, Herr HW, Zhang ZF, Soloway S, Sogani PC, Fair WR. The treated natural history of high risk superficial bladder cancer: 15-year outcome. J Urol. 1997;1997:62–7.

84. Shahin O, Thalmann G, Rentsch C, Mazzucchelli L, Studer U. A retrospective analysis of 153 patients treated with or without intravesical bacillus Calmette-Guerin for primary stage T1 grade 3 bladder cancer: recurrence, progression and survival. J Urol. 2003;169:96–100.

85. Nieder A, Simon M, Kim S. Radical cystectomy after bacillus Calmette-Guerin for high-risk Ta, T1 and carcinoma in situ: defining the risk of initial bladder preservation. Urology. 2006;67:737–41.

86. Herr HW. Tumour progression and survival in patients with T1G3 bladder tumours: 15-year outcome. Br J Urol. 1997;80:762–5.

87. Soloway MS, Hepps D, Katkoori D, Ayyathurai R, Manoharan M. Radical cystectomy for BCG failure: has the timing improved in recent years? BJU Int. 2010;108:182–6.

88. Herr HW, Sogani PC. Does early cystectomy improve the survival of patients with high risk superficial bladder tumors? J Urol. 2001;166:1296–9.

89. Lerner S, Tangen C, Sucharew H, Wood D, Crawford E. Patterns of recurrence and outcomes following induction Bacillus Calmette-Guerin for high risk Ta, T1 bladder cancer. J Urol. 2007;177:1727–31.

90. Palapattu GS, Haisfield-Wolfe ME, Walker JM, et al. Assessment of perioperative psychological distress in patients undergoing radical cystectomy for bladder cancer. J Urol. 2004;172:1814–7.

91. Crawford ED. Intravesical therapy for superficial cancer: need for more options. J Clin Oncol. 2002;20:3185–6.

92. Joudi FN, Smith BJ, O'Donnell MA, Konety BR. The impact of age on the response of patients with superficial bladder cancer to intravesical immunotherapy. J Urol. 2006;175:1634–9.

93. Resnick MJ, Bergey M, Magerfleisch L, Tomaszewski JE, Malkowicz SB, Guzzo TJ. Longitudinal evaluation of the concordance and prognostic value of lymphovascular invasion in transurethral resection and radical cystectomy specimens. BJU Int. 2011;107:46–52.

94. Solsona E, Iborra I, Dumont R, Rubio-Briones J, Casanova J, Almenar S. The 3-month clinical response to intravesical therapy as a predictive factor for progression in patients with high risk superficial bladder cancer. J Urol. 2000;164:685–9.

95. van Rhijn BW, van der Kwast TH, Alkhateeb SS, et al. A new and highly prognostic system to discern T1 bladder cancer substage. Eur Urol. 2012;61:378–84.

96. Gallagher BL, Joudi FN, Maymi JL, O'Donnell MA. Impact of previous bacille Calmette-Guerin failure pattern on subsequent response to bacille

Calmette-Guerin plus interferon intravesical therapy. Urology. 2008;71:297–301.

97. Masood S, Sriprasad S, Palmer J, Mufti G. T1G3 bladder cancer-indications for early cystectomy. Int Urol Nephrol. 2004;36:41–4.

98. Denzinger S, Otto W, Fritsche H. Bladder sparing approach for initial T1G3 bladder cancer: do multifocality, size of tumor or concomitant carcinoma in situ matter? A long-term analysis of 132 patients. Int J Urol. 2007;14:995–9.

99. Griffiths T, Charlton M, Neal D, Powell P. Treatment of carcinoma in situ with intravesical bacillus Calmette-Guerin without maintenance. J Urol. 2002;167:2408–12.

100. Solsona E, Iborra I, Rubio-Briones J, Casanova J, Almenar S. The optimum timing of radical cystectomy for patients with recurrent high-risk superficial bladder tumour. BJU Int. 2004;94:1258–62.

101. Denzinger S, Fritsche HM, Otto W, Blana A, Wieland WF, Burger M. Early versus deferred cystectomy for initial high-risk pT1G3 urothelial carcinoma of the bladder: do risk factors define feasibility of bladder-sparing approach? Eur Urol. 2008;53: 146–52.

102. Thomas F, Noon A, Rubin N, Goepel J, Catto J. Comparative outcomes of primary, recurrent and progressive high-risk non-muscle invasive bladder cancer. Eur Urol. 2012;63:145–54.

Clinical Scenario: Persistent CIS and High-Grade Ta Bladder Cancer After BCG

Clinical history: 79-Year-old man who has a persistent CIS despite induction and maintenance BCG for 6 months

Maurizio Brausi

21.1 How Much BCG Do You Give?

The original BCG induction therapy regimen was devised by Morales et al. in 1976 [1]. This regimen consisted of full-dose BCG administered intravesically once a week for 6 weeks together with a percutaneous dose.

Six years later, Brosman et al. reported their positive results with the same BCG schedule without the percutaneous dose and that scheme has become the standard of care treatment [2].

Although the optimal dose of BCG is unknown most clinical studies and meta-analyses have utilized the same schedule and this remains the standard of care. The question of how long BCG should be administered has been debated and is still controversial. Numerous randomized trials and subsequent meta-analyses have concluded that maintenance BCG therapy is superior to induction BCG alone for the prevention of recurrence and progression of NMIBC [3–9]. However, the definition of maintenance is controversial and the BCG maintenance schedule administered varies between institutions. Some centers use the

induction course followed by one instillation per month for 6 months, others use three instillations every 3 months for 1 year.

The current optimal maintenance schedule is based on the SWOG regimen used in the prospective, randomized study 8507 comparing maintenance versus no maintenance in intermediate- and high-risk patients with or without CIS. The induction course was followed by three instillations of BCG at month 3, 6, 12, 18, 24, 30, and 36. The results showed a significant improvement in the median recurrence-free survival that varied from 35.7 to 76.8 months in the standard and maintenance group, respectively [3].

The SWOG BCG maintenance schedule, although still empirical, has become the standard. Lamm et al. [10] reviewed the role of maintenance in intermediate- and high-risk disease.

In the EORTC trial 30911 comparing BCG versus BCG plus INH vs Epirubicin at a median follow-up of 9.2 years, time to first recurrence, time to distant metastases, and overall and disease-specific survival were all significantly prolonged in the BCG maintenance arms compared to epirubicin [9].

Further to the above two trials, a series of meta-analyses demonstrate the superiority of maintenance BCG in the reduction of recurrence and progression [10]. A large EORTC meta-analysis involving 4,683 patients showed BCG to be superior to other options (TURBT alone,

M. Brausi (✉)
Department of Urology Ausl Modena,
B. Ramazzini Hospital, Via G.Molinari 1,
Carpi-Modena 41012, Italy
e-mail: m.brausi@ausl.mo.it

B.R. Konety and S.S. Chang (eds.), *Management of Bladder Cancer:*
A Comprehensive Text With Clinical Scenarios, DOI 10.1007/978-1-4939-1881-2_21,
© Springer Science+Business Media New York 2015

TURBT with chemo, TURBT with other immunotherapy), and that maintenance was required for best outcome. In those trials that gave maintenance, progression was reduced [4].

Another EORTC meta-analysis including 700 patients with CIS compared BCG with other chemotherapy agents. A complete response was noted in 68.1 % of BCG patients versus 51.5 % of patients on chemotherapy [6].

This supports the use of BCG over chemotherapeutic alternatives, but leaves the regimen to be further explored. The maintenance regimen is recommended by AUA and IBCG guidelines while the EAU guidelines recommend BCG maintenance for at least 1 year [11].

21.2 What Dose to Give?

Since BCG produces significant side effects reducing the dose maintaining the same efficacy is a desirable goal. This question was answered by a large prospective randomized study from EORTC [12] including 1,355 patients with Ta-T1 intermediate and high risk tumors. The aim of this study was to examine whether 1/3 dose BCG was not inferior to full dose, and if 1 year maintenance was not inferior to 3 years, and if 1/3 strength for 1 year reduced toxicity. The final results of the study were published in early 2013. In 1,355 patients, with median follow-up of 7 years, there were no significant decreases in toxicity between 1/3 and FD, while 1/3 dose was found to be suboptimal.

After stratifying patients by risk group they showed that intermediate-risk patients receiving full-dose BCG for 1 year achieved equivalent results to patients receiving 3 years of treatment. In high-risk patients, 3 years of maintenance was associated with reduction in recurrence, but not progression or death. 1/3 dose in high-risk patients did not result in reduced recurrence. Finally, reducing the dose of BCG to 1/3 no reduction in toxicity was found.

In conclusion, the actual BCG schedule for patients with CIS should be: 1 vial (full dose) of BCG once weekly commencing 15–21 days after TUR followed by three instillations at month 3, 6, 12, 18, 24, 30, and 36 according to the SWOG schedule.

The 79-year-old patient presented with a persistent CIS after 6 months of BCG therapy. This scenario suggests two other important questions:
1. Does BCG maintain the same efficacy in the elderly as in young patients?
2. How can we define BCG failure?

21.3 The Role of BCG in the Elderly

Age-related changes that may impact on BCG functionality include deregulated immune and inflammatory responses.

Declining T-cell function is the most significant and best-characterized feature of immune-senescence [13, 14]. In a retrospective study of 805 patients with multiple of recurrent high-grade Ta or T1 tumors and/or CIS, Herr found that age did not impact on initial response to BCG therapy [15]. However, patients aged 70–79 years were 10 % less likely to sustain the response and remain free of tumor recurrence during a 5-year period (27 % vs. 37 %).

Joudi reported that patients older than 80 had a poor response to BCG + Interferon with a 22 % lower absolute disease-free rate for patients ≥80 years treated with BCG + Interferon, compared to patients 60–70 years of age [16]. There may also be a higher risk of BCG-related complications in patients older than 80 years as reported by Heiner [17].

21.4 When Do You Say That BCG Is Not Working? How Can We Define BCG Failure?

BCG failure is a heterogeneous term that encompasses a number of clinical scenarios. There are currently three published concepts to categorize a disease that appears during or following BCG instillations. The EAU defines BCG failure in these cases [18]:
1. Muscle-invasive bladder tumor is detected during follow-up.

2. High-grade NMIBC is present after 3–6 months.
3. Any worsening of disease occurring during BCG treatment, higher number of recurrences, higher T stage, higher grade, appearance of CIS despite an initial response.

The international bladder group (IBCG) tried to emphasize the importance of distinguishing recurrence from treatment failure. Recurrence refers to reappearance of disease, any grade, T category, or CIS after completion of therapy. Failure is any recurrence or progression that occurs during intravesical therapy [19].

There are four subgroup categories of BCG failure [20, 21]:
1. BCG intolerance: recurrent disease in an intolerant BCG patient and/or side effects.
2. BCG resistance: recurrence or persistence of lesser stage or grade after initial course which resolves with further BCG instillations.
3. BCG relapse: recurrence after initial resolution.
4. BCG refractory: non-improving or worsening disease despite BCG.

21.5 Predicting BCG Failure

There are no variables that can accurately predict response to BCG therapy, on an individual patient basis. Some clinico-pathological features can help urologists in predicting the risk of failure: female sex, older age, multifocality, recurrent tumors, associated CIS, lymphovascular invasion, recurrent disease cysto at 3 months, depth of lamina propria invasion, timing of failure (e.g. early vs. late) and two or more previous courses of BCG.

21.6 What Is Your Next Agent of Choice in Case of BCG Failure?

Treatment options for BCG failure.

Once a patient is deemed to have failed BCG there are two possible options:
1. Surgery, radical cystectomy.
2. Conservative treatment.

It is not uncommon for a uro-oncologic surgeon to be faced with a patient who after failing BCG therapy is not willing or not fit for RC.

The attitude of this author is to clearly explain to the patient and eventually relatives that any treatment other than RC must be considered oncologically inferior. Once a patient has decided to pursue a conservative approach, many options can be offered.

21.7 Interferon-alfa-BCG

Interferon-alfa (INF-alfa) is a cytokine produced by the immune system in response to insults such as tumor cell growth. It has been utilized in conjunction with BCG in patients with high-risk NMIBC who failed BCG therapy.

A US multicenter phase II study, involving 1,007 patients compared the effects of INF-alfa (50 millions) plus reduced dose BCG in BCG failure patients to a cohort of BCG naïve patients who received the same INF-alfa dose but with a standard-dose BCG protocol. The response rate in the group of patients who failed BCG was 45 % compared to 59 % in the BCG naïve group [16].

In conclusion, INF-alfa/BCG can be a reasonable option for patients who failed previous BCG therapy even if further studies have to confirm the results.

21.8 Gemcitabine

Gemcitabine is a nucleoside analog that causes defective DNA replication, leading to apoptosis of tumor cells. To date, some phase I and II studies in patients who failed BCG have been published. Although the number of patients treated in this setting is modest ($N=243$) some responses have been reported. Gemcitabine was administered intravesically at the dose of 2,000 mg a week for 6 weeks and then monthly in some protocols. The response rate varied from 40 to 70 % according to intermediate- or low-risk tumor characteristics [22]. In conclusion, intravesical gemcitabine is an alternative therapy for BCG-failure patients even if the reported follow-up is short (1–2 years).

21.9 Thermochemotherapy

Hyperthermia used in combination with intravesical MMC is defined as thermochemotherapy (TC). Synergo System is the name of the technology delivering hyperthermia. Inducing temperatures of approximately 42 °C in the bladder wall significantly improves the absorption of sequentially administered intravesical MMC compared to MMC alone. The role of Synergo in the treatment of BCG-failure patients has been studied by different authors. The schedule used was one instillation of MMC with Synergo a week for 6–8 weeks. The response rate varied from 50 to 56 % after 2 years with a progression rate of 8 % [22]. A bladder preservation rate of 87.6 % was reported in a recent systematic review allowing the authors to speculate that thermochemotherapy could become the standard of care in BCG-failure patients [23].

21.10 Aggressive Treatment

Radical cystectomy has been defined by different guidelines as the standard therapy for high-risk patients who failed BCG [11].

21.11 Is Your Choice of Proceeding with Cystectomy Influenced by How the Patient's Bladder Appears Cystoscopically?

The choice to proceed with cystectomy relies on the usual constellation of diagnostic tools available to the clinician. History, cystoscopy, and histology are going to be the key factors in making this complex clinical decision. A patient's response to previous treatment and knowledge of his/her disease will also strongly influence management. Bladder capacity should be evaluated during cystoscopy. A small bladder causing intense patient dysuria and pollachiuria determines a poor quality of life and sometimes is a very important feature affecting the decision-making process of further treatment. In these cases radical cystectomy should be seriously evaluated and discussed with our patients.

The cystoscopic appearance in our index patient "a 79-year-old who has persistent CIS despite induction and maintenance BCG for 6 months" may in fact be normal. However, this would not impact on our treatment decision, as he is known to have had a poor response to BCG, and has persistent CIS. White light cystoscopy may not be the most effective technique of diagnosing disease. In an attempt to improve the diagnostic yield of cystoscopy, additional techniques may be employed. A 2010 systematic review of photodynamic diagnosis showed this to be a superior technique when compared to white light cystoscopy. Twenty percent more tumor-positive patients were detected with PDD in all patients with non-invasive bladder tumors, and 39 % in patients when only CIS was analyzed.

Residual tumor was found less often, and recurrence-free survival was better at 12 and 24 months [18]. That said, it must be noted that PDD can cause a high number of false positives in patients who have received prior BCG.

Further, the appearance of the bladder may be misleading. Erythema, particularly in the setting of negative cytology may merely reflect post-BCG changes, rather than recurrent or persistent disease.

In summary, the appearance of the bladder may be misleading. It must be interpreted with caution, and an appreciation of the known history, response to treatment, cytology, and histology acquired at cystoscopy. While evidence of a tumor is self-evident, a normal appearing bladder, or an erythematous area requires further consideration, and cannot be accepted at face value. Finally, bladder capacity should be also evaluated and considered in the decision-making process.

References

1. Morales A, Edinger D, Bruce AW. Intracavitary Bacillus Calmette-Guerin in the treatment of superficial bladder tumours. J Urol. 1976;116(2):180–3.
2. Brosman SA. Experience with Bacillus Calmette-Guerin in patients with superficial bladder carcinoma. J Urol. 1982;128(1):27–30.
3. Lamm DL, Blumenstein BA, Cristmann JD, et al. Maintenance Bacillus Calmette-Guerin immunotherapy

for recurrent Ta-T1 and carcinoma in situ transitional cell carcinoma of the bladder: a randomized Southwest Oncology Group Study. J Urol. 2000;163:1124–9.

4. Sylvester RJ, van der Meijden AP, Lamm DL. Intravesical Bacillus Calmette-Guerin reduces the risk of progression in patients with superficial bladder cancer: a combined analysis of the published results of randomized clinical trials. J Urol. 2002;168:1964–70.

5. Bohle A, Jocham D, Bock PR. Intravesical bacillus Calmette-Guerin versus mitomycin C for superficial bladder cancer a formal meta-analysis of comparative studies on recurrence and toxicity. J Urol. 2003;169: 90–5.

6. Sylvester RJ, van der Meijden AP, Witjes JA, et al. Bacillus Calmette-Guerin versus chemotherapy for the intravesical treatment of patients with carcinoma in situ of the bladder: a meta-analysis of the published results of randomized clinical trials. J Urol. 2005;174:86–91.

7. Han RF, Pan JG. Can intravesical bacillus Calmette-Guerin reduce recurrence in patients with superficial bladder cancer? a meta- analysis of randomized trials. Urology. 2006;67:1216–23.

8. Malmstrom PU, Sylvester RJ, Crawford DE, et al. An individual patient data meta-analysis of the long term outcome of randomized studies comparing intravesical Mitomycin C versus bacillus Calmette-Guerin for non muscle invasive bladder cancer. Eur Urol. 2009;56:247–56.

9. Sylvester RJ, Brausi MA, Kirkels WJ, et al. Long-term efficacy results of EORTC Genito-urinary group randomized phase 3 study 30911 comparing intravesical instillations of epirubicin, bacillus Calmette-Guerin and bacillus Calmette-Guerin plus Isoniazid in patients with intermediate and high-risk stage TaT1 urothelial carcinoma of the bladder. Eur Urol. 2010;57(Suppl):766–70. 715–34.

10. Lamm DL, Persad R, Colombel M, et al. Maintenance bacillus Calmette-Guérin: the standard of care for the prophylaxis and management of intermediate- and high-risk non-muscle-invasive bladder cancer. Eur Urol. 2010;9(Suppl):715–34.

11. Brausi M, Witjes A, Lamm D, et al. A review of current guidelines and best practice recommendations for the management of non-muscle invasive bladder can-cer by the international bladder cancer group. J Urol. 2011;186:2158–67.

12. Oddens J, Brausi M, Sylvester R, et al. Final results of an EORTC-GU cancers group randomized study of mainte-nance bacillis Calmette-Guérin in intermediate-and high-risk Ta, T1 papillary carcinoma of the urinary blad-der: one-third dose versus full dose and 1 year versus 3 years of maintenance. Eur Urol. 2013;63:462–72.

13. Shariat S, Milowsky M, Droller M. Bladder cancer in the elderly. Urol Oncol. 2009;27:653–67.

14. Shariat S, Sfakianos J, Droller M, et al. The effect of age and gender on bladder cancer: a critical review of the literature. BJUI. 2009;105:300–8.

15. Herr H. Age and outcome of superficial bladder can-cer treated with bacille Calmette-Guérin therapy. Urology. 2007;70(1):65–8.

16. Joudi F, Smith B, O'Donnell A, et al. The impact of age on the response of patients with superficial blad-der cancer to intravesical immunotherapy. J Urol. 2006;175:1634–40.

17. Heiner J, Terris M. Effect of advanced age on the devel-opment of complications from intravesical bacillus Calmette-Guérin therapy. Urol Oncol. 2008;26:137–40.

18. Babjuk M, Oosterlinck W, Sylvester R et al. European Association of Urology guidelines on TaT1 non mus-cle invasive bladder cancer. Update march 2009. Arnhem, The Netherlands: European Association of Urology; 2009. Available from http://www.uroweb. org/professional-resources/guidelines/online.

19. Lamm D, Colombel M, Persad R, et al. Clinical recom-mendations for the management of non-muscle inva-sive bladder cancer. Eur Urol. 2008;7(Suppl):651–66.

20. Nieder AM, Brausi M, Lamm D, et al. Management of stage T1 tumors of the bladder: International Consensus Panel. Urology. 2005;66(Suppl 6A):108–25.

21. O'Donnell M. Optimizing BCG, therapy. Urol Onc. 2009;27:325–8.

22. Yates D, Brausi M, Catto J, et al. Treatment options available for bacillus Calmette-Guérin failure in non-muscle-invasive bladder cancer. Eur Urol. 2012;62: 1088–96.

23. Lammers RJM, Witjes JA, Innam BA, et al. The role of combined regimen with intravesical chemotherapy and hyperthermia in the management of non-muscle invasive bladder cancer: a systematic review. Eur Urol. 2011;60:81–93.

22

68-Year-old man previously treated years ago with BCG who has a high-grade Ta tumor with significant lower urinary tract symptoms after receiving his third dose of a planned 6-week BCG induction course

Donald L. Lamm and Nilay M. Gandhi

Bacillus Calmette-Guérin (BCG) immunotherapy very commonly produces symptoms of urinary frequency and dysuria that typically occur after the second or third instillation. These symptoms are so common that they are expected and generally not treated, but can herald severe, life-threatening, even fatal reactions. How can we reduce the risk of severe reactions? Can we identify those patients at risk for severe toxicity? How should mild, moderate, and severe toxicity be treated? Importantly, patients with recurrent high-grade urothelial carcinoma are at risk for disease progression and death. Can the benefits of BCG be provided safely to these high-risk bladder tumor patients who appear to be BCG intolerant?

The benefit of BCG is immunologic in nature [1] and the side effects can be both immunologic and infectious [2]. Unfortunately, the immunologic nature of BCG is often forgotten when treating patients and designing protocols. The concept that "more is better," which may generally apply to chemotherapy, can reduce the antitumor effect of BCG and has been shown to promote tumor growth and death in the animal model [3], while at the same time increasing the risk of severe toxicity. Classic immunology lectures given to first-year medical students teach that the second set reaction to an antigen is heightened and accelerated. Despite this common knowledge, as illustrated in the sample case, a second 6-week course of BCG (a time schedule commonly and appropriately seen with intravesical chemotherapy) is often used for patients with tumor recurrence after the initial course of BCG. This practice is based on small, uncontrolled historical series. The only randomized evaluation of repeat 6-week BCG immunotherapy failed to show any significant reduction of malignancy compared with induction alone [4]. In this scenario, the index patient should simply have his BCG stopped after his third instillation.

D.L. Lamm, M.D.
BCG Oncology, University of Arizona,
3815 E. Bell Road, Phoenix, AZ 85032, USA
e-mail: dlamm@bcgoncology.com

N.M. Gandhi, M.D. (✉)
James Buchanan Brady Urological Institute,
Johns Hopkins Medical Institutions, 600 N. Wolfe
Street, Marburg 134, Baltimore, MD 21287, USA
e-mail: nilaymgandhi@gmail.com

B.R. Konety and S.S. Chang (eds.), *Management of Bladder Cancer:
A Comprehensive Text With Clinical Scenarios*, DOI 10.1007/978-1-4939-1881-2_22,
© Springer Science+Business Media New York 2015

One cannot say, of course, that a second 6-week course of BCG should never be given. The immune stimulation and protection from bladder cancer recurrence, like the protection from tuberculosis, wanes with time and may be completely lost a decade after immunization [5]. A patient who has had no BCG for many years or a patient with an impaired immune response may benefit from a second full 6 weeks of BCG, but it is very unlikely that patients who develop strong symptomatic local adverse events benefit by continuing beyond the third instillation. DeBoer et al. documented that beneficial urinary cytokines induced by BCG peak after the sixth instillation during the first course, but with a second course they peak after the third instillation and are actually suppressed by the fourth, fifth and sixth instillation [6].

The correlation between benefit of BCG and side effects is not clear or reliable. It is reassuring to see patients exhibit mild frequency, dysuria, malaise, or fatigue as presumed evidence of an immune response. Fever has been reported to correlate with a reduction in the risk of recurrence. But many patients have no symptoms from BCG and remain free of tumor recurrence. Increasing side effects, on the other hand, do commonly precede a severe BCG reaction. What should be done in the face of increasing local symptoms of frequency and dysuria, which are often associated with malaise? First, diligence to continue intravesical treatment on schedule should be ignored. While 6 weekly instillations are thought to be optimal for induction of BCG immunity in most patients, the standard induction is an arbitrary schedule that does not necessarily fit everyone. If the side effects are tolerable (not increasing and not requiring medication), simply postponing treatment until all symptoms have resolved is the most appropriate approach. In some cases, the cause of the symptoms may be unclear, and the tumor risk remains high. If treatment is deemed necessary in the face of continuing symptoms, patients should be warned of the risks. In this case, one can consider BCG dose reduction and administration of ofloxacin or ciprofloxacin at 6 and 18 h after instillation. The number of viable colony forming units (CFU) in BCG is highly variable, ranging from 2 to 19×10^8 CFU per vial of TheraCys or from 2 to 8×10^8 CFU per vial of

Tice. Therefore to be effective, dose reduction of BCG must be aggressive. While the benefit of dose reduction is arguable and not universally found, experience with using the recommended logarithmic reduction to 1/3, 1/10, 1/30 and 1/100th dose now for decades has shown that most symptoms can be managed with no observable reduction in efficacy. In an effort to reduce BCG side effects, French investigators compared standard dose BCG with that plus ofloxacin 200 milligrams (mg) at 6 h post instillation and the following morning. They reported a significant reduction in local side effects with no reduction in efficacy [7]. Either dose reduction or prophylactic antibiotics can be given. Liberal use of BCG dose reduction to prevent escalating side effects is a recommended practice with the possible addition of fluoroquinolone antibiotic. A recent patient is a good example. He had received his fifth instillation elsewhere and had a fever to 102 °F with chills. Upon his sixth instillation, the patient was asymptomatic and started on 500 mg of ciprofloxacin immediately and the following morning, and should he develop a recurrent fever, a prescription was given for ciprofloxacin 500 mg twice daily and isoniazid 300 mg daily for 3 months. He again developed fever and chills, took his medicine as instructed, and avoided what could have been a life-threatening reaction.

Urologists who prescribe BCG should be familiar with the side effects and know how to best prevent and treat complications. We cannot expect every emergency room physician to know how to treat serious BCG reactions. While we would hope that infectious disease specialists would be well informed, experience has shown that the treatment of serious BCG reactions is sufficiently controversial, complicated and esoteric that even they must often review published recommendations.

22.1 Prevention of BCG Side Effects

All side effects cannot be prevented, and even with the best efforts, some serious side effects will occur but the majority of significant untoward reactions can be prevented. Experience in cooperative clinical trials has shown an impressive drop in side effects in more recent studies, now that urologists are more familiar with the treatment. Patients should be instructed to expect mild urinary frequency and dysuria beginning after the second or third instillation. These symptoms should last only a few days and should not be disabling. Mild malaise, fatigue, and "flu-like" symptoms similar to those following a vaccination are seen less frequently, likely a consequence of immune stimulation and not generally of concern. Patients destined to have worrisome side effects will often have increasing symptoms with successive instillations, and the progression of symptoms can generally be managed with dose reduction. Mild symptoms that are not increasing do not require treatment or dose adjustment. While fever has been associated with an improved response to BCG, experience has shown that mild fever or sensation of a chill are an indication to reduce the dose of BCG to 1/3 or less, with consideration into the addition of a fluoroquinolone 6 and 18 h after instillation. All side effects attributed to BCG should resolve, when possible, before additional BCG is given.

Isoniazid prophylaxis did not reduce the side effects of BCG in a large EORTC study [8], but giving ofloxacin 200 mg 6 and 18 h after the first urination post BCG instillation was studied in a double-blind multicenter trial in France. In 115 randomized patients, ofloxacin treatment reduced the incidence of class 2 and 3 adverse events by 22 % ($p<0.019$) and improved compliance with full BCG treatment from 66 to 81 % [7]. This benefit was seen without a reduction in tumor recurrence.

22.2 Treatment of Moderate BCG Side Effects

When BCG dose reduction and fluoroquinolone antibiotic prophylaxis fail to prevent significant side effects of BCG treatment, antitubercular antibiotics are needed. Mycobacteria such as BCG (*M. bovis*) grow slowly, typically respond slowly to antibiotics, and have a strong propensity to develop antibiotic resistance. The typical patient is one with persistent severe frequency, urgency and dysuria, characteristic of BCG cystitis. Less frequently, symptoms such as prolonged malaise, loss of appetite, night sweats and low-grade fever may occur, suggesting a systemic infection. As illustrated in Table 22.1, sites of infection, in addition to the bladder, may include the prostate (with prostatic-specific antigen [PSA] elevation and induration similar to that seen with prostate cancer), the epididymis (where prompt triple antibiotic therapy can prevent the need for surgical management), bone or joints (where the reaction is often immunologic, but can be prolonged by latent BCG infection), and when vesicoureteral reflux is present, renal parenchyma [9]. BCG can also induce ureteral obstruction as a result of cystitis or

Table 22.1 Complications of BCG therapy in 2,589 patients according to strain [9]

Side effect	Total	Armand frappier	Tice	Connaught	Pasteur	RIVM
Fever	75 (2.9 %)	3.8 %	4.7 %	4.7 %	0.6 %	2.1 %
G. Prost	23 (0.9 %)	1.8 %	1 %	0.2 %	0.6 %	0
Pneum/hep	18 (0.7 %)	0.4 %	0.8 %	0.6 %	1.2 %	0.8 %
Arthralgia	12 (0.6 %)	0.7 %	0.1 %	0.6 %	1.8 %	0
Hematuria	24 (1.0 %)	0.3 %	0.6 %	2.4 %	1 %	0.4 %
Rash	8 (0.3 %)	0.4 %	0	0.9 %	0	0
Ureteral obstruction	8 (0.3 %)	0.6 %	0.4 %	0.2 %	0	0
Epididymitis	10 (0.4 %)	0.4 %	0	0.2 %	1.2 %	0.8 %
Bladder contracture	6 (0.2 %)	0	0.3 %	0.2 %	0.6 %	0
Renal abscess	2 (0.1 %)	0	0	0.4 %	0	0
Sepsis	10 (0.4 %)	0.1 %	0.4 %	0.9 %	0.2 %	0
Cytopenia	2 (0.1 %)	0	0.3 %	0	0	0

ureteritis, the latter seen most commonly in patients with carcinoma in situ.

When treating these conditions, both the doctor and the patient must have patience. A common mistake is to give a 10-day course of antibiotics and then stop prematurely. Cystectomy inappropriately has also been recommended for patients with cancer-free bladders who have continued symptoms after inadequate courses of antibiotics. Using a two-drug combination of a fluoroquinolone such as ofloxacin (200–400 mg every 12 h), ciprofloxacin (500 mg every 12 h), or levofloxacin (500 mg every 24 h) plus isoniazid 300 mg daily is generally sufficient for milder reactions treated early. For more intense or prolonged symptoms, a three-drug combination is needed, adding rifampin 600 mg daily and/or ethambutol 1,200 mg daily. With ethambutol, monthly eye examinations are recommended to prevent ocular side effects such as optic neuritis which can be seen in about 6 % of patients [10]. Treatment is recommended for 3–6 months and symptoms may not even begin to improve for months after initiation of appropriate antibiotic therapy. The response to fluoroquinolones often occurs more promptly than the response to other types of antibiotics but should not be given for significant BCG infection as a single antibiotic. If bladder symptoms are unresponsive and intolerable, prednisone (30–60 mg daily, with a very gradual taper) may be used, but prednisone should not be given without appropriate antibiotic coverage due to the risk of increasing infection. If symptoms of frequency and dysuria are not treated effectively, bladder contracture may occur. Prevention of bladder contracture with long-term antibiotics is preferred, but if that is not effective, some patients will respond to bladder hydrodistension under anesthesia.

22.3 Treatment of Severe BCG Reactions

Patients with high fever and chills following BCG instillation are presumed to have BCG sepsis. They require prompt hospital admission and treatment for urosepsis and BCG reaction with broad spectrum antibiotic coverage including triple antitubercular antibiotics. Even with appropriate antibiotic treatment, hypotension followed by multisystem organ failure can occur. In these patients, treatment of the infection is essential but not sufficient, because a major component of the reaction is an overwhelming immune response. While the use of steroids in sepsis has been controversial [11], steroid administration to suppress this immune hypersensitivity response (methylprednisolone 60–100 mg or more IV daily) can be life-saving. It is important to taper steroids gradually to avoid recurrence of severe symptoms, and antibiotics must be continued even when the response to steroids is dramatic. Administration of steroids in the animal model of BCG sepsis significantly improves survival, but administration of steroids without concomitant antibiotics actually decreases survival [2].

Generally patients with severe BCG reactions should not receive BCG in the future, and fortunately the response to BCG is long term, so many of these patients will not require further treatment. But what about those who remain at high risk for progression of bladder cancer? What about those whose reaction to BCG was severe, but not abnormal? Primates injected with 1 g of BCG intravenously uniformly survive the infection, but a second intravenous injection in primates (like a second intraperitoneal BCG injection in rodents) is universally fatal. Sepsis resulting from a traumatic catheterization in a patient previously immunized to BCG is an expected response. These patients and those intolerant of BCG, who would benefit from the protection of BCG, may in the future be able to safely receive the benefit of immunotherapy.

22.4 Treatment of BCG Intolerant Patients

There are treatment options other than BCG, but comorbidity and advanced age make cystectomy prohibitively dangerous for many patients. Radiation therapy is demonstrated by randomized clinical trial to be ineffective in reducing the mortality of lamina propria invasive disease [12] and intravesical chemotherapy alone has not reduced disease progression or mortality. BCG clearly reduces recurrence, progression, metastasis, disease-specific survival and overall mortality, but only when the 3-week maintenance schedule is used. To provide the benefit of immunotherapy in patients who are unable to tolerate BCG despite dose reduction and prophylactic antibiotics, the use of heat-killed BCG immunotherapy can be administered. Initiation of optimal antitumor immune response requires the use of living BCG organisms. The dose of BCG is, in fact, based on the number of live bacteria as estimated by the colony forming units. However, in vitro animal and clinical studies have suggested that in BCG-immunized subjects, effective antitumor immune response can be recalled using non-viable BCG [13–15]. Since 2005, heat-killed BCG (sterilized in autoclave at 375 °F for 45 min) has been utilized in an experienced practice for 49 BCG intolerant patients. Twenty-nine consecutive patients treated with this heat-killed BCG preparation have been followed for 2 or more years. Comparing these patients with 30 age, sex and tumor grade-matched BCG tolerant patients treated with live TheraCys BCG, no significant difference in BCG tolerance or efficacy was found. BCG side effects were greatly reduced ($p<0.001$) and no severe toxicity was seen with heat-killed BCG [16].

22.5 Summary

BCG immunotherapy is very representative of the art and science of medicine. With education of patients and urologists, the incidence of side effects and withdrawal of treatment has markedly decreased. Patients are less anxious when they are taught to expect some increased frequency and mild discomfort with treatment, and side effects can be markedly reduced by logarithmic dose reduction and the use of fluoroquinolone antibiotics after instillation. Despite best efforts to reduce the risk, serious and even life-threatening side effects can occur. BCG is sensitive to appropriate antibiotics, and early treatment with effective combination antitubercular antibiotics resolves BCG infection. Techniques for

continuing the remarkable and highly significant benefit of 3-week maintenance BCG immunotherapy for intolerant patients using heat-killed organisms are being developed.

References

1. Gandhi NM, Morales A, Lamm DL. Bacillus Calmette-Guérin immunotherapy for genitourinary cancer. BJU Int. 2013;112:288–97.
2. Koukol SC, DeHaven J, Riggs DR, Lamm DL. Drug therapy of bacillus Calmette-Guérin sepsis. Urol Res. 1995;22(6):273.
3. Lamm DL, Reichert FD, Harris SC, Lucio RM. Immunotherapy of murine transitional cell carcinoma. J Urol. 1982;128(5):1104–8.
4. Palou J, Laguna P, Millan-Rodrıguez F, Hall RR, Salvador-Bayarri J, Vicente-Rodrıguez J. Control group and maintenance treatment with bacillus Calmette-Guérin for carcinoma in situ and/or high grade bladder tumors. J Urol. 2001;165:1488–9.
5. Weir RE, Gorak-Stolinska P, Floyd S, Lalor MK, Stenson S, Branson K, Blitz R, Anne Ben-Smith B, Fine PEM, Dockrell HM. Persistence of the immune response induced by BCG vaccination. BMC Infect Dis. 2008;8:9.
6. DeBoer EC, DeJong WH, Steerenberg PA, Aarden LA, Tetteroo E, DeGroot ER, et al. Induction of urinary interleukin-1 (IL-1), IL-2, IL-6, and tumor necrosis factor during intravesical immunotherapy with bacillus Calmette-Guérin in superficial bladder cancer. Cancer Immunol Immunother. 1992;34:306–12.
7. Colombel M, Saint F, Chopin D, Nicolas L, Rischmann P. The effect of ofloxacin on bacillus Calmette-Guérin induced toxicity in patients with superficial bladder cancer: results of a randomized, prospective, double-blind, placebo controlled, multicenter study. J Urol. 2006;176:935–9.
8. Sylvester RJ, Brausi MA, Kirkels WJ, et al. Long-term efficacy results of EORTC genito-urinary group randomized phase 3 study 30911 comparing intravesical instillations of epirubicin, bacillus Calmette-Guérin, and bacillus Calmette-Guérin plus isoniazid in patients with intermediate- and high-risk stage Ta T1 urothelial carcinoma of the bladder. Eur Urol. 2010;57(5):766–73.
9. Lamm DL. Complications of bacillus Calmette-Guérin immunotherapy. Urol Clin North Am. 1992;19:565–72.
10. Griffith DE, Brown-Elliott BA, Shepherd S, McLarty J, Griffith L, Wallace Jr RJ. Ethambutol ocular toxicity in treatment regimens for *Mycobacterium avium* complex lung disease. Am J Respir Crit Care Med. 2005;172(2):250–3.
11. Annane D, Bellissant E, Bollaert PE, Briegel J, Confalonieri M, De Gaudio R, Keh D, Kupfer Y, Oppert M, Meduri GU. Corticosteroids in the treatment

of severe sepsis and septic shock in adults: a systematic review. JAMA. 2009;301(22):2362–75.

12. Harland SJ, Kynaston H, Grigor K, Wallace DM, Beacock C, Kockelbergh R, Clawson S, Barlow T, Parmar MK, Griffiths GO. National Cancer Research Institute Bladder Clinical Studies Group: a randomized trial of radical radiotherapy for the management of pT1G3 NXM0 transitional cell carcinoma of the bladder. J Urol. 2007;178(3):807–13.

13. Shah G, Zhang G, Chen F, Cao Y, Kalyanaraman B, See W. Loss of BCG viability adversely affects the direct response of urothelial carcinoma cells to BCG exposure. J Urol. 2013;191:823–9.

14. Lamm DL, Harris SC, Gittes RF. Bacillus Calmette-Guérin and Dinitrochlorobenzene immunotherapy of chemically induced bladder tumors. Invest Urol. 1977;14:369.

15. De Boer EC, Rooijakkers SJ, Schamhart DH, Kurth KH. Cytokine gene expression in a mouse model: the first instillations with viable bacillus Calmette-Guérin determine the succeeding Th1 response. J Urol. 2003;170(5):2004–8.

16. Lamm DL, Gandhi NM, Iverson T, et al. Clinical experience with heat-inactivated bacillus Calmette-Guérin (BCG) immunotherapy. J Urol. 2013; 4:733.

Jeffrey C. Bassett, John D. Seigne, and Peter E. Clark

23.1 Introduction

In the treatment of non-muscle invasive bladder cancer (NMIBC), there are a number of different guidelines available to the clinician and the public to assist in the decision-making process. Included in these are the guidelines published by the American Urological Association (AUA), the European Association of Urology (EAU), the International Consultation on Urological Disease (ICUD), and National Comprehensive Cancer Network (NCCN) [1–7]. The purpose of the guidelines is to promote evidence-based decision-making, highlighting the clinical scenarios where good evidence regarding appropriate treatment already exists and providing direction for the scenarios where evidence is lacking.

J.C. Bassett, M.D., M.P.H.
Department of Urology, Kaiser Permanente Southern
California, 3430 E. La Palma Avenue,
Anaheim, CA 92806, USA
e-mail: Jeffrey.C.Bassett@kp.org

J.D. Seigne, M.B.
Division of Urology, Dartmouth-Hitchcock
Medical Center, Norris Cotton Cancer Center,
One Medical Center Drive, Lebanon, NH 03756, USA
e-mail: john.d.seigne@hitchcock.org

P.E. Clark, M.D. (✉)
Vanderbilt University Medical Center,
A-1302 Medical Center North, Nashville,
TN 37232-2765, USA
e-mail: peter.clark@vanderbilt.edu

Despite informing the same malignant process (i.e. NMIBC) and having comparable access to the available literature, the guidelines are not entirely interchangeable. For any one aspect in the treatment of NMIBC, the recommended next step may be different depending on the guideline referenced. There are a number of reasons for this, including the evidence available at the time of publication, the composition of the guideline panel, and the methodology used to interpret the available literature.

It is this last reason that may be the most salient. The methodologies used by the different guideline panels explain at least in part the differences in recommendations. As it pertains to the creation of the AUA, EAU, ICUD, and NCCN guidelines, each were authored by a panel of highly regarded experts in NMIBC. The first step by each panel was a literature search for the available evidence, followed by data extraction and analyses. Each panel then assigned a level of evidence to the manuscripts considered for inclusion, with priority being given to articles of the highest level per the Oxford Centre for Evidence-based Medicine Levels of Evidence [8]. Differences arise in the databases queried, the timeframe of the search, the method of data extraction and analysis, and the categorization of recommendations (see Table 23.1).

The methodology utilized by the most recent AUA guidelines appears the most rigorous. Articles relevant to NMIBC and published between January 1998 and December 2005 were

B.R. Konety and S.S. Chang (eds.), *Management of Bladder Cancer:*
A Comprehensive Text With Clinical Scenarios, DOI 10.1007/978-1-4939-1881-2_23,
© Springer Science+Business Media New York 2015

Table 23.1 Guideline panels' composition, evidence acquisition, and synthesis

	AUA	EAU	ICUD	NCCN
Publication year	2007	2013	2012	2013
Panel members	8	11	18	25
Database(s)	Medline	Medline Web of Science Embase	Medline 5 year major conference abstract review	–
Database search (yrs)	1998–2005	2010–2012	–	–
Methodology	Meta-analyses of extracted data	Prioritized by Oxford evidence level	Prioritized by Oxford evidence level	Prioritized by Oxford evidence level
Categorization of recommendations	Standard, recommendation, or option	Grade A–C	Grade A–D	Category 1–3

identified by four separate MEDLINE searches over the course of 18 months. Data were extracted from the articles to outcomes tables. Using the confidence profile method (where appropriate), three separate meta-analysis of the data were performed by the panel: (1) meta-analysis of the comparable randomized controlled trials, (2) meta-analysis of the individual arms of the randomized controlled trials, and (3) meta-analysis of the individual arms from all studies regardless of study design. Outcomes of interest included recurrence and progression. The final AUA guidelines on NMIBC were based on the results of the meta-analyses and, in some cases, the panel authors' opinions. Recommendations are assigned grades and separated into three levels based on how strongly the panel felt the recommendation should be followed, i.e. what the panel termed the "flexibility of the recommendation." The three levels are termed standard, recommendation, or option, each level having less of an evidence base and therefore more flexibility in application (see Table 23.2).

Similar to the AUA panels' approach, the EAU, ICUD, and NCCN guideline panels each performed literature searches using standard online data libraries, subsequently assigning levels of evidence to the data from the publications of good merit. Rather than generating independent meta-analyses, the data from the publications were combined with the clinical experience and knowledge of the panel members to determine recommendations. For the EAU and ICUD, recommendations were graded alphabetically,

the grade of the recommendation correlating with the level of evidence supporting it (see Table 23.2). As such, grade "A" recommendations were generally based on the highest level of evidence, grade "C" on the lowest level. The EAU guidelines graded recommendations A through C whereas the ICUD included a "D" grade when "no recommendation" was possible. The NCCN categorized recommendations numerically based on the level of evidence and degree of consensus amongst the panel members (see Table 23.2). Category 1 recommendations had high-level evidence and uniform consensus, Category 2a lower-level evidence with uniform consensus, Category 2b lower-level evidence with consensus (not uniform), and Category 3 recommendations had any level of evidence with no consensus amongst panel members.

The trade-off for approaching creation of guideline recommendations without the same methodological rigor as the AUA panel is the ability of the EAU, ICUD, and NCCN guidelines to take into account the more recent literature. The most recent AUA guidelines were published in 2007, the most current article included in their analyses published in 2005. In contrast, the EAU, ICUD, and NCCN guidelines each have been updated as of 2012 or later, each including publications as recent as 2012. In addition, there is a difference in scope. The AUA panel mostly limits their recommendations to those scenarios with enough data for meta-analyses to be performed, and as such, is relatively narrow in scope. In turn, the EAU, ICUD, and NCCN address many more

Table 23.2 Panels' categorization of recommendations definitions

Panel	Categorization	Definition
AUA	Standard	Health outcomes of the alternative interventions are sufficiently well known to permit meaningful decisions and virtual unanimity about which intervention is preferred.
	Recommendation	Health outcomes of the alternative intervention are sufficiently well known to permit meaningful decisions and appreciable but not unanimous majority agrees on which intervention is preferred.
	Option	Health outcomes of the interventions are not sufficiently well known to permit meaningful decisions or preferences are unknown or equivocal.
EAU	Grade A	Based on clinical studies of good quality and consistency that addressed the specific recommendations, including at least one randomized trial.
	Grade B	Based on well-conducted clinical studies, but without randomized clinical trials.
	Grade C	Recommendation made despite the absence of directly applicable clinical studies of good quality.
ICUD	Grade A	Usually depends on consistent level 1 evidence and often means that the recommendation is effectively mandatory and placed within a clinical care pathway.
	Grade B	Usually depends on consistent level 2 and or 3 studies, or "majority evidence" from RCT's.
	Grade C	Usually depends on level 4 studies or "majority evidence" from level 2/3 studies or expert opinion.
	Grade D	"No recommendation possible;" evidence is inadequate or conflicting and when expert opinion is delivered without a formal analytical process.
NCCN	Category 1	Based on high-level evidence, uniform consensus intervention is appropriate.
	Category 2a	Based on lower-level evidence, uniform consensus intervention is appropriate.
	Category 2b	Based on lower-level evidence, consensus that the intervention is appropriate.
	Category 3	Based on any level of evidence, major NCCN disagreement intervention is appropriate.

scenarios, albeit with the caveat that these recommendations are mainly based on expert opinion as opposed to high levels of evidence.

Regardless of the similarities and differences between the guidelines, each panel explicitly notes the dichotomy between best evidence and best outcome. While the guidelines strive to assimilate and disseminate the best evidence, they are not intended to replace the value of clinical expertise as it pertains to the individual patient. This should be kept in mind as we explore the following six clinical scenarios, vignettes that have been thematic throughout the NMIBC chapters preceding. The reader will note that while the clinical prompt includes the patient's age, the panels' recommendations are not age-adjusted, inherently relying on clinicians to integrate whether minor or major interventions are appropriate given the patient's age, medical co-morbidities, and treatment preferences (among others).

An additional consideration in the following vignettes is the format of the panels' recommendations. The AUA panel relies on individual case examples, and as such, the precision of the recommendation is dependent on the similarity between the vignette and one of the AUA panel's case examples. The EAU and ICUD guidelines are formatted as reviews, the reader responsible for synthesizing the relevant recommendations. The NCCN guidelines are presented as flow diagrams, i.e. decision trees that diverge at various diagnostic and therapeutic moments. As such, individuals with seemingly very different clinical courses may end up in the same group, and therefore with the same recommendation.

Finally, an additional notable inclusion in the EAU recommendations are risk tables from the European Organization for Research and Treatment of Cancer (EORTC) Genito-Urinary Cancer Group that allows for individualization of the likelihood of recurrence and progression [9].

The scoring system used to determine risk in these tables is based on independent predictors of recurrence and progression based on the number of tumors, tumor size, tumor grade, tumor depth of invasion, prior recurrence, and presence of concurrent carcinoma in situ (CIS). The EAU recommends clinicians use these tables to help stratify the patient into high, intermediate, or low risk (Grade B). Where appropriate, we have included these calculations in our interpretation of the EAU's recommendation for any one clinical vignette.

23.2 Clinical Vignettes

23.2.1 45-Year-Old Healthy Man with His First Large, High-Grade Ta Cancer

A synopsis of the panels' recommendations for an incident, large, HGTa tumor can be seen in Table 23.3.

23.2.1.1 AUA Guideline

This tumor is considered to be high risk in terms of recurrence (along with high grade T1 and CIS). Whereas the guidelines recommend that HG T1 lesions without muscularis in the specimen warrant a repeat resection (standard), in the case of HG Ta the guideline states "repeat resection may be appropriate." Subsequent to transurethral resection of the bladder tumor (TURBT), induction bacillus Calmette-Guerin (BCG) followed by maintenance BCG is suggested (recommendation), with maintenance consisting of three consecutive weeks of full-dose BCG at 3, 6, 12, 18, 24, 30, and 36 months if tolerated by the patient. The AUA guidelines do not make any specific recommendations regarding the components or timing of surveillance follow-up. The AUA panel recommends immediate, single-dose, postoperative intravesical chemotherapy to decrease recurrence for all non-muscle invasive tumors, the recommendation not specific either to grade or depth of invasion.

23.2.1.2 EAU Guideline

The EAU recommends re-resection for this tumor (Grade A). This is regardless of whether the TURBT was complete or incomplete and whether there was muscle in the original pathology specimen. This recommendation is due to the fact that the EAU recommended re-resection in all patients with a grade 3 (i.e. high-grade) tumors not involving the muscularis (Grade A), regardless of lamina propria involvement. Re-resection is recommended to be within 2–6 weeks (Grade C).

Per the EORTC risk tables, the EAU would estimate this man's likelihood of recurrence and progression to be 38 % and 5 % at 1 year, 62 %

Table 23.3 Recommendations for incident large, high-grade Ta tumor

	AUA	EAU	ICUD	NCCN
Re-staging TURBT				
Incomplete resection	NR[a]	Yes (A)	Yes (A)	Yes (2a)
No muscle in specimen	NR[a]	Yes (A)	NR	Yes (2a)
Intravesical therapy				
Agent	BCG (R)	BCG (A)	BCG (A)	BCG or MMC (2a)[b]
Duration, if response	I+M (R)	1–3 years (A)	NR	NR
Timing of surveillance				
Cystoscopy and urine cytology	NR	q3mo. for 2 yrs, then q6mo. for 3 yrs, then yearly (C)	q3mo. for 2 yrs, q4mo. for 1 yr, q6mo. for 2 yrs, then annually (NG)	q3-6mo. for 2 yrs. (2a)
Upper tract studies	NR	Yearly CT-IVU or IVU (C)	Periodic imaging by US, IVU, or CT (NG)	q1–2 years (2a)

BCG=bacillus Calmette-Guerin, I=induction, M=maintenance, NG=no specific grade, NR=no specific recommendation
Strength of recommendation indicated in () if applicable; refer to Table 23.2 for details
[a]AUA guidelines states "repeat resection may be appropriate"
[b]NCCN favors BCG over MMC in this setting and includes observation as an option

and 17 % at 5 years, respectively. He would be considered high risk, thus the recommendation for full-dose intravesical BCG for 1–3 years after re-resection (Grade A). The EAU only recommends a single postoperative dose of intravesical chemotherapy in patients with low- or intermediate-risk tumors (Grade A).

As it pertains to follow-up, the EAU assigns a Grade A recommendation to the follow-up being based on regular cystoscopy. For this patient, he would have cystoscopy and urine cytology every 3 months for the first 2 years, then every 6 months for three more years, then yearly (Grade C). In addition, yearly intravenous urogram (IVU) or CT-IVU is recommended (Grade C).

23.2.1.3 ICUD Guideline

Repeat resection is recommended if there is a question of completeness of the original TURBT (Grade A). Regarding an immediate, postoperative intravesical instillation of chemotherapy, the ICUD considers this to be an option, but not mandatory (Grade A). Intravesical BCG should follow TURBT (Grade A), the dose and duration not specified. The ICUD states that the likelihood of recurrence can be lowered with maintenance BCG, however the impact of BCG on progression "remains unclear." No specific recommendations are made regarding the timing of surveillance cystoscopy, urine studies, or imaging in high-grade Ta. The panel notes that follow-up schedules for HG Ta resemble those for CIS. Recommendations for CIS include cystoscopy and cytology every 3 months for 2 years, every 4 months in the third year, every 6 months in the fourth and fifth years, and once per year thereafter. Imaging by ultrasound, IVU, or CT is recommended "periodically."

23.2.1.4 NCCN Guideline

The panel recommends complete TURBT, with repeat resection if the resection is incomplete or if there is no muscularis propria in the specimen (Category 2a). This should be followed with induction mitomycin C (MMC) or BCG, the panel recommending BCG over MMC based on the available literature (Category 2a). Observation is also listed as an option. The NCCN only recommends a single, postoperative dose of intravesical

chemotherapy for LG Ta lesions and does not make any specific recommendations on maintenance intravesical therapy for incident HGTa.

Surveillance cystoscopy and urine cytology is recommended every 3–6 months for the first 2 years, then at increasing intervals "as appropriate" thereafter (Category 2a). Upper tract imaging is recommended every 1–2 years, the modality of imaging not specified (Category 2a). The panel considers use of urine molecular tests in follow-up a Category 2b recommendation.

23.2.2 Consensus

For the incident high-grade Ta tumor, the majority of the panels recommend re-resection if the original TURBT is incomplete, with the EAU and NCCN specifically advising re-resection if muscle is not present in the specimen. All panels favor at least an induction course of BCG. As it pertains to an immediate, single dose of intravesical chemotherapy postoperatively, none of the panels would specifically recommend it for this tumor. The AUA panel recommends it for all non-muscle invasive tumors, without differentiation based on risk. The EAU recommends it for low- and intermediate-risk tumors, the ICUD and NCCN guidelines for low risk only.

23.2.3 73-Year-Old Woman with Multiple, Recurrent High-Grade Ta Tumors That Has Received Perioperative MMC Chemotherapy and Has Significant Lower Urinary Tract Symptoms

Two factors related to this clinical scenario make determination of a guidelines-based treatment decision very difficult. One, the patient did not receive the consensus guideline recommendation for her incident tumor. As detailed in the clinical vignette above, induction BCG is the recommended treatment, with only the AUA guidelines supporting immediate postoperative MMC. Two, the patient's lower urinary tract symptoms after MMC introduce a variable not accounted for in the panels' recommendations. This omission does not imply that the woman's symptoms are irrelevant. Quite the opposite, it underscores the panel authors' admission that guidelines do not replace the value of clinical expertise, expertise relied upon both to alleviate the woman's symptoms and determine the next appropriate steps.

A revised clinical vignette that would allow for guideline interpretation might read:

23.2.4 73-Year-Old Woman with Multiple, Recurrent High-Grade Ta Tumors After MMC Chemotherapy

The recommendations per panel for this modified vignette would be as follows:

23.2.4.1 AUA Guideline

Per the panel, cystectomy should be considered a therapeutic alterative (recommendation), and in fact would be considered the "preferred treatment." The recommendation is based on the high likelihood of progression and the adverse consequences from an oncologic standpoint of delaying cystectomy. The panel considers further intravesical therapy an option, more so if it is a 6-week course of BCG in an individual whose recurrence can be classified as late. While noting the existence of alternative or combination intravesical regimens, the panel considers the data insufficient to draw any conclusions regarding appropriateness in this setting.

23.2.4.2 EAU Guideline

In the event of failed intravesical chemotherapy, the EAU recommends BCG instillations (no grade given to recommendation). This recommendation is based on the study by Malmstrom et al. [10], the panel noting "prior intravesical therapy has no impact of the effect of BCG." The guideline recommends holding BCG if patients have symptoms consistent with a UTI. In the event a patient has lower urinary tract symptoms secondary to BCG, the panel references the recommendations of the International Bladder Cancer Group (IBCG) and the publication by Rodriguez et al. for management [11, 12].

23.2.4.3 ICUD Guideline

The panel does not specifically address intravesical chemotherapy failures for HG Ta NMIBC. This is largely due to the fact that the panel considers intravesical BCG the standard in those with HG Ta (Grade A). The panel does note that "treatment and follow-up strategies generally resemble the strategies for CIS." In this context, if the patient's local symptomatology allowed for BCG, this would be the recommendation.

23.2.4.4 NCCN Guideline

The panel recommends that recurrence in this setting should be managed either with either cystectomy or an induction course of a different intravesical agent (in this case BCG given prior MMC) (grade 2a). The panel recommends withholding BCG if there are persistent severe local symptoms due to BCG.

23.2.5 Consensus

For recurrent, high-grade, multi-focal Ta tumor despite perioperative MMC, the guidelines would favor intravesical BCG. Extrapolating from the guideline text, failure of perioperative or induction intravesical chemotherapy does not affect the efficacy of subsequent BCG. The woman's local symptomatology post-MMC introduces a caveat outside the scope of the guidelines. And such, the initial management of these symptoms and subsequent treatment decisions require the clinician's expertise.

23.2.6 68-Year-Old Man with Rapidly Recurring Multiple, Low-Grade, Papillary Ta Tumors Despite Perioperative Mitomycin and One Induction Course of BCG

A synopsis of the panels' recommendations for multiple, low-grade Ta tumors after MMC and induction BCG can be seen in Table 23.4.

Table 23.4 Recommendations for rapidly recurring multiple, low-grade, papillary Ta tumors after perioperative MMC and induction BCG

	AUA	EAU	ICUD	NCCN
Continued Intravesical Rx	Yes (R)	Yes (C)	Yes (A)	Yes (2a)
Agent	MMC or BCG	BCG or chemoRx[a]	BCG	chemoRx[b]
Duration, if response	I+M (O)	1–3 years (C)[a]	NR	1–2 years (O)[b]
Cystectomy	NR	Yes (C)[a]	NR	Yes (2a)

BCG=bacillus Calmette-Guerin, I=induction, M=maintenance, MMC=mitomycin C, NR=no specific recommendation

Strength of recommendation indicated in () if applicable; refer to Table 23.2 for details

[a]If tumor ≥3 cm, BCG recommended by EAU for 1–3 years (Grade C). If tumor <3 cm, BCG, intravesical MMC, or intravesical epirubicin are options for 1 year EAU mentions intravesical MMC and epirubicin as options in this setting. Regardless of tumor size, continued intravesical therapy is favored option to cystectomy

[b]NCCN recommends a "change" in intravesical agents, and recommends adjuvant intravesical chemotherapy to prevent recurrent low-grade Ta. The optimal length of therapy is undetermined

23.2.6.1 AUA Guideline

For patients with recurrent low-grade Ta tumors, induction intravesical BCG or MMC is the next step (recommendation). The panels' meta-analyses found that TURBT+BCG induction decreases recurrences by 24 % (95 % CI: 3, 47) and TURBT+MMC induction decreased recurrences by 3 % (95 % CI: −10, 16) relative to TURBT alone. Due to the overlap in confidence intervals, the AUA states that the data "do not permit the conclusion" that induction BCG is superior to induction MMC in this setting. As such, induction MMC would likely be the next step for this man. The panel would also recommend maintenance therapy (option), as the meta-analyses found that TURBT+MMC maintenance decreased recurrence by 18 % (95 % CI: 6, 30) relative to TURBT alone. The panel does not discuss radical cystectomy in the setting of low-grade Ta disease.

23.2.6.2 EAU Guideline

Risk stratification of this patient would place him at intermediate or high risk of recurrence and progression, depending on the size of the tumors. If the patient had multiple, recurrent and "large (3 cm)" G1G2 Ta tumors, then by EAU definition the patient would be high risk. If not meeting the size criterion, the patient would be intermediate risk. Per the EAU risk tables and calculator, this patient would have between 38 and 61 % probability of recurrence at 1 year and between 62 and 78 % at 5 years. From the standpoint of progression, the patient would have a 1 and 6 % probability of progression at 1 and 5 years unless the tumor diameter was greater than or equal to 3 cm. In this setting, the patient would have a 5 and 17 % probability of progression at 1 and 5 years.

For treatment, the EAU recommends adjuvant intravesical chemotherapy instillations, repeat induction BCG, or radical cystectomy (Grade C). Intravesical chemotherapy or BCG would be appropriate if tumor size was less than 3 cm (i.e. intermediate risk), BCG if the tumor size was ≥3 cm. If intravesical chemotherapy was chosen, the provider is specifically encouraged to optimize the pH of the instillation and preserve the concentration by the limiting patient fluid intake (Grade B). Both MMC and epirubicin are mentioned as options. In order to optimize the effectiveness of intravesical chemotherapy, the panel suggests that the length of the instillation should be 1–2 h (Grade C). Additionally, the panel suggests that continued utilization of intravesical chemotherapy should not exceed 1 year (Grade C) as the available data does not demonstrate efficacy beyond this point. If intravesical BCG is chosen, the duration would be 1 year in the case of an intermediate risk tumor or 1–3 years if a high-risk tumor. Unlike recurrent of high-grade tumors, recurrent low-grade tumors after induction BCG does not render the patient the "highest-risk of the high-risk tumors," BCG-refractory, or a BCG failure. As such, the EAU recommendations favor continuing intravesical treatments over cystectomy (Grade C).

23.2.6.3 ICUD Guideline

The ICUD panel notes that in the case of incident HG Ta, BCG is usually overtreatment given the low risk of tumor progression and is not appropriate therapy (Grade B). However, the panel also notes that BCG is a superior "rescue therapy" compared to MMC for patients who have failed intravesical chemotherapy and should be used in this setting (Grade B). Given the details of the clinical vignette, this patient would be categorized as BCG resistant (persistence at 3 months after induction BCG) by the ICUD panel. Options for treatment include repeat BCG, salvage intravesical chemotherapy, intravesical interferon (either alone or in combination with low-dose BCG), and thermo-chemotherapy. Of these, the panel considers repeat TURBT and BCG the best option (Grade A), with the remaining options considered Grade C.

23.2.6.4 NCCN Guideline

For post-perioperative MMC plus induction BCG disease, the NCCN guidelines do not specifically alter the algorithm based on grade of recurrence. The panel's recommendation is a change in intravesical agent or proceeding with cystectomy (category 2a). If induction intravesical chemotherapy was pursued, maintenance intravesical chemotherapy in the event of a complete response is considered optional. The guidelines do specifically state that in the event of recurrence or persistence, no more than two consecutive induction cycles of an intravesical therapy agent should be given (category 2a).

23.2.7 Consensus

For recurrent, multi-focal, low-grade tumors despite MMC and induction BCG, the guidelines would favor bladder preservation with continued intravesical treatments. Notably, the next agent would vary depending on the guideline referenced, and in the case of the EAU recommendations, the size of the tumor. Adherence to the AUA and NCCN guidelines would result in the patient receiving MMC (induction±maintenance). The ICUD guidelines favors repeat BCG. From the viewpoint of the EAU panel,

either intravesical chemotherapy or BCG would be appropriate for if the tumor(s) were less than 3 cm (i.e. intermediate risk), BCG the appropriate choice if the tumor(s) were greater than or equal to 3 cm. The EAU, ICUD, and NCCN guidelines all include cystectomy as a possible option at this point, the NCCN guidelines are the most difficult to interpret as it pertains to the relative appropriateness of cystectomy compared to additional intravesical therapy.

23.2.8 72-Year-Old Woman with a 3 cm Low-Grade T1 Bladder Tumor Located in the Dome and Without Muscle Present in the Specimen

One important factor in this vignette is not accounted for in the panels' recommendations: tumor location. Obtaining muscularis while resecting tumors of the bladder dome increases the risk of perforation, particularly in bladders that have a relatively thin layer of muscle (as would likely be the case in this elderly woman). This is another example of a clinical caveat where the panels' recommendations must be considered in the context of the clinician's expertise as to whether it is technically possible to obtain muscle without perforation.

A synopsis of the panels' recommendations for an incident, large, LG T1 tumor irrespective of tumor location (i.e. assuming re-resection would yield muscularis without resulting in bladder perforation) can be seen in Table 23.5.

23.2.8.1 AUA Guideline

Repeat TURBT (standard) followed by induction and maintenance BCG (recommended) would be the guideline's recommendation. Cystectomy should be considered in select patients (option), with this patient meeting at least two of the factors listed for an increased risk of progression (large tumor size, tumor location in a site poorly accessible to complete resection, diffuse disease, presence of CIS, infiltration of lymphatic or vascular spaces, and prostatic urethral involvement). Random bladder biopsies are not recommended by the AUA.

Table 23.5 Recommendations for incident large, low-grade T1 tumor without muscle in specimen

	AUA	EAU	ICUD	NCCN
Re-staging TURBT	Yes (S)	Yes (A)	Yes (A)	Yes (2a)
Intravesical therapy	Yes (R)	Yes (A)	Yes (B)	Yes (2a)[a]
Agent	BCG (R)	BCG (A)	BCG (B)	BCG (1) or MMC (2a)
Duration, if response	I+M (R)	1–3 years (A)	NR	1–2 years (O)
Cystectomy	Yes (O)	NR	NR	Yes (2a)
Random bladder biopsies	NR	NR	NR	NR

BCG = bacillus Calmette-Guerin, I = induction, M = maintenance, MMC = mitomycin C, NR = no specific recommendation

Strength of recommendation indicated in () if applicable; refer to Table 23.2 for details

[a]If residual disease present at resection, NCCN recommends BCG (1) or cystectomy (2a). If no residual disease at re-resection, recommendation is BCG (1) or MMC (2a)

23.2.8.2 EAU Guideline

Repeat resection would be recommended (Grade A). Assuming a normal appearance of the remainder of the bladder, random bladder biopsies are not recommended. Given that the tumor is T1, it qualifies as a high-risk tumor and the recommendation would be for full-dose BCG for 1–3 years (grade A). Per the EAU risk tables and calculator, this patient would have between a 24 % and 46 % probability of recurrence at 1 year and 5 years respectively. From the standpoint of progression, the patient would have a 1 and 6 % probability of progression at 1 and 5 years.

23.2.8.3 ICUD Guideline

The ICUD does not distinguish between low- and high-grade T1 in terms of their recommended next steps. A re-staging TURBT is recommended regardless of the presence of muscle in the specimen. The authors note that tumor grade, multiplicity, size, concomitant CIS, involvement of the prostatic urethra, depth of lamina propia invasion, and early recurrence determine prognosis (Grade A). If a bladder-sparing approach was pursued, a re-staging TURBT should be followed by BCG (Grade B).

23.2.8.4 NCCN Guideline

The NCCN panel would strongly advise repeat TURBT (category 2a) followed by BCG (category 1) independent of the clinician's sense as to the completeness of the original resection. If residual disease is present at re-resection, cystectomy is an alternative option to BCG, however the panel considers BCG the preferred option as the next best step over cystectomy (category 1 vs. category 2a).

In the event of no residual disease at re-resection, MMC is also an option, albeit inferior to BCG (category 2a vs. category 1). Maintenance therapy would be optional and the NCCN does not recommend random bladder biopsies.

23.2.9 Consensus

For the incident, large, LG T1 tumor the consensus of the guidelines is repeat TURBT followed by induction intravesical BCG. While the duration of the BCG is not specified by all of the guidelines, the overall consensus is that maintenance BCG merits consideration. Random bladder biopsies are not recommended. If in the clinician's judgment muscle cannot be obtained without perforating the bladder, one can infer from the guidelines that cystectomy or a bladder-sparing approach would be a reasonable alternative.

23.2.10 79-Year-Old Man Who Has Persistent CIS Despite Induction and Maintenance BCG for 6 Months

A synopsis of the panels' recommendations for persistent CIS after 6 months of induction and maintenance BCG can be seen in Table 23.6.

23.2.10.1 AUA Guideline

Similar to the recommendation for the 73-year-old woman with multiple, recurrent high-grade Ta tumors outlined previously, the AUA guidelines

Table 23.6 Recommendations for persistent CIS after induction and maintenance BCG

	AUA	EAU	ICUD	NCCN
Continued Intravesical Rx	NR	Yes (C)	Yes (NG)	Yes (2a)
Agent		BCG (C)	valrubicin	valrubicin
Cystectomy	Yes (R)	Yes (C)	Yes (A)	Yes (2a)

BCG = bacillus Calmette-Guerin, NR = no specific recommendation
Strength of recommendation indicated in () if applicable; refer to Table 23.2 for details

state that cystectomy should be considered a therapeutic alterative (recommendation), stating that it is the "preferred treatment" given the patients exposure to BCG. The recommendation is based on the high likelihood of progression (meta-analyses showed benefit of BCG in terms of recurrence only and not progression) and the adverse consequences from an oncologic standpoint of delaying cystectomy. While noting the existence of alternative or combination intravesical regimens, the AUA considers the data insufficient to draw any conclusions.

23.2.10.2 EAU Guideline

Despite the persistence of CIS at 6 months, this patient does not meet the criteria of BCG-refractory or BCG-failure. In order to meet the criteria of BCG-refractory in the setting of CIS without concomitant Ta or T1 tumors, CIS would need to have been present at 3 and 6 months. The guidelines note that in patients with BCG present at 3 months, an "additional BCG course can achieve a complete response in >50 % of cases." Referenced is the publication by Babjuk et al. [2]. The options for treatment would be radical cystectomy and repeat induction BCG (Grade C). The guidelines also mention a "bladder-preserving strategy" as an option (Grade C). While this would include a combined chemo-radiation approach, it is doubtful that the EAU would specifically recommend chemo-radiation to this patient given the data demonstrating that radiation is not effective for CIS. The EAU does note that bladder-preserving strategies can yield responses, however "experience is limited other than radical cystectomy" and thus a bladder-preserving strategy "must be considered oncologically inferior at this time."

23.2.10.3 ICUD Guideline

This patient would be categorized as a BCG failure, i.e. disease at 6 months following BCG induction therapy and maintenance at 3 months. In this setting, the ICUD considers cystectomy to be the "gold standard" (Grade A). Other treatment options include intravesical chemotherapy, particularly valrubicin. However, the ICUD includes the caveat that it is approved for those who either refuse or are not fit for cystectomy, noting the small number of patients evaluated and the low success rates.

23.2.10.4 NCCN Guideline

Options for this patient include a change in intravesical agent or cystectomy (Category 2a). Intravesical chemotherapy would likely be valrubicin, as the guidelines note that it is approved for BCG-refractory CIS.

23.2.11 Consensus

For the persistent CIS after induction and maintenance BCG at 6 months, the strongest recommendations are for the patient to undergo a cystectomy. Repeat induction BCG (EAU, Grade C) or induction valrubicin (NCCN, Category 2a; ICUD) are options, however with the exception of the NCCN guidelines, they are considered inferior to bladder removal.

23.2.12 55-Year-Old Man with CIS and High-Grade Ta Tumors After Receiving a 6-Week Induction Course of BCG

A synopsis of the panels' recommendations for HGTa with CIS after 6 weeks of induction BCG can be seen in Table 23.7.

23.2.12.1 AUA Guideline

As was the case for the clinical vignette of persistent CIS after 6 months of induction and maintenance BCG, the AUA guidelines state that cystectomy should be considered a therapeutic alterative (recommendation) and is the "preferred treatment" given the patient's exposure to BCG. The guidelines do state that further intravesical therapy may be considered (option), particularly if the intravesical therapy is a 6-week course of BCG in an individual who is disease-free for a long enough period of time for the recurrence to be classified as "late." Given that this is not a late recurrence, cystectomy would be the guideline-based treatment.

Table 23.7 Recommendations for CIS and high-grade Ta after induction BCG

	AUA	EAU	ICUD	NCCN
Continued Intravesical Rx Agent	Yes (O) BCG or MMC (NG)[b]	NR[a]	Yes (A) BCG (A)	Yes (2a) chemoRx[c]
Cystectomy	Yes (R)	Yes (B)	NR	Yes (2a)

BCG = bacillus Calmette-Guerin, I = induction, M = maintenance, MMC = mitomycin C, NR = no specific recommendation

Strength of recommendation indicated in () if applicable; refer to Table 23.2 for details

[a]While cystectomy is the "preferred treatment," the AUA considers further intravesical treatment an option particularly if (1) it is repeat induction BCG and (2) a late recurrence

[b]The EAU recommends cystectomy. If the patient is not a suitable candidate, a bladder preserving approach is an option (C)

[c]NCCN recommends a "change" in intravesical agents

23.2.12.2 EAU Guideline

The presence of CIS and a high-grade tumor during BCG therapy renders the patient BCG-refractory and a BCG-failure. The patient should undergo radical cystectomy (Grade B), or, if the patient was not a suitable candidate for cystectomy, a bladder-preserving approach should be the next step (Grade C). The EAU does not make any further recommendations regarding the components of the bladder-preserving approach other than note that preservation strategies can be categorized as immunotherapy, chemotherapy, device-assisted therapy, and combination therapy.

23.2.12.3 ICUD Guideline

The patient would be categorized as BCG-resistant, and per the ICUD panel's recommendation, repeat TURBT and BCG are the best option (Grade A). Of note, the ICUD does not specifically differentiate how to proceed with post-induction BCG based on the pathologic characteristics of the recurrence (i.e. low grade vs. high grade, Ta vs. T1, concomitant CIS vs. CIS only).

23.2.12.4 NCCN Guideline

Per the NCCN, options for this patient would be similar to those for persistent CIS despite induction and maintenance BCG for 6 months above. Options include a change in intravesical agent (perhaps to valrubicin, although unclear due to the concomitant presence of HGTa) or cystectomy (category 2a). The NCCN recommendation would be the same regardless if this were Ta, CIS, or Ta with concomitant CIS after BCG.

23.2.13 Consensus

For the patient with HGTa and CIS after 6 weeks of induction BCG, there does not appear to be a consensus. The AUA and EAU guidelines both favor cystectomy (Recommendation and Grade B, respectively). The ICUD would recommend TURBT and BCG (Grade A), while the NCCN would recommend a cystectomy or a change to an intravesical chemotherapy agent (Category 2a).

23.3 Conclusion

Comparison of guidelines' recommendations for the clinical scenarios detailed above reveals consensus on a number of decision points in the treatment of NMIBC. For patients with incident, large, HGTa or LGT1 tumors, there is consensus regarding the importance of accurate pathologic staging and the utility of BCG. Yet other clinical vignettes result in very different treatment recommendations; there was a lack of consensus as to the next intravesical agent in the patient with multiple, LG Ta tumors after MMC and induction BCG. Similarly, for the patient with persistent CIS after induction and maintenance BCG at 6 months, and for the patient with HGTa and CIS after 6 weeks of induction BCG, there were marked differences in the next recommended treatment and the strength of the treatment recommendation.

The lack of consensus pertaining to some of the clinical vignettes underscores the limitations of any evidence-based guideline. Inherently, establishing the highest levels of evidence for any one step in a treatment paradigm requires both a critical mass of patients and a controlled environment in which the treatment can be administered and the response assessed. The more detailed the clinical scenario (i.e. recurrent, concomitant HGTa and CIS shortly after BCG vs. incident HGTa), the less likely a guideline panel will have the quality and consistency of evidence to make definitive recommendations. Furthermore, the greater number of non-tumor-specific considerations that merit integration into the treatment decision (i.e. age, comorbidity, patient preference, etc.), the less likely a guideline may be to dictate the next appropriate step. While the irony of this is not lost—the more complex the clinical scenario the more likely a clinician may be to consult outside sources to inform the appropriate next steps—it is not in and of itself surprising.

Instead, it speaks to the importance of interpreting guideline recommendations as the panels' authors intend; the weight or strength a panel ascribes to a treatment recommendation is likely as important as the recommendation itself. A clinical scenario that garners a standard, Grade A, or category 1 recommendation from the guidelines is likely based on level 1 evidence. As such, deviation should be the exception and not the rule. Conversely, recommendations with option, Grade C, or category 3 ratings are by definition based on more limited evidence, and are likely scenarios in which there are a number of different ways to proceed.

Going forward continued synthesis and interpretation of the best levels of evidence will likely remain the foundation on which guideline creation is based. However, panels need not be without guideposts. Guideline statements are not unique to urology, and tools are available to assess the evidence basis of the guidelines themselves. Authors on this subject have noted that panels should be more transparent both in their methods and disclosure of member bias [13]. Inclusion of patients as stakeholders, and integration of elements beyond the cancer-specific (i.e. age, comorbidity, and cost), is not without its challenges, but ultimately will be the criterion on which guideline panels themselves are judged [14].

As it pertains to the individual patient, clinical scenarios will always exist that are outside the scope of even the most detailed guideline. As such, the provision of the best care will always be reliant on the clinical expertise and judgment of the treating physicians.

References

1. Guideline for the Management of Nonmuscle Invasive Bladder Cancer: (Stages Ta, T1, and Tis): 2007 Update. American Urological Association. Accessed April 14, 2013, at https://www.auanet.org/education/guidelines/bladder-cancer.cfm
2. Guidelines on Non-muscle-invasive Bladder Cancer (TaT1 and CIS). European Assoication of Urology (EAU). Accessed April 14, 2013, at http://www.uroweb.org/guidelines/online-guidelines/
3. International Consultation on Urological Diseases (ICUD). Bladder cancer, 2nd edn. Accessed June 3, 2013, at http://www.icud.info/bladdercancer2nd.html
4. National Clinical Practice Guidelines in Oncology (NCCN Guidelines). Bladder cancer. Version 1. 2013. Accessed May 1st, 2013, at http://www.nccn.org/professionals/physician_gls/pdf/bladder.pdf

5. Hall MC, Chang SS, Dalbagni G, et al. Guideline for the management of nonmuscle invasive bladder cancer (stages Ta, T1, and Tis): 2007 update. J Urol. 2007;178:2314–30.
6. Babjuk M, Oosterlinck W, Sylvester R, et al. EAU guidelines on non-muscle-invasive urothelial carcinoma of the bladder, the 2011 update. Actas Urol Esp. 2012;36:389–402.
7. Burger M, Oosterlinck W, Konety B, et al. ICUD-EAU International Consultation on Bladder Cancer 2012: non-muscle-invasive urothelial carcinoma of the bladder. Eur Urol. 2013;63:36–44.
8. Oxford Centre for Evidence-based Medicine Levels of Evidence. March 2009. Accessed May 2013, at http://www.cebm.net/index.aspx?0=1025
9. Sylvester RJ, van der Meijden AP, Oosterlinck W, et al. Predicting recurrence and progression in individual patients with stage Ta T1 bladder cancer using EORTC risk tables: a combined analysis of 2596 patients from seven EORTC trials. Eur Urol. 2006;49:466–5. discussion 75–7.
10. Malmstrom PU, Sylvester RJ, Crawford DE, et al. An individual patient data meta-analysis of the long-term outcome of randomised studies comparing intravesical mitomycin C versus bacillus Calmette-Guerin for non-muscle-invasive bladder cancer. Eur Urol. 2009;56:247–56.
11. Rodriguez F, Palou J, Martinez R, et al. Practical guideline for the management of adverse events associated with BCG installations. Arch Esp Urol. 2008;61:591–6.
12. Witjes JA, Palou J, Soloway M, et al. Clinical practice recommendations for the prevention and management of intravesical therapy-associated adverse events. Eur Urol Suppl. 2008;7:667–74.
13. Dahm P, Chapple CR, Konety BR, et al. The future of clinical practice guidelines in urology. Eur Urol. 2011;60:72–4.
14. Brouwers MC, Kho ME, Browman GP, et al. AGREE II: advancing guideline development, reporting and evaluation in health care. J Clin Epidemiol. 2010;63:1308–11.

Open Radical Cystectomy

24

J. Joy Lee, Dipen J. Parekh, and Mark L. Gonzalgo

24.1 Background

In 1962, Drs. Whitmore and Marshall published their series of 230 cases of radical cystectomy for bladder cancer. Following their seminal work, the morbidity and mortality rate for radical cystectomy was reported to be approximately 35 % and 20 %, respectively [1]. Contemporary surgical experience with radical cystectomy is associated with an approximately 10 % early high-grade complication rate and mortality rate as low as 2.5 % [2, 3].

Open radical cystectomy with pelvic lymphadenectomy remains the gold standard for patients with clinically localized muscle-invasive bladder cancer. Other indications for radical cystectomy include carcinoma in-situ (cis) or high-grade tumors refractory to intravesical chemo- or immunotherapy, or recurrent multifocal superficial tumors unable to be managed adequately with repeat transurethral resection [4]. In several large series, the overall recurrence-free survival at 5 years for patients undergoing cystectomy approaches 70 %, ranging from 50 to 60 % for lymph-node positive stage 3 or 4 tumors to 89 % for stage 2 tumors [2, 5]. With the advent of laparoscopic/robotic technology, cystectomy can also be performed using minimally invasive surgical approaches. Robotic-assisted radical cystectomy (RARC) has been shown in retrospective and small prospective trials to be non-inferior to open radical cystectomy [6–10]. Ongoing multi-institutional randomized prospective trials are evaluating whether safety, oncologic control, clinical outcomes, and cost efficacy are comparable between the two techniques [11, 12].

J.J. Lee, M.D. (✉)
Department of Urology, Stanford University School of Medicine, 300 Pasteur Drive S287, Stanford, CA 94305, USA
e-mail: joylee1@stanford.edu; joylander@gmail.com

D.J. Parekh, M.D.
Department of Urology, University of Miami Miller School of Medicine, 1400 NW 10 Ave, Suite 510, Miami, FL 33136, USA
e-mail: parekhd@med.miami.edu

M.L. Gonzalgo, M.D., Ph.D.
Department of Urology, University of Miami Miller School of Medicine, 1120 NW 14th Street (M-814), Miami, FL 33101, USA
e-mail: m.gonzalgo@med.miami.edu

24.2 Preoperative Considerations

24.2.1 Staging

After the diagnosis of bladder cancer has been established, patients should undergo complete staging to evaluate for nodal spread and metastases (Fig. 24.1). Relevant laboratory tests include serum liver function tests and alkaline phosphatase to screen for liver and bone metastases. Guidelines vary on using chest X-ray versus

B.R. Konety and S.S. Chang (eds.), *Management of Bladder Cancer:*
A Comprehensive Text With Clinical Scenarios, DOI 10.1007/978-1-4939-1881-2_24,
© Springer Science+Business Media New York 2015

Fig. 24.1 Evaluation and staging for bladder cancer

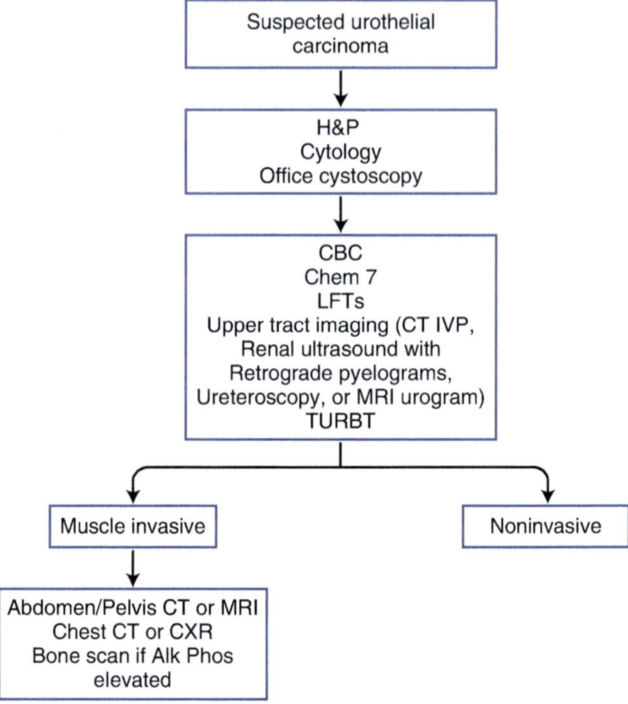

computed tomography (CT) for staging evaluation of the chest, but all agree that evaluation for lung metastases is indicated. CT of the abdomen and pelvis should always be obtained to determine whether extravesical extension or lymphadenopathy is present. Positron emission tomography (PET) CT or magnetic resonance imaging (MRI) may also be useful for bladder cancer staging, particularly in instances of non-muscle-invasive disease [13, 14]. Lastly, serum creatinine and calculated glomerular filtration rate (GFR) can provide important information regarding eligibility for certain chemotherapeutic regimens and diversions, as well as being important to obtain baseline values against which to compare long-term renal function post-diversion.

24.2.2 Neoadjuvant Treatment Considerations

Preoperative radiation therapy has not been shown to afford surgical candidates any survival benefit, and has not been routinely used since 1979 [15]. However, in instances of extensive comorbidity and poor performance status, endo-scopic resection with chemoradiation may be offered for muscle-invasive disease.

The indications for neoadjuvant chemotherapy are discussed in greater detail in "Chapter 30: Management of bladder cancer, role of chemotherapy and controversies surrounding its application" and/or "Chapter 35: Clinical scenario: The role of perioperative chemotherapy." Evidence favors a significant though modest survival benefit from neoadjuvant chemotherapy followed by radical cystectomy compared to radical cystectomy alone, but the optimal regimen, dosing, and schedule remains to be determined [16–19]. Neoadjuvant cisplatin-based chemotherapy combined with external beam radiation may also be useful when considering a bladder-sparing approach for disease management [20, 21]. In carefully selected patients, partial cystectomy has been shown to provide equivalent oncologic outcomes compared to radical cystectomy [22–25]. These patients generally have a solitary lesion located in a suitable location such as the dome of the bladder that can be excised with negative margins, adequate bladder capacity, and no evidence of carcinoma in situ on random bladder biopsies.

24.2.3 Type of Diversion

Following the decision to proceed with radical cystectomy, one of the foremost considerations for the patient is the type of diversion: ileal conduit, orthotopic bladder substitution/neobladder, or continent cutaneous reservoir. To date, there are no randomized controlled trials comparing the various types of diversions, and each has its unique sets of characteristics. A careful assessment of a patient's current quality of life and priorities should be weighed. Surgeons should accurately and honestly discuss their respective risks and benefits with the patient, including preoperative and intraoperative patient and tumor-related factors that would preclude one form of diversion or another (Table 24.1).

For instance, a preoperative glomerular filtration rate <35 mL/min is generally accepted as a contraindication to continent diversion due to prolonged contact of urine with bowel [26]. Gastrointestinal conditions, such as Crohn's disease or preexisting short gut syndrome, can be relative contraindications for continent diversion given the longer length of bowel necessary. Men with untreated urethral strictures should not undergo neobladder reconstruction. Tumor extending into the distal prostatic urethra or anterior vagina in females, often diagnosed intraoperatively, would also possibly rule out an orthotopic bladder substitution. Patients who prefer to know definitively what type of diversion they will be receiving can be offered preoperative transurethral biopsies of the bladder neck, prostate in men, and urethra, as this can help determine need for urethrectomy and potential suitability of

neobladder reconstruction. However, it is important to keep in mind that the final decision regarding feasibility of an orthotopic bladder substitution is made intraoperatively after frozen section analysis of the distal resection margin. Prior pelvic radiation, once thought to be a contraindication to orthotopic bladder substitution, should not preclude patients from pursuing this option, but patients should be informed that most series report a higher rate of complications in this setting [27, 28].

We recommend that all patients undergoing cystectomy meet with an enterostomal specialist to undergo further counseling regarding pros and cons of each type of diversion, as well as receiving education on postoperative management of specific diversions. All patients who desire continent cutaneous diversion must be able to maintain and perform a consistent schedule of catheterization. Patients undergoing neobladder reconstruction should also be counseled that they may require intermittent catheterization. An optimal stoma site from both a patient and technical perspective is marked before surgery even for patients who choose neobladders, as oncologic findings during surgery may dictate the ultimate form of diversion [29].

24.2.4 Preparation for Surgery

The day before surgery, patients are traditionally asked to undergo a mechanical bowel preparation using agents such as oral magnesium citrate or polyethylene glycol, with the goal of having clear stools by that evening to decrease bacterial load and expunge solid fecal contents. It should be noted however that over the last decade, an

Table 24.1 Contraindications for various forms of urinary diversion

Contraindications	Neobladder	Continent cutaneous pouch	Ileal conduit
Absolute	Creatinine clearance <35 mL/min Severe hepatic dysfunction TCC in urethral stump Severe urethral stricture	Creatinine clearance <35 mL/min Severe hepatic dysfunction	Short gut (use colon or stomach instead)
Relative	Unable/unwilling to self-catheterize Unwilling to follow up regularly Compromised intestinal function Inadequate external sphincter	Unable/unwilling to self-catheterize Unwilling to follow up regularly Compromised intestinal function	

increasing body of literature suggests that mechanical bowel preparation prior to colorectal and/or intestinal resections may not provide any significant advantage in perioperative outcomes, and may possibly increase the risk of anastomotic leakage, intra-abdominal abscesses and ileus [30]. Patients are also advised to take only a clear liquid diet starting the day before surgery. Patients are instructed to be strictly nil per os (NPO) after midnight, with the exception of routine morning medications. Maintaining hydration is paramount, and patients in whom volume status may be hard to manage at home can be pre-admitted to the hospital the day before surgery for IV hydration and closer monitoring of fluid balance. A type and cross-match is performed with 2 units of packed red blood cells available if needed. Alternate arrangements and contingencies should be made for patients who refuse potential transfusions in accordance with their religious or cultural beliefs. In addition to sequential compression devices, all patients are given subcutaneous heparin immediately prior to surgery for prophylaxis against thromboembolic events.

24.3 Surgical Technique and Anatomy

The patient is brought to the operating room and placed supine on the operating table. General anesthesia is induced, an arterial line is inserted, and a nasogastric tube is also placed to help decompress the bowel. The patient is positioned with the iliac crest over the break in the operating table such that flexion of the table allows for hyperextension of the abdomen. The arms may be tucked bilaterally or left abducted in as anatomical a position as possible. All pressure points are adequately padded with egg crate foam or gel pads. Reverse Trendelenburg positioning may also be used to help keep the bowel cephalad and out of the working field. The surgeon should take note of the previously marked stoma site, as a vigorous prep may sometimes wash off the marking. The patient is prepped from the nipples to the midthigh, including the genital region, and draped in sterile fashion. A Foley catheter is then placed sterilely to decompress the bladder.

A vertical midline incision is made from the pubic symphysis, curving at the umbilicus contralateral to the potential stoma site (and even further laterally if an umbilical catheterizable stoma is planned), extending at least 4 cm cephalad. The anterior rectus sheath is identified deep to Camper's and Scarpa's fascia, and incised in the midline. The decussation of fibers in the midline is identified, and the bellies of the rectus muscles are retracted laterally, obviating the need for any division of muscle. The posterior rectus fascia is incised, and the peritoneum entered sharply at the superior portion of the incision. This peritoneal window is carefully enlarged until one hand can be placed in the peritoneal cavity to help protect the bowel contents and assess for any adhesions. Next, the urachus is identified and its origin at the umbilicus is circumscribed. Identification of the lateral umbilical ligaments, through which the inferior epigastric vessels run, will help define the far lateral boundaries of the urachal dissection. A large Babcock or Kelly clamp is placed on this cephalad end for retraction, and the entire urachal remnant is dissected free to be removed en bloc with the cystectomy specimen (Fig. 24.2).

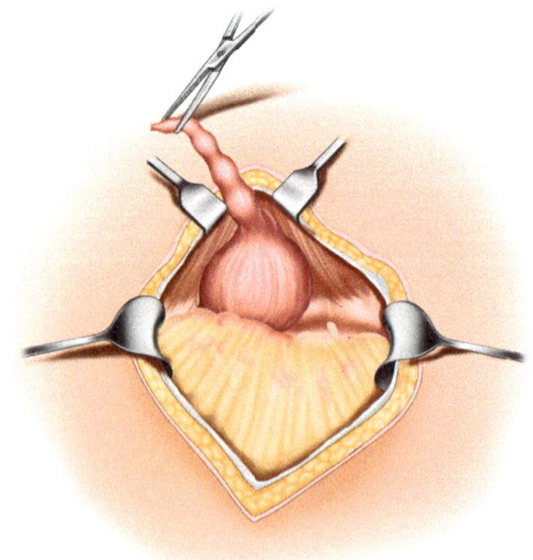

Fig. 24.2 Dissection of the urachus. Adapted from Weizer AZ, Lee CT. "16: Radical Cystectomy in Women." From Glenn's Urologic Surgery. Eds Graham SD, Keane TE. 7th ed. Lippincott Williams & Wilkins: Philadelphia, 2010; and Stein JP, Skinner DG. Surgical Atlas Radical Cystectomy. BJUI. 2004; 97: 197–221

The entire abdomen is systematically inspected to assess for any visceral metastases. Lysis of adhesions is performed if necessary. In patients undergoing cutaneous catheterizable diversions, inspection of the right colon, terminal ileum, and appendix can be made at this time. Similarly, in patients with a prior history of bowel resection, assessment can be made of prior anastomoses and the adequacy of bowel. At this time, a self-retaining Bookwalter retractor may be placed, and right-angle body wall retractors used to help with exposure.

The avascular white line of Toldt is identified and incised sharply beginning from the cecum and working cephalad, thereby allowing the ascending colon to be reflected medially. Near the hepatic flexure, care is taken to identify the duodenum while mobilizing the mesentery of the small bowel away from it. Similarly, the sigmoid and descending colon are reflected medially by dividing the white line of Toldt up toward the splenic flexure. At this point, a wide space should exist underneath the sigmoid and above the sacrum and iliac vessels, extending as far cephalad as the inferior mesentery artery, through which the left ureter will later be passed (Fig. 24.3). The small bowel and right colon are

then packed toward the epigastrum with moist laparotomy pads and malleable blade retractors.

Next, the ureters are identified at the level of their crossing over the iliac vessels. The ureters are each encircled with a vessel loop, and each is dissected free down toward the ureterovesical junction and cephalad as much as possible. Care is taken to preserve the periadventitial tissue and maintain a healthy vascular supply. As distally as possible, two metal clips are placed to prevent any possible tumor spillage, and the ureter is ligated in between. A cuff of the stay-side ureter distal to the clip may be excised and sent to pathology as a frozen section to assess for tumor or carcinoma in situ at the margin. If transitional cell carcinoma (TCC) or carcinoma in situ (cis) is found at the margin, additional cuffs of ureteral tissue are typically sent until a negative margin is achieved. It is worth noting, however, that the role of sequential ureteral resection for decreasing recurrence is debatable, especially when a pan-urothelial field defect theory is considered [31]. A recent meta-analysis estimates the rate of ureteral upper tract TCC in the setting of high grade muscle-invasive lower tract TCC to be between 0.75 % and 8 % [31, 32]. A clip is generally left on the ureter until the time of ureteroenteric anastomosis in order to allow for temporary passive dilation. In men, the gonadal vessels should be left intact, but in a female patient, the infundibulopelvic ligaments, through which the ovarian vessels run, are ligated at the level of the pelvic inlet. The vas deferens in men and round ligament in women are also clipped and divided.

24.4 Male Cystectomy

The lateral pedicle of the bladder is developed, using countertraction provided by a clamp on the urachal remnant to expose the ipsilateral pedicle. The lateral vascular pedicles can be divided using titanium clips, a stapling device with vascular loads, or the Ligasure device. The bladder is then retracted toward the pubis and the rectovesical pouch incised, thereby gaining access to Denonvillier's fascia and allowing for mobilization of the specimen off the rectum via blunt dissection (Fig. 24.4). The bladder, seminal vesicles,

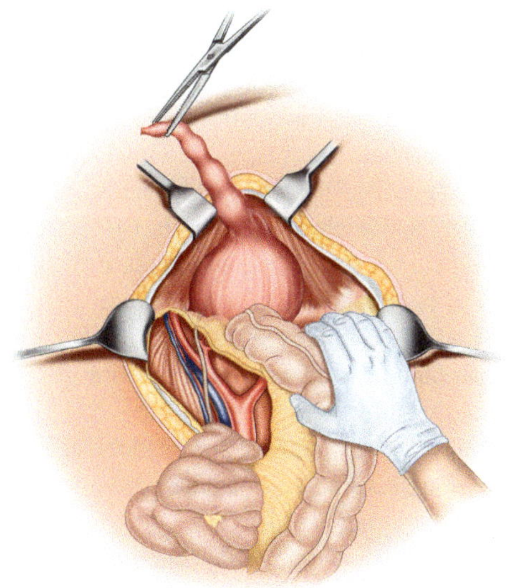

Fig. 24.3 Creation of mesenteric window for left ureter. Adapted from Stein JP, Skinner DG. Surgical Atlas Radical Cystectomy. BJUI. 2004; 97: 197–221

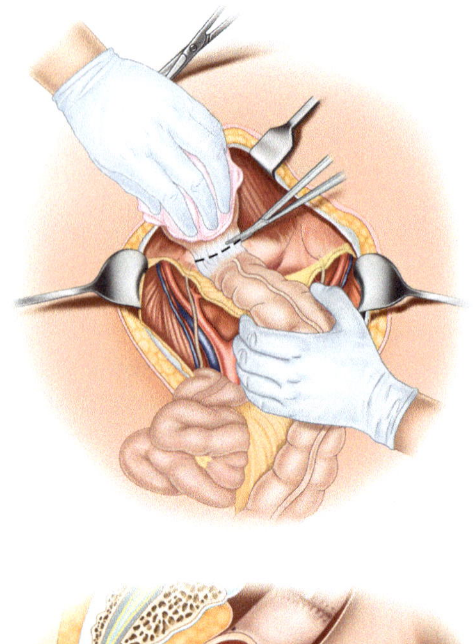

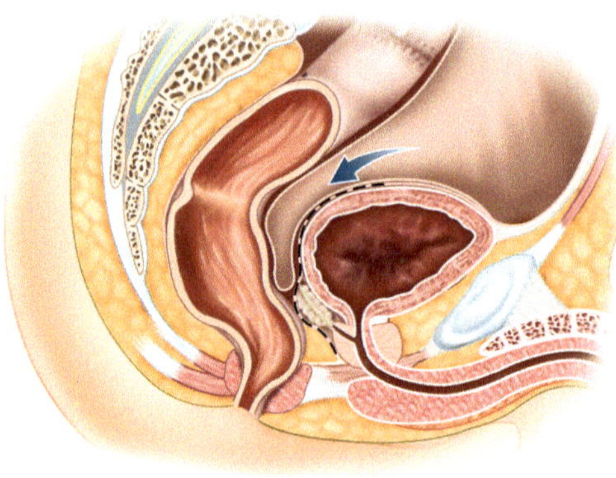

Fig. 24.4 Accessing Denonvillier's fascia and blunt dissection of the specimen from rectum. Adapted from Ghonheim MA. "15: Radical Cystectomy in Men." from Glenn's Urologic Surgery. Eds Graham SD, Keane TE. 7th ed. Lippincott Williams & Wilkins: Philadelphia, 2010; and Stein JP, Skinner DG. Surgical Atlas Radical Cystectomy. BJUI. 2004; 97: 197–221

and prostate are elevated away from the rectum as far distally as the urogenital diaphragm. The posterior pedicles are ligated using titanium clips or Ligasure. The space of Retzius is developed, and the endopelvic fascia is incised sharply to further expose the prostate (Fig. 24.5). A retropubic approach is used to excise the prostate en bloc with the cystectomy specimen. The dorsal venous complex can be ligated with an endovascular stapler or oversewn as necessary to achieve hemostasis. The urethra is sharply divided. If the patient is undergoing orthotopic substitution, leaving as much functional urethral length as oncologically permitted will improve continence [33]. The cystoprostatectomy specimen is removed en bloc and sent for pathologic analysis. A margin of the urethral stump should be excised and sent to pathology to verify absence of tumor. The pelvis is then carefully inspected for any evidence of rectal injury and bleeding.

24.5 Female Cystectomy

Anterior exenteration in a female patient proceeds in a similar fashion. The lateral pedicles of the bladder are defined and ligated. The incision at the pouch of Douglas enables the uterus to be swept anteriorly and the posterior vaginal wall to be separated from the rectum (Fig. 24.6). Posterior pedicles are divided with clips or the Ligasure device. The endopelvic fascia is incised near the posterior urethra. The bladder and uterus are mobilized anteriorly, and the urethra and vagina are divided. Again, a urethral cuff should be sent for frozen section to ensure a negative margin. As with a male cystectomy, preservation of the posterior hypogastric vessels and autonomic nerve fibers is believed to improve continence. Recent literature suggests that leaving the anterior vaginal wall and preservation of an intact vagina also has favorable implications for maintenance of the urethrovaginal sphincter mechanism without increasing positive margin rates [34, 35]. The vaginal cuff should be oversewn with absorbable sutures, providing a watertight closure (Fig. 24.7). Some surgeons may prefer to mobilize a pedicled omental flap to cover the vaginal stump suture line to decrease the possibility of neobladder fistulization. Some data suggest that an omental flap may also help support the neobladder and prevent posterior prolapse and urethro-pouch angulation [36].

Tumor involvement of the bladder neck was once thought to be an absolute contraindication to orthotopic neobladder due to the assumption that the bladder neck provided continence in females, as well as concern for urethral recurrence. However, neuroanatomical studies demonstrated that the rhabdosphincter, located in the distal two-thirds of the urethra, and preservation

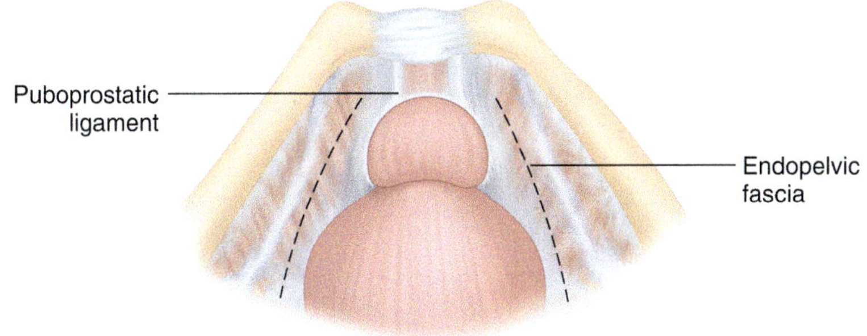

Fig. 24.5 Incising the endopelvic fascia. Adapted from Touijer K, Guillonneau B, Scardino P, Slawin K. Atlas of Clinical Urology, Volume 3, Chapter 12. LLC: Philadelphia, 2005

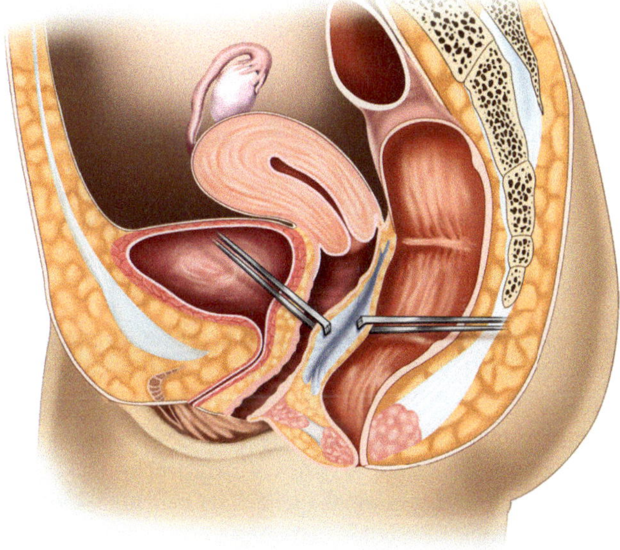

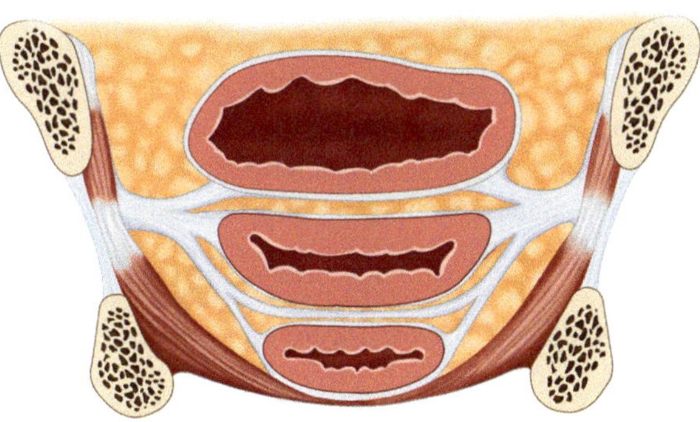

Fig. 24.6 Incising the pouch of Douglas. Adapted from Stein JP, Skinner DG. Surgical Atlas Radical Cystectomy. BJUI. 2004; 97: 197–221

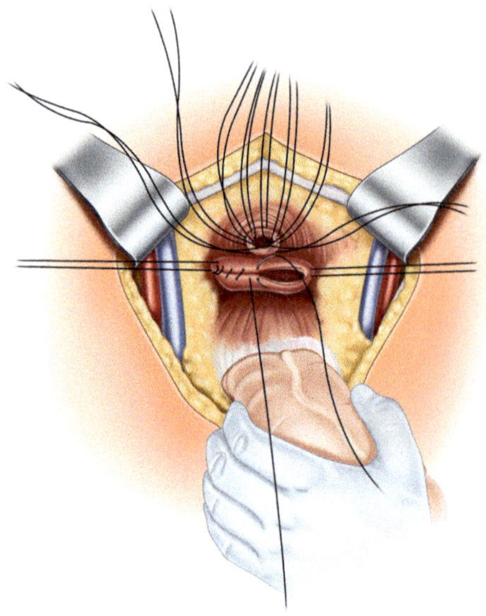

Fig. 24.7 Oversewing the vaginal stump

of its innervation were key to continence, and not the bladder neck [37]. Bladder neck involvement does however portend a higher risk of urethral recurrence [38].

24.6 Lymph Node Dissection

While controversy exists with regard to the anatomic limits of lymphadenectomy, evidence from multiple studies shows that thoroughness of the pelvic lymphadenectomy is associated with improved outcomes and survival vis-a-vis proper staging, but may also provide therapeutic benefit [39–43]. In contrast to colorectal cancer, in which consensus guidelines dictate a minimum yield of 12 lymph nodes, no such thresholds exist for bladder cancer [44]. A series of 322 patients by Herr et al. and a large series of Surveillance, Epidemiology, and End Results (SEER) registry patients suggested that at least ten lymph nodes should be evaluated to have prognostic significance [39, 45]. Stein and Skinner put forth the concept of lymph node density as a prognostic indicator, finding a 10-year recurrence-free survival of 43 % versus 17 % in patients with lymph node densities of 20 % or less and greater than 20 %, respectively [46].

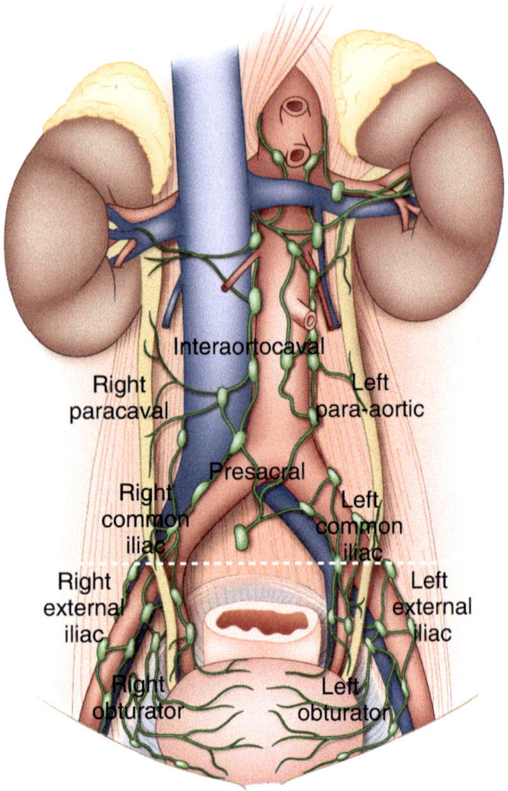

Fig. 24.8 Extent of standard and extended pelvic lymph node dissection (up to the inferior mesenteric artery)

The boundaries of the standard pelvic lymph node dissection are the bifurcation of the common iliac artery superiorly, the circumflex iliac vein inferiorly including the node of Cloquet, the genitofemoral nerve laterally, and the hypogastric vessels posteriorly. An extended lymph node dissection begins from the inferior mesenteric artery and proceeds caudad as with the standard template. Meticulous care should be taken to clip stay side lymphatic channels to prevent leak and lymphocele formation. Lymph node packets may be sent off separately as common iliac, external iliac, hypogastric, obturator, and presacral/presciatic packets, as studies have shown that individual packets are associated with increased node yield [47, 48]. An extended dissection would include left para-aortic, interaortocaval, and right paracaval packets up to the inferior mesenteric artery (Fig. 24.8) [47]. Further discussion may be found in Chapter 31: The role of pelvic lymphadenectomy at the time of radical cystectomy for bladder cancer.

24.7 Diversion

Following bilateral pelvic lymphadenectomy, the remainder of the operation is spent creating the urinary diversion.

24.7.1 Ileal Conduit

The previously created window underneath the sigmoid mesentery is located, and the left ureter is passed through toward the right side of the patient. The bowel is unpacked, and a 15-cm segment of terminal ileum, located at least 15 cm proximal to the ileocecal valve, is isolated and inspected to ensure the bowel appears well-vascularized and healthy. The mesentery of the isolated segment is inspected to find an appropriate spot in which division would provide a viable vascular arcade to the conduit segment. The mesentery is divided with the Ligasure device up to the border with the bowel. Two bowel clamps are placed on either end of the conduit segment to control spillage of bowel contents, and the bowel is divided using a GIA™ stapling device. Bowel continuity is then restored using the GIA™ stapler and TA™-60 stapling device to perform a side-to-side functional end-to-end anastomosis. It is our preference to reinforce the stapled anastomosis using non-absorbable sutures in an interrupted Lembert fashion. Mesenteric defects are also reapproximated to decrease the chance of an internal hernia.

The clipped ends of each ureter are trimmed and spatulated. A Bricker or Wallace technique is then used to create the ureteroenteric anastomosis at a site on the proximal end of the conduit, tension-free and without kinking of the ureter. The conduit should maintain an antegrade peristaltic direction toward the skin. Ureteral stents, using small caliber feeding tubes or single-J stents, are inserted retrograde just prior to complete closure of the ureteroenteric anastomoses to help facilitate healing. The ureteroenteric anastomoses may be tested by backfilling the ileal conduit with warm saline and inspecting for any leakage.

The conduit is then brought up to the abdominal wall at the site of previous marking. A fascial defect is created large enough to accommodate two fingers, but not too large so as to predispose to parastomal herniation. The staple line on the skin end of the conduit is excised sharply, and any creeping mesentery is trimmed back slightly to decrease tension. The stoma is matured by fixing the mucosa to the abdominal wall fascia in each quadrant, with additional absorbable interrupted tacking sutures from bowel mucosa to skin edge.

24.7.2 Neobladder

We have most commonly performed the Studer orthotopic neobladder [49]. The previously created window under the sigmoid mesentery is located, and the left ureter passed through this toward the right side of the patient. The bowel is unpacked, and a 60-cm segment of terminal ileum, located at least 15 cm proximal to the ileocecal valve, is isolated and inspected to ensure the bowel appears well-vascularized and healthy. The mesentery of the isolated segment is analyzed to find an appropriate spot in which division would provide a viable vascular arcade to the conduit segment. The mesentery and bowel are divided, and bowel continuity is then restored using the GIA™ stapler and TA™-60 stapling device to perform a side-to-side functional end-to-end anastomosis. Mesenteric defects are also reapproximated to decrease the chance of an internal hernia.

The bowel is reconfigured into a U-shape with a 20 cm afferent limb. The antimesenteric border of the segment is incised for approximately 40 cm from its distal end. The clipped ends of each ureter are trimmed and spatulated. A Bricker or Wallace technique is then used to create the end-to-side non-tunneled/Nesbit ureteroenteric anastomosis at a site on the afferent limb, tension-free and without kinking of the ureter. Ureteral stents are inserted retrograde just prior to complete closure of the ureteroenteric anastomoses to help facilitate healing. Distal periureteral tissue can be lightly tacked to the afferent limb and used to cover the anastomosis as well.

The opposite edges of the detubularized bowel are sewn together in either a single or double layer, creating a spherical pouch via four cross-folded segments. Just before completing the globularization, the most dependent portion of the pouch is determined and a through-and-through hole cut out for the urethro-enteric anastomosis. The pouch should reach the urethral stump in a tension-free manner. Additional length can be obtained by incising the mesentery and peritoneal surface, taking care not to injure the mesenteric vessels supplying the pouch.

After verifying that there is no tumor at the urethral margin frozen section, at least six absorbable sutures are placed from the pouch neourethra to the membranous urethra at 1, 3, 5, 7, 9, and 11 o'clock, to approximate the seromuscular layer of the pouch to the urethra. A large urethral catheter is inserted across the urethro-enteric anastomosis, and the ureteral stents are internalized and fixed to this catheter. The remainder of the orthotopic pouch is then closed. The six previously placed sutures are tied down. The reservoir is backfilled through the catheter to test for any leakage and to flush out any clots.

24.7.3 Continent Cutaneous Reservoir

Continent cutaneous diversions are much less common than orthotopic neobladders, and tend to be performed when urethrectomy precludes the possibility of neobladder but patients wish to avoid a stoma with external appliance. Some patients who are concerned about body image but do not want to run the risk of incontinence or have preexisting sphincteric insufficiency may also choose continent cutaneous diversion.

The Indiana pouch takes advantage of the intrinsic ileocecal valve and buttresses it to provide the continence mechanism. The ascending colon is mobilized along the white line of Toldt, and the adjacent terminal ileum approximately 10 cm long is isolated. The cecum is opened along the antimesenteric border and is augmented with an ileal segment to create the reservoir [50]. As with orthotopic substitutions, detubularization of the bowel is key to creating a compliant low-pressure reservoir that will protect the upper tracts. While the cecum is open, the ileocecal junction is imbricated.

Due to the inherent outlet obstruction provided by the continence mechanism, higher reservoir pressures are seen in continent cutaneous diversions compared to continent orthotopic diversions. For this reason, as well as colonization of the reservoir with bacteria, authors have advocated for antirefluxing ureteroenteric anastomoses using the Le Duc, Leadbetter, or Goodwin techniques [51–53]. Regardless of type of technique, the ureteroenteric anastomosis should remain tension-free and without angulation. Again, the left ureter is passed under the previously created window in the sigmoid mesentery, and bilateral uretero-tenial anastomoses are performed. Single J stents or feeding tubes should be used to stent the ureters, exteriorizing the distal ends either through a separate stab incision or attached to the irrigating catheter.

The pouch is closed in a Heineke-Mikulicz fashion to avoid bolus contractions. A stapler is used to taper the ileal segment that will serve as the catheterizable stoma. Similar to Mitrofanoff appendicovesicostomies, use of the appendix for continent cutaneous diversions has been described, especially as it carries a very high continence rate. However, rates of stenosis are much higher and reoperation rates can exceed 30 % [54, 55]. The stoma is then tunneled toward the umbilicus or right lower quadrant and matured. A Foley catheter is placed as a suprapubic tube into the pouch to help divert urine and allow for irrigation.

24.7.4 Closure

The pelvis is copiously irrigated with warm saline, and carefully inspected to ensure hemostasis. A Jackson-Pratt drain in the pelvis is recommended regardless of the type of diversion. The abdomen is then closed in multiple layers: rectus fascia, Camper's and Scarpa's fascia, and skin.

24.8 Postoperative Management

Our practice has been to remove the nasogastric tube prior to extubation of the patient, as both prospective and observational studies suggest decreased rates of ileus with early removal [56]. Evidence regarding the utility of gut promotility agents such as metoclopramide has been marginal, although the recently approved peripheral mu-opioid receptor antagonist almivopan has been shown decrease narcotic-induced postoperative ileus with reasonable cost efficacy [56, 57]. Some authors have advocated for placement of a gastrostomy tube during surgery as a means to circumvent the possibility of uncomfortable nasogastric tubes while providing a way of decompressing the stomach should the patient develop an ileus [58]. However, given that most series report rates of ileus in the 15–20 % range, our practice has not been to prophylactically place gastrostomies [35, 59, 60]. Patients may initiate limited oral liquid intake as early as the first postoperative day and are expected to ambulate as well. Other routine prophylactic measures such as sequential compression devices while in bed, subcutaneous Heparin, and regular incentive spirometry are ordered. Postoperative antibiotics such as a second-generation cephalosporin may also be given for 24 h following surgery.

For patients with an orthotopic or continent cutaneous constructions, the Foley catheter may be irrigated as early as the evening of surgery to minimize the risk of mucus plugging. Patients are maintained on thrice daily pouch irrigations while in the hospital, and are generally discharged on at least once daily irrigations. The ureteral catheters are typically removed between 7 and 14 days after surgery. It has not been our custom to evaluate for anastomotic leakage with a pouchogram prior to removing the Foley catheter, but if there is copious output from the Jackson-Pratt drain, a fluid creatinine level may be analyzed. The Jackson-Pratt drain is removed when there is low output and/or no urine leak.

Patients are generally seen in follow-up every 6 months for the first 2 years, and annually thereafter, with routine serum chemistries, urine cytology, and CT scan of the chest, abdomen, and pelvis to evaluate for local or upper tract recurrence, or metastasis. Patients with neobladders and continent cutaneous diversions additionally should have a serum vitamin B12 level checked annually given the larger bowel resection required

for the reservoir. High-risk patients (pathologic stage T3-4, positive nodes) should be considered for adjuvant chemotherapy if no neoadjuvant treatment was administered.

24.9 Complications

Radical cystectomy with urinary diversion is a major operation with significant morbidity. Complications, while generally minor, occur in approximately 60 % of patients within the first 90 days [59, 61]. It is important to keep in mind that complications may also occur decades after the initial surgery, and thus cystectomy patients require long-term follow-up not only from a purely oncologic point of view.

24.9.1 Short Term

All patients regardless of type of diversion are at risk for metabolic acidosis, though the risk is highest for those with continent diversions due to the increased surface area of bowel and longer contact time with urine. Symptoms may be fairly nonspecific: fatigue, nausea, anorexia, possible vomiting, and overall failure to thrive. A serum chemistry panel will reveal a hypochloremic hyperkalemic metabolic acidosis if ileum has been used. Treatment involves replacing bicarbonate. Patients with severe base deficits may need admission for fluids and IV sodium bicarbonate.

Patients with orthotopic neobladders often have incontinence after their Foley catheter is removed, and patients should be counseled preoperatively to expect this. It is important to have patients cycle their pouch by progressively increasing the time interval between urination in order to achieve full bladder capacity. Daytime continence recovers first, followed by nighttime incontinence [62]. Approximately 90 % of patients have daytime continence and 80 % have nighttime continence by 18 months [33, 63]. Bothersome nocturnal incontinence can be mitigated by timed voiding with the help of an alarm clock. Pelvic floor exercises, preservation of the rhabdosphincter, and nerve-sparing all influence time to recovery of continence [64]. Older patients generally have inferior continence [33]. Patients with intractable stress urinary incontinence may benefit from urethral bulking agents, slings, or artificial sphincter devices [65–67].

On the other hand, acute retention from mucus plugging may also occur, especially due to the relatively larger surface area of bowel used in orthotopic urinary diversion. It can be helpful to check a post-void residual at early follow-up visits to ensure adequate emptying, and to institute clean intermittent catheterization and pouch irrigations on an as needed basis. Retention and stasis also predispose to infection and calculus formation.

24.9.2 Long Term

Long-term complications can include obstruction at any level with subsequent renal impairment. Indeed, obstruction is the leading cause of long-term renal deterioration regardless of type of diversion [68]. Obstruction can also lead to recurrent bouts of pyelonephritis in the setting of infection. Ureteroenteric anastomotic strictures may require revision, either with open surgical resection of the stricture and neo-ureteroileal anastomosis, or through endoscopic methods such as balloon dilation and endoureterotomy [69]. A study of 85 ureteroileal strictures found that length of stricture was associated with outcome, and that strictures >1 cm had better success with open revision [70]. Late de novo urethral strictures or outlet obstruction can often be managed endoscopically. Stomal stenosis in the case of an ileal conduit or continent cutaneous diversion generally requires open revision.

Upper tract deterioration may also occur due to reflux of urine. It was initially believed that antireflux valves were necessary to preserve renal function, particularly in the case of orthotopic reconstruction. However, a properly formed spherical reservoir is compliant and thus allows for low-pressure voiding. Any straining is equally transmitted to both the reservoir and upper tracts. Additionally, the isoperistaltic afferent limb serves to diffuse some of the pressure. A prospec-

tive randomized study, though with limited follow-up, indeed found higher stricture rates and worse renal impairment with antireflux mechanisms in orthotopic bladder substitution [71]. However for continent cutaneous reservoirs, the outlet which provides continence also enables high pouch pressures. As such, the benefit of antirefluxing ureteric anastomoses must be weighed against higher rates of anastomotic strictures in continent cutaneous diversions [72].

Urinary retention can also be a late effect in orthotopic substitutions, seen even in the absence of identifiable outlet obstruction or dysfunctional voiding, and even in instances in which patients initially had excellent urinary function. For as yet unclear reasons, retention is more common in female patients and with an incidence of up to 50 % at 5 years [63]. Fixation of the neobladder, and supporting the posterior pelvis via omental flaps, sacrocolpopexy, or anchoring the vaginal apex to the round ligaments have been described to improve outcomes, but results are not conclusive [36, 73]. Retention is typically treated with intermittent catheterization, though reduction pouch-plasty and fixation have also been described [36].

24.9.3 Pouch-Vaginal Fistula

Despite even omental interposition flaps, fistulas between the neobladder and vaginal stump may occur in 1–10 % of female cystectomy cases [74, 75]. Depending on the location of the fistula, many of these may be repaired transvaginally with use of a Martius flap [76].

24.9.4 Urethral Recurrence

Several series have demonstrated an overall urethral recurrence rate of between 1.5 and 6 %, occurring even more than a decade after surgery [63]. In a series by Stein et al., prostatic involvement and continent cutaneous diversion were significant predictors for recurrence [77]. Tumor involvement of the bladder neck was once thought to be an absolute contraindication to orthotopic neobladder due to concern for urethral recurrence as well as the assumption that the bladder neck provided continence in females. However, neuroanatomical studies demonstrated that the rhabdosphincter, located in the distal two-thirds of the urethra, and preservation of its innervation were critical for preservation of continence [37]. Bladder neck involvement does however portend a higher risk of urethral recurrence [38].

24.10 Conclusions

Open radical cystectomy remains the gold standard for surgical management of muscle-invasive bladder cancer. Ongoing prospective randomized controlled trials comparing the safety and efficacy of open versus robotic cystectomy will help define the relevance of surgical technique to clinical outcomes. More studies, with standardized reporting of complications and validated instruments for assessing health-related quality of life will be necessary to help define the ideal populations for the various forms of urinary diversion. Improved diagnostics and imaging will allow for more accurate preoperative staging and maximum efficacy of radical cystectomy in the treatment and cure of bladder cancer.

References

1. Whitmore Jr WF, Marshall VF. Radical total cystectomy for cancer of the bladder: 230 consecutive cases five years later. J Urol. 1962;87:853–68.
2. Stein JP, Lieskovsky G, Cote R, Groshen S, Feng AC, Boyd S, et al. Radical cystectomy in the treatment of invasive bladder cancer: long-term results in 1,054 patients. J Clin Oncol. 2001;19(3):666–75.
3. Ghoneim MA, Abdel-Latif M, el-Mekresh M, Abol-Enein H, Mosbah A, Ashamallah A, et al. Radical cystectomy for carcinoma of the bladder: 2,720 consecutive cases 5 years later. J Urol. 2008;180(1):121–7.
4. Babjuk M, Oosterlinck W, Sylvester R, Kaasinen E, Böhle A, Palou-Redorta J, et al. EAU guidelines on non-muscle-invasive urothelial carcinoma of the bladder. Eur Urol. 2008;54(2):303–14.
5. Shariat SF, Karakiewicz PI, Palapattu GS, Lotan Y, Rogers CG, Amiel GE, et al. Outcomes of radical cystectomy for transitional cell carcinoma of the bladder: a contemporary series from the Bladder Cancer Research Consortium. J Urol. 2006;176(6 Pt 1):2414–22. discussion 2422.
6. Gondo T, Yoshioka K, Nakagami Y, Okubo H, Hashimoto T, Satake N, et al. Robotic versus open radical cystectomy: prospective comparison of perioperative and pathologic outcomes in Japan. Jpn J Clin Oncol. 2012;42(7):625–31.
7. Pruthi RS, Nielsen ME, Nix J, Smith A, Schultz H, Wallen EM. Robotic radical cystectomy for bladder cancer: surgical and pathological outcomes in 100 consecutive cases. J Urol. 2010;183(2):510–4.
8. Wang GJ, Barocas DA, Raman JD, Scherr DS. Robotic vs open radical cystectomy: prospective comparison of perioperative outcomes and pathological measures of early oncological efficacy. BJU Int. 2008;101(1): 89–93.
9. Smith AB, Raynor M, Amling CL, Busby JE, Castle E, Davis R, et al. Multi-institutional analysis of robotic radical cystectomy for bladder cancer: perioperative outcomes and complications in 227 patients. J Laparoendosc Adv Surg Tech A. 2012;22(1):17–21.
10. Styn NR, Montgomery JS, Wood DP, Hafez KS, Lee CT, Tallman C, et al. Matched comparison of robotic-assisted and open radical cystectomy. Urology. 2012;79(6):1303–8.
11. Parekh DJ, Messer J, Fitzgerald J, Ercole B, Svatek R. Perioperative outcomes and oncologic efficacy from a pilot prospective randomized clinical trial of open versus robotic assisted radical cystectomy. J Urol. 2013;189(2):474–9.
12. Nix J, Smith A, Kurpad R, Nielsen ME, Wallen EM, Pruthi RS. Prospective randomized controlled trial of robotic versus open radical cystectomy for bladder cancer: perioperative and pathologic results. Eur Urol. 2010;57(2):196–201.
13. Lawrentschuk N, Lee ST, Scott AM. Current role of PET, CT, MR for invasive bladder cancer. Curr Urol Rep. 2013;14(2):84–9.
14. Kibel AS, Dehdashti F, Katz MD, Klim AP, Grubb RL, Humphrey PA, et al. Prospective study of [18F] fluorodeoxyglucose positron emission tomography/computed tomography for staging of muscle-invasive bladder carcinoma. J Clin Oncol. 2009;27(26): 4314–20.
15. Skinner DG, Lieskovsky G. Contemporary cystectomy with pelvic node dissection compared to preoperative radiation therapy plus cystectomy in management of invasive bladder cancer. J Urol. 1984;131(6):1069–72.
16. Meeks JJ, Bellmunt J, Bochner BH, Clarke NW, Daneshmand S, Galsky MD, et al. A systematic review of neoadjuvant and adjuvant chemotherapy for muscle-invasive bladder cancer. Eur Urol. 2012;62(3): 523–33.
17. Grossman HB, Natale RB, Tangen CM, Speights VO, Vogelzang NJ, Trump DL, et al. Neoadjuvant chemotherapy plus cystectomy compared with cystectomy alone for locally advanced bladder cancer. N Engl J Med. 2003;349(9):859–66.

18. von der Maase H, Sengelov L, Roberts JT, Ricci S, Dogliotti L, Oliver T, et al. Long-term survival results of a randomized trial comparing gemcitabine plus cisplatin, with methotrexate, vinblastine, doxorubicin, plus cisplatin in patients with bladder cancer. J Clin Oncol. 2005;23(21):4602–8.

19. Advanced Bladder Cancer (ABC) Meta-analysis Collaboration. Neoadjuvant chemotherapy in invasive bladder cancer: update of a systematic review and meta-analysis of individual patient data advanced bladder cancer (ABC) meta-analysis collaboration. Eur Urol. 2005;8(2):202–5. discussion 205–206.

20. Koga F, Kihara K, Yoshida S, Yokoyama M, Saito K, Masuda H, et al. Selective bladder-sparing protocol consisting of induction low-dose chemoradiotherapy plus partial cystectomy with pelvic lymph node dissection against muscle-invasive bladder cancer: oncological outcomes of the initial 46 patients. BJU Int. 2012;109(6):860–6.

21. Shipley WU, Kaufman DS, Heney NM, Althausen AF, Zietman AL. An update of combined modality therapy for patients with muscle invading bladder cancer using selective bladder preservation or cystectomy. J Urol. 1999;162(2):445–50. discussion 450–451.

22. Knoedler JJ, Boorjian SA, Kim SP, Weight CJ, Thapa P, Tarrell RF, et al. Does partial cystectomy compromise oncologic outcomes for patients with bladder cancer compared to radical cystectomy? A matched case-control analysis. J Urol. 2012;188(4):1115–9.

23. Capitanio U, Isbarn H, Shariat SF, Jeldres C, Zini L, Saad F, et al. Partial cystectomy does not undermine cancer control in appropriately selected patients with urothelial carcinoma of the bladder: a population-based matched analysist. Urology. 2009;74(4):858–64.

24. Kassouf W, Swanson D, Kamat AM, Leibovici D, Siefker-Radtke A, Munsell MF, et al. Partial cystectomy for muscle invasive urothelial carcinoma of the bladder: a contemporary review of the M. D. Anderson Cancer Center experience. J Urol. 2006;175(6):2058–62.

25. Holzbeierlein JM, Lopez-Corona E, Bochner BH, Herr HW, Donat SM, Russo P, et al. Partial cystectomy: a contemporary review of the Memorial Sloan-Kettering Cancer Center experience and recommendations for patient selection. J Urol. 2004;172(3):878–81.

26. Davidsson T, Wullt B, Könyves J, Månsson A, Månsson K. Urinary diversion and bladder substitution in patients with bladder cancer. Urol Oncol. 2000;5(5):224–31.

27. Gschwend JE, May F, Paiss T, Gottfried HW, Hautmann RE. High-dose pelvic irradiation followed by ileal neobladder urinary diversion: complications and long-term results. Br J Urol. 1996;77(5):680–3.

28. Hautmann RE, de Petriconi R, Volkmer BG. Neobladder formation after pelvic irradiation. World J Urol. 2009;27(1):57–62.

29. Parekh DJ, Donat SM. Urinary diversion: options, patient selection, and outcomes. Semin Oncol. 2007;34(2):98–109.

30. Raynor MC, Lavien G, Nielsen M, Wallen EM, Pruthi RS. Elimination of preoperative mechanical bowel preparation in patients undergoing cystectomy and urinary diversion. Urol Oncol. 2013;31(1):32–5.

31. Picozzi S, Ricci C, Gaeta M, Ratti D, Macchi A, Casellato S, et al. Upper urinary tract recurrence following radical cystectomy for bladder cancer: a meta-analysis on 13,185 patients. J Urol. 2012;188(6): 2046–54.

32. Furukawa J, Miyake H, Hara I, Takenaka A, Fujisawa M. Upper urinary tract recurrence following radical cystectomy for bladder cancer. Int J Urol. 2007;14(6):496–9.

33. Casanova GA, Springer JP, Gerber E, Studer UE. Urodynamic and clinical aspects of ileal low pressure bladder substitutes. Br J Urol. 1993;72(5 Pt 2):728–35.

34. Hautmann RE, Paiss T, de Petriconi R. The ileal neobladder in women: 9 years of experience with 18 patients. J Urol. 1996;155(1):76–81.

35. Chang SS, Cole E, Cookson MS, Peterson M, Smith Jr JA. Preservation of the anterior vaginal wall during female radical cystectomy with orthotopic urinary diversion: technique and results. J Urol. 2002;168(4 Pt 1):1442–5.

36. Ali-El-Dein B, Gomha M, Ghoneim MA. Critical evaluation of the problem of chronic urinary retention after orthotopic bladder substitution in women. J Urol. 2002;168(2):587–92.

37. Colleselli K, Stenzl A, Eder R, Strasser H, Poisel S, Bartsch G. The female urethral sphincter: a morphological and topographical study. J Urol. 1998;160(1): 49–54.

38. Stein JP, Cote RJ, Freeman JA, Esrig D, Elmajian DA, Groshen S, et al. Indications for lower urinary tract reconstruction in women after cystectomy for bladder cancer: a pathological review of female cystectomy specimens. J Urol. 1995;154(4):1329–33.

39. Herr HW, Bochner BH, Dalbagni G, Donat SM, Reuter VE, Bajorin DF. Impact of the number of lymph nodes retrieved on outcome in patients with muscle invasive bladder cancer. J Urol. 2002;167(3):1295–8.

40. Herr HW. Extent of surgery and pathology evaluation has an impact on bladder cancer outcomes after radical cystectomy. Urology. 2003;61(1):105–8.

41. Stein JP, Skinner DG. The role of lymphadenectomy in high-grade invasive bladder cancer. Urol Clin North Am. 2005;32(2):187–97.

42. Stein JP. Lymphadenectomy in bladder cancer: how high is "high enough"? Urol Oncol. 2006;24(4):349–55.

43. Poulsen AL, Horn T, Steven K. Radical cystectomy: extending the limits of pelvic lymph node dissection improves survival for patients with bladder cancer confined to the bladder wall. J Urol. 1998;160(6 Pt 1):2015–9. discussion 2020.

44. Compton CC, Fielding LP, Burgart LJ, Conley B, Cooper HS, Hamilton SR, et al. Prognostic factors in colorectal cancer. College of American Pathologists Consensus Statement 1999. Arch Pathol Lab Med. 2000;124(7):979–94.

45. Wright JL, Lin DW, Porter MP. The association between extent of lymphadenectomy and survival among patients with lymph node metastases undergoing radical cystectomy. Cancer. 2008;112(11): 2401–8.

46. Stein JP, Cai J, Groshen S, Skinner DG. Risk factors for patients with pelvic lymph node metastases following radical cystectomy with en bloc pelvic lymphadenectomy: concept of lymph node density. J Urol. 2003;170(1):35–41.

47. Stein JP, Penson DF, Cai J, Miranda G, Skinner EC, Dunn MA, et al. Radical cystectomy with extended lymphadenectomy: evaluating separate package versus en bloc submission for node positive bladder cancer. J Urol. 2007;177(3):876–81. discussion 881–882.

48. Bochner BH, Cho D, Herr HW, Donat M, Kattan MW, Dalbagni G. Prospectively packaged lymph node dissections with radical cystectomy: evaluation of node count variability and node mapping. J Urol. 2004;172(4 Pt 1):1286–90.

49. Studer UE, Varol C, Danuser H. Orthotopic ileal neobladder. BJU Int. 2004;93(1):183–93.

50. Rowland RG, Mitchell ME, Bihrle R, Kahnoski RJ, Piser JE. Indiana continent urinary reservoir. J Urol. 1987;137(6):1136–9.

51. Le Duc A, Camey M, Teillac P. An original antireflux ureteroileal implantation technique: long-term followup. J Urol. 1987;137(6):1156–8.

52. Leadbetter WF, Clarke BG. Five years' experience with uretero-enterostomy by the combined technique. J Urol. 1955;73(1):67–82.

53. Goodwin WE, Harris AP, Kaufman JJ, Beal JM. Open, transcolonic ureterointestinal anastomosis; a new approach. Surg Gynecol Obstet. 1953;97(3):295–300.

54. Wiesner C, Stein R, Pahernik S, Hähn K, Melchior SW, Thüroff JW. Long-term follow-up of the intussuscepted ileal nipple and the in situ, submucosally embedded appendix as continence mechanisms of continent urinary diversion with the cutaneous ileocecal pouch (Mainz pouch I). J Urol. 2006;176(1):155–9. discussion 159–160.

55. Stein JP, Daneshmand S, Dunn M, Garcia M, Lieskovsky G, Skinner DG. Continent right colon reservoir using a cutaneous appendicostomy. Urology. 2004;63(3):577–80. discussion 580–581.

56. Ramirez JA, McIntosh AG, Strehlow R, Lawrence VA, Parekh DJ, Svatek RS. Definition, incidence, risk factors, and prevention of paralytic ileus following radical cystectomy: a systematic review. Eur Urol. 2013;64:688.

57. Hilton WM, Lotan Y, Parekh DJ, Basler JW, Svatek RS. Alvimopan for prevention of postoperative paralytic ileus in radical cystectomy patients: a cost-effectiveness analysis. BJU Int. 2013;111(7):1054–60.

58. Stein JP, Skinner DG. Surgical atlas. Radical cystectomy. BJU Int. 2004;94(1):197–221.

59. Hautmann RE, de Petriconi RC, Volkmer BG. Lessons learned from 1,000 neobladders: the 90-day complication rate. J Urol. 2010;184(3):990–4. quiz 1235.

60. De Nunzio C, Cindolo L, Leonardo C, Antonelli A, Ceruti C, Franco G, et al. Analysis of radical cystectomy and urinary diversion complications with the Clavien classification system in an Italian real life cohort. Eur J Surg Oncol. 2013;39(7):792–8.

61. Shabsigh A, Korets R, Vora KC, Brooks CM, Cronin AM, Savage C, et al. Defining early morbidity of radical cystectomy for patients with bladder cancer using a standardized reporting methodology. Eur Urol. 2009;55(1):164–74.

62. Hautmann RE, Abol-Enein H, Davidsson T, Gudjonsson S, Hautmann SH, Holm HV, et al. ICUD-EAU International Consultation on Bladder Cancer 2012: urinary diversion. Eur Urol. 2013;63(1):67–80.

63. Hautmann RE, Volkmer BG, Schumacher MC, Gschwend JE, Studer UE. Long-term results of standard procedures in urology: the ileal neobladder. World J Urol. 2006;24(3):305–14.

64. Kessler TM, Burkhard FC, Perimenis P, Danuser H, Thalmann GN, Hochreiter WW, et al. Attempted nerve sparing surgery and age have a significant effect on urinary continence and erectile function after radical cystoprostatectomy and ileal orthotopic bladder substitution. J Urol. 2004;172(4 Pt 1):1323–7.

65. Tchetgen MB, Sanda MG, Montie JE, Faerber GJ. Collagen injection for the treatment of incontinence after cystectomy and orthotopic neobladder reconstruction in women. J Urol. 2000;163(1):212–4.

66. Quek ML, Ginsberg DA, Wilson S, Skinner EC, Stein JP, Skinner DG. Pubovaginal slings for stress urinary incontinence following radical cystectomy and orthotopic neobladder reconstruction in women. J Urol. 2004;172(1):219–21.

67. Simma-Chiang V, Ginsberg DA, Teruya KK, Boyd SD. Outcomes of artificial urinary sphincter placement in men after radical cystectomy and orthotopic urinary diversions for the treatment of stress urinary incontinence: the University of Southern California experience. Urology. 2012;79(6):1397–401.

68. Jin X-D, Roethlisberger S, Burkhard FC, Birkhaeuser F, Thoeny HC, Studer UE. Long-term renal function after urinary diversion by ileal conduit or orthotopic ileal bladder substitution. Eur Urol. 2012;61(3): 491–7.

69. Lin DW, Bush WH, Mayo ME. Endourological treatment of ureteroenteric strictures: efficacy of Acucise endoureterotomy. J Urol. 1999;162(3 Pt 1):696–8.

70. Schöndorf D, Meierhans-Ruf S, Kiss B, Giannarini G, Thalmann GN, Studer UE, et al. Ureteroileal strictures after urinary diversion with an ileal segment - is there a place for endourological treatment at all? J Urol. 2013;190(2):585–90.

71. Shaaban AA, Abdel-Latif M, Mosbah A, Gad H, Eraky I, Ali-El-Dein B, et al. A randomized study comparing an antireflux system with a direct ureteric anastomosis in patients with orthotopic ileal neobladders. BJU Int. 2006;97(5):1057–62.

72. Pantuck AJ, Han KR, Perrotti M, Weiss RE, Cummings KB. Ureteroenteric anastomosis in continent urinary diversion: long-term results and complications of

direct versus nonrefluxing techniques. J Urol. 2000;163(2):450–5.

73. Stein JP, Ginsberg DA, Skinner DG. Indications and technique of the orthotopic neobladder in women. Urol Clin North Am. 2002;29(3):725–34. xi.

74. Stein JP, Grossfeld GD, Freeman JA, Esrig D, Ginsberg DA, Cote RJ, et al. Orthotopic lower urinary tract reconstruction in women using the Kock ileal neobladder: updated experience in 34 patients. J Urol. 1997;158(2):400–5.

75. Rapp DE, O'connor RC, Katz EE, Steinberg GD. Neobladder-vaginal fistula after cystectomy and orthotopic neobladder construction. BJU Int. 2004;94(7):1092–5. discussion 1095.

76. Tunuguntla HSGR, Manoharan M, Gousse AE. Management of neobladder-vaginal fistula and stress incontinence following radical cystectomy in women: a review. World J Urol. 2005;23(4): 231–5.

77. Stein JP, Clark P, Miranda G, Cai J, Groshen S, Skinner DG. Urethral tumor recurrence following cystectomy and urinary diversion: clinical and pathological characteristics in 768 male patients. J Urol. 2005;173(4):1163–8.

Michael Woods, Raj S. Pruthi, and Erik P. Castle

25.1 Introduction

The gold standard of treatment of muscle invasive bladder cancer is open radical cystectomy (ORC) and urinary diversion. While the procedure has well-established outcomes, it is associated with significant patient morbidity and mortality [1]. Laparoscopic surgery has been incorporated into various major urologic procedures such as nephrectomy and prostatectomy to decrease morbidity. However, the acceptance and implementation of laparoscopic techniques has been slower when it comes to radical cystectomy. The first laparoscopic simple cystectomy was reported in 1992 by Parra et al. describing the removal of a bladder for benign disease [2]. Since that publication, reports of laparoscopic radical cystectomy for malignant disease has followed but widespread acceptance within the urology community has been minimal. With the introduction of the daVinci™ surgical system (Intuitive Surgical, Sunnyvale, CA), the prevalence of robot-assisted radical cystectomies (RARC) has begun to rise over the past decade. In 2003, Menon et al. published the first RARC series [3]. Following that publication, we began to see small series of RARC with various factors analyzed such as operative outcomes, cystectomy in the female, and lymphadenectomy [4–7]. It was not until several years later that we began to see larger series reported. Within this chapter, we will describe the step-by-step approach to robot-assisted radical cystectomy and extracorporeal urinary diversion and briefly review the published clinical, pathologic, and oncologic outcomes of the procedure.

25.2 Indications

The indications for RARC are the same as those for ORC. There are no absolute preoperative contraindications specific to patients being considered for RARC. There are two intraoperative situations that are absolute contraindications to proceeding with RARC. The first situation is hypotension or compromised ventilation with positioning and abdominal insufflation. This may be encountered in the morbidly obese patient.

M. Woods, M.D. (⊠)
Department of Urology, The University of North Carolina Chapel Hill, 170 Manning Drive, Chapel Hill, NC 27599, USA
e-mail: Michael_woods@med.unc.edu

R.S. Pruthi, M.D.
Department of Urology, 170 Manning Drive, Chapel Hill, NC 27599, USA

UNC School of Medicine at Chapel Hill, 2105 Physicians Office Building, 170 Manning Dr., CB 7235, Chapel Hill, NC 27599-7235, USA
e-mail: raj_pruthi@med.unc.edu

E.P. Castle, M.D., F.A.C.S.
Department of Urology, Mayo Clinic Arizona, 5779 East Mayo Blvd., Phoenix, AZ 85054, USA
e-mail: castle.erik@mayo.edu

B.R. Konety and S.S. Chang (eds.), *Management of Bladder Cancer: A Comprehensive Text With Clinical Scenarios*, DOI 10.1007/978-1-4939-1881-2_25, © Springer Science+Business Media New York 2015

The second is CO_2 retention with insufflation that may manifest as unmanageable acidosis. Relative contraindications include abnormal anatomy, morbid obesity, prior radiation, and prior abdominal or pelvic surgery. Finally, as mentioned elsewhere throughout this book, urothelial carcinoma is a lethal disease requiring careful attention to surgical technique and if there is any concern that oncologic principles will be compromised a robot-assisted approach should not be used.

25.3 Patient and Preoperative Preparation

Patients being considered for RARC should undergo complete staging. Patients should be considered for neoadjuvant chemotherapy especially if there is suspicion of extravesical disease. For most patients, the authors currently do not use any form of mechanical or antibiotic bowel preparation unless there is a history of prior radiation, history of extensive prior abdominal surgery, or other similar extenuating circumstances. The patients should have nothing by mouth after midnight the day before surgery. All patients should be marked prior to surgery for the potential urostomy site. All patients should be educated preoperatively regarding care and maintenance of a urostomy, continent cutaneous diversion, or neobladder based on choice of urinary diversion.

25.3.1 Anesthesia and Patient Positioning

RARC is performed under general endotracheal anesthesia. Broad-spectrum antibiotics are administered within 1 h of surgical incision. Sequential compression devices are placed on the lower extremities and preoperative subcutaneous chemical prophylaxis for deep venous thrombosis is recommended. A nasogastric or orogastric tube is placed for decompression of the stomach. An arterial line may be inserted in order to monitor blood pressure and blood gases for the potential development of acidosis and hypercapnia.

A Foley catheter is placed after the patient is prepped and positioned.

The patient is placed in low lithotomy position with arms tucked to the side. Care must be taken to assure the patient's hands and elbows are adequately padded as they often lie between the patient's thigh and attachment of the stirrup. Alternatively, a split leg orthopedic bed can be used to avoid stir-ups. The patient will be placed in extreme/maximal trendelenburg during the case and consideration should be made to testing this prior to prepping and draping the patient. A chest strap may be used, however, patients rarely move on the bed with the arms tucked and the legs in low lithotomy position. Shoulder harnesses are not needed and should be avoided due to impingement complications.

25.3.2 Positioning of Operating Room Equipment and Personnel

A daVinci™ three- or four-arm system may be used (a four-arm unit is preferred as it allowed for better retraction during dissection). The robotic cart is docked between the patient's legs with the robotic instruments directed into the patient's pelvis, similar to the standard docking for a robotic prostatectomy. The primary assistant operates from the patient's right side and the fourth robotic arm is positioned on patient's left side. If a three-arm system is being used, then a second assistant should be used on the left side in order to assist with retraction. The control tower is placed just left of the patient's left leg. Adjacent to the control tower is the instrument table. This leaves ample room for the scrub nurse and a second assisted, if needed, on the left side of the patient. A viewing monitor is located on top of the control tower and additional monitors should be strategically placed for the assistant(s). This arrangement can easily be altered to accommodate a left side assistant. This is purely surgeon preference and a left side assistant may be advantageous if an intracorporeal urinary diversion is being performed. The surgeon console may be placed according to surgeon preference.

25.4 Technique

The technique of RARC can be generally divided into three parts:
- Extended Lymphadenectomy
- Radical Cystectomy
- Creation of the Urinary Diversion

Herein we will describe the step-by-step approach to the three parts of RARC. The authors currently perform RARC in the order they are listed above. However, some experienced groups will choose to perform the cystectomy portion of the procedure prior to the lymphadenectomy. Both techniques are felt to be equivalent. We feel that the benefit of performing the lymphadenectomy first is that it "sets up" the cystectomy. By skeletonizing the pelvic vasculature during the pelvic lymph node dissection (PLND), the pedicles to the bladder are exposed and in many cases ligated during the PLND and makes the cystectomy easier as well as allowing early identification of the obturator nerves. Nevertheless, it is ultimately up to the surgeon as long as standard oncologic principles are adhered to during the procedure.

There are a few procedural caveats and nuances when performing RARC in a female patient versus a male patient. For example, timing of the anterior vaginal dissection as well as management of the vaginal cuff makes the steps of the procedure slightly different. On the other hand, the remainder of the principles such as lymphadenectomy and ureteral dissection are no different. We will describe the general approach to RARC and make specific mention when appropriate about steps in the female patient.

25.4.1 Port Placement and Instruments

The ports are arranged in an "inverted-V" fashion (Fig. 25.1). Access and establishment of the pneumoperitoneum can be performed per surgeon preference. The camera port is placed in the midline cephalad to the umbilicus. If an extended lymphadenectomy is planned then placement of the camera port at least 3–4 cm to the cephalad

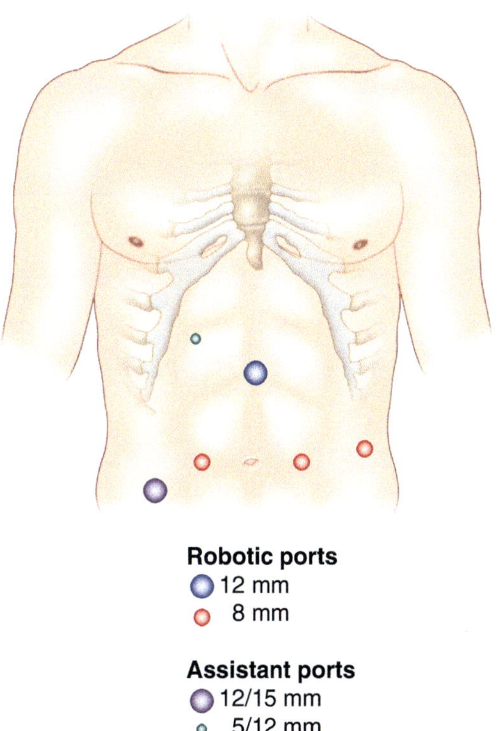

Fig. 25.1 Port placement for RARC with a right-sided assistant

will allow adequate proximal dissection on the great vessels. The two 8 mm robotic ports (right and left arms) are placed 10–11 cm lateral to midline just above the level of the umbilicus. Two assistant ports on the right (or left) are placed and the third working arm (the "fourth arm") port is placed lateral to the ipsilateral robotic port and on the opposite side of the assistant ports. If an intracorporeal diversion is planned, the assistant should be placed on the left side with the third robotic arm on the right side of the patient. We recommend using a 12 and 15 mm assistant ports. The 15 mm port will make extraction of lymph nodes easier as well as allow passage of a 15 mm specimen retrieval bag to be used for the bladder and prostate and the 12 mm port should be placed directly cephalad to the ipsilateral working arm which will allow direct access to the bladder pedicles with an endovascular stapler. It can be difficult to sufficiently articulate a stapler to divide the pedicles from the lateral assistant port. A list

Table 25.1 List of Instruments for RARC

Robotic instruments
Monopolar scissors
Fenestrated bipolar
Prograsp™ forceps
Large Needle drivers × 2
Robotic locking clip applier (*optional*)
Maryland bipolar (*optional*)
Cadiere forceps (*optional*)
Laparoscopic instruments (*bedside assistant*)
Suction/aspirator
Needle driver
Locking grasper
Atraumatic grasper
Locking clip applier (*small, medium and large*)
Suture
3-0 polyglactin cut to 20 cm for ureteral and bowel tags (*pre-tie the suture to the locking clips to be used on the ureters*)
0 polyglactin cut to 15 cm for ligation of the DVC
2-0 and 3-0 polyglactin cut to 20 cm for oversewing edges of the DVC and any bleeding sites from the neurovascular bundles and pedicles

of common robotic and laparoscopic instruments used during RARC can be found in Table 25.1.

25.4.2 Development of the Right Paravesical Space and Division of the Right Ureter

A 30° down lens can be used at the outset of the procedure. This allows for better visualization of the pelvis and retroperitoneum during the lymphadenectomy. With the right medial umbilical ligament identified, the peritoneum lateral to the ligament and medial to the right iliac vessels should be incised. Blunt dissection is employed to expose the endopelvic fascia. In male patients, dividing the vas deferens allows the bladder to be retracted medially and facilitates exposure of the pelvic vasculature. In female patients, ligation and division of the infundibulopelvic ligament as well as incision of the broad ligament and round ligament allows for access to the paravesical space. The identification of the obliterated umbilical artery and division of the vas deferens or round ligament are critical in avoiding inadvertent entry into the bladder or injury to the pelvic vasculature.

The right ureter is identified crossing over the iliac vessels after incision of the overlying peritoneum. The ureter should be dissected free of its underlying structures while preserving as much periureteral tissue as possible. The distal end can be dissected down to its insertion into the bladder. The right umbilical artery and/or right superior vesical artery should be seen just lateral to the insertion of the ureter into the bladder and can be clipped/ligated to allow for more length on the ureter. In female patients, the uterine artery is seen at this point and should be controlled and divided.

The ureter can be clipped distally with a locking clip. The proximal clip on the ureter should have a suture pre-tied to the clip (10–12 in.) so no additional "tagging" or marking of the ureter is required later in the procedure (Fig. 25.2). The ureter should be dissected free of its cephalad attachments. This should be done *before* dividing the ureter as proximal dissection can be difficult once the ureter is divided. Attempt should be made to preserve any vital blood supply to the ureter from the common iliac artery. The ureter can then be divided sharply. A margin can be sent for frozen section at this point if desired. It should be noted that too much or too aggressive dissection proximal on the ureter can result in devascularization of the ureter and may contribute to anastomotic stricture in the postoperative setting.

25.4.3 The Right Pelvic Lymphadenectomy

At this point the right pelvic lymphadenectomy is performed. It is the preference of the authors of this chapter to perform the lymphadenectomy at this time. In some cases, the lymphadenectomy can be deferred until after the cystectomy is performed. The procedure is performed using a "split-and-roll" technique. Currently, the proximal extent of our usual template is the bifurcation of the aorta. We recommend starting the dissection by splitting the lymphatic tissue over the

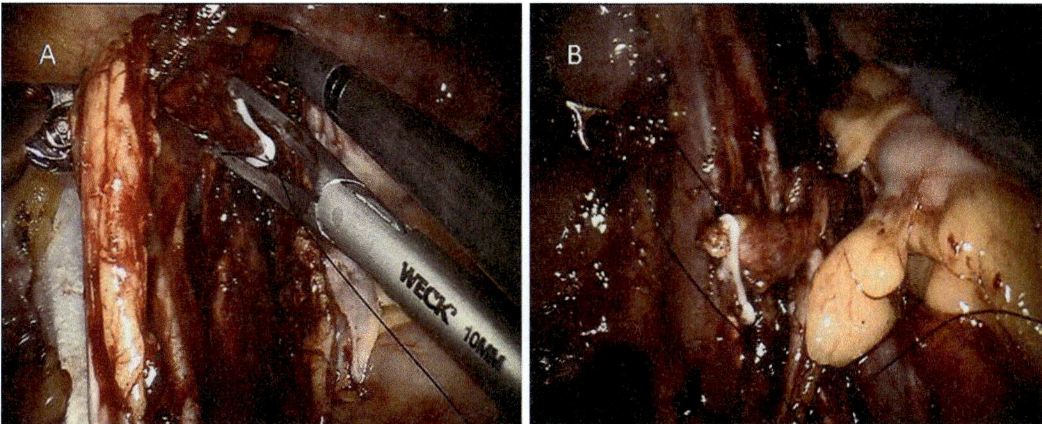

Fig. 25.2 (**a**) Tagging of ureter with a 15 mm Hem-o-lok clip with pre-placed tie. (**b**) Ureteral manipulation with clip/tie

entire extent of the right common iliac artery (Fig. 25.3a). The tissue is then dissected in a medial direction exposing the left common iliac vein and anterior surface of the sacrum (Fig. 25.3b). The authors find it beneficial to expose the left common iliac artery at this time (Fig. 25.3c). This allows for the right common iliac node packet to be easily ligated and divided at the bifurcation of the aorta and also starts to "set up" the left pelvic lymph node dissection by exposing known anatomy as a target for medial dissection after the left colon is reflected. The dissection is carried distally and divided at right internal iliac artery. After completion of the medial dissection, the lymphatic packet is mobilized laterally. The right common iliac vein and distal inferior vena cava (IVC) lie directly lateral to the right common artery. After the lateral edges of these venous structures have been exposed the lateral border the dissection at the genitofemoral nerve is defined (Fig. 25.3d). At this point the packet is divided at the distal extent of the dissection (bifurcation of common iliac) which will allow the packet to be easily isolated with blunt cephalad dissection.

The remainder of the right PLND is completed by splitting the lymphatic tissue over the right external iliac artery to the level of the circumflex iliac vein. After completing the external iliac lymph node dissection, we strongly recommend medial mobilization of the external iliac vessels and all associated lymphatic tissue exposing the pelvic side wall and origin of the obturator nerve (Fig. 25.4a, b). This maneuver will facilitate the removal of the obturator and hypogastric lymph nodes as these packets can generally be easily pulled from the underside or the external iliac vein (Fig. 25.4c). Additionally, this approach allows improved exposure of the internal iliac vein (Fig. 25.4d). The lymph nodes should be secured in a 10 mm specimen retrieval bag and can be removed in appropriate packets through the 15 mm port. In order to limit cost and use of too many bags, a reusable 10 mm bag can be used for all the different lymph node packets. While some have reported extracting the nodes with the bladder at the end of the procedure, one runs the risk of losing track of the node packets as well as orientation and identification of the respective packets.

25.4.4 Mobilization of the Sigmoid and Left Colon, Left Ureteral Dissection, and Left Pelvic Lymphadenectomy

This is begun by incising the peritoneum lateral to the left colon. The left colon and sigmoid colon should be released from the left sidewall to allow access to the left iliac vessels and left ureter. If the ureter is not readily visible it may be adherent to the backside of the sigmoid mesentery, this is

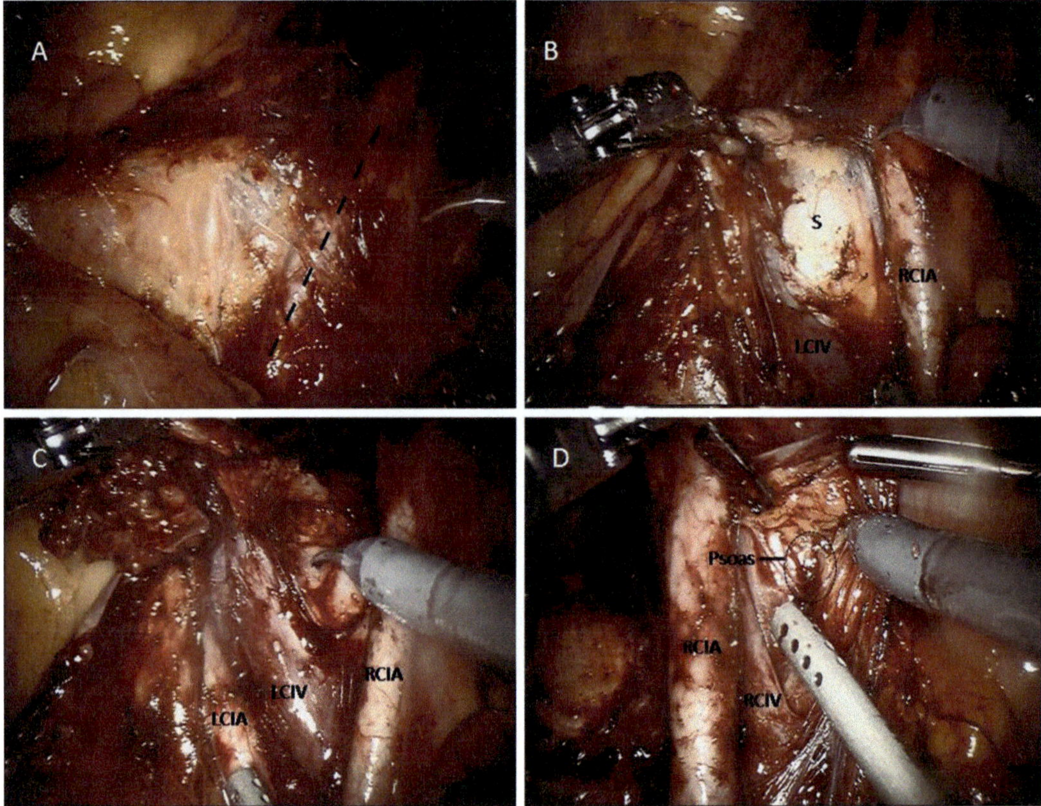

Fig. 25.3 Right common iliac lymph node dissection. (**a**) Exposure of right retroperitoneum, the *dashed line* represents location of the "split" of lymphatic tissue over the right common iliac artery (RCIA). (**b**) Medial dissection of lymphatic tissue exposes the left common iliac vein (LCIV) and sacrum (S). (**c**) By performing a second "split" over the left common iliac artery (LCIA) the packet can be divided at the bifurcation of the aorta and then dissected distally. (**d**) Lateral dissection of the packet demonstrating the edge of the right common iliac vein (RCIV) and right psoas muscle

especially common in obese patients. The ureter is dissected and tagged in the same manner as the right side. The left PNLD is completed at this point. The lymphatic tissue is split along the left common iliac artery. When splitting proximally toward the aortic bifurcation the space created by the right-sided PNLD is entered and the majority of medial aspect of the left common iliac node dissection has been completed. There will usually be only a small amount of medial lymphatic tissue remaining at the distal aspect of the left common iliac artery. This will simplify the left common iliac dissection. The remainder of the left PLND is completed in same manner at the right side dissection.

25.4.5 Transferring the Left Ureter Under the Sigmoid Mesentery

The left ureter can be transposed behind the sigmoid mesentery with the help of the right side assistant. The right side assistant should gently advance a blunt-tipped instrument below the mesentery along the anterior surface of the aorta. If the robotic "fourth arm" has been placed on the right side then it can be passed through very easily as well. The tag on the left ureter can be grasped and the ureter should easily pass through the mesenteric window. We recommend transferring the ureter prior to performing the cystectomy.

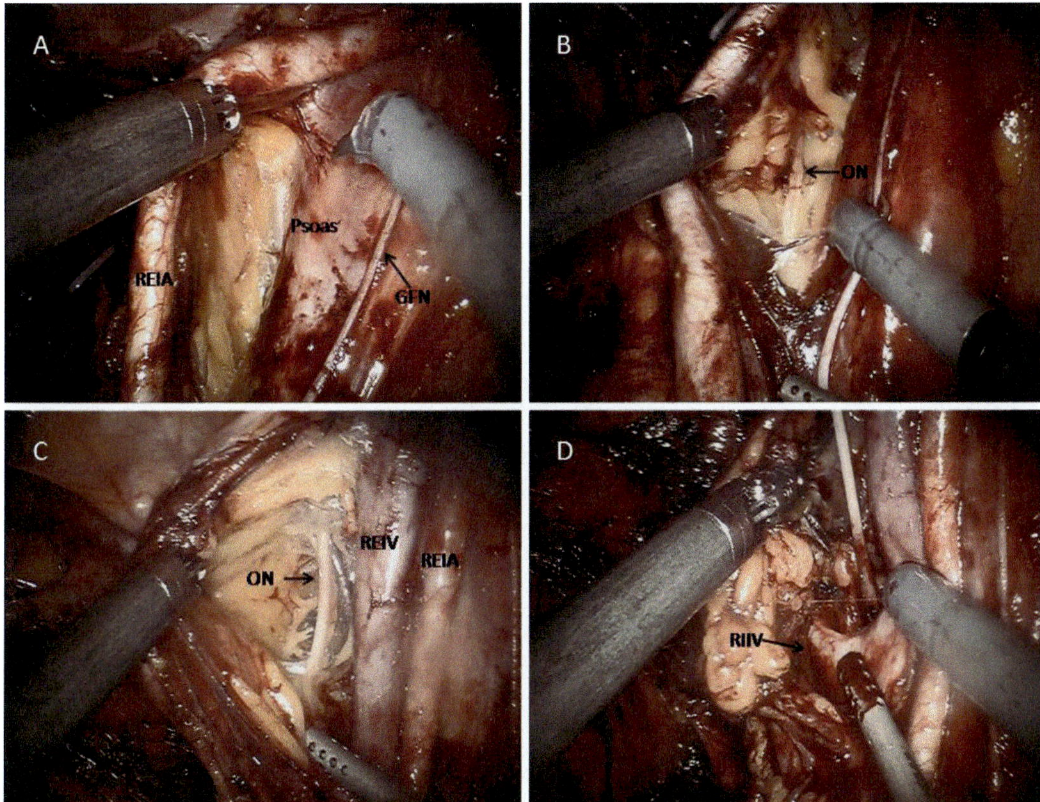

Fig. 25.4 Right obturator and hypogastric lymph node dissection. (**a, b**) Medial mobilization of the right external iliac vessels. (**c**) Removal of obturator lymph node packet from the underside of the external iliac artery and vein (REIA/REIV). (**d**) Dissection of right internal iliac vein (RIIV). (*ON* obturator nerve, *GFN* genitofemoral nerve)

25.4.6 Tagging the Distal Ileum and Preparing the Tags

The ileum should be tagged with a 3-0 absorbable suture. This should be left at least 10–12 in. in length. An additional short tag can be placed to orient the distal and proximal directionality of the ileum. The lateral attachments of the cecum can be mobilized to facilitate delivery of the ileum into the abdominal incision and make identification of the distal portion of the ileum easier. At this point, the suture tags on the ureters should be clipped with the suture tag on the ileum with a locking clip. The assistant can then grasp all three tags with one grasper and allow for easy externalization of the tags through the extraction incision. This step can also be performed after the ligation of the dorsal venous complex (DVC) when performing a male RARC, this will result in one less instrument exchange.

25.4.7 Identification, Ligation, and Division of the Superior Vesical Arteries

The obliterated umbilical and superior vesical arteries are clearly seen at the completion of the lymphadenectomy and are ligated with locking clips or divided with a vascular stapler.

25.4.8 Development of the Prerectal and Posterior Vesical Space

The camera lens can be changed to a 0° (degree) lens for optimal visualization. The peritoneum extending from the posterior bladder to the anterior sigmoid is incised. Using blunt and careful cautery dissection, the prerectal space is developed. One must employ the assistant(s) to retract the bladder and its posterior structures anteriorly.

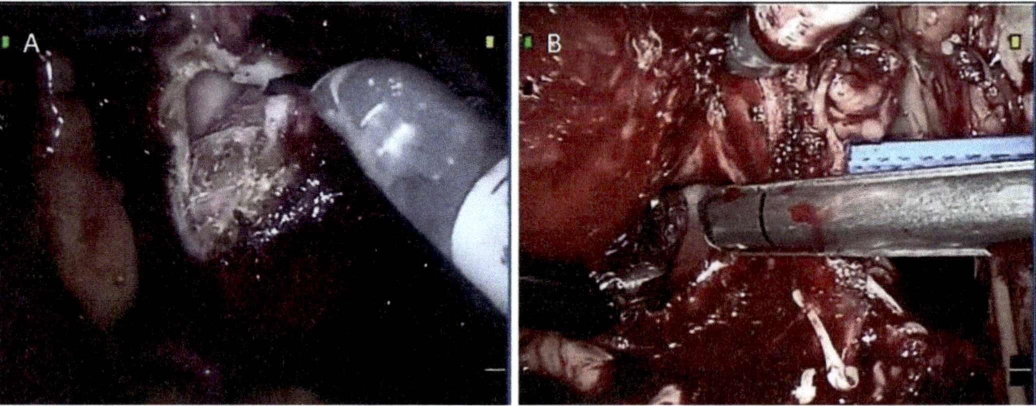

Fig. 25.5 (**a**) Incision of the vaginal cuff onto a sponge stick. (**b**) En bloc division of vagina and vascular pedicle to the bladder with an endovascular stapler

Alternatively, this can be accomplished by the fourth robotic arm. In male patients, Denonvillier's fascia needs to be incised to carry the dissection as far caudal as possible. The dissection should be carried down to the rectourethralis muscle. If a nerve sparing is desired then one should dissect anterior to Denonvillier's fascia and leave it on the anterior rectal surface staying close to the prostate.

In female patients, this dissection is aided with a sponge stick in the vagina. The bedside assistant or scrub tech can retract the vaginal cuff with manipulation of the sponge stick. If anterior vaginal wall sparing is planned then the dissection is carried between the posterior bladder and vagina. Much of the distal aspect of this dissection can be performed transvaginally at the start of the procedure before the robot is docked. If en bloc resection of the anterior vaginal wall is planned then the surgeon incises the vaginal cuff on the sponge stick and can then divide the lateral vagina and vascular pedicles en bloc with a stapler or an energy device of choice (Fig 25.5a, b).

25.4.9 Division of the Remaining Inferior Vesical Vessels

Once the limits of dissection are reached along the posterior aspect of the bladder, the lateral attachments of the bladder can be divided. For a non-nerve sparing procedure, this can be done with locking clips or a combination of the bipolar instrument and the monopolar instrument of choice. An endovascular stapler can be used as well but we recommend using locking clips near the distal aspect of dissection as it provides a more controlled division of the pedicle and will help avoid a rectal injury. It should be remembered that the dissection should be carried caudal through the endopelvic fascia thereby completely mobilizing the bladder from its lateral attachments and the rectum. Often a combination of lateral and posterior dissection is used in an alternating fashion to complete the dissection.

25.4.10 Preservation of the Neurovascular Bundles

In nerve-sparing procedures, the neurovascular bundles are encountered as they project off the posterior-lateral aspects of the prostate down to the anterior surface of the colon. The bundles can be mobilized by releasing the lateral fascia anterior to the bundles along the surface of the prostate. This should be done before ligating the inferior vesical pedicles in order to visualize them completely. This is particularly important in cases which energy devices and staplers are employed for vascular ligation. This dissection is connected to the incision anterior to Denonvillier's fascia that has already been performed during creation of the prerectal space. The inferior vesical pedicles and prostate pedicles should be clipped and divided with cold scissors to avoid neurovascular injury. The nerve sparing should be carried down to the genitourinary diaphragm to prevent injury during the apical and urethral dissection.

25.4.11 Mobilization of the Bladder and Completion of the Apical Dissection

The remaining bladder attachments should only be the urachus, anterior attachments, prostate in males, and urethra. The medial and median umbilical ligaments should be divided as far proximally as possible with electrocautery. The dissection and peritoneal incision is carried lateral to the medial umbilical ligaments caudal to the anterior surface of the bladder. If not already done, the endopelvic fascia should be incised bilaterally. The apical dissection of the prostate or vagina is then completed. At this point the dorsal venous complex can be ligated with a suture in a figure of eight fashion. Although an endovascular stapler can be employed for this step, we feel the suture ligation allows for better visualization and identification of the urethra.

25.4.12 Dissection, Ligation, and Division of the Urethra

It is very important to dissect out a generous urethral stump. This is important even in cases without a planned neobladder. A generous urethral stump allows for easier application of a locking clip or suture ligation to prevent tumor spillage during division. If the previous posterior dissection was adequate, there should be minimal posterior tissue other than some minor remnants of rectourethralis. The urethral catheter is removed by the bedside assistant and a locking clip is placed on the urethra by the bedside assistant or the robotic clip applier. The urethra is divided *distal* to the clip (Fig. 25.6a, b). A frozen section can be taken from the proximal portion of the divided urethra if needed.

Following division of the urethra the specimen is placed in a 15 mm specimen retrieval bag and retracted into the superior aspect of the abdomen. It is very important to ensure that there is excellent hemostasis in the pelvis. Often there is venous ooze from structures such as the dorsal venous complex, urethra, rectourethralis, and neurovascular bundles. Dropping the pneumoperitoneum to 5 mmHg can help identify potential bleeding areas. Strategic placement of "figure-of-eight" sutures or other hemostatic maneuvers will prevent postoperative pelvic bleeding. This is a key point, as many times this

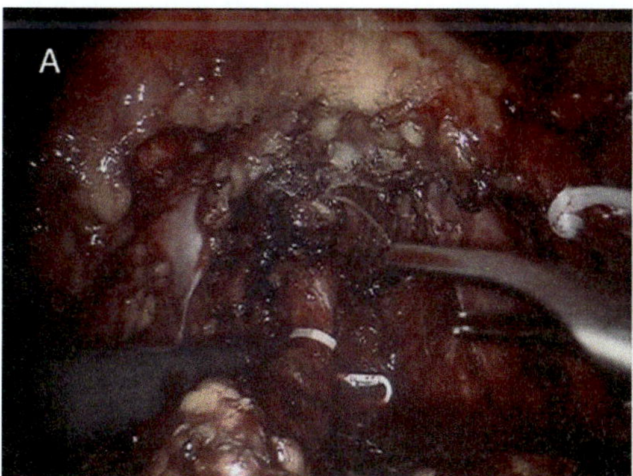
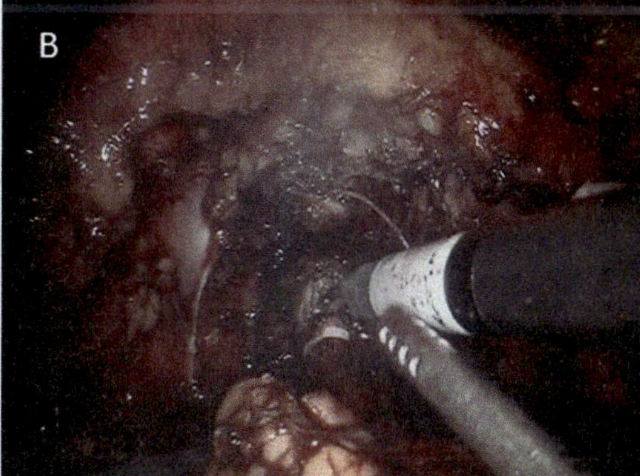

Fig. 25.6 (**a**, **b**) Occlusion of urethra with 15 mm Hem-o-lok clip with subsequent distal division of urethra

bleeding would otherwise go unnoticed until the diversion is being created and the pneumoperitoneum has been released.

In female patients, the urethra is removed en bloc with the bladder in most cases unless a neobladder is planned. The specimen in many cases can be removed through the opening of the vagina if the anterior wall is not spared. Closure of the vagina should be performed in a "clam shell" fashion. One must avoid the temptation to roll the vagina into a tube otherwise it may be too narrow for functional use and in some cases herniation of intraabdominal contents can be encountered. The vagina should be closed very meticulously with well placed absorbable suture. The closure should be checked externally through the vagina by palpation to ensure adequate closure. We also place permanent sutures at four points (two on each side) performing a paravaginal repair to provide some lateral support. While vaginal prolapse is not uncommon after a radical cystectomy, paravaginal fixation can help minimize lateral weakness postoperatively.

25.4.13 Specimen Extraction

The entire specimen can be entrapped in a 15 mm specimen retrieval bag. It will be extracted through a 6–8 cm infraumbilical or periumbilical incision. Prior to extraction, the tags on the ureters and the ileum should be grasped in a locking grasper by the bedside assistant to allow delivery into and through the extraction incision. The surgeon must avoid the temptation to try to incorporate the superior camera port into the extraction incision. If the incision is too high on the abdomen, the ureteroileal anastomosis may be difficult and traction of the left ureter may be necessary to deliver it into the wound. Therefore, we recommend that the incision be below the umbilicus.

25.4.14 Extracorporeal Urinary Diversion

The steps of performing an ileal conduit or neobladder through the extraction incision are the same for a standard ORC. The main caveat is that the surgeon avoids traction on the ureters at all costs. The surgeon should essentially perform the anastomosis at the level of the fascia and cut back on any devascularized ureter. In addition, one should make the extraction incision as large as is needed to perform a meticulous watertight anastomosis while not placing undue tension on the ureters. While tempting, too small of an incision can make the diversion difficult and the difference between a 5 and 10 cm incision is likely negligible when it comes to postoperative recovery.

Variations of technique for creation of the neobladder have been described. In some cases, it is easier to simply make the extraction incision very low and start at the pubic symphisis. This can allow for placement of anastomotic sutures in an "open" fashion through the extraction incision. The authors have found that this is a viable option in many patients. Placement of one or more of the urethral sutures can be performed robotically before extraction of the specimen and delivered into the wound for parachuting the neobladder down into the pelvis.

If the urethra-neobladder anastomosis is to be done robotically then a urethral catheter should be passed through the urethra and delivered through the extraction incision. The distal portion of the catheter can then be inserted into the anticipated urethral anastomotic site and the balloon inflated (Fig. 25.7a). Anastomotic sutures can be pre-placed in the posterior lip of the anticipated anastomotic site of the neobladder. The authors currently use two separate 2-0 absorbable sutures with UR-6 needles tied together and cut at a length of 7 in. (Fig. 25.7b). Gentle traction of the urethral catheter will allow for easier placement of the neobladder into the pelvis and down to the urethral stump. The urinary diversion stents can be left in the neobladder for removal cystoscopically later. Alternatively, one can bring them out through the abdominal wall as one would do in an open fashion. Another option is to bring the stents out the urethra alongside the catheter but may result in significant leakage. A final option is to tie it to the tip of the catheter but this can pose a problem if the catheter is dislodged early.

The fascia of the extraction incision can be closed and the pneumoperitoneum reestablished.

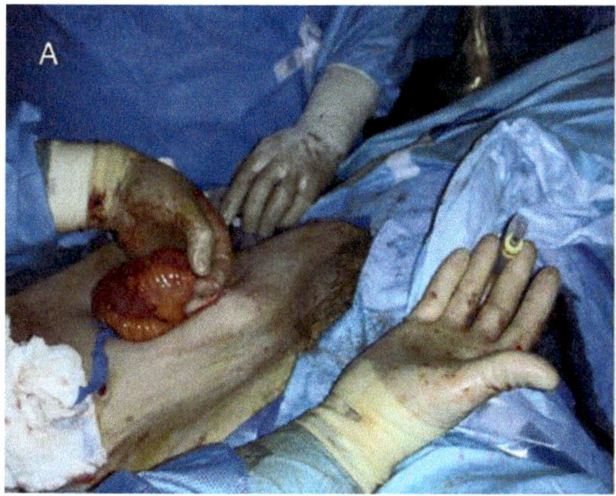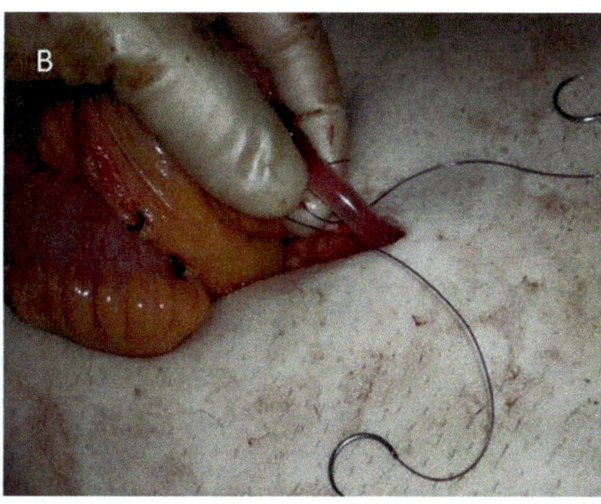

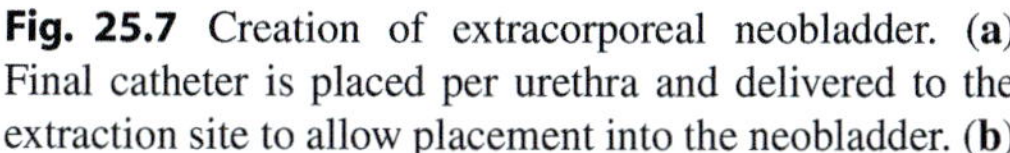

Fig. 25.7 Creation of extracorporeal neobladder. (**a**) Final catheter is placed per urethra and delivered to the extraction site to allow placement into the neobladder. (**b**) A double-armed suture is pre-placed at the 6 o'clock on the bladder neck to simplify a robotic anastomosis

During the remaining portion of the operation, less extreme trendelenberg should be used to decrease tension during suturing of the urethra-neobladder anastomosis. The anastomosis is completed in a running fashion starting at the 6 o-clock position. The balloon of the urethral catheter should be deflated during the anastomosis and the catheter moved as needed. Some surgeons have described placement of a traction suture on the neobladder for downward traction by the "fourth arm" during the anastomosis. Once completed the anastomosis is checked with irrigation. Abdominal drains, suprapubic tubes, and port site closures should be performed based on surgeon preference.

25.5 Postoperative Care

A nasogastric tube is not routinely left in place. The patients are maintained on broad-spectrum antibiotics for at least 24 h. Epidural catheters are not routinely used. Mechanical and medical prophylaxis of deep venous thrombosis is administered. Intravenous morphine and/or ketorolac are usually adequate for pain management and can be promptly switched to oral narcotics once the patient is tolerating a diet. Patients are encouraged to sit in a chair the same night of surgery. They are ambulated on the first postoperative day. Patients have nothing by mouth on postoperative day 1, but advance to 8 oz of non-carbonated clear liquids every 8 h on postoperative day 2, followed by unrestricted non-carbonated clear liquids on postoperative day 3, and finally a regular diet on postoperative day 4. Diet advancement is performed regardless of bowel function, and is only held or decreased in the setting of emesis or intractable nausea. Most patients do not seem to have significant third spacing and will rarely require additional fluid replacement other than standard maintenance fluids.

Ureteral stents and abdominal drains should be managed according to surgeon preference. Currently, the authors remove stents from a urostomy at 7–10 days. Foley catheters are removed from neobladders in 14–21 days. If the stents were not secured to the Foley during creation of the neobladder, then they are removed cystoscopically at the time of Foley removal in the office. The decision to perform a cystogram at the time of Foley removal is based on surgeon preference and is currently our standard practice.

The authors have found that some patients may have a continued leak of lymphatic fluid through a drain site up following removal. Consequently, a urostomy appliance can be placed over the drain site to collect the fluid until the incision heals and drainage ceases. We have found this drainage to be self-limiting and uniformly resolves spontaneously as the lymphatic fluid is absorbed intraperitoneally. If there is any concern of a urine leak, the fluid may be sent for creatinine analysis.

25.6 Review of Perioperative and Postoperative Complications

The existing literature on perioperative and postoperative complications of RARC is primarily compromised of single-center series. Kauffman et al. published their complication data on a series of 79 consecutive patients after RARC [8]. While 49 % of patients experienced complications within 90 days when using a standardized reporting system, a majority were minor, with infectious complications (41 %) occurring most commonly, followed by gastrointestinal (27 %) and thromboembolic events (10 %). Another series by Treiyer and colleagues evaluated 84 consecutive RARC patients with overall and major 30-day Clavien complication rates of 53 % and 12 %, respectively [9]. Khan and colleagues reported outcomes of their first 50 robotic cystectomies [10]. The Clavien 90-day complication rate was 34 %, with major complications occurring in 10 % of this cohort.

Hayn et al. studied 156 consecutive patients undergoing RARC and reported an overall complication rate of 52 % within 90 days, including a 33 % major complication and a 21 % readmission rate [11]. The authors classified all complications using the Memorial Sloan Kettering Cancer Center (MSKCC) system. The most common complications reported in Hayn's series were gastrointestinal (31 %), infectious (25 %), and genitourinary (13 %). The study is noteworthy in that all cystectomies at this institution were performed robotically decreasing selection bias. However, limitations of single institution studies are well known, and have led to multi-institutional analyses, which provide more robust and generalizable data.

Kang et al. describes a multi-institutional evaluation of complications during and after robotic cystectomy in seven participating Korean institutions [12]. Retrospectively analyzing data

from 104 patients, the authors reported an overall complication rate of 27 % using the modified Clavien system, with 7.7 % considered major complications and 19 % minor complications. Intraoperative complications represented 3.8 % of the total number of complications, with three conversions to open surgery. Two were secondary to adhesions with one due to an external iliac vein injury. Our own multi-institutional study evaluated a larger sample size of 227 patients spread between four institutions [13]. The overall complication rate was 30 % with 7 % having a major complication as defined by the Clavien classification system, with no perioperative deaths. Interestingly, younger patients in this series were more likely to experience complications.

There are several recent reports comparing outcomes of robotic and open radical cystectomies. Ng et al. performed a prospective cohort study of 187 consecutive patients (104 ORC and 83 RARC) who underwent radical cystectomy [14]. Thirty-day Clavien complications revealed a higher overall rate in the open group at 30 days (59 % vs. 41 %, $p = 0.04$), as well as a significant increase in major complications (30 % vs. 10 %; $p = 0.007$). At 90 days, the overall complication rate, while greater in the open cohort, was not statistically significantly different. However, there did appear to be more major complications in the open cohort at 90 days (31 % vs 17 %; $p = 0.03$). In a multivariate analysis controlling for a variety of comorbidities, RARC remained an independent predictor of fewer overall and major complications at both 30 and 90 days. The types of complications observed were similar to those in contemporary open series, including gastrointestinal, infectious, and thromboembolic events. Although this study was strengthened by prospective data collection, a large sample size, and procedures performed by a single surgeon, it remains limited by its observational methodology and lack of randomization.

There are now two single-center randomized trials comparing ORC and RARC that have published. Nix et al. reported results of our prospective, randomized study, including 20 patients undergoing ORC and 21 in the RARC cohort [15]. Although designed as a non-inferiority study comparing lymph node yield, several secondary endpoints were evaluated, including complication rate. Comparing those undergoing open and robotic procedures, no difference in complication rates was noted (50 % vs. 33 %, respectively; $p=0.28$). In a multivariate analysis controlling for age, body mass index, and pathologic stage there was a trend toward a lower complication rate in the robotic group, but it did not reach statistical significance ($p=0.0503$). Parekh et al. recently published results of their single-center prospective randomized trial of ORC and RARC. There was 20 patients in each arm and there was no significant difference in positive surgical margin rates, lymph node yield, or complication rate (5 % vs. 5 %, 23 % vs. 11 %, and 25 % vs. 25 %, respectively) [16]. A multi-institutional, randomized study is currently in the recruitment phase, the results of which will clarify these questions (the RAZOR trial, NCT01157676).

25.7 Pathologic and Oncologic Outcomes of RARC

Two important pathologic issues are incidence of positive surgical margins (PSM) and an adequate pelvic lymph node dissection (PLND). The importance of achieving negative surgical margins during radical cystectomy is critical considering the fact that patients with positive soft tissue margins have increased recurrence rates and almost a threefold decrease in survival [17, 18]. The reported rate of PSM for RARC ranges from 0 to 7.6 % [8, 10, 11, 19–21]. Novara et al. provided a benchmark from the open radical cystectomy literature in a multi-institutional series of over 4,000 patients where the PSM rate was 6.3 % [22]. The inclusion of a pelvic lymphadenectomy at the time of cystectomy provides both prognostic information and potential therapeutic benefit [23, 24]. Furthermore, the number of lymph nodes removed has been shown to have prognostic significance by several authors and it is also well established that an extended template will improve lymph node yield [23–26]. The retrospectively reported lymph node yield for PLND during RARC range from 17 to 43 [10, 21, 27–

29]. Nix et al. demonstrated no difference in lymph node yield between robotic and open cystectomy in a randomized trial [15]. In a unique study by Davis et al., robotic lymph node dissections had a yield of 93 % compared to open lymphadenectomy when a "second look open dissection" was used following the robotic PLND [28]. The take home message is that a meticulous pelvic lymphadenectomy should be performed and is certainly possible, including extended templates, if the surgeon is dedicated to this goal.

While there are no reports on long-term (>5 years) oncologic outcomes, there are several reports of short and intermediate-term follow-up that have emerged. Pruthi and Wallen reported short-term cancer outcomes in 50 patients [30]. They had a mean follow-up 13.2 months and experienced an overall and disease-specific survival of 90 % and 94 %, respectively. Dasgupta et al. published their RARC experience in 20 patients with >6 months follow-up [31]. They reported with a median follow-up of 23 months an overall and disease-free survival of 95 and 90 %. Martin et al. reported outcomes in series of 80 patients with the longest mean follow-up to date from Mayo Clinic in Arizona [32]. Fifty-nine patients had >6 months follow-up with a mean follow-up of 25 months (range 6–49). The overall survival at 12 months, 24 months, and 36 months was 82 %, 69 %, and 69 %, respectively, and recurrence-free survival at 12 months, 24 months, and 36 months was 82 %, 71 %, and 71 %, respectively. Kauffman et al. reported a 2-year disease-free, cancer-specific, and overall survival of 74 %, 85 %, and 79 %, respectively. [33] When compared to historical ORC, oncologic outcomes for RARC as measured by survival are equivalent in the intermediate-term. Additional data from Mayo Clinic Arizona and University of North Carolina were published for node-positive patients having undergone RARC [34]. A total of 275 patients were reviewed with focus on 50 patients with lymph node-positive disease. With a mean follow-up of 42 months the oncologic outcomes compared favorably to open cohorts reported in the literature. In summary, the current literature demonstrates the fact that at 2–3 years the oncologic outcomes of RARC compare favorably to historical controls.

25.8 Recommendations for Getting Started and Avoidance of Complications

First, appropriate patient selection cannot be overemphasized during the primary stages of transition to robotic cystectomy. As an initial case, we would recommend beginning with a thin male patient and non-bulky tumor. Because of several parallels drawn from the maneuvers used during robotic prostatectomy, a male patient will provide familiarity and comfort during the initial, most challenging steps involved in the procedure. Furthermore, patient size is often an important factor in the level of difficulty, with some of the most challenging robotic cystectomy cases occurring in morbidly obese patients. Technical issues are often more challenging in obese patients, due to the need for appropriate retraction, which is especially difficult during left ureteral identification due to the large amount of epiploic, mesenteric, and retroperitoneal fat.

We recommend avoiding locally advanced and large tumors early in your experience. Bulky tumors can produce significant challenges with anterior retraction of the bladder during the posterior dissection. This particular problem will place the surgeon at risk for inadvertent entry into the bladder or rectal injury secondary to the lack of a posterior working space.

There are several intraoperative techniques that may help avoid complications. To start with, ureteral dissection is an important part of robotic cystectomy. Ureteral strictures represent an extremely troubling late complication of urinary diversions, and the majority of these can be attributed to ischemia of the distal ureter, in some cases resulting from poor surgical technique during ureteral mobilization. Care must be taken to avoid tension during dissection. During dissection, a robotic arm is often employed to elevate the ureter, and due to the lack of tactile feedback, excessive tension may be unintentionally placed on the ureter. It is therefore essential to use visual cues to constantly assess this degree of tension. Additionally, it is important to leave peri-ureteral tissue surrounding the ureter,

which can be easily scraped away by aggressive manipulation with the robotic instruments. As mentioned earlier, a technique which we have found effective and efficient to minimize ureteral trauma involves the use of a pre-tied Hem-o-lok clip. We place a 15 mm clip with a 20 cm silk tie proximal to the site of ureteral transection. Once divided, the tie/clip functions as a secure stay for all future manipulation without direct handling of the ureter (Fig 25.2a, b).

An additional technique we utilize to minimize ureteral ischemia, limitation of proximal mobilization to just above the common iliac vessels allows for mobilization of the ureter away from the working field during extended pelvic lymphadenectomy while maintaining perforating vessels to the ureter above the aortic bifurcation. Although tempting, additional proximal dissection is rarely needed to complete the urinary diversion, even if done through a limited incision during extracorporeal reconstruction.

While a small extraction incision is possible, it is important to make it large enough to safely accommodate construction of the urinary diversion. This allows for creation of the ureteroenteric anastomosis without additional ureteral tension aggravated by a small incision. We believe that the benefits of a robotic approach will not be undone through limited extension of this incision.

A rectal injury can be a disastrous complication resulting in a colostomy, rectal fistula, and even death if unrecognized. When performing the posterior dissection in male patients, particular attention should be paid to careful and thorough mobilization of the rectum to avoid injury during division of the vascular pedicles. Our preference for division of these pedicles is with use of a vascular stapler. The posterior dissection usually becomes more difficult as one progresses distally, and it should be kept in mind that the rectum lies in a more anterior location when approaching the prostatic apex. We recommend allotting adequate time to fully mobilize the distal aspect of the rectum away from the prostate in much the same fashion as one prepares for neurovascular bundle preservation during a robot-assisted radical prostatectomy. Once this is

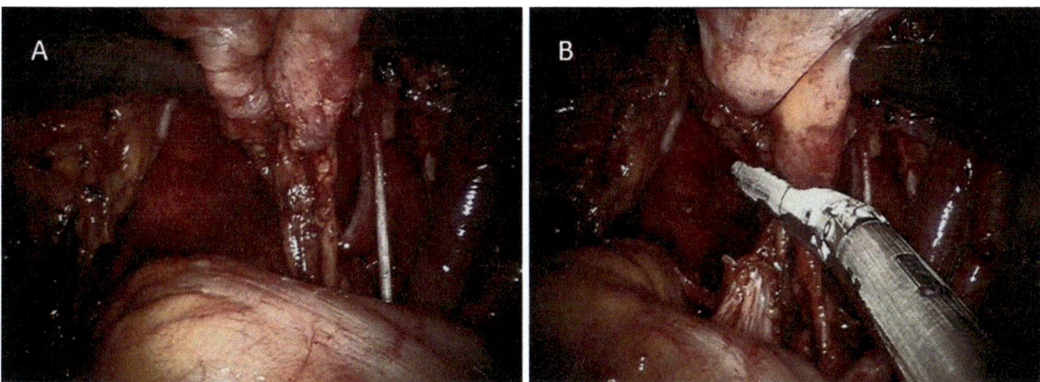

Fig. 25.8 (**a**) Appearance of right bladder pedicle after thorough mobilization of the rectum. (**b**) Division of bladder pedicle with an endovascular stapler

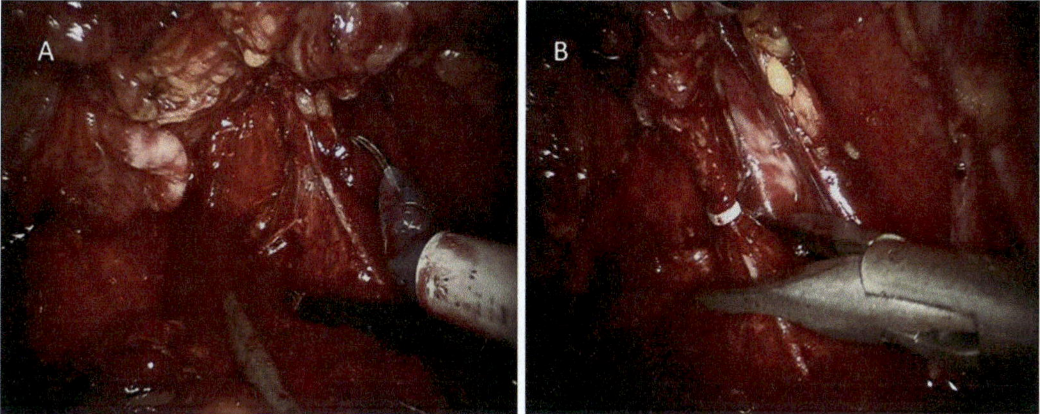

Fig. 25.9 (**a**, **b**) Control of the distal bladder pedicle with a Hem-o-lok clip

accomplished, the surgeon will be left with a narrow column of vascular tissue from the superior vesical artery to the prostatic apex. This will allow safe application of the vascular stapler above all rectal tissue as shown in Fig. 25.8a, b. When employing the stapler, we recommend the larger, more blunt blade be positioned medially to avoid inadvertent placement of the sharper, thinner blade into the rectum; also helpful is upward (anterior) articulation of the stapler away from the rectum.

If the separation of the bladder/prostate and rectum is difficult, we would then recommend proceeding cautiously through isolation of individual pedicles as one progresses distally, using Hem-o-lok (weck) clips for vascular control (Fig. 25.9a, b). If at any point a bulky tumor impedes visualization of the posterior plane, use of a 30° upward-facing lens may be warranted, which may improve visualization of the underside of the bladder.

The ability to perform an adequate pelvic lymph node dissection during RARC has been a popular target for opponents of the robotic approach. However, this has been refuted by several authors [15, 28, 29], and we uphold that a meticulous dissection of any template can be performed robotically if the surgeon is committed to this goal. One of the most challenging aspects of the PLND is performing an adequate and safe dissection of the lymphatic tissue in the bifurcation of the common iliac vessels. The difficulty of dissection can be decreased by medial mobilization of the external iliac vessels and all associated lymphatic tissue. This will expose the medial aspect of the psoas muscle and the most proximal aspect of the obturator nerve while releasing all lateral attachments of this nodal packet as shown in Fig. 25.4a, b. It will further allow the surgeon to return to the medial side of the vessels and easily withdraw the entire lymph node packet from the bifurcation of the vessels (Fig. 25.4c). Overall, this will not only help decrease the risk of a vascular injury to the hypogastric vessels and alleviate the anxiety associated with dissection in this challenging area but also allow excellent access for the hypogastric vein dissection (Fig. 25.4d).

25.9 Conclusion

Robot-assisted radical cystectomy is a feasible and reproducible procedure for the management of bladder cancer. There have been an increasing number of publications reporting outcomes of RARC over the past decade. There appears to be equivalent pathologic outcomes to the gold standard ORC and intermediate-term oncologic outcomes look promising. Fortunately, the results of a large multicenter, randomized trial will be available in the near future. We are optimistic this procedure will continue to become standardized and increasingly utilized in the practicing urologist armamentarium.

References

1. Lowrance WT, Rumohr JA, Chang SS, Clark PE, Smith Jr JA, Cookson MS. Contemporary open radical cystectomy: analysis of perioperative outcomes. J Urol. 2008;179:1313–8.
2. Parra RO, Andrus CH, Jones JP. Laparoscopic cystectomy: initial report on a new treatment for the retained bladder. J Urol. 1992;148:1140–4.
3. Menon M, Hemal AK, Tewari A, Shrivastava A, Shoma AM, El-Tabey NA, et al. Nerve-sparing robot-assisted radical cystoprostatectomy and urinary diversion. BJU Int. 2003;92:232–6.
4. Guru KA, Kim HL, Piacente PM, Mohler JL. Robot-assisted radical cystectomy and pelvic lymph node dissection: initial experience at Roswell Park Cancer Institute. Urology. 2007;69:469–74.
5. Lowentritt BH, Castle EP, Woods M, Davis R, Thomas R. Robot-assisted radical cystectomy in women: technique and initial experience. J Endourol. 2008;22:709–12.
6. Pruthi RS, Stefaniak H, Hubbard JS, Wallen EM. Robot-assisted laparoscopic anterior pelvic exenteration for bladder cancer in the female patient. J Endourol. 2008;22:2397–402.
7. Woods M, Thomas R, Davis R, Andrews PE, Ferrigni RG, Cheng J, et al. Robot-assisted extended pelvic lymphadenectomy. J Endourol. 2008;22:1297–302.
8. Kauffman EC, Ng CK, Lee MM, Otto BJ, Portnoff A, Wang GJ, et al. Critical analysis of complications after robotic-assisted radical cystectomy with identification of preoperative and operative risk factors. BJU Int. 2010;105:520–7.
9. Treiyer A, Saar M, Kopper B, Kamradt J, Siemer S, Stockle M. Robotic-assisted laparoscopic radical cystectomy: evaluation of functional and oncological results. Actas Urol Esp. 2011;35:152–7.
10. Khan MS, Elhage O, Challacombe B, Rimington P, Murphy D, Dasgupta P. Analysis of early complications of robotic-assisted radical cystectomy using a standardized reporting system. Urology. 2011;77:357–62.
11. Hayn MH, Hellenthal NJ, Hussain A, Stegemann AP, Guru KA. Defining morbidity of robot-assisted radical cystectomy using a standardized reporting methodology. Eur Urol. 2011;59:213–8.
12. Kang SG, Kang SH, Lee YG, Rha KH, Jeong BC, Ko HM, et al. Robot-assisted radical cystectomy and pelvic lymph node dissection: a multi-institutional study from Korea. J Endourol. 2010;24:1435–40.
13. Smith AB, Raynor M, Amling CL, Busby JE, Castle E, Davis R, et al. Multi-institutional analysis of robotic radical cystectomy for bladder cancer: perioperative outcomes and complications in 227 patients. J Laparoendosc Adv Surg Tech A. 2012;22:17–21.
14. Ng CK, Kauffman EC, Lee MM, Otto BJ, Portnoff A, Ehrlich JR, et al. A comparison of postoperative complications in open versus robotic cystectomy. Eur Urol. 2010;57:274–81.
15. Nix J, Smith A, Kurpad R, Nielsen ME, Wallen EM, Pruthi RS. Prospective randomized controlled trial of robotic versus open radical cystectomy for bladder cancer: perioperative and pathologic results. Eur Urol. 2010;57:196–201.
16. Parekh DJ, Messer J, Fitzgerald J, Ercole M, Svatek R. Perioperative outcomes and oncologic efficacy from a pilot prospective randomized clinical trial of open versus robotic assisted radical cystectomy. J Urol. 2013;189:474–9.
17. Dotan ZA, Kavanagh K, Yossepowitch O, Kaag M, Olgac S, Donat M, et al. Positive surgical margins in soft tissue following radical cystectomy for bladder cancer and cancer specific survival. J Urol. 2007;178:2308–12.

18. Hadjizacharia P, Stein JP, Cai J, Miranda G. The impact of positive soft tissue surgical margins following radical cystectomy for high-grade, invasive bladder cancer. World J Urol. 2009;27:33–8.

19. Hellenthal NJ, Hussain A, Andrews PE, Carpentier P, Castle E, Dasgupta P, et al. Surgical margin status after robot assisted radical cystectomy: results from the international robotic cystectomy consortium. J Urol. 2010;184:87–91.

20. Schumacher MC, Jonsson MN, Wiklund NP. Robotic cystectomy. Scand J Surg. 2009;98:89–95.

21. Pruthi RS, Nielsen ME, Nix J, Smith A, Schultz H, Wallen EM. Robotic radical cystectomy for bladder cancer: surgical adn pathological outcomes in 100 consecutive cases. J Urol. 2010;183:510–5.

22. Novara G, Svatek RS, Karakiewicz PI, Skinner E, Ficarra V, Fradet Y, et al. Soft tissue surgical margin status is a powerful predictor of outcomes after radical cystectomy: a multicenter study of more than 4,400 patients. J Urol. 2010;183:2165–70.

23. Leissner J, Hohenfellner R, Thuroff JW, Wolf HK. Lymphadenectomy in patients with transitional cell carcinoma of the urinary bladder: significance for staging and prognosis. BJU Int. 2000;85:817–23.

24. Poulsen AL, Horn T, Steven K. Radical cystectomy: extending the limits of pelvic lymph node dissection improves survival for patients with bladder cancer confined to the bladder wall. J Urol. 1998;160: 2015–20.

25. Herr H, Lee C, Chang S, Lerner S, Bladder Cancer Collaborative Group. Standardization of radical cystectomy and pelvic lymph node dissection for bladder cancer: a collaborative group report. J Urol. 2004;171:1823–8.

26. Herr HW, Faulkner JR, Grossman HB, Natale RB, deVere White R, Sarosdy MF, et al. Surgical factors influence bladder cancer outcomes: a cooperative group report. J Clin Oncol. 2004;22:2781–9.

27. Hellenthal NJ, Hussain A, Andrews PE, Carpentier P, Castle E, Dasgupta P, et al. Lymphadenectomy at the time of robot-assisted radical cystectomy: results from the international robotic cystectomy consortium. BJU Int. 2010;107:642–6.

28. Davis JW, Gaston K, Anderson R, Dinney CP, Grossman HB, Munsell MF, et al. Robot assisted extended pelvic lymphadenectomy at radical cystectomy: lymph node yield compared with second look open dissection. J Urol. 2010;185:79–84.

29. Lavery HJ, Martinez-Suarez HJ, Abaza R. Robotic extended pelvic lymphadenectomy for bladder cancer with increased nodal yield. BJU Int. 2010;107:1802–5.

30. Pruthi RS, Wallen EM. Is robotic radical cystectomy an appropriate treatment for bladder cancer? Short-term oncologic and clinical follow-up in 50 consecutive patients. Urology. 2008;72:617–22.

31. Dasgupta P, Rimington P, Murphy D, Challacombe B, Hemal A, Elhage O, et al. Robotic assisted radical cystectomy: short to medium term oncologic and functional outcomes. Int J Clin Pract. 2008;62:1709–14.

32. Martin AD, Nunez RN, Pacelli A, Woods ME, Davis R, Thomas R, et al. Robot-assisted radical cystectomy: intermediate survival results at a mean follow-up of 25 months. BJU Int. 2010;105:1706–9.

33. Kauffman EC, Ng CK, Lee MM, Otto BJ, Wang GJ, Scherr DS. Early oncologic outcomes for bladder urothelial carcinoma patients treated with robotic-assisted radical cystectomy. BJU Int. 2010;107:628–35.

34. Mmeje CO, Nunez-Nateras R, Nielsen ME, Pruthi RS, Smith A, Wallen EM, et al. Oncologic outcomes for lymph node-positive urothelial carcinoma patients treated with robot assisted radical cystectomy: with mean follow-up of 3.5 years. Urol Oncol. 2013;31:1621.

48-year-old healthy man with 4 cm,
T2 urothelial carcinoma and negative
metastatic evaluation who desires
immediate cystectomy without neoadjuvant
chemotherapy, erectile function
preservation, and an ileal neobladder

Richard E. Hautmann

26.1 Talk to the Patient

First of all I would tell him: no hectic actions!

Patients diagnosed with cancer often want to schedule an operation as soon as possible, even the next day. Others may delay surgery while they obtain additional opinions, search the Internet, and try to decide about treatment. How long does the window of opportunity to cure a cancer remain open?

In patients with muscle invasion at diagnosis, a delay in surgery is associated with a more advanced pathologic stage, especially when the delay is longer than 90 days. Although an appropriate time should be given for consideration of options and pre-treatment evaluation, undue delay may compromise cancer control. Once the diagnosis of muscle-invasive disease is made, proceeding with radical cystectomy (RC) expeditiously would seem to be in the patient's best interest. Next, I would confirm the correctness of the patient's decision and tell him, that there is—as always—good news and bad news.

R.E. Hautmann, M.D., M.D. hon (✉)
University of Ulm, Boschstrasse 4a, 89231,
Neu-Ulm, Germany
e-mail: richard.hautmann@uni-ulm.de

26.2 Decision for Immediate Radical Cystectomy: The Good News and the Bad News

Good news is that he has selected the best available treatment. Recently, a Dutch population-based study confirmed the relative survival rate after RC to be superior to the relative survival after all other treatment modalities [1]. Bad news is that his chances of cure are not 100 %, due to unrecognized micro-metastasis at the time of surgery.

For detailing the chances of cure I would use the postoperative nomogram predicting risk of recurrence after RC for bladder cancer (BC) of the International Bladder Cancer Nomogram Consortium [2], if his final pathologic stage proves to be pT2, pNO, G3.

Nomograms are predictive tools that are more complex than simple risk group models and provide a tailored assessment of a given patient's risk. An accurate predictive model provides a clinical tool that can be used by both patients and clinicians in evaluating options after cystectomy. A prognostic tool that provides improved individual risk assessment compared with conventional risk models will facilitate patient's decision making because treatment choice can be influenced strongly by risk prediction. This may play a particularly relevant role in the management of BC patients, given the data supporting a possible benefit for perioperative chemotherapy. At present, the option of receiving adjuvant chemotherapy on or off a clinical protocol is a reasonable consideration for BC patients at high risk of postoperative recurrence (P3, P4, or N+tumors). A patient faced with a decision to choose adjuvant chemotherapy with its potential adverse effects will base the choice on an understanding of the inherent risk that the tumor has for jeopardizing long-term health and survival [2].

For a pT2, NO, MO, G3 tumor, the nomogram has a 60-month progression-free rate prediction of 80 %.

26.3 Understaging: The Patient Must Be Informed

The reported discordance between staging on transurethral bladder resection and on RC pathology in the literature ranges from 20 to 80 %. Correct staging in BC has direct implications for its management. The upstaging from organ-confined to non-organ-confined disease has been reported in up to 40 % of cases. Specifically, Mitra et al. developed a pre-cystectomy decision model to predict pathologic upstaging and oncologic outcomes in clinical stage T2 BC. The study describes a cross-validated decision tree generated using pre-cystectomy variables aiming to stratify patients with cT2 tumors based on the risk of pathologic upstaging and adverse oncologic outcomes. This model can be potentially employed as a tool for making clinical decisions with respect to neoadjuvant chemotherapy (NACT) in these patients [3].

- Age, presence of hydronephrosis, evidence of deep muscularis propria invasion and lymphovascular invasion on transurethral resection specimen, as well as tumor growth pattern and count, were significantly associated with upstaging.
- When these factors were included in a decision tree model, 70.6 % of patients with

hydronephrosis experienced upstaging and had the worst outcome ($P<0.001$).

- In patients without hydronephrosis, tumor growth pattern was a second-tier discriminator ($P<0.001$); in patients with non-papillary tumors, 71.7 % cases with evidence of deep muscularis propria involvement experienced upstaging compared to 53.8 % of cases with no deep muscle involvement ($P=0.012$), whereas, among patients with combined papillary and non-papillary features, 33 % of cases aged ≤ 65 years were upstaged compared to 47 % of cases aged >65 years ($P=0.036$).

26.4 Decision Against Neoadjuvant Chemotherapy: Not Every Muscle Invasive Bladder Cancer (MIBC) Needs Neoadjuvant Chemotherapy

The number need to treat (NNT) represents the number of patients, on average, that must be treated to result in one additional outcome. In this scenario, the NNT for the given patient is approximately 9–10, which is rather high and constitutes a strong argument against NACT in his case. We have to acknowledge that neoadjuvant treatment (chemotherapy, radiation) does not benefit every patient and delays curative treatment for a significant percentage of patients with MIBC (40 %). Patients may receive chemotherapy unnecessarily because a more-complete operation may have indicated a greater likelihood of surgical cure. It is also unlikely that NACT will compensate for a poor operation in which significant tumor volume has been left behind in the pelvis.

An improved risk stratification of clinical stage T2 (cT2) patients can potentially identify candidates who may derive maximal benefit from this approach. Clinical stage T2 patients, who are pathologically upstaged at cystectomy have significantly worse prognosis than their counterparts who are not upstaged. The identification of such candidates who may be subsequently upstaged represents a strategy for selecting those patients who may benefit the most from NACT, whereas other patients can undergo early RC [3].

Despite evidence supporting perioperative chemotherapy, few randomized studies compare neoadjuvant and adjuvant chemotherapy for bladder cancer [4]. Consequently, the standard of care regarding the timing of chemotherapy for locally advanced BC remains controversial. In this study, there was no statistically significant difference in OS and DSS between patients receiving neoadjuvant versus adjuvant systemic platinum-based chemotherapy for locally advanced BC. In addition, there was no significant difference between neoadjuvant and adjuvant cisplatin- or carboplatin-based chemotherapy. Chemotherapy sequence relative to surgery appeared less important than whether or not a patient actually received perioperative chemotherapy.

Level I evidence supports the use of NACT for clinical (c) T2-T4aNOMO UCB. A recent multi-institutional study reported that only 12 % of patients with cT2-T4aNOMO received NACT, whereas 22 % received adjuvant systemic chemotherapy. The exact reasons for these practice patterns remain unclear [4].

In addition, the SWOG study [5] had a myriad of weaknesses that cannot be overlooked. A few examples to mention are: (1) A total of 317 patients were accrued over an 11-year period (1987–1998)! Of these, 307 patients had complete records available for review. Thirty-nine patients with available records did not have a cystectomy, 22 had RC aborted because of unresectable tumor or positive nodes, and four experienced tumor progression while receiving MVAC. Of the 268 patients who had a RC, nine had surgery performed outside of protocol; (2) 24 patients had no node dissection, 98 patients had limited node sampling and 146 patients had a standard bilateral PLND. The median number of nodes removed from all patients was 10. Twenty-four percent of the patients had 0–4 nodes removed, 25 % had 5–9 nodes, 25 % had 10–15 nodes, and 26 % had more than 15 nodes removed. The median number of nodes after none, limited, or standard PLND was zero, 7, and 15, respectively. Node

status was positive for 21 % patients. Of the 242 patients with status of surgical margins reported, 25 (10 %) had positive margins. Local recurrence occurred in 41 (15 %) of the 268 patients after RC and was balanced between treatment arms [5]; (3) Study patients were operated on by 106 different surgeons in 109 institutions. Fourteen surgeons performed five or more cystectomies on this study and two did fewer than five operations. All but one of the high-volume surgeons were urologic oncologists. Of the 109 institutions represented, 50 were community hospitals ($n = 84$ patients), 36 were academic medical centers ($n = 137$ patients), and 23 were VA/military hospitals ($n = 47$ patients), of which half had academic affiliations. Of the 268 cystectomies, 115 were performed by urologic oncologists and 153 were performed by general urologists; urologic oncologists were only responsible for 9 % of patients who received surgery at VA/military and community institutions combined [5].

26.5 Impact of Surgical Quality

Even more compelling evidence of the importance of surgical quality was provided by an analysis of INT-0080 in the United States involving multiple institutions and surgeons. Negative surgical margins and ten or more lymph nodes removed were associated with better overall survival independent of patient's age, pathologic stage, nodal status and whether chemotherapy was given. These surgical factors also predicted pelvic relapse, which is a death knell in most patients. Of the patients 15 % had local recurrence and all eventually died of disease. Local recurrence developed in 68 % of cases with positive surgical margins compared to 6 % with negative margins, while high vs. low volume urologists had a positive margin rate of 4 % vs. 14 % [6].

This cooperative group trial shows that the quality of RC and PLND directly impacts the chances of survival, and it is surgeon-dependent. Irrespective of the positive result of the Grossman study these flaws make it difficult to accept level I evidence for NACT.

26.6 Capsule or Prostate Sparing RC

Studies from the last two decades include the result from 13 centers worldwide. Many of them report a pattern of failure (local versus distant) that is highly unusual. Although a local recurrence rate of 7 of 252 patients is to be expected in this combined series the distant failure rate of 34 of 252 patients is at least twice as high as expected for the given series of superficial or organ-confined TCC. The observed distant failure rate of sexuality-preserving RC in this potentially lethal disease is more than 5 % higher as compared with standard RC. The precise underlying mechanism of this unexpected pattern of failure following sexuality-sparing cystectomy is not fully understood. Furthermore, surgeons considering procedures that preserve a portion of the prostatic urethra, the prostatic capsule, or the entire prostate should recognize a 6 % risk of significant prostatic cancer in any residual tissue, and the potential risk of urethral tumor involvement with TCC.

Daytime continence following radical versus sexuality-sparing cystectomy is identical. Data on night-time continence of sexuality-sparing cystectomy are inconclusive. The continuous intermittent catheterization rate following sexuality-sparing cystectomy, however, seems to be higher than after standard cystectomy.

The only advantage sexuality-preserving cystectomy has is, indeed, preservation of these functions in a much higher percentage than following standard or nerve-sparing cystectomy. This is at the cost of "radicality," however, and results in a 10–15 % higher oncologic failure rate [7].

Currently, the role of prostate sparing RC (PSRC) in treating bladder cancer remains controversial, and can be considered from both sides of a counterbalanced argument. One point of view underscores valid concerns regarding occult malignancy in the prostate at the time of surgery, and the potentially increased risks of local or systemic recurrence that may be associated with this procedure. To some extent, PSRC violates one of the basic oncologic principles of en bloc excision of the organ(s) at risk, and the literature does not currently support oncologic equivalence when compared with classic RC. The other point of view emphasizes the substantial improvements in functional outcomes described for PSRC which undoubtedly weighs heavily for many patients when deciding about appropriate treatment pathways. Through earlier acceptance of cystectomy, PSRC may indirectly provide a potential oncologic benefit, as well as facilitate minimally invasive approaches, further reducing the morbidity of this procedure.

Above all, the oncologic efficacy of this procedure should be considered controversial, and it is considered heresy by some. In addition, there are still many important limitations to this literature [8].

26.7 Improved Technique of RC with Erectile Function Preservation

We have described a new technique for nerve-sparing RC with preservation of vasa deferentia, seminal vesicles, and neurovascular bundles (NVB) (Fig. 26.1a–e). *No prostatic tissue is left behind, thus eliminating the risk of local recurrence from BC as well as de novo prostate cancer.*

The indication for this seminal vesicle sparing RC is limited to high-risk NMIBC, MIBC including

Fig. 26.1 (continued) Urology Supplements 9 (2010) 428–432. (**d**) The RC is begun as a standard nerve-sparing radical prostatectomy, with high release of the neurovascular bundles. Gentle traction is exerted on the balloon catheter to extrude the vesical neck. Denonvillier's fascia is opened with a short transverse incision over the ampullae of the vases and the base on the vesicles. After transaction of vesicles and ampullae, an easy cleavage plane is developed between the trigone and catheter balloon anteriorly and the vesicles posteriorly until the cul-de-sac has been reached. Adapted from Richard E. Hautmann, Oliver Hautmann, Björn G. Volkmer, Stefan Hautmann. Nerve-sparing Radical Cystectomy: A New Technique European. Urology Supplements 9 (2010) 428–432. (**e**) Posterior view of the NVBs, ampullae of the vases, seminal vesicles inferiorly and prostate, bladder, and ureters anteriorly. Transsection of the inferior pedicle of the bladder 2 cm anterior of the NVB

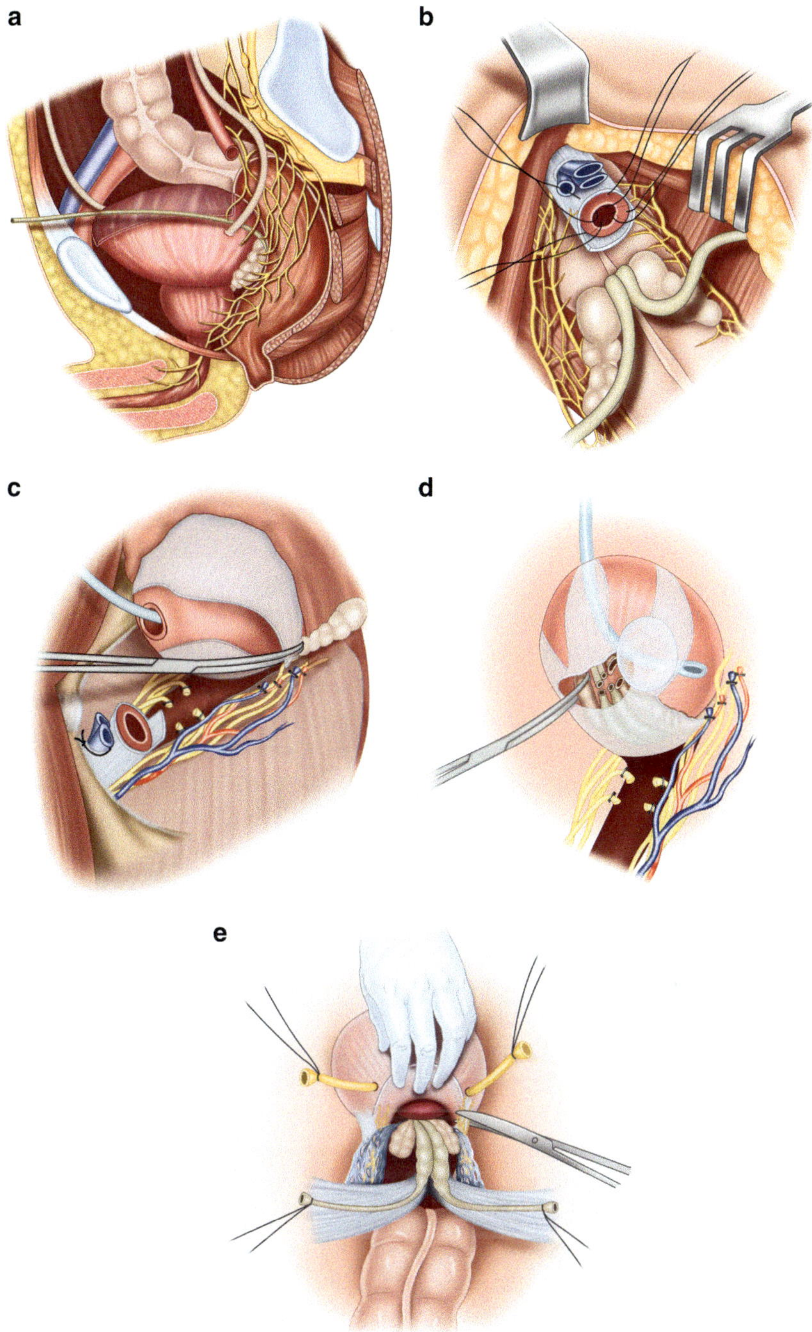

Fig. 26.1 (**a**) Fibers of the pelvic plexus surround the lateral aspect of the bladder neck, the proximal prostate, and the seminal vesicles in a cage-like fashion, whereas relatively few nerve fibers are found on the purely anterior surfaces of these organs. Branches designated as cavernous nerves and destined for the urinary sphincter are mainly located posteriorly in the pelvic plexus. Those nerves are located posterolateral to the seminal vesicles and course very close to their tips. A gentle dissection of the seminal vesicles or a seminal vesicle-sparing technique during RC may reduce the risk of injury to these nerves and, in consequence, may improve postoperative continence and potency rates. (**b**) Final situation after RC has been completed: Seminal vesicles protect > air bag < like the NVBs by moving the cleavage plain 2 cm anterior of the nerves. (**c**) Standard dissection laterally to the prostatic fascia to free the NVBs from the prostate and the lateral surface of the seminal vesicles (*dotted line*) carries a high risk to ruin the erectile function by injuring these nerves. Adapted from Richard E. Hautmann, Oliver Hautmann, Björn G. Volkmer, Stefan Hautmann. Nerve-sparing Radical Cystectomy: A New Technique European.

stage pT2 and all T3 stages away from the trigone. Using this technique preservation of erectile function can almost be guaranteed (see Fig. 26.1a–e) [9].

The sympathetic fibers and lymph tissue overlying the bifurcation of the aorta extending to the sacral promontory are also preserved. The limits of lymph node dissection include the level of the ureter as it crosses the common iliac artery proximally, the genitofemoral nerve laterally, and the lymph node of Cloquet and circumflex iliac vein distally. The external iliac artery and vein are skeletonized, and the obturator fossa, pelvic side wall, and hypogastric branches are cleared of lymph node tissue.

RC is begun with an intrafascial prostatectomy, which is done in a retrograde fashion. For optimal protection of the NVB and to avoid damage to the autonomic nerves running into the membranous urethra, a "high-release" approach with incision of the endopelvic and periprostatic fascia and bunching of Santorini plexus at the level of the prostate and not distal to it is of utmost importance. The dorsolateral NVB can be separated from the prostatic capsule. The prostatic apex is approached laterally directly along the prostatic capsule, and the membranous urethra is delivered sharply out of the donut-shaped prostatic apex to avoid nerve damage on the dorsolateral side of the urethra and to maintain maximum urethral length. Despite the intrafascial approach, Denonvillier's fascia very often remains on the posterior surface of the prostate specimen where it is fused with the prostatic capsule in the midline. At the base of the prostate, a 2–3-cm transverse incision of Denonvillier's fascia is carried out, and both the vases and the seminal vesicles are transacted. A cleavage plane is easily developed anterior to the ampullae/seminal vesicles and dorsal to the trigone. The balloon of the transurethral catheter serves a control, because it is easily palpated. In this fashion, most of the NVB are spared. The ascending cleavage plane easily reaches the cul-de-sac, with the inferior bladder pedicles still intact. The remainder of the RC can be done in an ascending or descending fashion. The latter seems to offer better control of the bundles. The vasa are identified and left on the pelvic peritoneum. The peritoneum is incised transversely 5 cm anterior to the cul-de-sac. Care is taken to enter the plane between posterior bladder wall ventrally and the vases and seminal vesicles dorsally. The ureters are traced down into the pelvis, where the umbilical and superior vesicle arteries are clipped and divided as they branch anteriorly off the hypogastric artery. The ureters are then divided distally near the entrance to the bladder. The vasa deferentia are traced to the area of the peritoneal cul-de-sac, and the peritoneum is divided. A plane of dissection is sharply developed between the anterior surface of the vasa and the posterior surface of the bladder. Identification of the seminal vesicles posteriorly marks the appropriate plane of dissection. The pelvic plexus can be preserved by sectioning the dorsomedial pedicle along its ventral aspect, anterolateral to the seminal vesicles and then terminating the dissection at the base of the prostate. Care should be taken to avoid even minimal trauma to the pelvic plexus through clamping pinching of the tissue located on the dorsolateral aspect of the seminal vesicles. Because there is no need to dissect posterior to these structures, the NVB remain untouched [9].

26.8 Complications to Consider

RC and subsequent urinary diversion has been assessed the most difficult surgical procedure in the field of urology. The surgical morbidity following RC is significant and when strict reporting guidelines are used, much higher than previously published. Accurate reporting of postoperative complications is essential for patient counseling, combined-modality treatment planning, clinical trial design, assessment of surgical success and for perioperative patient education. RC and urinary diversion are two steps of one operation, and almost 75 % of all complications stem from the diversion.

We have recently reported the 90-day morbidity of the ileal neobladder in a large contemporary, homogenous series of patients who underwent radical cystectomy at a tertiary academic referral centre using a standard approach

[10]. Between January 1986 and September 2008 we performed 1,540 radical cystectomies. Of these patients 66 % finally received a neobladder. All complications within 90 days of surgery were defined, categorized and classified by an established 5 grade and 11 domain modification of the original Clavien system. Of 1,013 patients 58 % experienced at least one complication within 90 days of surgery. Infectious complications were most common (24 %) followed by genitourinary (17 %), gastrointestinal (15 %) and wound-related complications (9 %). The 90-day mortality rate was 2.3 %. Of the patients 36 % had minor (grade 1–2) and 22 % had major (grade 3–5) complications. On univariate analysis the incidence and severity of the 90-day complications rate correlate highly significantly with age, tumor stage, American Society of Anesthesiologists score, and preoperative comorbidity [10].

We also analyzed the long-term complications of this series. Only the 923 patients with follow-up longer than 90 days (median 72 months, range 3–267) were included in the analysis. The complication rate was calculated using the Kaplan–Meier method [11].

The overall long-term complication rate was 40.8 % with three neobladder-related deaths. Hydronephrosis, incisional hernia, ileus or small bowel obstruction and feverish urinary tract infection were observed in 16.9, 6.4, 3.6, and 5.7 % of patients, respectively, 20 years postoperatively. Subneovesical obstruction in 3.1 % of cases was due to local tumor recurrence in 1.1 %, neovesicourethral anastomotic stricture in 1.2 %, and urethral stricture in 0.9 %. Chronic diarrhea was noted in nine patients, Vitamin B12 was substituted in two patients. Episodes of severe metabolic acidosis occurred in 11 patients and 307 of 923 required long-term bicarbonate substitution. Rare complications included cutaneous neobladder fistulas in two cases, and intestinal neobladder fistulas, iatrogenic neobladder perforation, spontaneous perforation and necrotizing pyocystis in one each.

Even in experienced hands the long-term complication rate of RC and neobladder formation are not negligible. Most complications are diversion-related, and the challenge of optimum care for these elderly patients with comorbidities is best mastered at high volume hospitals by high volume surgeons [11].

26.9 Postoperative Care

Critical components for good long-term results require not only surgical finesse but also patient compliance and meticulous postoperative care. Immediate postoperative management should include the following steps:

- Subcutaneous heparin prophylaxis into the arm instead of the thigh to prevent lymphoceles.
- Bladder substitute rinsed every 6 h with aspiration of mucus.
- Bowel stimulation with parasympathomimetics from day 2 or 3 and following.
- Withdrawal of ureterral stents at day 5–7 after resumed bowel activity.
- First removal of the suprapubic tube on day 8–10 (cystogram).
- Withdrawal of urethral catheter on day 10–12.

Following catheter withdrawal, patients are carefully instructed on how to void. Initially, they are taught to empty the neobladder in a sitting position every 2 h during the day by relaxing the pelvic floor and increasing the intra-abdominal pressure. The following points must be observed:

- Voiding without residual urine.
- Sterile urine.
- Alarm clock at night.
- Venous blood gas analysis every second day.
- Supplement of bicarbonate (2–6) and salt.

Additional instructions to patients include: Increase fluid intake; check body weight regularly; increase reservoir capacity by adhering to regular voiding intervals: at first, 2 h; thereafter, 3 h and later, 4 h with the goal capacity of 500 ml.

Meticulous long-term follow-up is essential regarding metabolism (vitamin B12, electrolytes, base excess), continence, volume of voided urine (400–500 ml), sterile urine, residual urine (if yes—check regular voiding intervals), and bladder neck obstruction (if yes—perform incision or resection) [12].

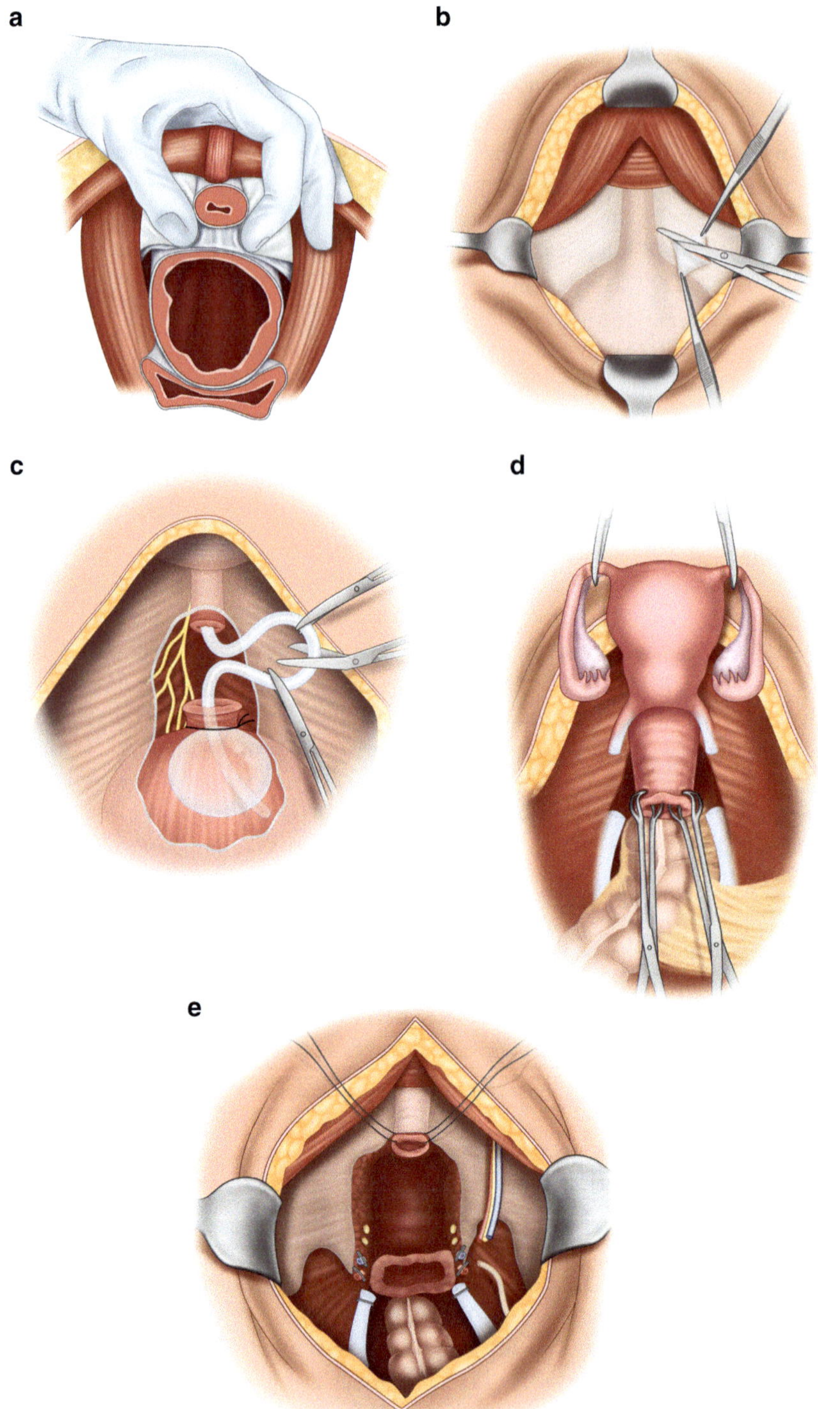

Fig. 26.2 (**a**) Packed vagina gives ideal exposure to urethra and pelvic support structures. A povidone-iodine pack is placed into the vagina and the urethra rides on top of the anterior vaginal wall. Without that trick, the urethra falls back into the pelvic cavity, and mobilization of the urethra results in bleeding and jeopardizes the urethral support. (**b**) Urethral support-sparing cystectomy in women. Incision of endopelvic fascia is parallel to posterior urethra and urethravesical junction. Preparation of the urethra requires special attention to surgical detail to avoid damage to the proximal urethra, anterior vaginal wall, and urethral support, which could jeopardize the continence mechanism and micturition. (**c**) Transsection of posterior urethra after ligation of bladder neck including Foley catheter.

26.10 Robotic Versus Open Surgical Approach

There is increasing interest in laparoscopic and robotic cystectomy, with either intra-corporeal or extra-corporeal formation of conduit or the orthotopic substitute. Whether reports with intermediate follow-up suggesting equivalent pathologic and oncologic outcome will be confirmed remains to be determined. But there are advantages in terms of blood loss, transfusion rate, postoperative pain, and return of bowel function. In most reported series, cases were highly selected. There are a number of reports of intra-corporeal surgery for diversion; most surgeons currently prefer an extra-corporeal technique because it is faster. However, the ureters must be kept long, and there is concern about an increased risk of ureteroileal stenosis. Technology will probably need to improve before intra-corporeal reconstruction becomes standard practice [13].

When stage distribution (organ-confined versus non-organ-confined) and survival rates of laparoscopic and open RC are cross-checked against surrogate markers (LN+, margin+, distant failure, local recurrence rate, etc.), it becomes evident that the laparoscopic RC and open cohorts reported in the literature are not identical. To explain the observed discrepancy, there must be a selection bias. Data on overall, disease-specific and recurrence-free survival on laparoscopic RC are still immature compared with the standard of care that must remain in open RC. To prove the non-inferiority of laparoscopic compared with open surgery regarding outcome, multicenter prospective trails are urgently needed, and are currently underway in the U.S. Until then, I consider laparoscopic RC as experimental surgery [14].

Supporting this opinion, a randomized trial comparing robotic and open cystectomy was presented as a late-breaking abstract in the plenary session of the 2013 AUA.

The investigators found no differences in complications, oncologic outcomes or LOS between the two procedures and, thus, closed the study early. The results of the trial call into question the usefulness of robotic cystectomy and highlight the importance of comparative effectiveness studies before the dissemination of new technologies [15].

26.11 Differences with a Female Patient

While indications, contraindications, complications, postoperative care are the same as in female patients, the operative technique of RC with sexuality preservation in females is obviously different. Figure 26.2a–e presents the most important tricks that are helpful to obtain good results [16].

26.12 Conclusion

Urothelial carcinoma of the bladder is a highly aggressive malignancy that causes significant morbidity and mortality. In T2 patients acceptable cure rates (80 %) may be obtained by immediate cystectomy thus sparing the patient the morbidity of neoadjuvant chemotherapy: A seminal vesical sparing cystectomy technique and

---

Fig. 26.2 (continued) To guarantee completeness of resection of the bladder neck the Foley is under traction and is filled with 50 cc. Upward traction of specimen facilitates dissecting the specimen off the anterior vaginal wall while saving the urethral support structures and the nerves. (**d**) Uterosacral ligaments on both sides are divided. Edges of transverse incision in posterior fornix of vagina are held under gentle traction with Allis clamps. Posterior bladder wall is dissected off anterior vaginal wall down to bladder neck. Autonomic nerve fibers (inferior hypogastric plexus), which run laterally to vessels, are separated from lateral wall of bladder and vagina. (**e**) Final result of a precise modified anterior exenteration with maximum preservation of the urethral support structures. The bottom of this amazingly small defect being the anterior vaginal wall. As compared with standard cystectomy, a maximum of urethral and vaginal support structures including the nerves have been saved

reconstruction using an ileal neobladder further helps to stimulate patient and physician decision toward early cystectomy.

References

1. Goossens-Laan CA, Visser O, Hulshof MC, Wouters MW, Bosch JL, Coebergh JW, Kil PJ. Survival after treatment for carcinoma invading bladder muscle: a Dutch population-based study on the impact of hospital volume. BJUI. 2011;110:226–32.
2. International Bladder Cancer Nomogram Consortium. Postoperative nomogram predicting risk of recurrence after radical cystectomy for bladder cancer. J Clin Oncol. 2006;24:3967–72.
3. Mitra AP, Skinner EC, Miranda G, Daneshmand S. A precystectomy decision model to predict pathological upstaging and oncological outcomes in clinical stage T2 bladder cancer. BJU Int. 2012;111:240–8.
4. Wosnitzer MS, Hruby GW, Murphy AM, Barlow LJ, Cordon-Cardo C, Mansukhani M, Petrylak DP, Benson MC, McKiernan JJ. A comparison of the outcomes of neoadjuvant and adjuvant chemotherapy for clinical T2-T4aNO-N2MO bladder cancer. Cancer. 2012;118:358–64.
5. Herr HW, Faulkner JR, Grossman HB, Natale RB, deVere White R, Sarosdy MF, Crawford ED. Surgical factors influence bladder cancer outcomes: a cooperative group report. J Clin Oncol. 2004;22:2781–9.
6. Herr HW, Dotan Z, Donat SM, Bajorin DF. Defining optimal therapy for muscle invasive bladder cancer. J Urol. 2007;177:437–43.
7. Hautmann RE, Stein JP. Neobladder with prostatic capsule and seminal-sparing cystectomy for bladder cancer: a step in the wrong direction. Urol Clin N Am. 2005;32:177–85.
8. Kiefer JC, Cherullo EE, Jones JS, Gong MC, Campbell SC. Prostate-sparing cystectomy: has Pandora's box been opened? Expert Rev Anticancer Ther. 2007;7(7):1003–14.
9. Hautmann RE, Hautmann O, Volkmer BG, Hautmann S. Nerve-sparing radical cystectomy: a new technique. Eur Urol Suppl. 2010;9:428–32.
10. Hautmann RE, de Petriconi RC, Volkmer BG. Lessons learned from 1,000 neobladders: the 90-day complication rate. J Urol. 2010;184:990–4.
11. Hautmann RE, de Petriconi RC, Volkmer BG. 25 Years of experience with 1,000 neobladders: long-term complications. J Urol. 2011;185:2207–12.
12. Hautmann RE, Botto H, Studer UE. How to obtain good results with orthotopic bladder substitution: the 10 commandments. Eur Urol Suppl. 2009;8:712–7.
13. Hautmann RE, Abol-Enein H, Davidsson T, Gudjonsson S, Hautmann SH, Holm HV, Lee CT, Liedberg F, Madersbacher S, Manoharan M, Mansson W, Mills RD, Penson DF, Skinner EC, Stein R, Studer UE, Thueroff JW, Turner WH, Volkmer BG, Abai X. ICUD-EAU international consultation on bladder cancer 2012: urinary diversion. Eur Urol. 2013;63:67–80.
14. Hautmann RE. The oncologic results of laparoscopic radical cystectomy are not (yet) equivalent to open cystectomy. Curr Opin Urol. 2009;19:522–6.
15. Laudone V. Late breaking news: interim analysis of a prospective randomized trial comparing robotic and open cystectomy at memorial sloan-kettering cancer center. J Urol. 2013: 116.
16. Hautmann RE. The Ileal Neobladder. Atlas Urol Clin North Am. 2001;9(2):85.

Norm D. Smith, Gary D. Steinberg, and Cheryl T. Lee

27.1 Introduction

Radical cystectomy with pelvic lymphadenectomy and urinary diversion is the standard of care for muscle-invasive urothelial bladder cancer [1, 2], yet an extremely complex operation associated with considerable postoperative morbidity, oftentimes directly related to the urinary diversion [3–5]. Robot-assisted radical cystectomy is a less invasive technique with radical cystectomy and pelvic lymphadenectomy performed

via a robot-assisted laparoscopic approach [6]. After completion of the radical cystectomy and pelvic lymphadenectomy, urinary diversion is then performed by extracorporeal, intracorporeal, or hybrid techniques. Reported advantages of robotic cystectomy from small, single-institution series are decreased estimated blood loss, lower blood transfusion rates, lessened pain and opioid requirements, earlier time to oral intake, shorter hospital stay, fewer wound complications, and faster perioperative and postoperative convalescence and recovery [7–9]. Nonetheless, robotic cystectomy and urinary diversion are still associated with significant complications. Johar et al. [10] described complications in 939 patients after robotic cystectomy from the International Robotic Cystectomy Consortium database, with complications analyzed and graded according to the Memorial Sloan-Kettering Cancer Center system. Forty-one and Forty-eight percent of patients experienced complications within 30 days and 90 days of surgery, respectively. Nearly 20 % of patients had a grade 3 or higher complication after robotic cystectomy and 90-day mortality was 4.2 %. Yuh and colleagues [11] reported on 196 patients who underwent robotic cystectomy, extended pelvic lymph node dissection, and urinary diversion (continent diversions performed in 68 % of cases). Complications within 90 days of surgery were defined and categorized by the modified

At the Forefront of Medicine®
http://www.uchospitals.edu
http://www.uchicagokidshospital.org
http://www.facebook.com/UChicagoMed

N.D. Smith, M.D. (✉)
The University of Chicago Medicine,
5841 S. Maryland Ave., MC 6038, Chicago,
IL 60637, USA
e-mail: nsmith1@surgery.bsd.uchicago.edu

G.D. Steinberg, M.D., F.A.C.S.
Department of Surgery, Section of Urology,
The University of Chicago Medicine,
5841 South Maryland Avenue, MC 6038,
Room J-653, Chicago, IL 60637, USA
e-mail: gsteinbe@surgery.bsd.uchicago.edu

C.T. Lee, M.D.
Department of Urology, University of Michigan,
1500 E. Medical Center Dr., 7303 CCGC, Ann Arbor,
MI 48109-5946, USA
e-mail: ctlee@umich.edu

B.R. Konety and S.S. Chang (eds.), *Management of Bladder Cancer:*
A Comprehensive Text With Clinical Scenarios, DOI 10.1007/978-1-4939-1881-2_27,
© Springer Science+Business Media New York 2015

Clavien system. Eighty percent of patients experienced a complication within 90 days after radical cystectomy and urinary diversion; 35 % experienced a major complication, with 90-day mortality of 4.1 %. Thus, postoperative complications and morbidity following robotic cystectomy are considerable but generally comparable to contemporary open radical cystectomy series, and in many cases directly related to the urinary diversion component of the surgery.

There are myriad urinary diversions with nuances regarding intestinal segment utilized and various technical considerations, but all diversions can be generally categorized as non-continent cutaneous diversions, continent cutaneous diversions, and continent orthotopic diversions [12]. The ideal urinary diversion does not exist but would theoretically match functions of the native bladder including low pressure filling and storage, high compliance, intact sensation, continence and voluntary emptying to completion [12–15]. Once a urinary diversion is selected, operative technique and surgeon experience can lead to improved outcomes for patients undergoing radical cystectomy and urinary diversion, regardless of open or robotic approaches. Optimal outcomes are influenced by preoperative, intraoperative, and postoperative factors but particular surgical attention to detail regarding the bowel anastomosis and ureterointestinal anastomoses are critical to urinary diversion. Overall, perioperative mortality for radical cystectomy and urinary diversion is higher for patients treated by low-volume surgeons in low-volume hospitals [16, 17]. The history of urinary diversion is complex like the procedure itself, from the first recorded radical cystectomy performed in 1887 in Cologne, Germany by Bardenheuer without urinary diversion [18], through the first publication of long-term outcomes of radical cystectomy and urinary diversion in 1962 by Whitmore [19] to the most recent complex intracorporeal robotic neobladder reconstructions. In this chapter, we will review contemporary urinary diversion via open and robotic approaches.

27.2 Preoperative Concerns [18]

27.2.1 Patient Optimization and Education

Potentially reversible and/or treatable medical conditions should certainly be addressed prior to radical cystectomy and urinary diversion. The American College of Cardiology/American Heart Association Guidelines on Perioperative Cardiovascular Evaluation and Care for Noncardiac Surgery recommend preoperative testing only for select patients, including those with significant atrial or ventricular arrhythmias, severe valvular disease, unstable coronary syndromes and/or decompensated heart failure [20]. Almost 20 % of patients undergoing radical cystectomy and urinary diversion present with poor nutritional status defined as preoperative albumin <3.5 g/dl, preoperative weight loss >5 % of body weight, or body mass index <18.5 kg/m^2. When using this definition by Greg and colleagues, nutritional deficiency was an independent predictor of both 90-day perioperative mortality and all-cause mortality [21]. Similarly, Lambert and associates reported significantly higher disease-specific and all-cause mortality, as well as increased complications in patients undergoing radical cystectomy with preoperative hypoalbuminemia compared to patients with normal serum albumin [22]. Early studies suggested use of preoperative gastrointestinal hyperalimentation in malnourished patients prior to radical cystectomy in efforts to reduce complications [23], but it is unclear whether this strategy has any effect on either postoperative morbidity or mortality. Furthermore, total parenteral hyperalimentation has not proven advantageous for malnourished cystectomy patients either pre- or perioperatively [18].

Structured patient education prior to radical cystectomy and urinary diversion is sound medical practice and has potential to decrease morbidity after surgery. Koch et al. implemented a collaborative care pathway for patients undergoing radical cystectomy and urinary diversion including preoperative instruction for patients and family regarding surgery, plan of care, and hospital orientation, with subsequent decrease in average hospital stay from 12.7 to 10.3 days and concomitant decrease in postoperative morbidity [24]. Preoperative counseling regarding early ambulation, incentive spirometry and enterostomal therapy has potential to limit morbidity in the early postoperative period, and further development of patient education materials describing the procedure, patient preparation prior to surgery, description of the expected hospital course, and detailed discharge instructions may also be valuable [25].

27.2.2 Bowel Preparation

Historically, mechanical bowel preparation prior to radical cystectomy and urinary diversion has been the standard of care with potential advantages of reducing wound complications, enteric anastomotic leaks, and intra-abdominal infections [18]. However, more recently, Large and colleagues reported use of GoLYTELY® mechanical bowel preparations in patients undergoing radical cystectomy with an ileal conduit urinary diversion did not alter rates of perioperative infectious, wound, and bowel complications [26]. Similarly, Hashad and associates randomized 40 consecutive patients undergoing radical cystectomy and ileal conduit urinary diversion to a standard 3-day mechanical bowel preparation versus overnight fasting prior to surgery and found no significant differences in complications between the two groups [27]. Thus, mechanical bowel preparation is likely unnecessary for small bowel segment urinary diversions. However, full mechanical bowel preparation should be strongly considered for colonic urinary diversions to minimize stool contamination of the wound and operative field.

27.2.3 Parenteral Antibiotics

Postoperative infectious complications following radical cystectomy and urinary diversion occur in up to 25 % of patients [4], so perioperative administration of prophylactic antimicrobials is a standard of care in efforts to prevent surgical site infections, despite a paucity of evidence regarding optimal agents and duration of use [28, 29]. The American Urological Association (AUA) developed a Best Practice Policy Statement on Urologic Surgery Antimicrobial Prophylaxis with most recent review and update in 2012, recommending antimicrobial prophylaxis for all patients undergoing open, laparoscopic or robotic surgery involving entry into the urinary or gastrointestinal tracts, preferably with a second- or third-generation cephalosporin [30]. Alternatively, an aminoglycoside plus metronidazole or clindamycin can be substituted for patients with severe beta-lactam allergies. The duration of antimicrobial prophylaxis should be ≤24 h as prolonged administration can potentially increase risks of antimicrobial resistance and *Clostridium difficile* colitis [18].

27.2.4 Venous Thromboembolism (VTE) Prophylaxis

Deep venous thrombosis (DVT) is common after radical cystectomy with urinary diversions with possible devastating consequence of pulmonary thromboembolism (PE), which is a major cause of mortality in this patient population [31]. Clément and others prospectively evaluated incidence and risk factors for VTE in 583 consecutive patients undergoing urologic cancer surgery managed with early ambulation, graduated compression stockings or intermittent pneumatic compression, and either low-molecular-weight heparin or low-dose unfractionated heparin daily for 15 days as VTE prophylaxis [32]. All patients underwent bilateral lower extremity venous Doppler ultrasound on postoperative day 7 with DVT and PE in 7.4 % and 2.2 % of patients, respectively. Radical cystectomy and urinary diversion was independently associated with VTE on multivariable analysis (OR 3.47, $p = 0.002$). Aside from potential mortality from PE, long-term morbidity from VTE can significantly increase health care costs [33, 34].

In 2009, the AUA published a Best Practice Statement for prevention of DVT in patients undergoing urologic surgery which was reviewed and confirmed for validity in 2011, recommending intermittent pneumatic compression devices for laparoscopic or robotic surgery with either low-molecular-weight heparin or low-dose unfractionated heparin reserved only for high-risk groups. Both intermittent pneumatic compression devices and pharmacologic prophylaxis should be strongly considered in patients undergoing open urologic surgery [35]. As patients embarking on radical cystectomy and urinary diversion are by definition high-risk, combination VTE prophylaxis (early ambulation, intermittent pneumatic compression, and pharmacologic prophylaxis) should be employed as routine. Continued anticoagulation with daily low-molecular-weight heparin or aspirin for up to 3 months after surgery is worth consideration based on risk/benefit and cost analyses [18].

27.2.5 Urinary Diversion Considerations

27.2.5.1 Selection of Bowel Segment [12]

Although any segment of bowel can be potentially utilized for urinary diversion, several factors including renal function, previous abdominal surgery and/or bowel resection, history of pelvic radiation therapy and type of diversion affect the intestinal segment ultimately employed. Each segment of bowel has specific and potentially significant electrolyte abnormalities, as well as acid/base disturbances which impact the particular bowel type used for any given patient.

27.2.5.1.1 Stomach

Stomach has both advantages and disadvantages compared to other bowel segments for urinary diversion, including the lowest permeability to urinary solutes and decreased risk of bacteriuria due to acidification of the urine [36]. However, the stomach acidifies the urine due to proton and chloride secretion with resultant hypochloremic metabolic alkalosis and increased risk of the hematuria-dysuria syndrome due to excess acid production. Stomach should thus be avoided in patients with renal insufficiency due to impairment of bicarbonate excretion and difficulties correcting hypochloremic metabolic alkalosis [12].

27.2.5.1.2 Jejunum

Jejunum for urinary diversion is very uncommon due to significant side effects including severe electrolyte imbalances from increased sodium and chloride excretion coupled with potassium and hydrogen ion reabsorption. Sodium and chloride loss is also associated with water and volume loss, often with severe dehydration as a consequence. Use of jejunum thus leads to hyponatremic, hypochloremic, hyperkalemic metabolic acidosis and is generally a poor urinary diversion choice for patients after radical cystectomy [12].

27.2.5.1.2 Ileum and Colon

The ileum and colon are most often utilized for urinary diversion as both segments have good mesenteric blood supply with straightforward mobilization of the segment and minimal acid, base, and electrolyte disturbances. Use of either ileum or colon is associated with ammonium chloride reabsorption and resultant hyperchloremic metabolic acidosis [37]. The metabolic acidosis can be problematic for patients with renal insufficiency (serum creatinine >2.0 mg/dl) and may cause loss of appetite, lethargy and weight loss. Conservative treatments include maintaining adequate hydration and minimizing urinary stasis, but some patients require alkalinizing medications or chloride transport blockers [12]. Potential complications specific to use of ileum for urinary diversion include fat and vitamin B12 malabsorption, as well as diarrhea. Patients with urinary diversions utilizing colon segments do not usually experience nutritional problems unless the ileocecal valve is excluded from bowel continuity (such as Indiana Pouch), with subsequent increased risk of diarrhea, bacterial colonization of the ileum, and associated fluid and bicarbonate losses [12].

27.3 Radical Cystectomy, PLND

Radical cystectomy with bilateral pelvic lymph node dissection via open and robotic techniques is well-described in this textbook and elsewhere. Surgical quality and technique matter in muscle-invasive bladder cancer and benchmarks of radical cystectomy and pelvic lymph node dissection regardless of approach include soft tissue margin status, extent of lymphadenectomy and experience of the surgeon [38]. Positive surgical margins and extent of lymphadenectomy both have significant impact on bladder cancer oncologic outcomes and higher volume surgeons have both lower operative mortality and positive margin rate compared to lower volume surgeons [38]. These surgical benchmarks for radical cystectomy are critical regardless of open or robotic techniques.

27.4 Types of Urinary Diversion

Urinary diversions are classified into three major categories: non-continent cutaneous diversions, continent cutaneous diversions, and continent orthotopic diversions.

27.4.1 Non-continent Cutaneous Diversions

Non-continent cutaneous urinary diversions [12] utilize a short segment of either ileum or colon (the conduit) in isoperistaltic orientation, with the ureters anastomosed to the proximal end of the conduit and the distal end serving as a cutaneous stoma for drainage of urine from the intestinal segment to an external collection device attached to the skin by adhesive to prevent leakage of urine. Non-continent cutaneous urinary diversions are the most common with advantages of shorter operative times and ease of construction compared to other urinary diversions, as well as decreased risk of postoperative complications. Non-continent cutaneous diversions are preferred in patients with impaired renal function, inability to care for a continent reservoir, locally advanced disease, or significant comorbidities to shorten operative time and simplify postoperative recovery. Pre- and postoperative enterostomal therapy helps a patient select the optimal stoma site, improve understanding of their urinary diversion and more readily adapt to new body image. Selection of the stoma site is critical as improper positioning can promote urinary leakage, skin problems, and decreased quality of life.

Complications associated with non-continent cutaneous diversions include febrile urinary tract infection and pyelonephritis, parastomal hernia, stomal stenosis or retraction, and long-term deterioration of the upper tracts. Factors potentially contributing to upper tract deterioration include chronic bacteruria and reflux nephropathy, significant metabolic acidosis, stomal stenosis, ureterointestinal strictures or even preexisting renal dysfunction from obstruction due to locally advanced disease [12]. Although significant care goes toward maintenance of the urinary drainage device, this appliance can be changed once every few to several days, greatly reducing the overall burden of care to the patient and family compared to other forms of urinary diversion.

27.4.2 Ileal Conduit (Fig. 27.1)

The ileal conduit has been the most common urinary diversion since introduction by Bricker in 1950 [39]. An ileal conduit is fashioned either open or robotically using 15–20 cm of ileum at least 15 cm from the ileocecal valve to prevent vitamin B12 and bile salt malabsorption. The segment for the ileal conduit is taken out of continuity from the bowel and the two ends of ileum are anastomosed back together to re-establish small bowel continuity, usually in stapled fashion. The conduit is opened on its distal or stomal side and irrigated free of succus material. The proximal or "butt" end of the ileal conduit is typically sutured closed (to avoid stone formation on staple line) and the ureters anastomosed in an end to side fashion to that end of the conduit segment using a refluxing technique, usually over a feeding tube or single-J ureteral stent. The open distal or stomal end of the ileal conduit is brought to the skin level through the rectus fascia of the anterior abdominal wall and anastomosed, usually as an end or "rosebud" stoma [40, 41]. The rosebud technique can be difficult in the markedly obese patient due to a combination of a thick abdominal wall and tethering of the bowel mesentery. As an alternative in this situation, a loop or modified Turnbull stoma may be technically easier but is associated with a higher rate of parastomal hernia.

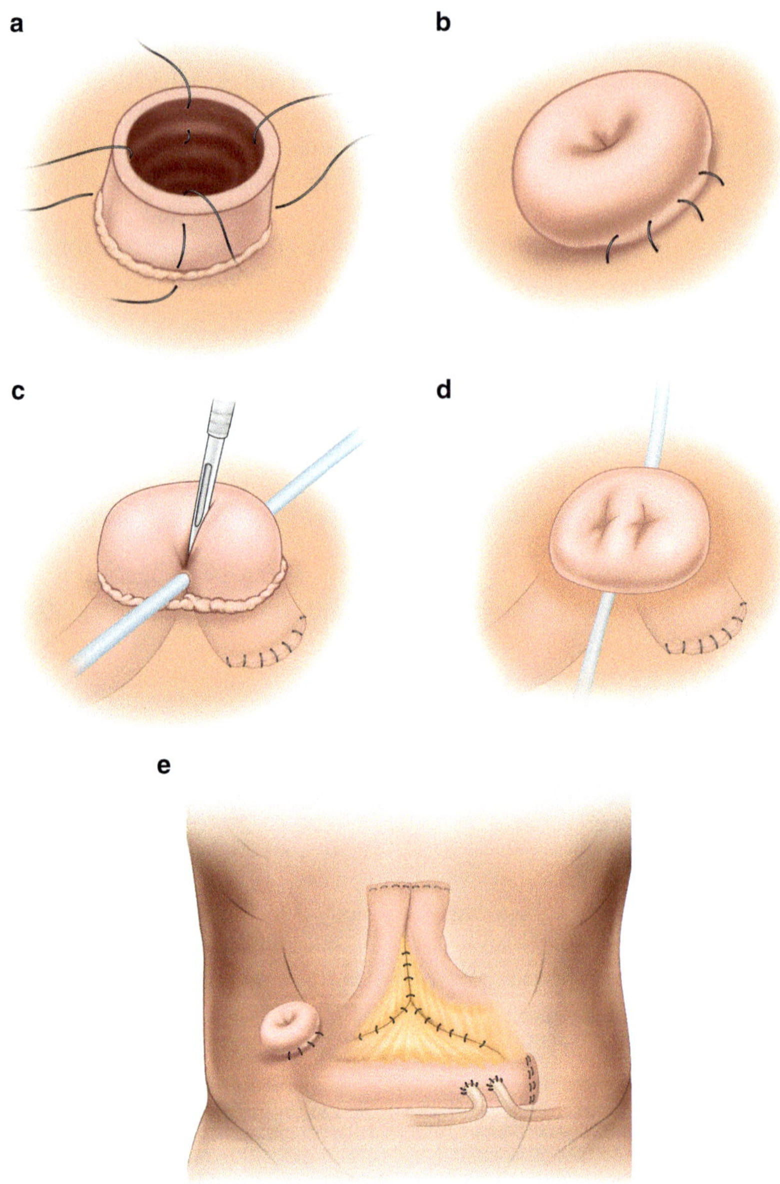

Fig. 27.1 Ileal conduit—a 15–20 cm segment of ileum is isolated and oriented in isoperistaltic fashion. Bowel continuity is re-established utilizing a staples anastomosis. The stoma is brought through the anterior abdominal wall with eversion via a "rosebud" (**a, b**) or "Turnbull" (**c, d**) stoma. Adapted from Hemal AK, Abol-Enein H, Tewari A et al. Robotic radical cystectomy and urinary diversion in the management of bladder cancer. Urol Clin North Am 2004; 31(4): 719

27.4.3 Colon Conduit

A colon conduit is a reasonable alternative for patients when the ileum is not a safe or viable option for urinary diversion. For instance, patients who have had extensive pelvic radiation may have radiation damage to small bowel, precluding ileum as the ideal choice for urinary diversion due to increased risk of postoperative complications, including bowel anastomotic leak or stricture. In this relatively rare population, the transverse colon is generally a radiation-spared segment of bowel and provides an excellent alternative for urinary diversion. Electrolyte abnormalities are similar between ileal and colon conduits, but non-refluxing ureterointestinal anastomoses (using taenia) are easier in colonic segments [12]. In summary for non-continent cutaneous urinary diversions, ileal and colon conduits are comparable segments and provide both a safe and reliable method of urinary diversion for patients after radical cystectomy for bladder cancer [42]. Despite safety and efficacy of both ileal and colon conduits, the need for an external collection appliance remains an inconvenience and may significantly alter body image, particularly in younger patients.

27.4.4 Continent Cutaneous Urinary Diversions

The second broad category of urinary diversion is the continent cutaneous urinary diversion consisting of a larger internal reservoir made from various bowel segments with a continent stoma at the level of the skin. The basic concepts of a continent cutaneous diversion include a detubularized bowel segment to destroy peristaltic integrity and maximize volume per surface area of intestine [40], as well as a leak proof stoma that requires intermittent catheterization (usually every 4–6 h) to effectively drain urine from the reservoir. A continent catheterizable diversion was first described by Gilchrist in the 1950s [43], but increased interest in continent diversion in the early 1980s led to various techniques of fashioning bowel reservoirs for urinary storage. There are various techniques for creation of the continent catheterizable stoma, but all are generally based on three main categories of stoma, using either the small caliber appendix or a tapered length of bowel (Mitrofanoff or Monti technique), the terminal ileum to exploit the non-refluxing ileocecal valve, or lastly a nipple or flap valve (Kock or Mainz pouch) [44]. The catheterizable stoma is brought out through either the anterior abdominal wall or umbilicus, depending

on both patient factors (obesity) and/or surgeon preference. Despite the advent and increased utilization of continent orthotopic urinary diversion, continent cutaneous diversions are an excellent alternative for patients who do not want a non-continent cutaneous diversion but have absolute or relative contraindications for use of the native urethra such as previous surgery, radiation to the pelvis, or cancer at the bladder neck and/or prostatic urethra [12]. Although many forms of continent cutaneous urinary diversion exist, the Indiana Pouch is technically the easiest to perform and by far the most popular.

27.4.5 Indiana Pouch (Fig. 27.2)

The Indiana Pouch was first described by Rowland in 1985 [45], but has been significantly modified over time. The most recent iteration includes a plicated terminal ileum to the level of the ileocecal valve which serves as the continent catheterizable stoma and a detubularized right colon fashioned into a low-pressure reservoir [46]. Clinical outcomes coupled with relative technical ease have made the Indiana Pouch the mainstay for continent cutaneous urinary diversion. Bihrle reported 98 % continence with overall low re-operative and complication rates in long-term follow-up of 150 patients with Indiana Pouch urinary diversions [47]. Blute and colleagues described a 15 % re-operative rate, as well as a late complication rate of 17 %, including stomal stenosis and hernia, pouch calculi, incontinence, small bowel obstruction, and renal insufficiency in a series of 194 women managed with Indiana Pouch urinary diversions [48].

27.4.6 Koch Pouch

The Koch pouch was first described in 1982 and employed both the ileocecal valve in creating a continent catheterizable stoma, as well as an intussuscepted nipple valve for urine continence and an anti-reflux mechanism. The Koch pouch has historical significance as it increased interest in continent urinary diversions, but has diminished

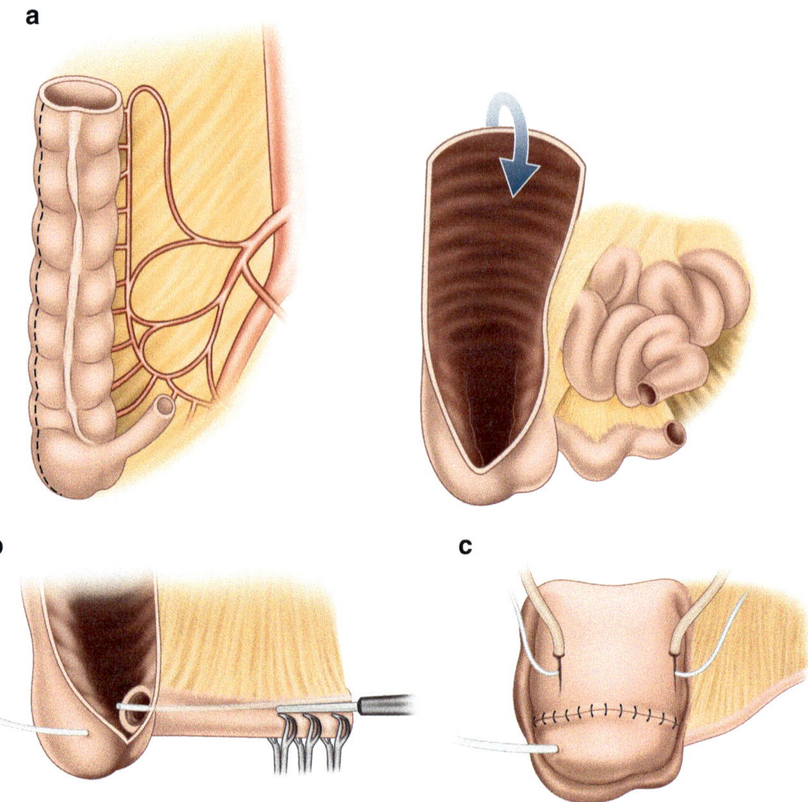

Fig. 27.2 Indiana pouch—(**a**) The right colon and roughly 10 cm of terminal ileum are isolated and then the right colon segment is detubularized along the antimesenteric border and folded upon itself in "clamshell" fashion. (**b**) The continent catheterizable limb is created by tapering the efferent limb using a stapling device. (**c**) The ureters are implanted into the Indiana pouch in either refluxing or non-refluxing fashion. Adapted from Hemal AK, Abol-Enein H, Tewari A et al. Robotic radical cystectomy and urinary diversion in the management of bladder cancer. Urol Clin North Am 2004; 31(4): 719

significantly in utilization due to high complication and re-operation rates coupled with technical challenges of creating the pouch [44].

27.4.7 Orthotopic Continent Diversions

The catheterizable stoma of a continent cutaneous urinary diversion was a significant advance over the external urinary drainage appliance, yet patients still have to perform frequent clean intermittent catheterization to empty the urinary reservoir. Like continent cutaneous urinary diversions, continent orthotopic diversions have a larger, internal reservoir but the continence mechanism is derived from the orthotopic location of the diversion with utilization of the native urethral sphincter. The orthotopic neobladder most closely resembles the native bladder, maintaining relatively normal voiding also with improved sexuality, body image and global sense of well-being [49]. Since the 1980s, several reconstructive techniques and procedures have been reported to create various orthotopic continent diversions (the most common are discussed below), yet there is no consensus regarding the best orthotopic diversion.

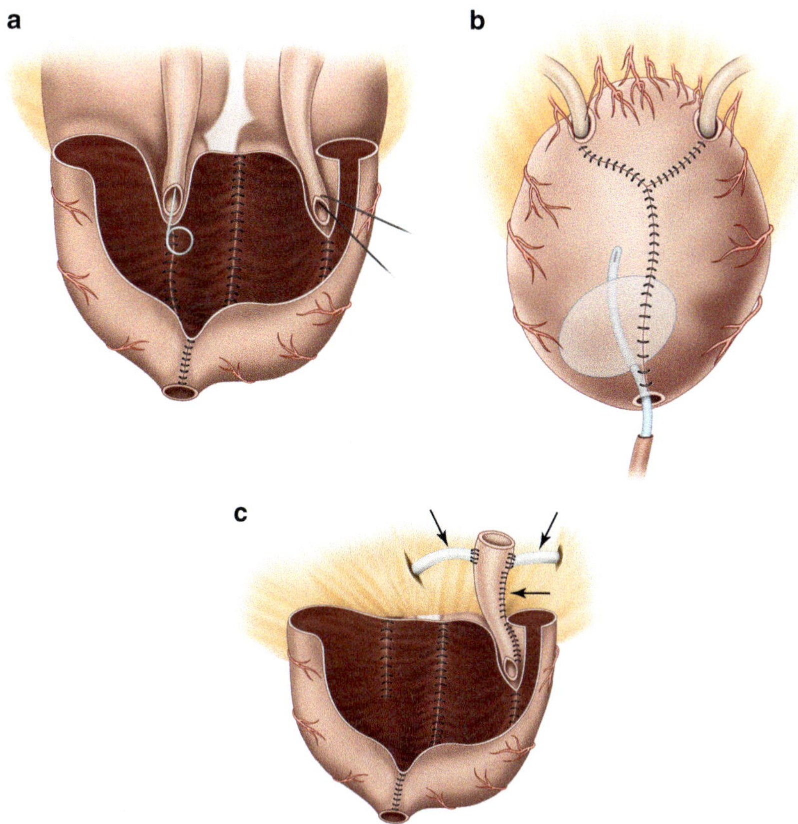

Fig. 27.3 Hautmann neobladder and chimney modification—(**a**) a 40 cm segment of distal ileum is folded into a "W" configuration and the ureters are embedded in serosa-lined troughs. Mucosa to mucosa ureterointestinal anastomoses are performed over ureteral stents. (**b**) Closed neobladder after the ureterointestinal anastomoses with urethral catheter inferiorly. (**c**) Chimney modification with 6–8 cm long ileal segment isolated to serve as the antireflux "chimney" in addition to the "W" segment of ileum. The ureters (*arrowheads*) are anastomosed to the chimney segment (*arrow*). Adapted from Hemal AK, Abol-Enein H, Tewari A et al. Robotic radical cystectomy and urinary diversion in the management of bladder cancer. Urol Clin North Am 2004; 31(4): 719

27.4.8 Hautmann Neobladder and Chimney Modification (Fig. 27.3)

Hautmann (University of Ulm, Germany) first described this neobladder [50], utilizing 60–80 cm of detubularized ileum oriented in a "W" shape and then reconstructed into a spherical pouch with the ureters reimplanted directly into the pouch or into an isoperistaltic chimney of tubularized ileum [51, 52]. The chimney modification to the Hautmann neobladder simplifies the ureterointestinal anastomoses with laudable goals of decreasing ureterointestinal strictures and preventing neobladder-ureteral reflux. Extending the chimney toward the kidneys favors a tension-free ureteral anastomosis with minimal ureteral ischemia, less mobilization, and more proximal resection of the ureters. The chimney also prevents competition of the ureters with the bowel mesentery for space near the posterior wall of the neobladder, decreases the risk of ureteral angulation and obstruction during periods of distention of the neobladder, allows for easier repair and revision of ureteral strictures, and assists with prevention of neobladder-ureteral reflux given the isoperistaltic nature of the chimney segment [12]. Following reconstruction of the neobladder into a low pressure, high compliance reservoir and the ureterointestinal anastomoses, the neobladder is then anastomosed to the urethra with the native urethral sphincter providing the continence mechanism. Voiding with an orthotopic neobladder occurs via relaxation of the external urinary sphincter, with coordinated Valsalva and/or Crede maneuvers. Hautmann reported data from the first 290 patients with early and late neobladder-related complications in 15.4 % and 23.4 % of patients, respectively. Early and late re-operation rates were 0.3 % and 4.4 %, respectively. Over 95 % of patients were continent with roughly 4 % requiring clean intermittent catheterization to empty the neobladder effectively [50]. Generally, the need for clean intermittent catheterization increases with longer follow-up.

27.4.9 Studer Neobladder (Fig. 27.4)

Studer (University of Bern, Switzerland) first reported this neobladder, utilizing a 60 cm segment of ileum with the distal 40 cm detubularized and oriented into a "U" shape and then reconstructed into a spherical pouch with the ureters reimplanted into the proximal 20 cm of the ileal segment which remains as a tubularized, isoperistaltic chimney [53]. Like the Hautmann neobladder chimney modification, the Studer neobladder chimney promotes a tension-free ureteral anastomosis with minimal ureteral ischemia, less mobilization, more proximal resection of the ureters,

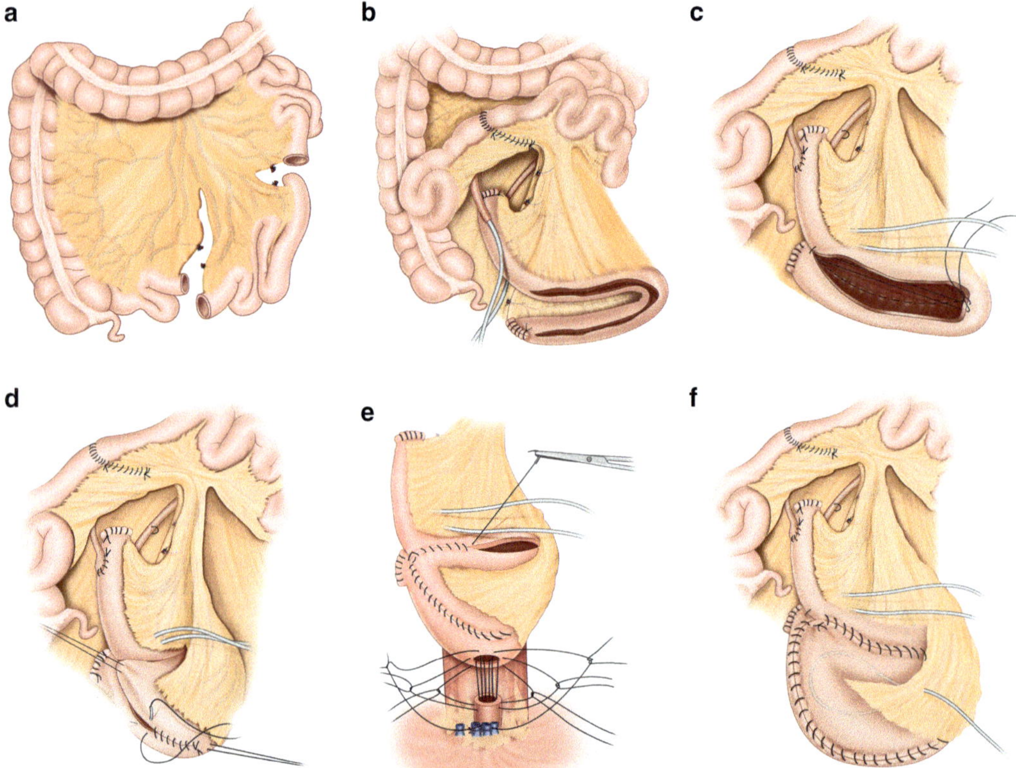

Fig. 27.4 Studer orthotopic neobladder—(**a**) An ileal segment roughly 60 cm in length is isolated approximately 20 cm proximal to the ileocecal valve and bowel continuity re-established via stapled anastomosis. (**b**) The distal 40–45 cm of the isolated ileal segment is opened along its antimesenteric border and folded into a "U" configuration, leaving 15 cm of the proximal ileal segment as the anti-reflux "chimney." (**c**) The ureters are implanted into the chimney and the backwall of the "U" configuration is closed with a 2-0 polyglycolic acid or Vicryl running suture. (**d**) The bottom of the "U" is folded over and closed in "clamshell" fashion. (**e**) The most dependent portion of the neobladder is selected for the neobladder-urethral anastomosis, performed with five or six interrupted 2-0 absorbable sutures. (**f**) In addition to a Foley catheter, a cystostomy or "suprapubic" tube is placed into the neobladder anteriorly prior to final closure of the reservoir to enhance postoperative irrigation of mucus in the neobladder. Adapted from Hemal AK, Abol-Enein H, Tewari A et al. Robotic radical cystectomy and urinary diversion in the management of bladder cancer. Urol Clin North Am 2004; 31(4): 719

allows for easier repair and revision of ureteral strictures if necessary, and assists with prevention of neobladder-ureteral reflux given the isoperistaltic nature of the long chimney segment [12]. Studer and colleagues described daytime continence rates of over 90 % at 1 year and nighttime continence of approximately 80 % after 2 years, with complication rates comparable to other urinary diversions including roughly 15 % of patients having major complications [53].

27.4.10 Sigmoid Pouch (Reddy)

Reddy (University of Minnesota, United States) first reported the sigmoid pouch [54], using a 30 cm detubularized sigmoid segment oriented into a "U" shape and then reconstructed into a spherical pouch with the ureters reimplanted directly into the pouch utilizing the tenaie of the sigmoid for non-refluxing anastomoses. A sigmoid pouch allows for a simpler urethral anastomosis because of inherent anatomic proximity of the pouch to the urethra but tends to have a higher rate of incontinence and uninhibited contractions compared to ileal neobladders. Contraindications to use of the sigmoid colon for a urinary reservoir include diverticulosis, colon polyps, inflammatory large bowel disease, and colon cancer. As such, the colon must be thoroughly evaluated by barium enema and/or colonoscopy prior to use for urinary diversion [52].

27.5 Selection of Diversion Type

Specific selection of urinary diversion type is a complicated process impacted by several factors such as renal function, bladder cancer stage and prognosis, previous surgical and radiation therapy, goals of surgery, overall patient physical and mental status, patient and family preferences, as well as surgeon training and experience. Patients adapt well to all forms of urinary diversion with proper selection and planning [55]. Bladder cancer stage and goals of surgery are important factors in selection of the specific urinary diversion. The simplest surgical procedure is logically the best option when palliation is the primary goal of surgery [56], but any diversion is reasonable when cure is the goal and cancer outcome is not compromised by selection of diversion type [13]. In women, urethral and/or anterior vaginal wall involvement with cancer is a contraindication to orthotopic neobladder reconstruction. Further, Stein and colleagues found bladder neck involvement with cancer is a significant risk factor for concomitant urethral and anterior vaginal wall involvement in a large single-institution histopathologic review [57]. Frozen-section analysis of the distal surgical margin is reasonable to assess urethral involvement with cancer at the time of radical cystectomy and urinary diversion and subsequent risk of urethral recurrence [58]. In men, a positive urethral margin at the time of cystectomy, as well as prostatic stromal involvement with cancer are contraindications for orthotopic neobladder due to the increased risk of urethral disease and recurrence [59].

Most patients appreciate the concept of continent orthotopic urinary diversion, but there are several absolute and relative contraindications. Absolute contraindications include malignant involvement of the urethra, impaired renal and/or hepatic function, inability to perform self-catheterization (quadriplegia or severe multiple sclerosis), and the inability to understand or comply with patient responsibilities or potential complications of a continent orthotopic urinary diversion. Relative contraindications include advanced age, previous pelvic radiation, need for postoperative chemotherapy, inflammatory bowel disease, impaired functional status, body habitus, and a noncancerous but abnormal urethra [12]. Patients must have the physical and mental ability to perform self-catheterization with continent urinary diversions, which seems obvious for patients with catheterizable stomas, but patients with orthotopic neobladders have increased risk of requiring long-term intermittent catheterization (especially women) and must be agreeable to this preoperatively [60]. Absorption of urinary solutes and free water loss occur in any urinary diversion with a bowel segment reservoir, and thus renal reserve and urine concentrating ability must be able to compensate. As such, the minimum creatinine clearance for continent diversion is considered 40–50 ml/min and patients with a serum creatinine greater than 2.0 mg/dl should be further evaluated with a more detailed assessment of renal function prior to continent urinary diversion [44]. Patients with renal impairment may still be candidates for continent diversion with retained ability to produce a urinary pH<5.8 following an ammonium chloride load, urinary concentrating ability to >600 mOsm/kg in response to water restriction, the presence of minimal proteinuria, and a glomerular filtration rate >35 ml/min [12].

Advanced patient age (>70 years old) is no longer considered in and of itself a relative contraindication to continent cutaneous or orthotopic urinary diversions, and consideration must be given to potential differences between physiologic and chronologic age when selecting urinary diversion in the elderly. Data suggest age is not a significant predictor of continence after orthotopic neobladder [61] but inability to void to completion and nighttime incontinence may be increased in patients older than 70 years of age. Continent orthotopic urinary diversions were initially only performed in male patients as it was presumed women were at increased risk of urinary incontinence and local tumor recurrence, but interestingly, urinary retention is a greater risk in women and cancer involvement of the urethra is rare in the absence of bladder neck involvement. The etiology of hypercontinence in women with orthotopic neobladders is not well-understood but may be due to angulation of the neobladder-urethral junction from increased pelvic floor descent with neobladder filling [12]. Regardless, up to 20–40 % of women require clean intermittent catheterization with orthotopic neobladders [62]. Overall, female continent orthotopic urinary diversion provides reasonable long-term functional results given appropriate selection criteria. Finally, regarding selection of urinary diversion type, the selection criteria for continent cutaneous and continent orthotopic diversions are essentially the same, unless urethral abnormalities including involvement with cancer are an issue. Under these circumstances, a continent cutaneous urinary diversion is more appropriate [12].

27.5.1 Comparison of Urinary Diversions

Despite significant efforts to create and modify urinary diversions to resemble the native bladder, there is a paucity of data to support benefits of any specific urinary diversion over others. Most studies suggest morbidity and mortality rates of non-continent and continent urinary diversions are similar [55, 63–65], with urinary diversion-related complications in the majority of patients after radical cystectomy [66]. As such, assessment of quality of life after urinary diversion is increasingly important.

27.5.2 Continence

Perhaps the most important factor of urinary diversion to patients is the prevention of urinary leakage. Non-continent cutaneous diversions can leak usually due to improperly positioned stomas or poorly fitting external urinary collection appliances. These risks can be minimized with pre- and postoperative enterostomal therapy, as well as adherence to sound surgical techniques during creation of the stoma. Continent urinary diversions are also associated with episodes of urinary leakage. The Indiana Pouch has a low risk of incontinence from the stoma, but is associated with occasional catheterization difficulties and a 15–20 % re-operation rate for all complications [12]. The efferent or catheterizable limb of the Indiana pouch should be as short in length as technically feasible and a straight shot from the skin to the pouch in efforts to avoid kinking and redundancy of the limb and minimize risk of problems with catheterization. The orthotopic neobladder has low rates of urinary leakage with daytime continence rates of over 90 %, but nocturnal incontinence is more problematic and occurs in up to 25 % of patients. The etiology of nighttime incontinence is likely multifactorial and potentially includes surgical injury to the external urinary sphincter, pelvic floor relaxation during sleep, uninhibited contractions of the neobladder, medications taken at night, decreased urethral closing pressure and/or loss of spinal reflexes controlling sphincteric contraction during sleep, increased urine output at night associated with aging, and increased urine output due to reabsorption of hypertonic acidic urine [12]. The majority of patients need to void 2–3 times per night to maintain nocturnal continence. Aside from risk of incontinence with orthotopic neobladders, approximately 4–10 % of males and up to 40 % of female patients develop significant urinary retention and require clean intermittent catheterization [50]. Significant mucus production from the bowel segment used to create the urinary diversion can occasionally cause urethral obstruction or impede conduit or pouch emptying. Mucus production decreases over time but still the majority of neobladder patients experiences some degree of mucus obstruction and occasionally need surgical procedures for mucus-related complications [67]. Mucus-related complications are rare in non-continent cutaneous urinary diversions.

27.5.3 Quality of Life (QOL)

It is important the surgeon personalize care for the patient undergoing radical cystectomy and urinary diversion as the procedure adversely affects many aspects of QOL. Myriad factors go toward measuring a patient's post-treatment satisfaction after radical cystectomy and urinary diversion with no general consensus on optimal methodology to measure QOL. Currently, no validated questionnaire specifically measures QOL in patients with urinary diversion but several generic validated questionnaires measure QOL after radical cystectomy and urinary diversion, including the general health SF-36 Quality of Life Survey and Sickness Impact Profile (SIP) surveys, as well as cancer-specific QLQ-C30 and Functional Assessment of Cancer Therapy general score (FACT-G) surveys [68–71]. Mansson and Mansson introduced a bladder cancer-specific questionnaire, but it remains unclear whether this will yield different results compared to previous studies with more generic questionnaires [72]. Since urinary leakage is such a significant complaint after cystectomy and urinary

diversion, continent diversions would potentially have less impact on a patient's lifestyle and health-related satisfaction [73]. The literature is mixed on QOL after radical cystectomy and non-continent versus continent diversions. Several studies comparing ileal conduit with orthotopic neobladder show no significant differences in health-related QOL [74, 75]. Other studies have shown significant benefit in QOL with an orthotopic neobladder compared to an ileal conduit. Dutta and colleagues reported only a trend toward improved QOL scores for patients with orthotopic neobladders, but emotional and functional well-being were improved with a neobladder compared to an ileal conduit [76]. Hobisch and associates described significantly higher QOL for patients with orthotopic neobladder compared to ileal conduit using the QLQ-C30 questionnaire and further reported 97 % of neobladder patients would recommend the same urinary diversion to other patients, compared to only 36 % of patients with an ileal conduit urinary diversion [63].

27.5.4 Sexual Function

Inherent to cystoprostatectomy in men is the risk of erectile dysfunction caused by damage to autonomic nerves from the sacral parasympathetic plexus supplying the corpora cavernosa of the penis. Although the risk of erectile dysfunction has decreased since the description of nerve-sparing cystectomy by Schlegel in 1987 [77], sexual dysfunction remains a significant QOL issue after radical cystectomy and urinary diversion [66]. Patients experience diminished sexual desire, decreased interaction with one's partner, and less frequent sexual activity, all of which are more significant in patients with ileal conduits compared to continent cutaneous diversions [78]. Nerve-sparing techniques can preserve sexual function in the majority of men and have not been associated with greater risk of cancer recurrence with proper patient selection [79]. In patients with erectile dysfunction after radical cystectomy and urinary diversion, significant improvements in sexual function and satisfaction are demonstrated in patients who received penile implants [66].

Anterior pelvic exenteration with urinary diversion in women can cause decreased vaginal vault size, scarring and reduced lubrication, all potentially resulting in painful intercourse and loss of sexual function [12].

27.6 Perioperative Considerations

27.6.1 Anesthetic Considerations

General anesthesia is most commonly used for radical cystectomy and urinary diversions, but combined general anesthesia and epidural may have impact on intraoperative bleeding and postoperative analgesia [80]. Regardless of anesthesia type, close intraoperative monitoring of cardiac and respiratory status is essential to reduce postoperative morbidity in patients undergoing cystectomy and urinary diversion. Cardiac optimization during surgery is a critical task for the anesthesia team but challenging due to typical significant comorbidities, blood loss, fluid shifts and loss of urine output as an indicator of volume status. Pillai et al. performed a randomized, prospective, double-blind clinical trial evaluating use of esophageal Doppler-guided cardiovascular optimization ($n=32$) vs. standard intraoperative management ($n=34$) in patients undergoing radical cystectomy and urinary diversion, and found patients with esophageal Doppler-guided optimization had earlier return of flatus, less nausea/vomiting, decreased ileus, fewer wound infections, and higher volume fluid resuscitation compared to standard management [81]. Anesthetic management can certainly impact recovery and morbidity in the cystectomy patient population.

27.6.2 General Postoperative Strategies

Despite a paucity of scientific evidence, postoperative early ambulation, incentive spirometry and aggressive physical therapy may decrease morbidity with minimal risk to the patient. Benefits of postoperative respiratory exercises on reduction of pulmonary complications were observed in patients undergoing major abdominal surgery in a recent meta-analysis [82]. Early ambulation and physical therapy attempt to minimize the potential harmful effects of prolonged immobility including ileus, pulmonary complications, DVT/PE, and overall weakness/deconditioning [83]. Fast-track rehabilitation programs have also been implemented in efforts to accelerate postoperative recovery and reduce morbidity. Saar and colleagues implemented fast-track rehabilitation for robotic cystectomy and urinary diversion including omission of mechanical bowel preparation, postoperative antimicrobials and nasogastric tubes, as well as early mobilization within a few hours of surgery, oral nutrition within 24 h, and minimization of narcotics. Fast-track rehabilitation was associated with use of fewer morphine equivalents and earlier time to mobilization and regular diet [84], but further studies are clearly necessary to determine if fast-track rehabilitation can decrease postoperative morbidity.

27.6.3 Nasogastric Tube

Routine postoperative nasogastric tube (NGT) decompression after radical cystectomy and urinary diversion is controversial. Historically, an NGT was maintained until either low outputs and/or return of flatus but this practice has undergone scrutiny due to patient discomfort, as well concerns that the NGT may actually be detrimental to recovery. Inman and associates discovered return of bowel sounds, flatus and length of hospital stay were significantly improved in almost 200 cystectomy patients without an NGT compared to over 200 with an NGT without significant differences in postoperative ileus between groups [85]. Further, early NGT removal with administration of intravenous metoclopramide appears to reduce postoperative atelectasis and promote early return of bowel function in patients after radical cystectomy and urinary diversion [86].

27.6.4 Nutrition

Postoperative nutrition after radical cystectomy and urinary diversion is a significant issue as almost 20 % of patients have nutritional deficiencies prior to surgery [21], with postoperative ileus a major compounding factor [87]. Oral nutrition is preferred if possible compared to total parenteral nutrition (TPN). Roth et al. performed a prospective clinical trial randomizing 157 consecutive radical cystectomy patients to either TPN during the first five postoperative days compared to oral nutrition alone with a primary outcome of postoperative complications, and discovered a significantly higher complication rate in the TPN group (69 % vs. 49 %, $p=0.013$), with a threefold higher risk of infectious complications in patients receiving TPN [88]. Another small study evaluated early artificial enteral feeding via percutaneous jejunostomy tube placed at the time of cystectomy and urinary diversion but demonstrated poor tolerability and relatively high complication rates with minimal impact on early return of bowel function [89].

Although chewing gum after radical cystectomy and urinary diversion facilitates slightly earlier return of bowel function [87, 90], Alvimopan (Entereg®) likely has significantly greater impact. Alvimopan, a peripherally acting μ-opioid receptor antagonist, was approved by the United States Food and Drug Administration in 2008 to accelerate gastrointestinal recovery following partial bowel resection with primary bowel anastomosis. Vora and colleagues studied the utility of alvimopan in 50 consecutive patients that underwent radical cystectomy and urinary diversion and found time to flatus, bowel movements, and regular diet, as well as rate of postoperative ileus and length of hospital stay were significantly improved with alvimopan ($N=23$) compared to controls ($N=27$) [91]. A recent cost-analysis evaluated the possible cost-effectiveness of alvimopan in cystectomy patients and determined alvimopan has potential for cost savings given the assumptions that postoperative ileus occurs in ≥ 14 % of radical cystectomy patients and extends hospital stay ≥ 3.5 days, as well as the assumption alvimopan results in a relative risk reduction of ≥ 44 % for postoperative ileus [92]. A randomized, placebo-controlled, double-blind, phase 4 clinical trial evaluating alvimopan in patients undergoing radical cystectomy with urinary diversion has been completed with eagerly anticipated, but as yet unpublished results (www.clinicaltrials.gov NCT00708201).

27.7 Open Techniques

Techniques for radical cystectomy via open and robotic approaches are well-described elsewhere, including separate chapters in this textbook. Further, certain technical aspects of urinary diversion are previously addressed in this chapter when discussing the specific diversion types. Attention will now be given to specific and critically important technical aspects of both open and robotic urinary diversions.

27.7.1 Bowel Anastomosis

The bowel anastomosis is a crucial step of urinary diversion as postoperative bowel leak results in significant morbidity and even mortality. Gastrointestinal complications occur in almost 30 % of patients undergoing radical cystectomy and urinary diversion with roughly 1 % of patients having an anastomotic bowel leak [4]. Leung and colleagues performed a meta-analysis comparing stapled versus hand sewn bowel anastamoses showing no statistical differences in bowel obstruction, wound infection, or anastomotic complications, with two of the studies showing shorter operative times with the stapled anastomosis [93]. No trials to date have reported significantly different bowel anastomosis techniques specifically for patients undergoing radical cystectomy with urinary diversion.

27.7.2 Ureterointestinal Anastomoses

Proper tissue handling, preservation of peri-ureteral adventitia and blood supply, lack of thermal energy near the ureters, and overall sound surgical technique may help decrease the risk of morbidity due to ureterointestinal anastomoses [18]. Regarding ureteral stents, some studies show stents to decrease the risk of urine leaks and ureteral stricture, whereas other studies suggest the opposite [94–96]. Mullins and associates reported ureteral stents had no effect on postoperative ureterointestinal stricture rates but were associated with lower rates of postoperative ileus in almost 200 patients after radical cystectomy and urinary diversion [97]. There is also uncertainty regarding the impact of running versus interrupted ureterointestinal anastomoses on the rates of ureteral stricture. Large and colleagues identified a stricture rate of 8.5 % in 149 consecutive patients with interrupted ureterointestinal anastomoses versus 12.7 % in 109 consecutive patients with running ureterointestinal anastomoses. Postoperative urinary tract infection and running technique were associated with ureterointestinal stricture on multivariate analysis [98].

27.8 Robotic Techniques

Robotic radical cystectomy is generally performed with the patient in modified lithotomy position with steep Trendelenberg (Fig. 27.5). This particular positioning unquestionably facilitates the operation but may also be associated with complications such as neuropraxia and compartment syndrome [99, 100]. For extracorporeal urinary diversion, immediate repositioning into the supine position after the robotic cystectomy and pelvic lymph node dissection can minimize risk of these dreaded complications. For robotic radical cystectomy with intracorporeal urinary

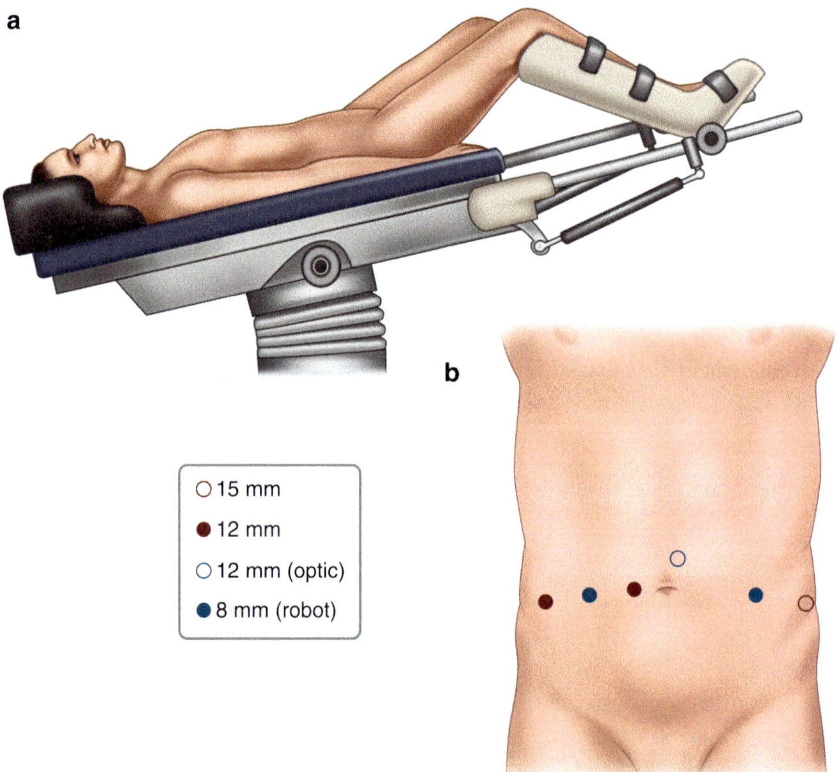

Fig. 27.5 (**a**) Robotic radical cystectomy is performed with the patient in modified lithotomy position with steep Trendelenberg. (**b**) Port placement for robotic cystectomy is similar to robotic prostatectomy except the ports are 3–5 cm higher, depending on patient body habitus. Adapted from Hemal AK, Abol-Enein H, Tewari A et al. Robotic radical cystectomy and urinary diversion in the management of bladder cancer. Urol Clin North Am 2004; 31(4): 719

diversion, patient positioning is similar to robotic prostatectomy except the ports are 3–5 cm higher, depending on patient body habitus. The operating room table is generally in maximum Trendelenberg and ports consist of the camera port, three 8 mm robotic ports, two 12 mm assistant ports (one for bowel anastomosis), and one 5 mm suction port [101]. Many surgeons incorporate the "technique of spaces" into robotic cystectomy including dissection of the periureteral space, lateral pelvic space, anterior rectal space, and the retropubic space [102]. Regarding urinary diversion, the periureteral space is paramount to proper ureteral dissection. Dissection of the periureteral space starts with incision of the posterior peritoneum above the iliac vessels and identification of the ureters bilaterally. The robotic fourth arm is useful for this part of the dissection to retract the sigmoid colon medially [101]. After ureteral identification, the ureters are dissected carefully to the level of the bladder with care to avoid excessive retraction or devascularization and then divided between clips. Frozen section analysis of the distal ureter is generally at surgeon discretion. Due to the importance of meticulous surgical technique during ureteral dissection, some concern exists regarding possible increased ureterointestinal stricture rates during robotic cystectomy and urinary diversion because of loss of haptic feedback. However, Anderson and colleagues reported no significant difference in ureterointestinal stricture rates between open and robotic cystectomy, 8.5 % versus 12.6 %, respectively [103].

27.9 Intracorporeal Urinary Diversion

Following completion of the robotic radical cystectomy and pelvic lymph node dissection, the left ureter is passed beneath the sigmoid mesentery into the right lower quadrant. Attention is then turned to the small bowel and the segment of ileum is selected for the conduit or neobladder, at least 15 cm proximal to the ileocecal valve, as in the open technique. The bowel is divided using either the EndoGIA stapler (Covidien, Mansfield, MA, USA) or 60-mm laparoscopic stapler (Echelon Stapler; Ethicon

Endo-Surgery Inc., Cincinnati, OH, USA) and the ileal segment isolated for the conduit or neobladder. Extreme care must be taken to keep orientation of the small bowel during isolation of the conduit, as well as division of the bowel and mesentery to preserve blood supply to both the urinary diversion and the bowel anastomosis. Guru and colleagues initially described the "Marionette technique" in 2010 [104] to assist with handling of the ileum and retraction, which at times can be difficult robotically. Briefly, after isolation of the bowel segment, a Keith needle silk suture is passed through the anterior abdominal wall, then through the distal end of the selected bowel segment and then back out through the same location in the anterior abdominal wall. The stitch is kept in position with a surgical instrument but not tied, which allows raising and lowering of the ileal segment during creation of the ileal conduit (like a puppet on a string), hence the "Marionette technique" (Fig. 27.6). Collins and associates recently reported evolving techniques of robotic cystectomy, pelvic lymph node dissection and totally intracorporeal urinary diversion in a large series of patients from Karolinska University Hospital, Stockholm, Sweden [105]. Robotic cystectomy and intracorporeal urinary diversion was performed in 113 patients, including 43 with ileal conduit and 70 with orthotopic neobladder. Median operating room time was 292 min with robotic ileal conduit urinary diversion but 420 min with robotic neobladder [105]. The authors detail specific measures and evolved techniques in efforts to avoid complications during robotic cystectomy, PLND and intracorporeal urinary diversion (Table 27.1). Hybrid techniques have also been described, such as robotic cystectomy and pelvic lymph node dissection, followed by extracorporeal ureterointestinal anastomoses and creation of neobladder, then closing fascia, redocking the robot and finishing the neobladder-urethral anastomosis robotically [6]. Robotic urinary diversion generally follows the same surgical principles as open urinary diversion [106], with critically important technical aspects of both open and robotic urinary diversions including the bowel anastomosis and ureterointestinal anastomoses, as previously discussed.

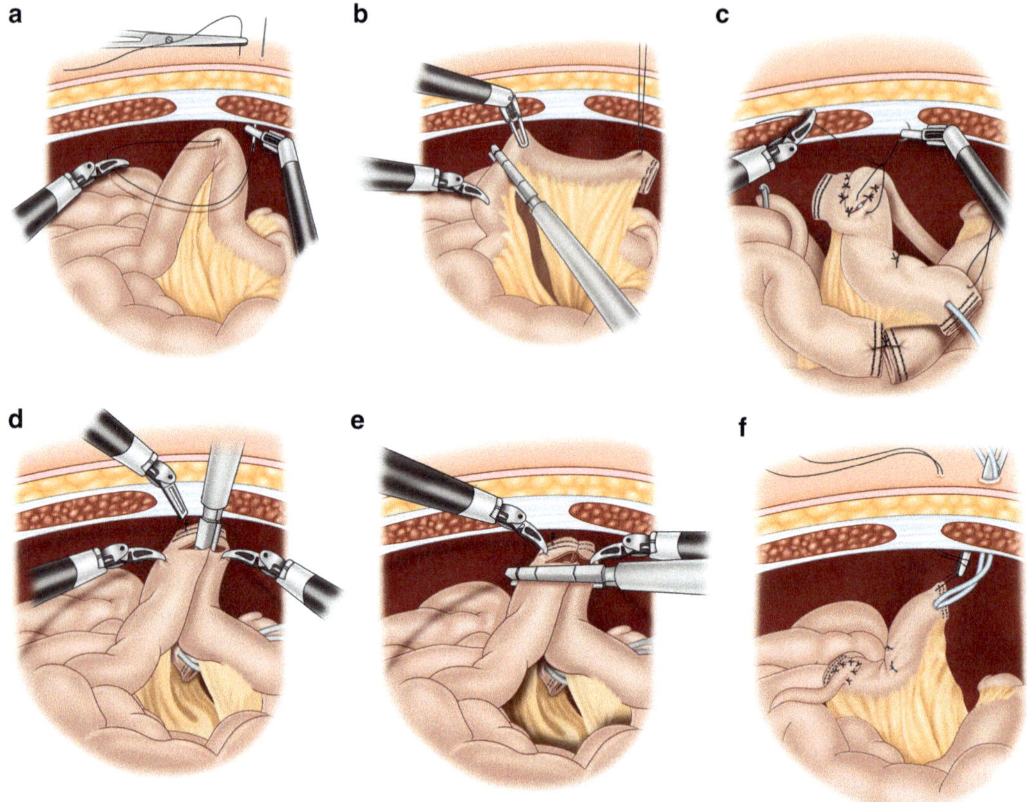

Fig. 27.6 The Marionette technique of robotic intracorporeal ileal conduit—(**a**) After isolation of the ileal segment for the conduit, a long silk suture using a Keith needle is brought through the anterior abdominal wall, passed full-thickness through the marked distal end of the ileal conduit segment and then brought back through the abdominal wall. The suture is not tied but rather controlled with an instrument to allow for raising and lowering of the conduit like a "puppet on a string" during the procedure. (**b**) An Endo-GIA 45-mm stapler is used through a right-sided assistant port to divide the bowel on both ends of the ileal conduit segment. The marionette is raised and lowered as needed for traction. (**c**) The ureterointestinal anastomoses are then performed via Bricker technique with interrupted 4-0 suture over ureteral stents. Again, the marionette is raised and lowered as needed for traction to facilitate the anastomoses. (**d**) Stapled bowel anastomosis performed first in side-to-side fashion along the antimesenteric border. (**e**) Stapled bowel anastomosis completed with Endo-GIA stapler in end-fashion. (**f**) Creation of the stoma—The previously marked stoma site is incised and dissected to the level of the anterior rectus fascia. The fascia is open with a cruciate incision and a hemostat passed through the muscle into the peritoneum. The distal end of the conduit and stents are extracted using the marionette suture and the stoma is fashioned via standard open techniques. Adapted from Hemal AK, Abol-Enein H, Tewari A et al. Robotic radical cystectomy and urinary diversion in the management of bladder cancer. Urol Clin North Am 2004; 31(4): 719

27.10 Conclusions

Radical cystectomy, bilateral pelvic lymph node dissection and urinary diversion is an extremely complex operation with relatively high complication rates. Many forms of urinary diversion exist but certainly the ileal conduit, Indiana pouch, and orthotopic neobladder are most commonly utilized. Open techniques for urinary diversion are well-established and robotic urinary diversion generally follows the same surgical principles. Regardless of open versus robotic approach or diversion type, meticulous attention to surgical detail during the bowel anastomosis and ureterointestinal anastomoses is essential in efforts to diminish postoperative morbidity.

Table 27.1 Avoiding complications during robotic radical cystectomy and urinary diversion (Reprinted from European Urology, 64, JW Collins et al. Robot-assisted Radical Cystectomy: Description of an Evolved Approach to Radical Cystectomy, 655, copyright 2013, with permission from Elsevier.)

Stage of operation	Complications to avoid	Evolved Technique
Patient selection	Inappropriate case selection for RARC	Avoid patients with decreased pulmonary compliance who cannot tolerate the Trendelenburg position. Avoid previous extensive abdominal surgery and patients with bulky disease
1. Port placement	Trauma to bowel adhesions Leakage from port sites	First port placed with Hasson technique. Camera port secured with purse string suture to prevent air leakage Maintain adequate periureteral tissue on the mobilized ureters
2. Dissection of ureters	Ureteric strictures	Good surgical planes; stay anterior to rectal fat
3. Development of anterior rectal space	Rectal injury	Avoid injury to the obturator nerve by identifying it early in the dissection. If transected, it should be repaired with tension-free end-to-end anastomosis using 9.0 Prolene interrupted sutures
4. Development of lateral pelvic space	Injury to the obturator nerve in elderly patients, atherosclerotic external iliac vessels may be tortuous in the pelvis	Tortuous vessels should be identified
5b(male). Nerve-sparing dissection	PSM on the prostate	Review imaging prior to operation. Intrafascial dissection can be used for T2 prostate tumors
5(female). Mobilization of bladder and transection of urethra	Urethrovaginal or vesicovaginal fistula	With both organ-sparing and non-organ-sparing approaches, to avoid the potential of a vesicovaginal fistula, make sure that the vaginal closure is not aligned with the cut urethra when an orthotopic neobladder is planned
6. Bladder take-down	Injury to the inferior epigastric vessels. Bleeding from the DVC	Avoid inferior epigastric vessels Increase pneumoperitoneum to 20 mmHg prior to dissection. Then, oversew with 3.0 V-Loc or Biosyn suture
7. PLND	Damage to collapsed walls of the iliac and hypogastric veins	Careful dissection. If veins are damaged, a small cut is often controlled with pressure with or without Surgicel. Suturing a cut vein may result in a tear and a larger hole in the vein
8a. Removing the specimen	Ruptured specimen bag	Specimen is removed through an extended camera port in men, vagina in women. Make sure the incision is large enough. The specimen can be removed under direct vision, with the camera placed in a 15-mm hybrid port
8b. Formation of the ileal conduit	Damage to the mesentery of the ileal conduit Leakage from uretero-ileal anastomoses	The camera can be placed through a 15-mm hybrid port after removal of the specimen to verify that the mesentery is not malrotated and anastomoses are not under tension Single J stents, with the end of the stent brought through the stoma, prevents temporary occlusion at the level of the abdominal wall caused by postoperative edema The ileal stoma should be formed after removal of the specimen and decompression of pneumoperitoneum

RARC = robot-assisted radical cystectomy; PSM = positive surgical margin; DVC = dorsal vein complex; PLND = pelvic lymph node dissection

References

1. Stein JP, Lieskovsky G, Cote R, et al. Radical cystectomy in the treatment of invasive bladder cancer: long-term results in 1,054 patients. J Clin Oncol. 2001;19(3):666.
2. Stein JP, Skinner DG. Results with radical cystectomy for treating bladder cancer: a 'reference standard' for high-grade, invasive bladder cancer. BJU Int. 2003;92(1):12.
3. Cookson MS, Chang SS, Wells N, et al. Complications of radical cystectomy for nonmuscle invasive disease: comparison with muscle invasive disease. J Urol. 2003;169(1):101.
4. Shabsigh A, Korets R, Vora KC, et al. Defining early morbidity of radical cystectomy for patients with bladder cancer using a standardized reporting methodology. Eur Urol. 2009;55(1):164.
5. Konety BR, Allareddy V, Herr H. Complications after radical cystectomy: analysis of population-based data. Urology. 2006;68(1):58.
6. Hemal AK, Abol-Enein H, Tewari A, et al. Robotic radical cystectomy and urinary diversion in the management of bladder cancer. Urol Clin North Am. 2004;31(4):719.
7. Wang GJ, Barocas DA, Raman JD, et al. Robotic vs open radical cystectomy: prospective comparison of perioperative outcomes and pathological measures of early oncological efficacy. BJU Int. 2008;101(1):89.
8. Guru KA, Kim HL, Piacente PM, et al. Robot-assisted radical cystectomy and pelvic lymph node dissection: initial experience at Roswell Park Cancer Institute. Urology. 2007;69(3):469.
9. Dasgupta P, Rimington P, Murphy D, et al. Robotically assisted radical cystectomy. BJU Int. 2008;101(12):1489.
10. Johar RS, Hayn MH, Stegemann AP, et al. Complications after robot-assisted radical cystectomy: results from the International Robotic Cystectomy Consortium. Eur Urol. 2013;64(1):52.
11. Yuh BE, Nazmy M, Ruel NH, et al. Standardized analysis of frequency and severity of complications after robot-assisted radical cystectomy. Eur Urol. 2012;62(5):806.
12. Gong EM, Steinberg GD. Urinary diversions and reconstructions. In: Vogelzang NJ, Scardino PT, Shipley WU, Debruyne FMJ, Linehan WM, editors. Comprehensive textbook of genitourinary oncology. 3rd ed. Philadelphia, PA: Lippincott, Williams and Wilkins; 2006. p. 507–16. Chapter 28A.
13. Hautmann RE, Bachor R. Bladder substitutes for continent urinary diversion. Monogr Urol. 1994;15:47–59.
14. Benson MC, Olsson CA. Urinary diversion. Urol Clin North Am. 1992;19:779–95.
15. Wein AJ. Pathophysiology and categorization of voiding dysfunction. In: Walsh PC, Retik AB, Vaughan ED, Wein AJ, editors. Campbell's urology. 8th ed. Philadelphia, PA: WB Saunders; 2002. p. 887–99.
16. Birkmeyer JD, Stukel TA, Siewers AE, et al. Surgeon volume and operative mortality in the United States. N Engl J Med. 2003;349:2117–27.
17. Birkmeyer JD, Siewers AE, Finlayson EV, Stukel TA, Lucas FL, Batista I, Welch HG, et al. Hospital volume and surgical mortality in the United States. N Engl J Med. 2002;346(15):1128–37.
18. Richards KA, Steinberg GD. Perioperative outcomes in radical cystectomy: how to reduce morbidity? Curr Opin Urol. 2013;23(5):456–65.
19. Whitmore WF, Marshall VF. Radical total cystectomy for cancer of the bladder: 230 consecutive cases five years later. J Urol. 1962;87:853–68.
20. Fleisher LA, Beckman JA, Brown KA, et al. ACC/AHA 2007 guidelines on perioperative cardiovascular evaluation and care for noncardiac surgery: Executive summary: a report of the American college of cardiology/American heart association task force on practice guidelines (writing committee to revise the 2002 guidelines on perioperative cardiovascular evaluation for noncardiac surgery): developed in collaboration with the American society of echocardiography, American society of nuclear cardiology, heart rhythm society, society of cardiovascular anesthesiologists, society for cardiovascular angiography and interventions, society for vascular medicine and biology, and society for vascular surgery. Circulation. 2007;116(17):1971–96.
21. Gregg JR, Cookson MS, Phillips S, et al. Effect of preoperative nutritional deficiency on mortality after radical cystectomy for bladder cancer. J Urol. 2011;185:90–6.
22. Lambert JW, Ingham M, Gibbs BB, et al. Using preoperative albumin levels as a surrogate marker for outcomes after radical cystectomy for bladder cancer. Urology. 2013;81(3):587–92.
23. Terry WJ, Bueschen AJ. Complications of radical cystectomy and correlation with nutritional assessment. Urology. 1986;27:229–32.
24. Koch MO, Seckin B, Smith Jr JA. Impact of a collaborative care approach to radical cystectomy and urinary reconstruction. J Urol. 1995;154:996–1001.
25. Golden TM, Ratliff C. Development and implementation of a clinical pathway for radical cystectomy and urinary system reconstruction. J Wound Ostomy Continence Nurs. 1997;24:72–8.
26. Large MC, Kiriluk KJ, DeCastro JG, et al. The impact of mechanical bowel preparation on postoperative complications for patients undergoing cystectomy and urinary diversion. J Urol. 2012;188:1801–5.
27. Hashad MM, Atta M, Elabbady A, et al. Safety of no bowel preparation before ileal urinary diversion. BJU Int. 2012;110:1109–13.
28. Amin M. Antibacterial prophylaxis in urology: a review. Am J Med. 1992;92:114S–7.
29. Hara N, Kitamura Y, Saito T, et al. Perioperative antibiotics in radical cystectomy with ileal conduit urinary diversion: efficacy and risk of antimicrobial prophylaxis on the operation day alone. Int J Urol. 2008;15:511–5.

30. Wolf Jr JS, Bennett CJ, Dmochowski RR, et al. Best practice statement on urologic surgery antimicrobial prophylaxis. J Urol. 2008;179:1379–90.

31. Quek ML, Stein JP, Daneshmand S, et al. A critical analysis of perioperative mortality from radical cystectomy. J Urol. 2006;175:886–90.

32. Clément C, Rossi P, Aissi K, et al. Incidence, risk profile and morphological pattern of lower extremity venous thromboembolism after urological cancer surgery. J Urol. 2011;186:2293–7.

33. Prandoni P, Lensing AW, Cogo A, et al. The long term clinical course of acute deep vein thrombosis. Ann Intern Med. 1996;125:1–7.

34. Bergqvist D, Jendteg S, Johansen L, et al. Cost of long term sequelae of deep vein thrombosis of the lower extremities: an analysis of a defined patient population in Sweden. Ann Intern Med. 1997;126:454–7.

35. Forrest JB, Clemens JQ, Finamore P, et al. AUA best practice statement for the prevention of deep vein thrombosis in patients undergoing urologic surgery. J Urol. 2009;181:1170–7.

36. Kurzrock EA, Baskin LS, Kogan BA. Gastrocystoplasty: is there a consensus? World J Urol. 1998;16(4):242–50.

37. McDougal WS, Stampfer DS, Kirley S, Bennett PM, Lin CW. Intestinal ammonium transport by ammonium and hydrogen exchange. J Am Coll Surg. 1995;181(3):241–8.

38. Skinner EC, Stein JP, Skinner DG. Surgical benchmarks for the treatment of invasive bladder cancer. Urol Oncol. 2007;25(1):66–71.

39. Bricker E. Bladder substitution after pelvic evisceration. Surg Clin North Am. 1950;30:1511.

40. Hinman F. Selection of intestinal segments for bladder substitution: physical and physiological characteristics. J Urol. 1988;139:519.

41. Persky L. Large and small bowel urinary conduits. In: Glenn JF, editor. Urologic surgery. 4th ed. Philadelphia, PA: JB Lippincott; 1991. p. 1004–12.

42. Bachor R, Hautmann R. Options in urinary diversion: a review and critical assessment. Semin Urol. 1993;11:235–50.

43. Gilchrist RK, Merricks JW, Hamlin HH, Rieger IT. Construction of a substitute bladder and urethra. Surg Gynecol Obstet. 1950;90:752–60.

44. Benson MC, Olsson CA. Cutaneous continent urinary diversion. In: Walsh PC, Retik AB, Vaughan ED, Wein AJ, editors. Campbell's urology. 8th ed. Philadelphia, PA: WB Saunders; 2002. p. 3789–834.

45. Rowland RG, Mitchell ME, Bihrle R, et al. The cecoileal continent urinary reservoir. World J Urol. 1985;3:185.

46. Rowland RG, Kropp BP. Evolution of the Indiana continent urinary reservoir. J Urol. 1994;152:2247–51.

47. Bihrle R. The Indiana Pouch continent urinary reservoir. Urol Clin North Am. 1997;24:773–9.

48. Steinberg GD, Rinker-Schaeffer CW, Sokoloff MH, Brendler CB. Highlights of the urologic oncology meeting, June 2, 2001. J Urol. 2002;168:653–9.

49. Weijerman PC, Schurmans JR, Hop WC, Schroder FH, Bosh JL. Morbidity and quality of life in patients with orthotopic and heterotopic continent urinary diversion. Urology. 1998;51(1):51–6.

50. Hautmann RE, Depetriconi R, Gottfried H, Kleinschmidt K, Mattes R, Paiss T. The ileal neobladder: complications and functional results in 363 patients after 11 years of follow-up. J Urol. 1999;161:422–8.

51. Lippert CM, Theodorescu D. The Hautmann neobladder with chimney: a versatile modification. J Urol. 1997;158:1510–2.

52. Hollowell CM, Steinberg GD, Rowland RG. Current concepts of urinary diversion in men. In: Droller MJ, editor. Current clinical urology: bladder cancer: current diagnosis and treatment. Totowa, NJ: Humana Press Inc.; 2001. p. 343–66.

53. Studer UR, Danuser H, Merz VW, Springer JP, Zingg EJ. Experience in 100 patients with an ileal low pressure bladder substitute combined with an efferent tubular isoperistaltic segment. J Urol. 1995;154:49–56.

54. Reddy PK. Detubularized sigmoid reservoir for bladder replacement after cystoprostatectomy. Urology. 1987;29(6):625–8.

55. Carlin BI, Rutchik SD, Resnick MI. Comparison of the ileal conduit to the continent cutaneous diversion and orthotopic neobladder in patients undergoing cystectomy: a critical analysis and review of the literature. Semin Urol Oncol. 1997;15(3):189–92.

56. Montie JE, Pontes JE, Smyth EM. Selection of the type of urinary diversion in conjunction with radical cystectomy. J Urol. 1987;137:1154–5.

57. Stein JP, Cote RJ, Freeman JA, Esrig D, Elmajian DA, Groshen S, Skinner EC, Boyd SD, Lieskovsky G, Skinner DG. Indications for lower urinary tract reconstruction in women after cystectomy for bladder cancer: a pathological review of female cystectomy specimens. J Urol. 1995;154(4):1329–33.

58. Stein JP, Esrig D, Freeman JA, Grossfeld GD, Ginsberg DA, Cote RJ, Groshen S, Boyd SD, Lieskovsky G, Skinner DG. Prospective pathologic analysis of female cystectomy specimens: risk factors for orthotopic diversion in women. Urology. 1998;51(6):951–5.

59. Iselin CE, Robertson CN, Webster GD, Vieweg J, Paulson DF. Does prostate transitional cell carcinoma preclude orthotopic bladder reconstruction after radical cystoprostatectomy for bladder cancer? J Urol. 1997;158(6):2123–6.

60. Steven K, Poulsen AL. The orthotopic Kock ileal neobladder: functional results, urodynamic features, complications and survival in 166 men. J Urol. 2000;164:288.

61. Elmajian DA, Stein JP, Esrig D, Freeman JA, Skinner EC, Boyd SD, Lieskovsky G, Skinner DG. The Kock ileal neobladder: updated experience in 295 male patients. J Urol. 1996;156(3):920–5.

62. Stein JP, Stenzl A, Grossfeld GD, Freeman JA, Esrig D, Boyd SD, Lieskovsky, Bartsch G, Skinner

DG. The use of orthotopic neobladders in women undergoing cystectomy for pelvic malignancy. World J Urol. 1996;14(1):9–14.

63. Hobisch A, Tosun K, Kinzl J, Kemmler G, Bartsch G, Holtl L, Stenzl A. Quality of life after cystectomy and orthotopic neobladder versus ileal conduit urinary diversion. World J Urol. 2000;18:338–44.

64. Laven BA, O'Connor RC, Steinberg GD, Gerber GS. Long-term results of antegrade endoureterotomy using the holmium laser in patients with ureterointestinal strictures. Urology. 2001;58(6):924–9.

65. Gburek B, Lieber M, Blute M. Comparison of Studer ileal neobladder and ileal conduit urinary diversion with respect to perioperative outcome and late complications. J Urol. 1998;160(3–1):721–3.

66. Hart S, Skinner E, Meyerowitz B, Boyd S, Lieskovsky G, Skinner D. Quality of life after radical cystectomy for bladder cancer in patients with an ileal conduit, or cutaneous or urethral kock pouch. J Urol. 1999;162(1):77–81.

67. N'Dow J, Robson CN, Matthews JN, Neal DE, Pearson JP. Reducing mucus production after urinary reconstruction: a prospective randomized trial. J Urol. 2001;165(5):1433–40.

68. Ware JE. SF-36 health status questionnaire. Boston, MA: Quality Quest, Inc.; 1989.

69. Aaronson NK, et al. J Natl Cancer Inst. 1993; 85(5):365.

70. Da Silva FC, Fossa SD, Aaronson NK, Serbouti S, Denis L, et al. The quality of life of patients with newly diagnosed prostate cancer: experience with EORTC clinical trial 30853. Eur J Cancer. 1996;32A:72.

71. Bergner M, Bobbitt RA, Carter WB, et al. The sickness impact profile: development and final revision of a health status measure. Med Care. 1981;19(8): 787–805.

72. Mansson A, Mansson W. When the bladder is gone: quality of life following different types of urinary diversion. World J Urol. 1999;17:211–8.

73. Sullivan LD, Chow VDW, Ko DSC, Wright JE, McLoughlin MG. An evaluation of quality of life in patients with continent urinary diversions after cystectomy. Br J Urol. 1998;81:699–704.

74. Hara I, Miyake H, Hara S, Gotoh A, Nakamura I, Okada H, Arakawa S, Kamidona S. Health-related quality of life after radical cystectomy for bladder cancer: a comparison of ileal conduit and orthotopic bladder replacement. BJU Int. 2002;89:10–3.

75. Fugisawa M, Isotani S, Gotoh A, Okada H, Arakawa S, Kamidono S. Health-related quality of life with orthotopic neobladder versus ileal conduit according to the SF-36 survey. Urology. 2000;55(6):862–5.

76. Dutta SA, Chang SS, Coffey CS, Smith Jr JA, Jack G, Cookson MS. Health related quality of life assessment after radical cystectomy: comparison of ileal conduit with continent orthotopic neobladder. J Urol. 2002;168:164–7.

77. Schlegel PN, Walsh PC. New anatomical approach to radical cystoprostatectomy with preservation of sexual function. J Urol. 1987;138:1402.

78. Boyd SD, Feinberg SM, Skinner DG, Lieskovsky G, Baron D, Richardson J. Quality of life survey of urinary diversion patients: comparison of ileal conduits versus continent Kock ileal reservoirs. J Urol. 1987;138(6):1386–9.

79. Brendler CB, Steinberg GD, Marshall FF, et al. Local recurrence and survival following nerve sparing radical cystoprostatectomy. J Urol. 1990;144:1137.

80. Ozyuvaci E, Altan A, Karadeniz T, et al. General anesthesia versus epidural and general anesthesia in radical cystectomy. Urol Int. 2005;74:62–7.

81. Pillai P, McEleavy I, Gaughan M, et al. A double-blind randomized controlled clinical trial to assess the effect of Doppler optimized intraoperative fluid management on outcome following radical cystectomy. J Urol. 2011;186:2201–6.

82. Grams ST, Ono LM, Noronha MA, et al. Breathing exercises in upper abdominal surgery: a systematic review and meta-analysis. Rev Bras Fisioter. 2012;16:345–53.

83. Patel BK, Hall JB. Perioperative physiotherapy. Curr Opin Anaesthesiol. 2013;26(2):152–6.

84. Saar M, Ohlmann CH, Siemer S, et al. Fast-track rehabilitation after robot-assisted laparoscopic cystectomy accelerates postoperative recovery. BJU Int. 2013;112(2):E99–106.

85. Inman BA, Harel F, Tiguert R, et al. Routine nasogastric tubes are not required following cystectomy with urinary diversion: a comparative analysis of 430 patients. J Urol. 2003;170:1888–91.

86. Donat SM, Slaton JW, Pisters LL, Swanson DA. Early nasogastric tube removal combined with metoclopramide after radical cystectomy and urinary diversion. J Urol. 1999;162:1599–602.

87. Ramirez JA, McIntosh AG, Strehlow R, et al. Definition, incidence, risk factors, and prevention of paralytic ileus following radical cystectomy: a systematic review. Eur Urol. 2013;64(4):588–97.

88. Roth B, Birkhäuser FD, Zehnder P, et al. Parenteral nutrition does not improve postoperative recovery from radical cystectomy: results of a prospective randomized trial. Eur Urol. 2013;63:475–82.

89. Maffezzini M, Gerbi G, Campodonico F, Parodi D. A multimodal perioperative plan for radical cystectomy and urinary intestinal diversion: effects, limits, and complications of early artificial nutrition. J Urol. 2006;176:945–9.

90. Choi H, Kang SH, Yoon DK, et al. Chewing gum has a stimulatory effect on bowel motility in patients after open or robotic radical cystectomy for bladder cancer: a prospective randomized comparative study. Urology. 2011;77:884–90.

91. Vora AA, Harbin A, Rayson R, et al. Alvimopan provides rapid gastrointestinal recovery without nasogastric tube decompression after radical cystectomy and urinary diversion. Can J Urol. 2012;19:6293–8.

92. Hilton WM, Lotan Y, Parekh DJ, et al. Alvimopan for prevention of postoperative paralytic ileus in radical cystectomy patients: a cost-effectiveness analysis. BJU Int. 2013;111(7):1054–60.

93. Leung TT, MacLean AR, Buie WD, et al. Comparison of stapled versus handsewn loop ileostomy closure: a meta-analysis. J Gastrointest Surg. 2008;12:939–44.

94. Regan JB, Barrett DM. Stented versus non-stented ureteroileal anastomoses: is there a difference with regard to leak and stricture? J Urol. 1985;134:1101–3.

95. Faulknier B, Chaksupa D, Malas A, et al. Persistent candiduria complicating intraureteral stenting: a case report and review of the literature. W V Med J. 2003;99:25–7.

96. Keane PF, Bonner MC, Johnston SR, et al. Characterization of biofilm and encrustation on ureteric stents in vivo. Br J Urol. 1994;73:687–91.

97. Mullins JK, Guzzo TJ, Ball MW, et al. Ureteral stents placed at the time of urinary diversion decrease postoperative morbidity. Urol Int. 2012;88:66–70.

98. Large MC, Cohn JA, Kiriluk KJ, Dangle P, Richards KA, Smith ND, et al. The impact of running versus interrupted anastomosis on ureterointestinal stricture rate after radical cystectomy. J Urol. 2013;190(3):923–7.

99. Manny TB, Gorbachinsky I, Hemal AK. Lower extremity neuropathy after robot assisted laparoscopic radical prostatectomy and radical cystectomy. Can J Urol. 2010;17:5390–3.

100. Galyon SW, Richards KA, Pettus JA, et al. Three-limb compartment syndrome and rhabdomyolysis after robotic cystoprostatectomy. J Clin Anesth. 2011;23:75–8.

101. Poch MA, Raza J, Nyquist J, Guru KA. Tips and tricks to robot-assisted radical cystectomy and intracorporeal diversion. Curr Opin Urol. 2013;23(1):65–71.

102. Hayn MH, Agarwal PK, Guru KA. Robot-assisted radical cystectomy in male: technique of spaces. robotics in genitourinary surgery. London: Springer; 2011.

103. Anderson CB, Morgan TM, Kappa S, et al. Ureteroenteric anastomotic strictures after radical cystectomy – does operative approach matter? J Urol. 2013;189:541–7.

104. Guru KA, Seixas-Mikelus SA, Hussain A, et al. Robot-assisted intracorporeal ileal conduit: marionette technique and initial experience at Roswell Park Cancer Institute. Urology. 2010;76(4):866–71.

105. Collins JW, Tyritzis S, Nyberg T, et al. Robot-assisted radical cystectomy: description of an evolved approach to radical cystectomy. Eur Urol. 2013;64(4):654–63.

106. Goh AC, Gill IS, Lee DJ, et al. Robotic intracorporeal orthotopic ileal neobladder: replicating open surgical principles. Eur Urol. 2012;62(5):891–901.

Christian Weiss and Claus Rödel

28.1 Introduction

The standard of care for transitional-cell carcinoma of the bladder with invasion to the muscularis propria is radical cystectomy. Sophisticated techniques for urinary diversion have been developed to improve patients' quality of life. Even the construction of a neobladder with continent urinary diversion, however, cannot substitute for the patient's original bladder. Attempts to obtain organ preservation are only justified when they have a high likelihood of achieving local cure with no compromise in survival rates. Adequate local control cannot be achieved with TUR, chemotherapy, or radiotherapy, when used alone. Several groups have reported the value of combining all three modalities, with salvage cystectomy being reserved for patients with incomplete response or local relapse [1–3].

28.2 Series of Combined Modality Treatment in the United States and Europe

The centers that pioneered modern bladder preservation therapy included Harvard University in the US; the University of Paris in France; and the University of Erlangen in Germany [4–6]. In the 1980s, studies under the auspices of the US National Bladder Cancer Group showed that irradiation of the bladder tumor could be safely combined with cisplatin in patients who were considered not to be candidates for cystectomy [4]. In 1988, Housset et al. from Paris began a prospective trial of preoperative chemoradiotherapy, using 5-fluorouracil and cisplatin with concomitant radiation therapy, followed by cystectomy or additional chemoradiotherapy. Histopathological examination of the cystectomy specimen revealed complete pathologic response in the first 18 patients after induction therapy. Complete responders were considered candidates for bladder preservation and salvage cystectomy was restricted to patients with an incomplete response after induction therapy. This treatment strategy resulted in a 5-year survival of 63 % [5]. In 1990, Sauer et al. from Erlangen reported the results of a phase II study of cisplatin with concomitant radiotherapy after TURBT in 67 patients with muscle-invasive bladder cancer. Complete response was obtained in 75 % of patients and 3-year overall survival was 66 % [6]. Over the past 20 years, the concept of organ preservation by

C. Weiss, M.D. (✉) • C. Rödel, M.D.
Department of Radiotherapy and Oncology,
University Hospital, Goethe University,
Theodor-Stern-Kai 7, 60590 Frankfurt, Germany
e-mail: Christian.Weiss@kgu.de;
Claus.Roedel@kgu.de

B.R. Konety and S.S. Chang (eds.), *Management of Bladder Cancer:*
A Comprehensive Text With Clinical Scenarios, DOI 10.1007/978-1-4939-1881-2_28,
© Springer Science+Business Media New York 2015

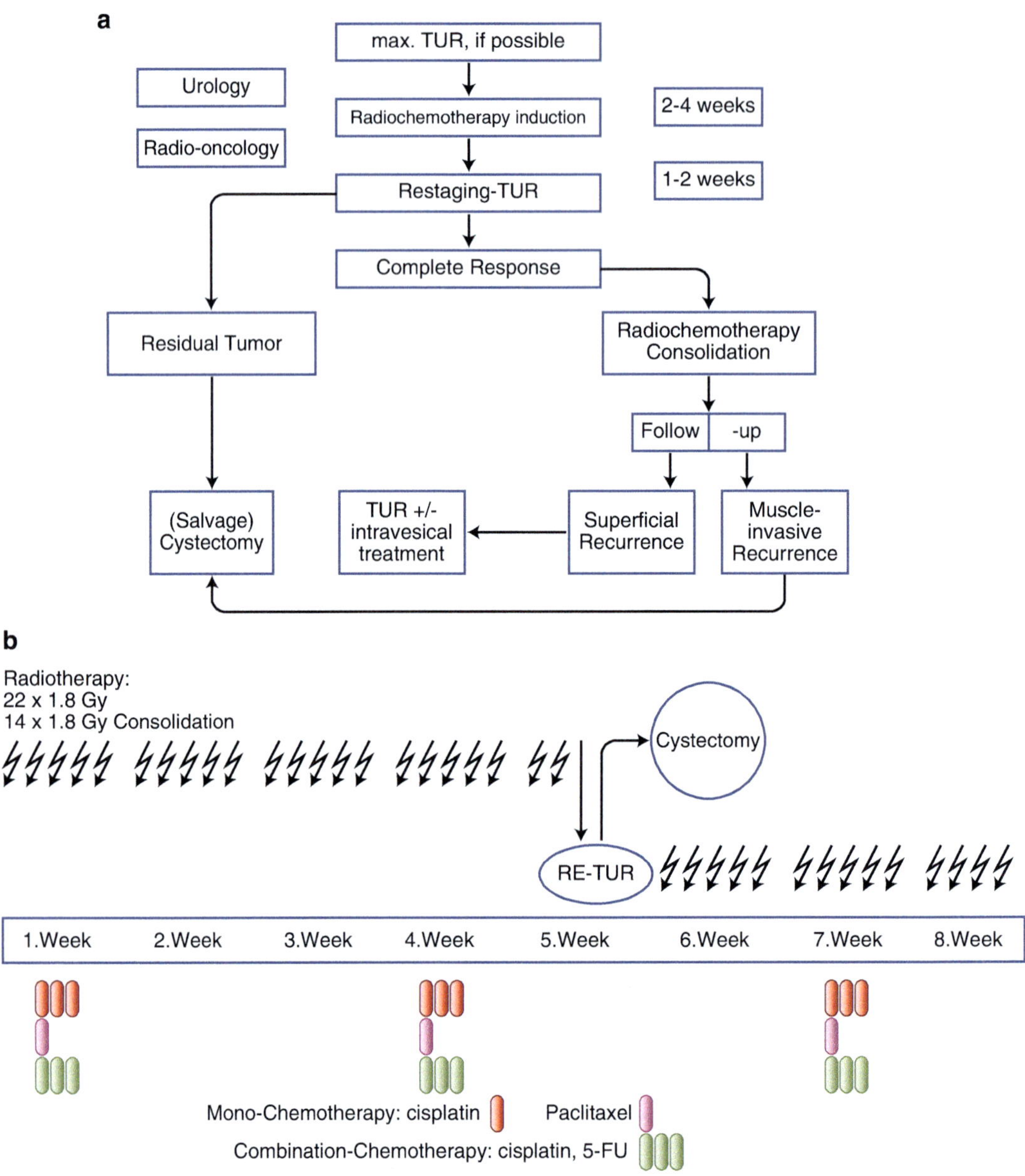

Fig. 28.1 (**a**) Massachusetts General Hospital Boston: Schedule of combined modality therapy. (**b**) Radiochemotherapy regimen

conservative surgery and combined radiotherapy and chemotherapy has been investigated in several prospective series from single centers and cooperative groups, with more than 1,000 patients included [7–29]. The actual concepts of bladder preservation trimodality therapy from Boston and Erlangen are displayed in Figs. 28.1a, b and 28.2a, b [1, 2].

With these concepts, including the updated long-term experiences of Boston and Erlangen, 5-year overall survival rates in the range of 50–60 % have been reported and about three-quarters of the surviving patients maintained their own bladder (Table 28.1 and 28.2) [23, 30–32].

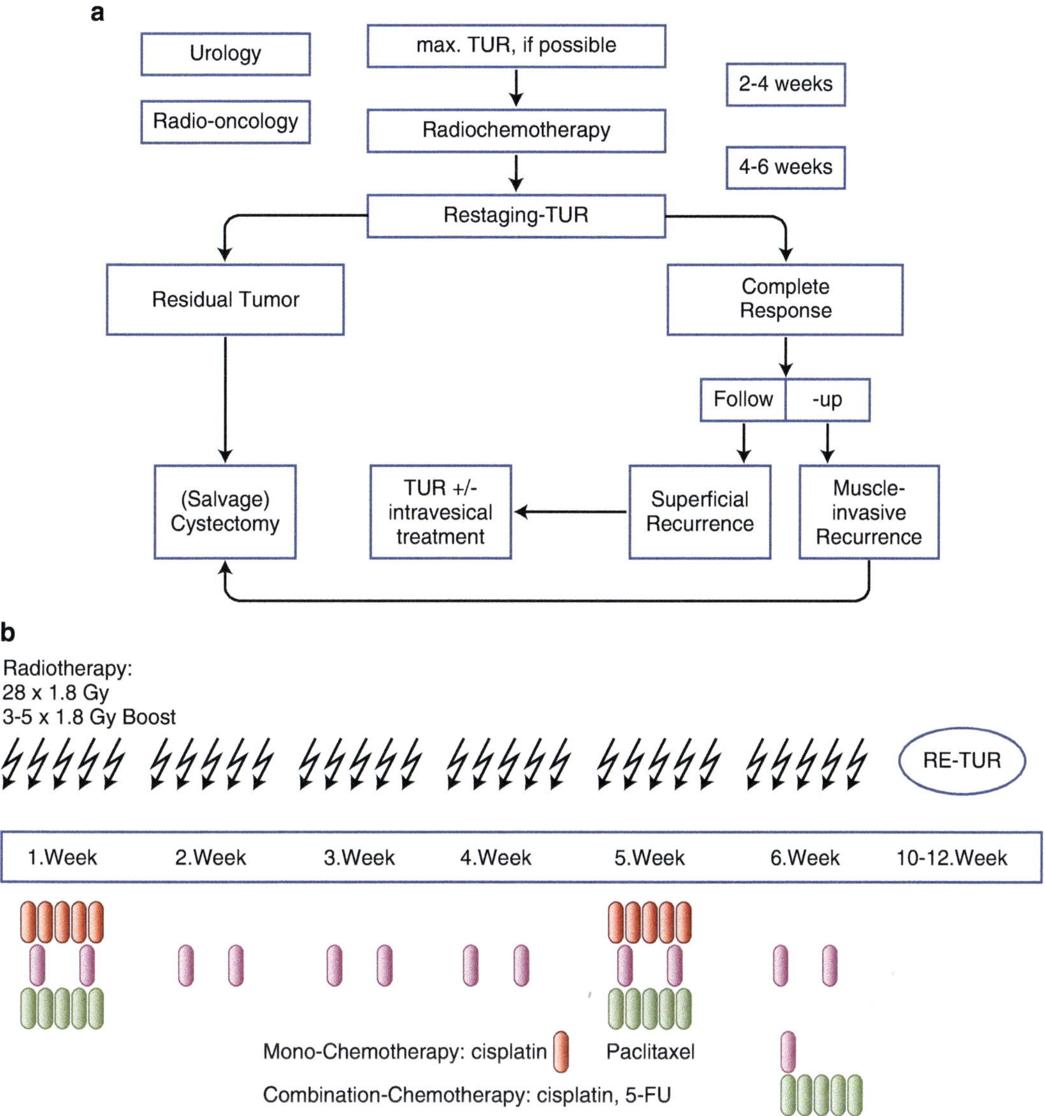

Fig. 28.2 (**a**) University Erlangen: schedule of combined modality therapy. (**b**) Radiochemotherapy regimen

28.3 Optimization of the Components of the Trimodality Approach

As more experience is acquired with organ-sparing treatment in bladder cancer, it is clear that future directions of clinical and basic research will focus on two main topics: (a) the optimization of the respective treatment components, including optimization of radiation techniques and fractionation schedules as well as incorporation of novel cytotoxic and biologic agents, and (b) the proper selection of patients who will most probably benefit from the respective treatment alternatives.

28.3.1 Radiation Fractionation Regimens and Doses

With standard fractionation (1.8–2 Gy per fraction) the total radiation dose is typically in the range of 45–50 Gy to treat the pelvic lymph nodes, and between 55 to 70 Gy to the bladder.

Table 28.1 MGH and RTOG: Series of combined-modality treatment and selective bladder preservation

Series	n	Clinical stage	Treatment	Complete response (%)	Overall survival 5-Year (%)	Overall survival with bladder 5-Year (%)
MGH 1986–1993 [7]	106	T2-4a	TUR + 2 cycles MCV + RT 39.6Gy á 1.8Gy + RT Boost 24.8Gy á 1.8Gy for responder	66	52	43
RTOG 85-12 1986–1988 [8]	42	T2-4a	TUR + RCT 40Gy á 2Gy with concurrent Cis + RCT Boost 24Gy á 2Gy for responder	66	52	42
RTOG 88-02 1988–1990 [9]	91	T2-4a	TUR + 2 cycles MCV + RCT 39.6Gy á 1.8Gy with concurrent Cis + RCT Boost 24.8Gy á 1.8Gy for responder	75	62 (4 years)	44 (4 years)
RTOG 89-03 1990–1993 [10]	123	T2-4a	TUR + 2 cycles MCV vs. no chemotherapy + RCT 39.6Gy á 1.8Gy with concurrent Cis + RCT Boost 24.8Gy á 1.8Gy for responder	61 vs. 55	49 vs. 48	36 vs. 40
MGH 1993–1994 [11]	18	T2-4a	TUR + RCT 42.5Gy split á 1.25/1.5Gy bid with concurrent Cis/5FU + RCT Boost 55Gy split á 1.25/1.67Gy bid for responder	78	83 (3 years)	78 (3 years)
MGH 1986–2000 [30]	190	T2-4a	TUR + RCT different agents/schedules/mainly Cis based	60	54	
RTOG 95-06 1995–1997 [12]	34	T2-4a	TUR + RCT 24Gy split á 3Gy bid with concurrent Cis/5FU + RCT Boost 20Gy split á 1.25Gy bid for responder	67	83 (3 years)	66 (3 years)
RTOG 97-06 1997–1999 [13]	47	T2-4a	TUR + RCT 40.8Gy split á 1.8/1.6Gy bid with concurrent Cis + RCT Boost 24Gy split á 1.5Gy bid for responder	74	61 (3 years)	48 (3 years)
MGH 1986–2006 [31]	348	T2-4a	TUR + RCT different agents/schedules/mainly Cis based	72	52	42
MGH and RTOG: Series of combined-modality treatment and selective bladder preservation integrating newer radiosensitizing drugs						
RTOG 99-06 [33]	80	T2-4a	TUR + RCT with Pac/Cis + adjuvant Gem/Cis	81	56	47
RTOG 0233 2002–2008 [34]	93	T2-4a	TUR + RCT with Pac/Cis vs. 5FU/Cis + adjuvant Gem/Cis/Pac	46 vs. 47	71 vs. 75	67 vs. 71

MGH Massachusetts General Hospital; *RTOG* Radiation therapy oncology group; *TUR* Transurethral resection; *RT* Radiotherapy; *RCT* Radiochemotherapy; *bid* Bis in die; *MCV* Methotrexate, cisplatin, vinblastine; *Cis* cisplatin; *5FU* 5-fluorouracil; *Pac* Paclitaxel; *Gem* Gemcitabine; *pCR* Pathologic complete response; *OS* Overall survival; *vs* Versus

Table 28.2 Further series of combined modality treatment for bladder cancer

Series	N	Clinical stage	Treatment	Complete response (%)	Overall survival 5-Year (%)	Overall survival with bladder 5-Year (%)
Russell et al. (1990) [14]	34	T1-4	TUR+RCT 44 Gy á 2 Gy with concurrent 5FU+RCT Boost 16 Gy á 2 Gy for responder	81	64 (4 years)	n.g. (overall rate of cystectomy: 10/34)
Rotman et al.(1990) [15]	20	T1-4	TUR+RCT 60–65 Gy á 1.8 Gy with concurrent 5FU	74	39	n.g. (19/20 maintained bladder)
Given et al. (1995) [16]	93	T2-4	TUR+2 or three cycles MVAC or MCV+RCT 64.80 Gy á 1,8 Gy with concurrent Cis (in 49 patients)	63	39	n.g.
Housset et al. (1997) [17]	120	T2-4	TUR+RCT 24 Gy á 3 Gy with concurrent Cis /5FU+RCT Boost 20 Gy á 2.5 Gy for responder	77	63	n.g.
Varveris et al. (1997) [18]	42	T1-4	TUR+RCT 68-74 Gy at 1.8–2 Gy with concurrent Cis/Doc	62	78 (median f/u of 25 mo)	n.g.
Fellin et al. (1997) [19]	56	T2-4	TUR+2 cycles of MCV+RCT 40 Gy á 1.8 Gy with concurrent Cis+RCT Boost 24 Gy á 2 Gy for responder	50	55	41
Cervek et al. (1998) [20]	105	T2-4	TUR+2-4 cycles MCV+RT 50 Gy á 2 Gy	52	58 (4 years)	45 (4 years)
Zapatero et al. (2000) [21]	40	T2-4	TUR+3 cycles MCV+RT 60 Gy á 2 Gy	70	84 (4 years)	82.6 (4 years)
Arias et al. (2000) [22]	50	T2-4	TUR plus two cycles MVAC+RCT 45 Gy á 1.80 Gy with concurrent Cis+RCT Boost 20 Gy á 2.0 Gy for patients responder	68	48	-
Rödel et al. (2002) [23]	415	T1-4	TUR+RT/RCT 50.4–59.4 Gy á 1.8 Gy with or without concurrent Carbo or Cis (±5FU)	72	50	42
Chen et al. (2003) [24]	23	T3-4	TUR+RCT 60–61.2 Gy á 1.8/2 Gy with concurrent Cis/5FU/ leucovorin	89	69 (3 years)	n.g.
Peyromaure et al. (2004) [25]	43	T2	TUR+RCT 24 Gy á 3 Gy with concurrent Cis/5FU+RCT Boost 20 Gy á 2.5 Gy for responder	74	60 (cancer specific)	n.g. (overall rate o f cystectomy: 25.6 %)
Danesi et al. (2004) [26]	77	T2-4	TUR+2 cycles of MCV (42 pts)+RCT 69 Gy á 1 Gy tid with concurrent Cis/5FU	90	58	47
Hussain et al. (2004) [27]	41	T2-4	TUR+RCT 55 Gy á 2.75 Gy with concurrent 5FU/MMC	69	36 %	n.g. (overall rate of cystectomy: 12 %)
Kragelj et al. (2005) [28]	84	T1-4	TUR+RCT 64 Gy á 1.8–2.2 Gy with concurrent Vin	78	25 % (9 years)	n.g.
Dunst et al. (2005) [29]	68	T1-4	TUR+RCT 50.4–59.4 Gy á 1.8 Gy with concurrent Cis or Pac	87	45	n.g.
Müller et al. (2007) [35]	42	T1-4	TUR+RCT 50.4–59.4 Gy á 1.8 Gy with concurrent Pac (+Cis in five patients)	86 (for 28 patients)	–	–

(continued)

Table 28.2 (continued)

Series	N	Clinical stage	Treatment	Complete response (%)	Overall survival 5-Year (%)	Overall survival with bladder 5-Year (%)
Wittlinger et al. (2009) [36]	45	T1-4	TUR+RCT 55.8–59.4 Gy á 1.8 Gy with concurrent Cis+RHT	96	80 (3 years)	43 patients retained their own bladder
Caffo et al. (2003/2011) [37, 38]	26	T2-4	TUR+RCT 54 Gy á 1.8/2 Gy with concurrent Cis/Gem	100	70.1	73.8
Kent and Oh et al. (2004/2009) [39, 40]	24		TUR+RCT 60 Gy á 2 Gy+Gem	91	76	62
Sangar and Choudhury et al. (2005/2011) [41, 42]	50	T2-3	TUR+RCT 52.5 Gy á 2.625 Gy+Gem	88	65	64
Zapatero et al. (2012) [43]	41	T2-4	TUR+3 cycles MCV+RT 60 Gy á 2 Gy for responder	71	73	83
	39		TUR+RCT 64.8 Gy varying fractionations+concurrent Cis (or Pac in five patients)	80		
James et al. (2012) [44]	182	T2-4	TUR+RCT 55 Gy á 2.75 or 64 á 2 Gy+concurrent MMC/5Fu	–	48	–
	178	T2-4	TUR+RT 55 Gy á 2.75 or 64 á 2 Gy	–	35	–
Tunio et al. (2012) [45]	120	T2-4	TUR+RCT 55 Gy á 2.75 or 64 á 2 Gy+concurrent Cis (whole pelvis RT)	93.1	52.9	58.9
	110	T2-4	TUR+RCT 55 Gy á 2.75 or 64 á 2 Gy+concurrent Cis (bladder only RT)	92.8	51	57.1

TUR Transurethral resection; *RT* Radiotherapy; *RCT* Radiochemotherapy; *bid* Bis in die; *tid* Thrice in die; *RHT* Regional deep hyperthermia; *MCV* Methotrexate, cisplatin, vinblastine; *MVAC* Methotrexate, vincristine, adriamycin, cisplatin; *Cis* Cisplatin; *Carbo* Carboplatin; *5FU* 5-fluorouracil; *MMC* Mitomycin C; *Doc* Docetaxel; *Pac* Paclitaxel; *Vin* Vinblastine; *Gem* Gemcitabine; *pCR* Pathologic complete response; *NG* Not given; *OS* Overall survival; *f/u* follow-up; *vs* versus

At least four retrospective analyses have suggested improved local control with doses greater than 55–60 Gy,[46–49] however, others have found no evidence to support such a relationship [50, 51]. Phase III randomized studies comparing different conventionally fractionated dose schedules have never been undertaken. In a recent meta-analysis of 15 radiation series with different fractionation schedules and total doses (five combined with brachytherapy), Pos et al. found evidence for an overall dose–response relationship with an increase in local control by a factor of 1.44–1.47 for an increment in dose of 10 Gy [52]. This indicates that a dose escalation could significantly improve local control.

Hyperfractionated regimens, defined as the delivery of a larger number of smaller fractions with no increase in overall treatment time, have been examined in an effort to exploit differences in the molecular repair capacity of tumor and normal tissues. This may allow an increase in total dose with no increase in the risk of late complications. Naslund et al. randomized 168 patients to receive 1 Gy three times daily to a total dose of 84 Gy versus 2 Gy once daily to a total dose of 66 Gy [53]. Goldobenko et al. reported a four-arm randomized study in 177 patients comparing conventional radiotherapy (60 Gy in 2 Gy fractions) to three hyperfractionated strategies (60 and 70 Gy in 1 Gy twice daily, 67.2 Gy in 1.2 Gy fractions twice daily) [54]. Clinical complete response and local control were improved in the hyperfractionated arms relative to conventional fractionation. A meta-analysis based on the pooled data of these studies indicated a significant improvement in local control and overall survival with hyperfractionated treatment and higher total doses [55].

Given the short potential doubling time for most transitional cell cancers of the bladder (in the range of 5–8 days), accelerated radiation therapy (designed to deliver the same total dose in a shorter interval relative to conventionally fractionated radiotherapy) may overcome radioresistance due to tumor cell repopulation. A retrospective analysis by Maciejewsky and Majewski suggested that tumor clonogenic repopulation in bladder cancer accelerates after a lag period of 5–6 weeks after start of treatment and that a dose increment of 0.36 Gy per day is required to compensate for this repopulation [56]. Horwich et al. recently reported the results of a randomized study in 229 patients with bladder cancer that either received 60.8 Gy in 32 fractions over 26 days or 64 Gy in 32 fractions over 45 days [57]. The accelerated schedule, however, did not improve local control or survival rates and was associated with increased acute bowel complications.

Hypofractionated radiation schedules (with larger daily doses in the range of 2.5–6 Gy) have also been used to treat bladder cancer patients, usually in the palliative setting. There has been only one small phase III study reporting on curative radiotherapy where increased doses per fraction (30 Gy in 3 Gy daily fractions, 4 weeks break, than 30 Gy in 1.5 Gy daily fractions) were compared with 60 Gy in 1.5 Gy fractions [58]. Survival was inferior (39 vs. 52 %) in the hypofractionated arm.

Another way to improve the therapeutic ratio is to reduce the volume irradiated with the aim to minimize toxicity and simultaneously to escalate the total dose to the tumor region. To achieve this goal the implementation of new technical developments like image-guided adaptive radiotherapy on the one and optimizing general target volume definition on the other hand are necessary. Actually several groups reported the feasibility to integrate the newer techniques into clinical practice and were able to document that the volume of normal tissue irradiated can be significantly smaller without reducing the clinical target volume [59–61]. Furthermore, an interesting pilot study by Sondergaard et al. reported a more precise demarcation of the bladder tumor by injecting lipiodol in the suspected region [62]. Nevertheless it still remains unclear, if pelvic lymph nodes have to be treated in all patients, if the total dose should always be prescribed for the whole bladder, or if partial bladder irradiation is a viable option. Two recent studies suggest that irradiation of the pelvic lymph nodes or even the whole bladder is not associated with a survival benefit. Tunio et al. randomized 230 patients to receive whole-pelvis ($n=120$) or bladder-only radiotherapy ($n=110$). No difference was found for bladder preservation, disease-free survival, and overall survival [45]. An even more restrictive volume was irradiated within the bladder cancer 2001 trial (BC 2001). The trial had a partial 2-by-2 factorial design. Patients were randomly assigned (in a 1:1 ratio) to undergo radiotherapy with or without synchronous chemotherapy with fluorouracil and mitomycin C and either whole-bladder radiotherapy or modified-volume radiotherapy to uninvolved bladder. Remarkably, pelvic lymph node relapse was documented only in 9 patients (4.9 %) in the chemoradiotherapy group and 12 (6.7 %) in the radiotherapy group, though detailed data are not yet available [44].

In summary, the available data indicate that differences in local control between different radiation schedules are more related to the total dose than to the fractionation regimens. Reduction of overall treatment time and large fraction sizes should be avoided, especially when radiotherapy is combined with concomitant chemotherapy. New treatment techniques, such as image-guided and intensity modulated radiotherapy as well as interstitial radiotherapy in selected cases (unifocal, small bulk disease) or the use of particle therapy, in particular protons, may allow dose escalation with the expectation to further improve tumor response and long-term local control. This has to be supported by further investigations on target volume definition [44, 45, 59–61, 63–66].

28.3.2 Induction, Concurrent, and Adjuvant Chemotherapy

The rationale for combining radiation therapy with chemotherapy after conservative surgery of the bladder tumor is twofold. First, certain cytotoxic agents may have the potential of sensitizing tumor cells to radiation and to inhibit repopulation during radiotherapy, thus increasing local cure rates. Second, the high rate of occult metastases necessitates an attempt to eradicate occult metastases that have already developed in as many as 50 % of muscle-invasive tumors [67, 68].

Until recently, the only prospective, randomized comparison of radiotherapy alone versus concomitant chemoradiotherapy in bladder cancer demonstrated an improved local control rate when cisplatin was given in conjunction with radiotherapy [69]. However, this was a small study (99 patients) and was not powered to detect even a 15 % improvement in survival. Over the past decades cisplatin-based chemoradiotherapy was the backbone of organ preserving regimen, especially in Boston and Erlangen. The intensification of the Erlangen concurrent chemotherapy protocols over the past 20 years yielded an increasing rate of complete response rates with 61 % for patients treated with radiotherapy alone, 66 % after chemoradiotherapy (CRT) with carboplatin, 82 % after CRT with cisplatin, and 87 % after CRT with 5-FU and cisplatin [23]. This was also associated with a significant improvement in overall survival.

As a landmark study, the above-mentioned BC 2001 trial confirmed the superiority of concurrent chemoradiotherapy to radiotherapy alone. At 2 years, rates of locoregional disease-free survival were 67 % in the chemoradiotherapy group and 54 % in the radiotherapy group. Five-year rates of overall survival were 48 % in the chemoradiotherapy group and 35 % in the radiotherapy group. Toxicity grade 3 or 4 was slightly more common in the chemoradiotherapy group during treatment but not during follow-up. In conclusion concurrent chemoradiotherapy with 5FU and mitomycin-C was effective and tolerated well in this elderly, relatively frail group of patients [44]. In our opinion, the most effective agent for concurrent therapy remains cisplatin. Nevertheless, 5-floururacil with mitomycin C, paclitaxel or docetaxel alone are valid alternatives for patients not able to receive cisplatin. However, the optimal regimen and combination of radiotherapy with chemotherapy remains to be established.

In the Radiation Therapy Oncology Group (RTOG) series, a major effort was undertaken to determine the role of induction chemotherapy in studies 88-02 and, in a randomized design, in 89-03 (Table 28.1) [9, 10]. In the latter study, treating patients with two cycles of induction MCV (methotrexate, cisplatin, vinblastine), failed to improve complete response, local tumor control and survival. Moreover, due to toxicity, only 67 % of patients completed the MCV induction chemotherapy. As a result, subsequent studies employed adjuvant rather than neoadjuvant chemotherapy. However, in RTOG 97-06, again only 40 % of patients went on to receive a full three cycles of adjuvant MCV chemotherapy [13].

Newer chemotherapeutic agents, particularly gemcitabine and the taxanes, have shown significant single agent activity against urothelial tumors and both have exhibited higher response rates and acceptable toxicity when used in combination with cisplatin or even as triplet regimen in metastatic disease. Moreover, both paclitaxel and gemcitabine are potent radiation sensitizers. Recent phase I/II studies established gemcitabine in combination with radiotherapy as a feasible regimen in bladder-sparing treatment. Long-term results, meanwhile available, show high rates in terms of overall, disease-specific and bladder intact survival [37–42]. Series of concurrent chemoradiotherapy regimen using platinum and paclitaxel or docetaxel, respectively, have also recently been published [18, 70, 71]. The RTOG started a trial using paclitaxel and cisplatin concomitantly with twice-daily irradiation followed by either selective bladder preservation or radical cystectomy and four cycles of adjuvant chemotherapy with gemcitabine and cisplatin (RTOG 99-06). In 2009 the results from this trial have been reported: the complete response rate after induction therapy was 81, 70 % completed all treatment per protocol or with minor variation, and the 5-year rate of overall survival 56 % [33]. Recently, the successor trial, a randomized multicenter phase II trial, compared the same regimen of RTOG 99-06 with twice-daily radiation plus 5-fluorouracil-cisplatin (RTOG 0233). The 5-year overall survival was almost identical in both groups with 71 % for patients receiving paclitaxel-cisplatin and 75 % for patients with 5-fluorouracil-cisplatin. No major differences in toxicity regarding both schedules were found [34].

Another new component to enhance efficacy of trimodality therapy is of more technical origin. The University of Erlangen launched a phase II trial to evaluate the safety and efficacy of adding concurrent deep regional hyperthermia to their well-established trimodality bladder-preserving treatment approach [36]. The rationale came from two recent randomized clinical trials reported improved clinical results when adding hyperthermia to chemotherapy [72] or radiotherapy [73] for bladder cancer patients, respectively. The first one added hyperthermia to intravesical mitomycin-C instillation after TUR for intermediate- and high-risk superficial T1 bladder cancer, and demonstrated a significantly reduced local failure rate at 2 years (17.1 vs. 57.5 %, $p = 0.0002$) [72]. In the second trial, hyperthermia combined with radiotherapy significantly increased the complete response rate (73 vs. 51 %, $p = 0.01$) for muscle-invasive bladder cancer, and was associated with a non-significant trend toward improved local control rates (42 vs. 33 %, $p = $ n.s.). The Erlangen group reported within their quadrimodal approach a complete response rate of 96 % (43 of 45 patients). Local recurrence-free survival was 85 %, overall survival was 80 %, disease-specific survival was 88 %, metastasis-free survival was 89 % and thus all with a bladder-preserving rate of 96 % at 3 years [36].

Modification of tumor hypoxia, either with hyperbaric oxygen or hypoxic cell sensitizers, during radiotherapy may be another avenue of improving radiosensitivity. Hoskin et al. used nicotinamide together with carbogen (95 % O_2 with 5 % CO_2) and radical radiotherapy in a phase III study for bladder cancer (ARCON-study). The primary end point defined as local control after cystoscopy at 6 months was not significantly different between radiotherapy with carbogen and nicotinamide compared to radiotherapy alone (81 % vs. 76 %). However, just more than half of patients underwent cystoscopy at that time. In contrast 3-year estimates of overall survival were 59 and 46 % ($p = 0.04$) and 3-year estimates of recurrence-free survival 54 and 43 % ($p = 0.06$) in favor of radiotherapy with carbogen and nicotinamide [74].

Future aspects of radiosensitization relate to the potential inhibition of oncogene products frequently activated and overexpressed in bladder cancer, such as H-ras and c-erbB-1. Treatment of mice expressing activated H-ras bladder cancer cell line tumors with farnesyltransferase inhibitors

Table 28.3 Role of molecular markers in predicting favorable or unfavorable outcome in bladder cancer series treated with radiotherapy alone or with radiotherapy as a treatment component

	Favorable			No effect	Unfavorable		
	TR/LC	DFS/DSS	OS		TR/LC	DFS/DSS	OS
High-AI	X [96], X [89], X [81], X [98]	X [84]	X [84]		X [87]		X [87]
bcl-2 overexpr.				X [96], X [82]	X [91], X [94]	X [91]	X [85]
bax overexpr.				X [102]			
p53 overexpr.	X [97]	X [97]	X [97]	X [23], X [85], X [99], X [82], X [95], X [92], X [86], X [93], X [80], X [90, 103, 104]	X [89], X [91]	X [91], X [83]	X [83]
Loss of pRb	X [79], X [93], X [94]	X [79]	X [79]	X [89], X [86], X [83], X [80]			
Cyclin D1 overexpr.				X [89]			
p21 overexpr.			X [92]	X [105], X [95], X [91]		X [83]	X [83]
p16 overexpr.				X [80], X [105]		X [106]	
p27 overexpr.				X [105]			
mdm2 overexpr.				X [97]			
High-Ki67	X [96], X [98, 107]	X [98]		X [92, 104]	X [88]	X [89], X [102]	
High-MI	X [81]			X [87]			
DNA aneuploidy			X [108]	X [109]	X [110]	X [110]	
GLUT1/CAIX				X [111]		X [100]	X [100]
EGFR overexpr.		X [80]	X [80]				
Her2/neu overexpr.					X [80, 103]		
High – XRCC1		X [101]					
High – APE1		X [101]					
Survivin overexpr.				X [103]	X [112]		
MRE 11 high						X [104, 106]	

TIP 60	X [106]		
NFκB pos	X	X [103]	
VEGF B/C/R2 overexpr.		X [113]	X [113]

TR Tumor response, *LC* Local control, *DFS* Disease-free survival, *DSS* Disease-specific survival, *OS* Overall survival

Glossary: *AI* Apoptotic index; *bcl-2* Antiapoptotic protein, prevents activation of proapoptotic caspase proteins; *bax* Homo- or heterodimers of proapototic bax repress the antiapototic activity of bcl-2; *p53* Transcriptional activator of genes with a p53-binding site, associated with cell cycle arrest and apoptosis; *Rb* Retinoblastoma protein, its phosphorylation state has important implications for cell cycle progression; *Cyclin D* Pairs with cyclin-dependent kinases CDK 4 and 6 and acts in the G1 phase of the cell cycle; *p16, p21* and *p27* Cyclin-dependent kinase inhibitors, bind to cyclin-CDK-complexes, leading to cell cycle arrest in the G1-phase; *mdm2* (Mouse double minute 2), induction of mdm2 transcription is induced by p53 and results in p53 degradation; *Ki67* Marker of proliferation, expressed in the nucleus of proliferating cells; *MI* Mitotic index; *GLUT1/CAIX* Glucose transporter-1 protein and carbonic anhydrase IX are both regulated by hypoxia inducible factor-1 (HIF-1), intrinsic cellular markers of hypoxia; *EGFR* Epidermal growth factor receptor; *HER2/neu* Human epithelial growth factor receptor-2, belongs to the EGFR family, activation leads to proliferative signals within the cells; *XRCC1* and *APE1* X-ray repair cross complement group 1 and human AP endonuclease: DNA repair proteins of the base excision repair pathway. *MRE11* Meiotic recombination 11 homolog, *TIP 60* Tat-interactive protein; *VEGF* Vascular endothelial growth factor

(which inhibit the posttranslational modifications of H-ras) before irradiation significantly decreased tumor cell clonogenicity and tumor regrowth [75]. Inhibition of EGF receptor activity with small molecule tyrosine kinase inhibitors or antibodies against receptors may also markedly increase tumor radiosensitization in bladder cancer [76].

28.3.3 Patient Selection: Predictive and Prognostic Factors

Clinical criteria helpful in determining patients for bladder preservation include variables such as small tumor size (less than 5 cm), early tumor stage, a visibly and microscopically complete TUR, absence of ureteral obstruction, and no evidence of pelvic lymph node metastases. On multivariate analysis, the completeness of TUR was found to be one of the strongest prognostic factors for overall survival [23]. Thus, a TUR as thorough as safely possible should always be attempted. Patients at greater risk of new tumor development after initial complete response are those with multifocal disease and extensive associated carcinoma in situ at presentation. Anemia has also been shown to predict reduced local control as well as a higher rate of distant metastases and death from bladder cancer [77]. Recently, the group at the MGH developed nomograms predicting the response to bladder preserving treatment. The final nomograms included information on clinical T stage, presence of hydronephrosis, whether a visibly complete transurethral resection of bladder tumor was performed, age, sex, and tumor grade. With these nomograms individualized estimates of complete response, disease-specific survival, and bladder intact disease-specific survival became possible [78].

Translational research to identify molecular markers that may better identify a tumor's true malignant potential as well as its response to specific cytotoxic therapies are sorely needed. Overall, the findings on molecular markers do not yet confirm that abnormal expression of any of these proteins unequivocally predicts tumor response—with possibly one exception: higher rates of spontaneous apoptosis were significantly related to better initial response and better local control with bladder preservation in most studies (Table 28.3) [79–101]. Apoptosis represents a biological endpoint regulated by many factors, including p53, bcl-2 and bax, pRb, among others. It is now becoming increasingly clear that the inability to undergo apoptosis due to overexpression of bcl-2 or overexpression of survivin, a member of the inhibitor of apoptosis family, may predict local failure after irradiation and chemotherapy. The RTOG Genitourinary Translational Research Group has recently published results from 73 patients treated within the RTOG trials: Her-2 expression was significantly associated with reduced tumor response, whereas the epidermal growth factor receptor (EGFR) expression intriguingly predicted for improved overall and disease-specific survival [80]. Based on these findings, a recently activated RTOG trial (RTOG 05-24) uses chemoradiation with paclitaxel and trastuzumab for Her-2 overexpressing tumors (2+ or greater immunohistochemical staining), whereas patients with less than 2+ Her-2 staining will receive radiotherapy with weekly paclitaxel but not trastuzumab.

References

1. Rodel C, Weiss C, Sauer R. Trimodality treatment and selective organ preservation for bladder cancer. J Clin Oncol. 2006;24:5536–44.
2. Kaufman DS, Shipley WU, Feldman AS. Bladder cancer. Lancet. 2009;374:239–49.
3. Rodel C. Current status of radiation therapy and combined-modality treatment for bladder cancer. Strahlenther Onkol. 2004;180:701–9.
4. Shipley WU, Prout Jr GR, Einstein AB, et al. Treatment of invasive bladder cancer by cisplatin and radiation in patients unsuited for surgery. JAMA. 1987;258:931–5.
5. Housset M, Maulard C, Chretien Y, et al. Combined radiation and chemotherapy for invasive transitional-cell carcinoma of the bladder: a prospective study. J Clin Oncol. 1993;11:2150–7.
6. Sauer R, Dunst J, Altendorf-Hofmann A, et al. Radiotherapy with and without cisplatin in bladder cancer. Int J Radiat Oncol Biol Phys. 1990;19:687–91.
7. Kachnic LA, Kaufman DS, Heney NM, et al. Bladder preservation by combined modality therapy for invasive bladder cancer. J Clin Oncol. 1997;15:1022–9.

8. Tester W, Porter A, Asbell S, et al. Combined modality program with possible organ preservation for invasive bladder carcinoma: results of RTOG protocol 85-12. Int J Radiat Oncol Biol Phys. 1993;25:783–90.

9. Tester W, Caplan R, Heaney J, et al. Neoadjuvant combined modality program with selective organ preservation for invasive bladder cancer: results of Radiation Therapy Oncology Group phase II trial 8802. J Clin Oncol. 1996;14:119–26.

10. Shipley WU, Winter KA, Kaufman DS, et al. Phase III trial of neoadjuvant chemotherapy in patients with invasive bladder cancer treated with selective bladder preservation by combined radiation therapy and chemotherapy: initial results of Radiation Therapy Oncology Group 89-03. J Clin Oncol. 1998;16:3576–83.

11. Zietman AL, Shipley WU, Kaufman DS, et al. A phase I/II trial of transurethral surgery combined with concurrent cisplatin, 5-fluorouracil and twice daily radiation followed by selective bladder preservation in operable patients with muscle invading bladder cancer. J Urol. 1998;160:1673–7.

12. Kaufman DS, Winter KA, Shipley WU, et al. The initial results in muscle-invading bladder cancer of RTOG 95-06: phase I/II trial of transurethral surgery plus radiation therapy with concurrent cisplatin and 5-fluorouracil followed by selective bladder preservation or cystectomy depending on the initial response. Oncologist. 2000;5:471–6.

13. Hagan MP, Winter KA, Kaufman DS, et al. RTOG 97-06: initial report of a phase I-II trial of selective bladder conservation using TURBT, twice-daily accelerated irradiation sensitized with cisplatin, and adjuvant MCV combination chemotherapy. Int J Radiat Oncol Biol Phys. 2003;57:665–72.

14. Russell KJ, Boileau MA, Higano C, et al. Combined 5-fluorouracil and irradiation for transitional cell carcinoma of the urinary bladder. Int J Radiat Oncol Biol Phys. 1990;19:693–9.

15. Rotman M, Aziz H, Porrazzo M, et al. Treatment of advanced transitional cell carcinoma of the bladder with irradiation and concomitant 5-fluorouracil infusion. Int J Radiat Oncol Biol Phys. 1990;18:1131–7.

16. Given RW, Parsons JT, McCarley D, et al. Bladder-sparing multimodality treatment of muscle-invasive bladder cancer: a five-year follow-up. Urology. 1995;46:499–504.

17. Housset M, Dufour B, Maulard-Durdux C, Chretien Y, Mejean A. Concomitant fluorouracil (5-FU)-cisplatin (CDDP) and bifractionated split course radiation therapy (BSCRT) for invasive bladder cancer. Proc Am Soc Clin Oncol. 1997;16:319a. Abstract.

18. Varveris H, Delakas D, Anezinis P, et al. Concurrent platinum and docetaxel chemotherapy and external radical radiotherapy in patients with invasive transitional cell bladder carcinoma. A preliminary report of tolerance and local control. Anticancer Res. 1997;17:4771–80.

19. Fellin G, Graffer U, Bolner A, et al. Combined chemotherapy and radiation with selective organ preservation for muscle-invasive bladder carcinoma. A single-institution phase II study. Br J Urol. 1997;80:44–9.

20. Cervek J, Cufer T, Zakotnik B, et al. Invasive bladder cancer: our experience with bladder sparing approach. Int J Radiat Oncol Biol Phys. 1998;41:273–8.

21. Zapatero A, Martin de Vidales C, Marin A, et al. Invasive bladder cancer: a single-institution experience with bladder-sparing approach. Int J Cancer. 2000;90:287–94.

22. Arias F, Dominguez MA, Martinez E, et al. Chemoradiotherapy for muscle invading bladder carcinoma. Final report of a single institutional organ-sparing program. Int J Radiat Oncol Biol Phys. 2000;47:373–8.

23. Rodel C, Grabenbauer GG, Kuhn R, et al. Combined-modality treatment and selective organ preservation in invasive bladder cancer: long-term results. J Clin Oncol. 2002;20:3061–71.

24. Chen WC, Liaw CC, Chuang CK, et al. Concurrent cisplatin, 5-fluorouracil, leucovorin, and radiotherapy for invasive bladder cancer. Int J Radiat Oncol Biol Phys. 2003;56:726–33.

25. Peyromaure M, Slama J, Beuzeboc P, et al. Concurrent chemoradiotherapy for clinical stage T2 bladder cancer: report of a single institution. Urology. 2004;63:73–7.

26. Danesi DT, Arcangeli G, Cruciani E, et al. Conservative treatment of invasive bladder carcinoma by transurethral resection, protracted intravenous infusion chemotherapy, and hyperfractionated radiotherapy: long term results. Cancer. 2004;101:2540–8.

27. Hussain SA, Stocken DD, Peake DR, et al. Long-term results of a phase II study of synchronous chemoradiotherapy in advanced muscle invasive bladder cancer. Br J Cancer. 2004;90:2106–11.

28. Kragelj B, Zaletel-Kragelj L, Sedmak B, et al. Phase II study of radiochemotherapy with vinblastine in invasive bladder cancer. Radiother Oncol. 2005;75:44–7.

29. Dunst J, Diestelhorst A, Kuhn R, et al. Organ-sparing treatment in muscle-invasive bladder cancer. Strahlenther Onkol. 2005;181:632–7.

30. Shipley WU, Kaufman DS, Zehr E, et al. Selective bladder preservation by combined modality protocol treatment: long-term outcomes of 190 patients with invasive bladder cancer. Urology. 2002;60:62–7. discussion 67-68.

31. Efstathiou JA, Spiegel DY, Shipley WU, et al. Long-term outcomes of selective bladder preservation by combined-modality therapy for invasive bladder cancer: the MGH experience. Eur Urol. 2012;61:705–11.

32. Krause FS, Walter B, Ott OJ, et al. 15-year survival rates after transurethral resection and radiochemotherapy or radiation in bladder cancer treatment. Anticancer Res. 2011;31:985–90.

33. Kaufman DS, Winter KA, Shipley WU, et al. Phase I-II RTOG study (99-06) of patients with muscle-invasive bladder cancer undergoing transurethral surgery, paclitaxel, cisplatin, and twice-daily radiotherapy followed by selective bladder preservation or radical cystectomy and adjuvant chemotherapy. Urology. 2009;73:833–7.

34. Mitin T, Hunt D, Shipley WU, et al. Transurethral surgery and twice-daily radiation plus paclitaxel-cisplatin or fluorouracil-cisplatin with selective bladder preservation and adjuvant chemotherapy for patients with muscle invasive bladder cancer (RTOG 0233): a randomised multicentre phase 2 trial. Lancet Oncol. 2013;14(9):863–72.

35. Muller AC, Diestelhorst A, Kuhnt T, et al. Organ-sparing treatment of advanced bladder cancer: paclitaxel as a radiosensitizer. Strahlenther Onkol. 2007;183:177–83.

36. Wittlinger M, Rodel CM, Weiss C, et al. Quadrimodal treatment of high-risk T1 and T2 bladder cancer: transurethral tumor resection followed by concurrent radiochemotherapy and regional deep hyperthermia. Radiother Oncol. 2009;93(2):358–63.

37. Caffo O, Fellin G, Graffer U, et al. Gemcitabine and radiotherapy plus cisplatin after transurethral resection as conservative treatment for infiltrating bladder cancer: long-term cumulative results of 2 prospective single-institution studies. Cancer. 2011;117:1190–6.

38. Caffo O, Fellin G, Graffer U, et al. Phase I study of gemcitabine and radiotherapy plus cisplatin after transurethral resection as conservative treatment for infiltrating bladder cancer. Int J Radiat Oncol Biol Phys. 2003;57:1310–6.

39. Kent E, Sandler H, Montie J, et al. Combined-modality therapy with gemcitabine and radiotherapy as a bladder preservation strategy: results of a phase I trial. J Clin Oncol. 2004;22:2540–5.

40. Oh KS, Soto DE, Smith DC, et al. Combined-modality therapy with gemcitabine and radiation therapy as a bladder preservation strategy: long-term results of a phase I trial. Int J Radiat Oncol Biol Phys. 2009;74:511–7.

41. Sangar VK, McBain CA, Lyons J, et al. Phase I study of conformal radiotherapy with concurrent gemcitabine in locally advanced bladder cancer. Int J Radiat Oncol Biol Phys. 2005;61:420–5.

42. Choudhury A, Swindell R, Logue JP, et al. Phase II study of conformal hypofractionated radiotherapy with concurrent gemcitabine in muscle-invasive bladder cancer. J Clin Oncol. 2011;29:733–8.

43. Zapatero A, Martin De Vidales C, Arellano R, et al. Long-term results of two prospective bladder-sparing trimodality approaches for invasive bladder cancer: neoadjuvant chemotherapy and concurrent radio-chemotherapy. Urology. 2012;80:1056–62.

44. James ND, Hussain SA, Hall E, et al. Radiotherapy with or without chemotherapy in muscle-invasive bladder cancer. N Engl J Med. 2012;366:1477–88.

45. Tunio MA, Hashmi A, Qayyum A, et al. Whole-pelvis or bladder-only chemoradiation for lymph node-negative invasive bladder cancer: single-institution experience. Int J Radiat Oncol Biol Phys. 2012;82:e457–62.

46. Greven KM, Solin LJ, Hanks GE. Prognostic factors in patients with bladder carcinoma treated with definitive irradiation. Cancer. 1990;65:908–12.

47. Smaaland R, Akslen LA, Tonder B, et al. Radical radiation treatment of invasive and locally advanced bladder carcinoma in elderly patients. Br J Urol. 1991;67:61–9.

48. Moonen L, vd Voet H, de Nijs R, et al. Muscle-invasive bladder cancer treated with external beam radiation: influence of total dose, overall treatment time, and treatment interruption on local control. Int J Radiat Oncol Biol Phys. 1998;42:525–30.

49. Quilty PM, Kerr GR, Duncan W. Prognostic indices for bladder cancer: an analysis of patients with transitional cell carcinoma of the bladder primarily treated by radical megavoltage X-ray therapy. Radiother Oncol. 1986;7:311–21.

50. Pollack A, Zagars GK, Swanson DA. Muscle-invasive bladder cancer treated with external beam radiotherapy: prognostic factors. Int J Radiat Oncol Biol Phys. 1994;30:267–77.

51. Shipley WU, Rose MA, Perrone TL, et al. Full-dose irradiation for patients with invasive bladder carcinoma: clinical and histological factors prognostic of improved survival. J Urol. 1985;134:679–83.

52. Pos FJ, Hart G, Schneider C, et al. Radical radiotherapy for invasive bladder cancer: what dose and fractionation schedule to choose? Int J Radiat Oncol Biol Phys. 2006;64:1168–73.

53. Naslund I, Nilsson B, Littbrand B. Hyperfractionated radiotherapy of bladder cancer. A ten-year follow-up of a randomized clinical trial. Acta Oncol. 1994;33:397–402.

54. Goldobenko GV, Matveev BP, Shipilov VI, et al. Radiation treatment of bladder cancer using different fractionation regimens. Med Radiol (Mosk). 1991;36:14–6.

55. Stuschke M, Thames HD. Hyperfractionated radiotherapy of human tumors: overview of the randomized clinical trials. Int J Radiat Oncol Biol Phys. 1997;37:259–67.

56. Maciejewski B, Majewski S. Dose fractionation and tumour repopulation in radiotherapy for bladder cancer. Radiother Oncol. 1991;21:163–70.

57. Horwich A, Dearnaley D, Huddart R, et al. A randomised trial of accelerated radiotherapy for localised invasive bladder cancer. Radiother Oncol. 2005;75:34–43.

58. Kob D, Arndt J, Kriester A, et al. Results of percutaneous radiotherapy of bladder cancer using 1 and 2 series of irradiation. Strahlenther Onkol. 1985;161:673–7.

59. Foroudi F, Wong J, Kron T, et al. Online adaptive radiotherapy for muscle-invasive bladder cancer:

results of a pilot study. Int J Radiat Oncol Biol Phys. 2011;81:765–71.

60. McDonald F, Lalondrelle S, Taylor H, et al. Clinical implementation of adaptive hypofractionated bladder radiotherapy for improvement in normal tissue irradiation. Clin Oncol (R Coll Radiol). 2013;25(9):549–56.

61. Pos FJ, Hulshof M, Lebesque J, et al. Adaptive radiotherapy for invasive bladder cancer: a feasibility study. Int J Radiat Oncol Biol Phys. 2006;64:862–8.

62. Sondergaard J, Olsen KO, Muren LP, et al. A study of image-guided radiotherapy of bladder cancer based on lipiodol injection in the bladder wall. Acta Oncol. 2010;49:1109–15.

63. Henry AM, Stratford J, McCarthy C, et al. X-ray volume imaging in bladder radiotherapy verification. Int J Radiat Oncol Biol Phys. 2006;64:1174–8.

64. Pos F, Horenblas S, Dom P, et al. Organ preservation in invasive bladder cancer: brachytherapy, an alternative to cystectomy and combined modality treatment? Int J Radiat Oncol Biol Phys. 2005;61:678–86.

65. Hata M, Miyanaga N, Tokuuye K, et al. Proton beam therapy for invasive bladder cancer: a prospective study of bladder-preserving therapy with combined radiotherapy and intra-arterial chemotherapy. Int J Radiat Oncol Biol Phys. 2006;64:1371–9.

66. Foroudi F, Wilson L, Bressel M, et al. A dosimetric comparison of 3D conformal vs intensity modulated vs volumetric arc radiation therapy for muscle invasive bladder cancer. Radiat Oncol. 2012;7:111.

67. Hautmann RE, de Petriconi RC, Pfeiffer C, et al. Radical cystectomy for urothelial carcinoma of the bladder without neoadjuvant or adjuvant therapy: long-term results in 1100 patients. Eur Urol. 2012;61:1039–47.

68. Stein JP, Lieskovsky G, Cote R, et al. Radical cystectomy in the treatment of invasive bladder cancer: long-term results in 1,054 patients. J Clin Oncol. 2001;19:666–75.

69. Coppin CM, Gospodarowicz MK, James K, et al. Improved local control of invasive bladder cancer by concurrent cisplatin and preoperative or definitive radiation. The National Cancer Institute of Canada Clinical Trials Group. J Clin Oncol. 1996;14:2901–7.

70. Nichols Jr RC, Sweetser MG, Mahmood SK, et al. Radiation therapy and concomitant paclitaxel/carboplatin chemotherapy for muscle invasive transitional cell carcinoma of the bladder: a well-tolerated combination. Int J Cancer. 2000;90:281–6.

71. Dunst J, Weigel C, Heynemann H, et al. Preliminary results of simultaneous radiochemotherapy with paclitaxel for urinary bladder cancer. Strahlenther Onkol. 1999;175 Suppl 3:7–10.

72. Colombo R, Da Pozzo LF, Salonia A, et al. Multicentric study comparing intravesical chemotherapy alone and with local microwave hyperthermia for prophylaxis of recurrence of superficial transitional cell carcinoma. J Clin Oncol. 2003;21:4270–6.

73. van der Zee J, Gonzalez Gonzalez D, van Rhoon GC, et al. Comparison of radiotherapy alone with radiotherapy plus hyperthermia in locally advanced pelvic tumours: a prospective, randomised, multicentre trial. Dutch Deep Hyperthermia Group. Lancet. 2000;355:1119–25.

74. Hoskin PJ, Rojas AM, Bentzen SM, et al. Radiotherapy with concurrent carbogen and nicotinamide in bladder carcinoma. J Clin Oncol. 2010;28:4912–8.

75. Cohen-Jonathan E, Muschel RJ, Gillies McKenna W, et al. Farnesyltransferase inhibitors potentiate the antitumor effect of radiation on a human tumor xenograft expressing activated HRAS. Radiat Res. 2000;154:125–32.

76. Bellmunt J, Hussain M, Dinney CP. Novel approaches with targeted therapies in bladder cancer. Therapy of bladder cancer by blockade of the epidermal growth factor receptor family. Crit Rev Oncol Hematol. 2003;46(Suppl):85–104.

77. Gospodarowicz MK, Hawkins NV, Rawlings GA, et al. Radical radiotherapy for muscle invasive transitional cell carcinoma of the bladder: failure analysis. J Urol. 1989;142:1448–53. discussion 1453–4.

78. Coen JJ, Paly JJ, Niemierko A, et al. Nomograms predicting response to therapy and outcomes after bladder-preserving trimodality therapy for muscle-invasive bladder cancer. Int J Radiat Oncol Biol Phys. 2013;86:311–6.

79. Agerbaek M, Alsner J, Marcussen N, et al. Retinoblastoma protein expression is an independent predictor of both radiation response and survival in muscle-invasive bladder cancer. Br J Cancer. 2003;89:298–304.

80. Chakravarti A, Winter K, Wu CL, et al. Expression of the epidermal growth factor receptor and Her-2 are predictors of favorable outcome and reduced complete response rates, respectively, in patients with muscle-invading bladder cancers treated by concurrent radiation and cisplatin-based chemotherapy: a report from the Radiation Therapy Oncology Group. Int J Radiat Oncol Biol Phys. 2005;62:309–17.

81. Chyle V, Pollack A, Czerniak B, et al. Apoptosis and downstaging after preoperative radiotherapy for muscle-invasive bladder cancer. Int J Radiat Oncol Biol Phys. 1996;35:281–7.

82. Cooke PW, James ND, Ganesan R, et al. Bcl-2 expression identifies patients with advanced bladder cancer treated by radiotherapy who benefit from neoadjuvant chemotherapy. BJU Int. 2000;85: 829–35.

83. Garcia del Muro X, Condom E, Vigues F, et al. p53 and p21 expression levels predict organ preservation and survival in invasive bladder carcinoma treated with a combined-modality approach. Cancer. 2004;100:1859–67.

84. Harada S, Sato R, Nakamura R, et al. The correlation between spontaneous and radiation-induced apoptosis in T3B bladder cancer (histological grade G3), and the precedence between the two kinds of apopto-

sis for predicting clinical prognosis. Int J Radiat Oncol Biol Phys. 2000;48:1059–67.

85. Hussain SA, Ganesan R, Hiller L, et al. BCL2 expression predicts survival in patients receiving synchronous chemoradiotherapy in advanced transitional cell carcinoma of the bladder. Oncol Rep. 2003;10:571–6.

86. Jahnson S, Risberg B, Karlsson MG, et al. p53 and Rb immunostaining in locally advanced bladder cancer: relation to prognostic variables and predictive value for the local response to radical radiotherapy. Eur Urol. 1995;28:135–42.

87. Lara PC, Perez S, Rey A, et al. Apoptosis in carcinoma of the bladder: relation with radiation treatment results. Int J Radiat Oncol Biol Phys. 1999;43:1015–9.

88. Lara PC, Rey A, Santana C, et al. The role of Ki67 proliferation assessment in predicting local control in bladder cancer patients treated by radical radiation therapy. Radiother Oncol. 1998;49:163–7.

89. Moonen L, Ong F, Gallee M, et al. Apoptosis, proliferation and p53, cyclin D1, and retinoblastoma gene expression in relation to radiation response in transitional cell carcinoma of the bladder. Int J Radiat Oncol Biol Phys. 2001;49:1305–10.

90. Ogura K, Habuchi T, Yamada H, et al. Immunohistochemical analysis of p53 and proliferating cell nuclear antigen (PCNA) in bladder cancer: positive immunostaining and radiosensitivity. Int J Urol. 1995;2:302–8.

91. Ong F, Moonen LM, Gallee MP, et al. Prognostic factors in transitional cell cancer of the bladder: an emerging role for Bcl-2 and p53. Radiother Oncol. 2001;61:169–75.

92. Osen I, Fossa SD, Majak B, et al. Prognostic factors in muscle-invasive bladder cancer treated with radiotherapy: an immunohistochemical study. Br J Urol. 1998;81:862–9.

93. Pollack A, Czerniak B, Zagars GK, et al. Retinoblastoma protein expression and radiation response in muscle-invasive bladder cancer. Int J Radiat Oncol Biol Phys. 1997;39:687–95.

94. Pollack A, Wu CS, Czerniak B, et al. Abnormal bcl-2 and pRb expression are independent correlates of radiation response in muscle-invasive bladder cancer. Clin Cancer Res. 1997;3:1823–9.

95. Qureshi KN, Griffiths TR, Robinson MC, et al. Combined p21WAF1/CIP1 and p53 overexpression predict improved survival in muscle-invasive bladder cancer treated by radical radiotherapy. Int J Radiat Oncol Biol Phys. 2001;51:1234–40.

96. Rodel C, Grabenbauer GG, Rodel F, et al. Apoptosis, p53, bcl-2, and Ki-67 in invasive bladder carcinoma: possible predictors for response to radiochemotherapy and successful bladder preservation. Int J Radiat Oncol Biol Phys. 2000;46:1213–21.

97. Rotterud R, Berner A, Holm R, et al. p53, p21 and mdm2 expression vs the response to radiotherapy in transitional cell carcinoma of the bladder. BJU Int. 2001;88:202–8.

98. Weiss C, Rodel F, Wolf I, et al. Combined-modality treatment and organ preservation in bladder cancer. Do molecular markers predict outcome? Strahlenther Onkol. 2005;181:213–22.

99. Wu CS, Pollack A, Czerniak B, et al. Prognostic value of p53 in muscle-invasive bladder cancer treated with preoperative radiotherapy. Urology. 1996;47:305–10.

100. Hoskin PJ, Sibtain A, Daley FM, et al. GLUT1 and CAIX as intrinsic markers of hypoxia in bladder cancer: relationship with vascularity and proliferation as predictors of outcome of ARCON. Br J Cancer. 2003;89:1290–7.

101. Sak SC, Harnden P, Johnston CF, et al. APE1 and XRCC1 protein expression levels predict cancer-specific survival following radical radiotherapy in bladder cancer. Clin Cancer Res. 2005;11:6205–11.

102. Matsumoto H, Wada T, Fukunaga K, et al. Bax to Bcl-2 ratio and Ki-67 index are useful predictors of neoadjuvant chemoradiation therapy in bladder cancer. Jpn J Clin Oncol. 2004;34:124–30.

103. Koga F, Yoshida S, Tatokoro M, et al. ErbB2 and NFkappaB overexpression as predictors of chemoradiation resistance and putative targets to overcome resistance in muscle-invasive bladder cancer. PLoS One. 2011;6:e27616.

104. Choudhury A, Nelson LD, Teo MT, et al. MRE11 expression is predictive of cause-specific survival following radical radiotherapy for muscle-invasive bladder cancer. Cancer Res. 2010;70:7017–26.

105. Rotterud R, Pettersen EO, Berner A, et al. Cell cycle inhibitors and outcome after radiotherapy in bladder cancer patients. Acta Oncol. 2002;41:463–70.

106. Laurberg JR, Brems-Eskildsen AS, Nordentoft I, et al. Expression of TIP60 (tat-interactive protein) and MRE11 (meiotic recombination 11 homolog) predict treatment-specific outcome of localised invasive bladder cancer. BJU Int. 2012;110:E1228–36.

107. Weiss C, Rodel F, Ott O, et al. Pretreatment proliferation and local control in bladder cancer after radiotherapy with or without concurrent chemotherapy. Strahlenther Onkol. 2007;183:552–6.

108. Hug EB, Donnelly SM, Shipley WU, et al. Deoxyribonucleic acid flow cytometry in invasive bladder carcinoma: a possible predictor for successful bladder preservation following transurethral surgery and chemotherapy-radiotherapy. J Urol. 1992;148:47–51.

109. Jenkins BJ, Martin JE, Baithun SI, et al. Prediction of response to radiotherapy in invasive bladder cancer. Br J Urol. 1990;65:345–8.

110. Wijkstrom H, Tribukait B. Deoxyribonucleic acid flow cytometry in predicting response to radical radiotherapy of bladder cancer. J Urol. 1990;144:646–50.

111. Sherwood BT, Colquhoun AJ, Richardson D, et al. Carbonic anhydrase IX expression and outcome

after radiotherapy for muscle-invasive bladder cancer. Clin Oncol (R Coll Radiol). 2007;19:777–83.

112. Weiss C, von Romer F, Capalbo G, et al. Survivin expression as a predictive marker for local control in patients with high-risk T1 bladder cancer treated with transurethral resection and radiochemotherapy. Int J Radiat Oncol Biol Phys. 2009;74:1455–60.

113. Lautenschlaeger T, George A, Klimowicz AC, et al. Bladder preservation therapy for muscle-invading bladder cancers on radiation therapy oncology group trials 8802, 8903, 9506, and 9706: vascular endothelial growth factor B overexpression predicts for increased distant metastasis and shorter survival. Oncologist. 2013;18:685–6.

Albert J. Chang, Maurice Marcel Garcia, and Mack Roach III

29.1 Introduction

Radical cystectomy with bilateral pelvic lymph node dissection is the standard of care for localized muscle invasive bladder cancer (cT2N0M0) or locally advanced bladder cancer (cT3-4N0M0). The standard approach includes the removal of the bladder, prostate, seminal vesicles, and distal ureters in men although partial or total prostate-sparing procedures are being evaluated by some investigators. In women, the bladder, urethra, adjacent vagina, uterus, and distal ureters are removed. Many patients with muscle invasive bladder cancer are not candidates for cystectomy due to poor performance status and medical comorbidities. Radical cystectomy is also associated with significant morbidity, risk of perioperative mortality, and decreased quality of life.

The multi-modality bladder preservation approach is becoming increasingly popular. Patients choosing the bladder preservation therapy undergo maximal transurethral resection of the bladder tumor (TURBT) followed by definitive chemoradiation therapy. This treatment approach offers similar survival outcomes to radical cystectomy with 5-year overall survival rates ranging from 40 to 60 % [1–4]. In addition, approximately two-thirds of patients undergoing this approach are alive with a functional bladder at 5 years [2].

29.2 Patient Work-Up

Patients must be carefully selected for bladder preservation to ensure the success of the treatment. To select patients for bladder preservation therapy, a comprehensive work-up should include (1) a detailed history and physical exam focusing on symptoms of hematuria, flank pain, urinary function, and bowel function; (2) routine bloodwork with a complete blood count evaluating for anemia and comprehensive metabolic panel with creatinine level for kidney function; (3) urinalysis with urine cytology; (4) office cystoscopy with biopsy; (5) CT or MR imaging of

A.J. Chang, M.D., Ph.D. (✉) • M. Roach III, M.D.
Department of Radiation Oncology, Helen Diller Family Comprehensive Cancer Center, University of California, San Francisco, 1600 Divisadero Street, Box 1708, San Francisco, CA 94115, USA
e-mail: changaj@radonc.ucsf.edu; mroach@radonc.ucsf.edu

M.M. Garcia, M.D., M.A.S.
Department of Urology, (Moffit-Long, Mount Zion), San Francisco General Hospital and The San Francisco Veteran's Adminstration Hospital, University of California San Francisco, 400 Parnassus Avenue, Box A-633, San Francisco, CA 94143, USA
e-mail: MGarcia@urology.ucsf.edu

B.R. Konety and S.S. Chang (eds.), *Management of Bladder Cancer: A Comprehensive Text With Clinical Scenarios*, DOI 10.1007/978-1-4939-1881-2_29,
© Springer Science+Business Media New York 2015

the abdomen and pelvis to evaluate for hydronephrosis, lesions in the upper urinary tract, extent of bladder involvement, lymph node involvement, and distant metastasis; and (6) chest x-ray or CT to rule out pulmonary metastasis. Also, an exam under anesthesia (EUA) should be performed with a maximally safe transurethral resection of the tumor. Bladder mapping with random biopsies of the bladder and prostatic urethra should be performed during the EUA to evaluate for multifocal disease.

29.3 Prognostic Factors

Positive prognostic factors for patients undergoing definitive chemoradiation are young age, good performance status, unifocal T2/T3a disease, absence of nodal disease, absence of CIS, low grade, small tumors with a maximal diameter of 5 cm in greatest dimension, normal kidney function with absence of hydronephrosis, good urinary function, and visibly complete TURBT. Patients with these factors should undergo a maximally safe TURBT in order to eliminate any gross disease. Bladder biopsies and prostatic urethra biopsies should be negative to rule out multifocal disease. Any hydronephrosis should be relieved with stent or nephrostomy tube placement. Adequate renal function is ideal as patients often receive platinum-based chemotherapy. Alternative chemotherapy options for patients with poor renal function include 5-fluorouracil/mitomycin-C and paclitaxel.

An important factor for the success of patients undergoing bladder preservation is the completeness of TURBT. Often patients may present to a radiation oncologist and medical oncologist after incomplete TURBT for consideration bladder preservation therapy. If there is any uncertainty regarding the completeness of TURBT, a discussion with the urologist performing the initial TURBT or a repeat cystoscopy with TURBT is indicated. Patients with incomplete TURBT are less likely to attain a complete response with chemoradiation and have decreased survival when compared with patients undergoing complete TURBT as highlighted in a recent study [5].

Some but not all studies suggest that the presence of carcinoma in situ (CIS) has been demonstrated to be a poor prognostic factor for failure of chemoradiation therapy. In a study involving 40 patients, CIS was identified to be the most significant factor associated with bladder local control. Patients with CIS were at ninefold increased risk of bladder recurrence than patients without CIS [6]. Patients with CIS also have lower CR rates suggesting that CIS may be associated with relative resistance to chemoradiation therapy [6, 7]. Although a poor prognostic factor for local recurrence, the presence of CIS should not be an absolute contraindication for bladder preservation therapy as approximately 50–60 % of patients with CIS still remain free from bladder recurrence [6].

Other poor prognostic factors include advanced T stage and tumor size >5 cm, which have been associated with decreased response rate, decreased relapse-free survival, and increased distant metastasis [8, 9]. Several series have demonstrated that patients with large T3 and T4 tumors have increased local recurrence and distant relapse rates compared to patients with T2 and small T3 tumors [9, 10]. Also, patients with tumors >5 cm have nearly a tenfold increased risk of developing distant metastases compared to patients with tumors less than 5 cm [6].

Patients with small capacity bladders and poor bladder function are less than ideal candidates for bladder preservation. Decreased bladder compliance and bladder irritation is a recognized effect of radiation therapy. As a result, patients with already poor bladder function and small capacity may experience further urgency, frequency, involuntary detrusor contractions, incontinence, and reduction in capacity after radiation treatment making their quality of life miserable. If medically fit, patients with poor bladder function should undergo radical cystectomy rather than bladder preservation therapy. After cystectomy and urinary diversion, these patients report good overall quality of life [11].

29.4 Evidence Supporting Bladder Preservation

Bladder preservation therapy was initially reserved for patients who were not candidates for surgery. The initial studies were performed in an unselected population of patients receiving radiotherapy alone without chemotherapy. In these series [9, 12–15], radiation was delivered to a total treatment dose of 55–65 Gy in five daily treatments per week with a resulting complete clinical response rate (cCR) of 40–52 % with approximately 41 % of patients free from an invasive recurrence. Patients who did not obtain a clinical complete response or experienced a local recurrence underwent salvage cystectomy [16].

Several studies were performed to compare the results of radical cystectomy with external beam radiotherapy. When evaluating these studies, it is important to note that the patients undergoing cystectomy were more likely to have earlier stage and smaller tumors, better performance status, and younger age than patients undergoing radiation therapy indicating a selection bias [17–19]. Another important point to consider when evaluating these studies is that patients undergoing bladder preservation were clinically staged while patients undergoing cystectomy were pathologically staged. Because clinical staging underestimates the stage in 50 % of patients [20], patients undergoing bladder preservation therapy were likely to have more advanced stage disease at presentation than reported. An additional source of bias includes the fact that delays in the initiation of therapy have been shown to negatively impact outcomes. Substantial delays may stem from the decision-making for surgical candidacy, the patients' refusal for surgery, the referral process, and the simulation and planning process.

The Danish National Bladder Cancer Group performed a study including 183 patients randomizing them to 40 Gy neoadjuvant radiotherapy followed by cystectomy or 60 Gy external beam radiotherapy alone arm. Patients in the radiotherapy alone arm experiencing local recurrence underwent salvage cystectomy. Again, no significant differences in OS were observed (29 vs. 23 %), but an increase in pelvic recurrences was reported in patients receiving radiotherapy alone (35 vs. 7 %) [19]. This study demonstrates the effectiveness of salvage cystectomy for local recurrences.

Subsequent reports suggested that administration of concurrent systemic treatment with radiation therapy after maximal TURBT improved clinical complete response (CR) rate and local control compared with radiotherapy alone. The National Cancer Institute of Canada randomized patients to radiation therapy alone or radiation with concurrent cisplatin. An improvement in pelvic failure was observed with chemoradiation (40 vs. 59 %). A similar studied was performed in 45 centers from the United Kingdom demonstrating improved bladder and pelvic control rates (67 vs. 54 %) with addition of 5-fluorouracil and mitomycin C to radiation compared with radiation alone. Thus trimodality treatment with maximal TURBT followed by concurrent chemoradiation therapy is the standard of care for patients with muscle invasive disease undergoing bladder preservation therapy.

The role of radiation has also been investigated in earlier stage, high-grade T1 bladder cancer. Following maximal TURBT, high-grade T1 bladder cancer has a 69–80 % chance of recurrence and a 33–48 % chance of progression to muscle invasive disease [21]. The Medical Research Council evaluated the role of radiation therapy in 210 patients with pT1 Grade 3 transitional cell bladder cancer after maximal TURBT. Patients with unifocal disease and no CIS were randomized to observation or 60 Gy radiotherapy. Patients with mutifocal disease were randomized to intravesical therapy (mitomycin C—MMC) or the Bacille Calmette-Guérin (BCG) vaccine or 60 Gy radiotherapy. No statistical differences in 5-year PFS (52 control vs. 41 % radiotherapy) or OS (61 control vs. 52.5 % radiotherapy) were observed. The investigators concluded that addition of radiotherapy is not better than more conservative treatment of intravesical MMC or BCG. However, a large weakness of this trial is the lack of concurrent chemotherapy with radiotherapy [22]. As mentioned above, concurrent chemoradiation is more effective in eradicating muscle invasive bladder cancer than radiation alone. Extending from this, a study out of Erlangen, Germany has demonstrated favorable results with concurrent chemoradiation in patients with high-grade T1 tumors [23]. A phase II trial (RTOG 0926) is currently evaluating this approach of concurrent chemoradiation in patients with Grade 2–3, T1 bladder cancer.

29.5   Radiation Therapy Technique

Bladder preservation therapy involves a multidisciplinary approach. The schema for this approach is depicted in Fig. 29.1. As mentioned above, patients undergo a rigid cystoscopy in the operating room followed by maximal TURBT. After maximal TURBT, the patients proceed to induction chemoradiotherapy, usually with cisplatin-based chemotherapy. The radiation treatment volume encompasses the bladder, prostate, and the pelvic lymph nodes to an initial dose of 40 Gy. The decision on whether to irradiate the lymph nodes has not been studied in a randomized setting. However, support for irradiation of the lymph nodes may be extrapolated from surgical studies demonstrating that the extent of lymph node dissection improves survival rates, even in node-negative patients [24, 25]. The improvement in survival may reflect the presence of microscopic lymph node disease and the ability to be eradicated to prevent future distant metastatic disease.

After 40 Gy, a repeat cystoscopy and biopsy is usually performed to evaluate treatment response in patients who might be deemed surgical candidates. Incomplete responders proceed with cystectomy. Patients with a complete response continue with radiation treatment. The treatment volume at this point is reduced to include the whole bladder to a total dose of 54 Gy. Then, a second cone-down volume is incorporated to treat the bladder tumor volume to 64–65 Gy. For very elderly patients and others unfit for salvage surgery post chemotherapy, cystoscopy may be omitted with the commitment to pursue definitive chemoradiation.

With administration of high dose of radiation therapy, there is concern for rectal and bowel toxicity. This toxicity is minimized by conformal delivery of radiation therapy and accurate, reproducible patient setup. For example, with intensity-modulated radiotherapy (IMRT), a high dose of radiation can be delivered to the target volume while sculpting undesirable dose away from the rectum, bowel, and pelvic bones. IMRT utilizes inverse computer optimization to create a highly conformal dose distribution matching the shape of the tumor and target by modulating multiple beam intensities.

With the tight conformality of IMRT, accuracy of patient setup becomes critical. Imprecise patient setup and organ motion can negate the benefits of IMRT and lead to undertreatment of the target and unintended dose to normal tissue. Significant variations in bladder filling and motion up to 2.7 cm have been noted [26, 27].

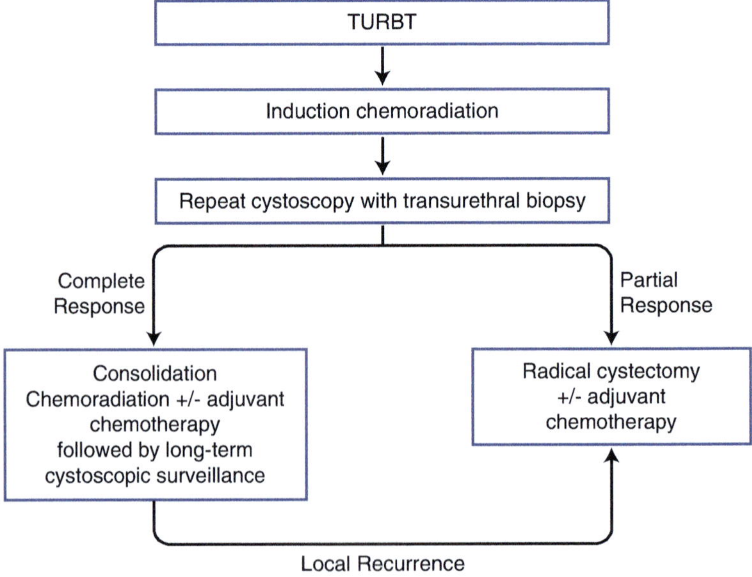

Fig. 29.1 Schema of trimodality treatment for bladder preservation therapy

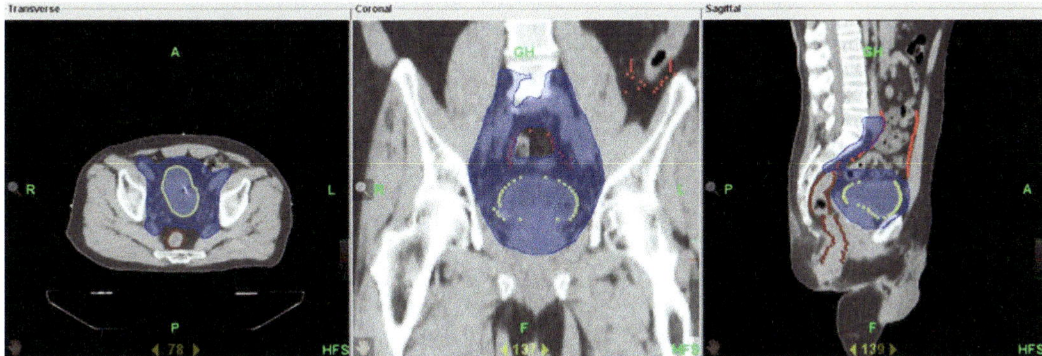

Fig. 29.2 Intensity modulated radiation therapy: Shaded in *blue* is the volume including the bladder (*yellow*), prostate, and lymph nodes receiving the initial prescription dose of 40 Gy. Depicted is a highly conformal dose delivery matching the target while minimizing the dose to the rectum (*brown*), and bowel (*red*)

Patient setup has been improved with rigid immobilization techniques and image-guided radiotherapy (IGRT). IGRT includes the use of three-dimensional imaging with on-board CT imaging. With on-board CT imaging, an imager rotates around the patient in the treatment position to acquire volumetric images which are reconstructed three-dimensionally to depict the patient's anatomy. These images can be utilized to verify that the bladder is in the same position as that at the time of treatment planning to ensure adequate treatment delivery. If variations in bladder filling and motion are noted, treatment delivery can be adapted. With increased precision in patient setup, smaller treatment fields with less margin for setup error can be utilized, resulting in decreased normal tissue irradiation and toxicity. An example of an intensity-modulated radiation treatment plan delivered by Tomotherapy (Madison, Wisconsin), which has on-board CT imaging capabilities, is depicted in Fig. 29.2.

Target delineation is critical for IMRT. The target must be identified with accuracy to ensure treatment adequacy while minimizing toxicity. However, after maximal TURBT, tumor bed delineation on the treatment planning CT is technically challenging. Recent work at UCSF has shown that custom designed gold fiducials can be placed to mark the borders of the tumor bed. The urologist can cystoscopically implant gold-seed markers directly at the borders of the tumor bed at the time of TURBT (Fig. 29.2). These markers can be readily identified on CT. With the bladder map, identification of gold seed marker position, and open communication to the urologist, the radiation oncologist can accurately define the tumor bed volume.

These fiducial markers can also improve the accuracy of treatment delivery. For example, these markers can be used for gating of radiation treatment and/or tracking of tumor and bladder movement. With gated radiotherapy based on marker position, radiation is delivered only when the target (as defined by the gold markers) is localized within the treatment field. The gold markers can also be used for tracking on the CyberKnife (Accuray, CA) System. CyberKnife allows for real-time organ position and motion correction during radiotherapy. Thariat et al. demonstrated the feasibility of re-irradiating bladder cancer using Cyberknife. The use of gold fiducial markers has been implemented for tracking on Cyberknife at UCSF (Fig. 29.3) [28].

29.6 Surveillance

Following bladder preservation therapy, close follow-up is necessary. Repeat cystoscopy and urine cytology are performed every 3 months during the first year, every 4 months during the second year, every 6 months up to 5 years, then annually until year 10. CT of the chest, abdomen, and pelvis should be performed every 6 months.

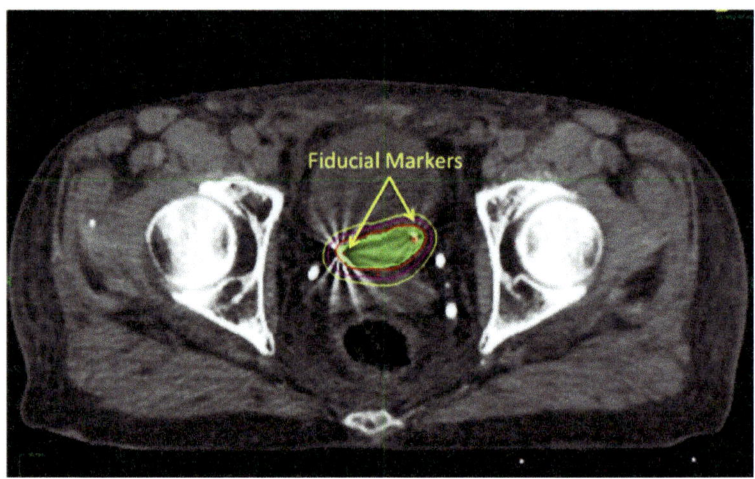

Fig. 29.3 Cyberknife treatment: Shaded in *green* is the target volume. The prescription isodose is indicated by the *red line*. The 70 and 50 % isodose lines are indicated by the *purple* and *yellow lines*, respectively. Also seen are the fiducial markers used for tracking (*yellow arrows*)

The disease-specific survival at 5 years is approximately 66 % with approximately 80 % of those alive retaining their bladder. Patients that experience a local recurrence or have persistent disease undergo a salvage cystectomy. The importance of close surveillance is underscored by the cure rate of 45 % following salvage cystectomy with no increased morbidity compared with primary cystectomy [29].

29.7 Quality of Life

A common misconception of bladder preservation is the notion of a poorly functioning bladder after chemoradiation therapy. Several studies have demonstrated acceptable toxicity and low complication rates with chemoradiaton therapy. In one prospective study utilizing patient reported urinary quality of life questionnaires, no significant differences were observed between patients who underwent radiotherapy in comparison to a matched control group [30]. Another study demonstrated that approximately 75 % of patients have a functioning urinary bladder with little or no distress from the urinary tract [31]. Zietman et al. performed urodynamics study along with quality of life questionnaire in patients undergo bladder preservation therapy at the Massachusetts General Hospital. With adequate long-term follow up of 6.3 years, 78 % patients retained compliant bladders with normal capacity and flow

parameters. 85 % of patients did not experience any urgency and 50 % of patients retained normal erectile function. A recent study evaluating late pelvic toxicity in 157 patients treated on multiple RTOG trials for bladder preservation demonstrated late Grade 3 or greater toxicity in 12 patients (7 %) with symptoms resolving in all but one patient [32].

29.8 Conclusion

Bladder preservation is a multidisciplinary effort that involves experienced urologists, medical oncologists, and radiation oncologists. The treatment involves a maximal TURBT followed by chemoradiotherapy for bladder preservation is a reasonable alternative to cystectomy for treatment of muscle invasive bladder cancer. The majority of patients undergoing this approach will retain a normally functioning bladder with no compromise in survival. Cystectomy can be reserved as a salvage option in patients with local failure.

The above mentioned, 53-year-old gentleman with a solitary, 2 cm T2 tumor is a candidate for bladder preservation. Although many studies were performed in the elderly, his young age and high performance status are positive prognostic factors. Also patients with excellent urinary function are likely to maintain satisfactory urinary function. This patient should undergo maximal

TURBT along with random biopsies of the bladder to ensure that he has solitary disease. Although diffuse CIS is associated with an increased rate of local recurrence, the unifocal CIS does not preclude him from undergoing bladder preservation therapy. He will have to be followed closely with routine surveillance cystoscopy and urine cytology along with CT imaging of his chest, abdomen, and pelvis. If local recurrence is detected, salvage cystectomy can be performed without significantly increased morbidity and detriment in survival.

References

1. Efstathiou JA, Spiegel DY, Shipley WU, Heney NM, Kaufman DS, Niemierko A, et al. Long-term outcomes of selective bladder preservation by combined-modality therapy for invasive bladder cancer: the MGH experience. Eur Urol. 2012;61(4):705–11. PubMed PMID: 22101114.
2. Shipley WU, Prout Jr GR, Einstein AB, Coombs LJ, Wajsman Z, Soloway MS, et al. Treatment of invasive bladder cancer by cisplatin and radiation in patients unsuited for surgery. JAMA. 1987;258(7):931–5. PubMed PMID: 3613023.
3. James ND, Hussain SA, Hall E, Jenkins P, Tremlett J, Rawlings C, et al. Radiotherapy with or without chemotherapy in muscle-invasive bladder cancer. N Engl J Med. 2012;366(16):1477–88. PubMed PMID: 22512481.
4. Shipley WU, Winter KA, Kaufman DS, Lee WR, Heney NM, Tester WR, et al. Phase III trial of neoadjuvant chemotherapy in patients with invasive bladder cancer treated with selective bladder preservation by combined radiation therapy and chemotherapy: initial results of Radiation Therapy Oncology Group 89–03. J Clin Oncol. 1998;16(11):3576–83. PubMed PMID: 9817278.
5. Rodel C, Grabenbauer GG, Kuhn R, Papadopoulos T, Dunst J, Meyer M, et al. Combined-modality treatment and selective organ preservation in invasive bladder cancer: long-term results. J Clin Oncol. 2002;20(14):3061–71. PubMed PMID: 12118019.
6. Fung CY, Shipley WU, Young RH, Griffin PP, Convery KM, Kaufman DS, et al. Prognostic factors in invasive bladder carcinoma in a prospective trial of preoperative adjuvant chemotherapy and radiotherapy. J Clin Oncol. 1991;9(9):1533–42. PubMed PMID: 1875217.
7. Coppin C, Gospodarowicz M. The NCI-Canada trial of concurrent cisplatin and radiotherapy for muscle invasive bladder cancer. Prog Clin Biol Res. 1990;353:75–83. PubMed PMID: 2217429.
8. George L, Bladou F, Bardou VJ, Gravis G, Tallet A, Alzieu C, et al. Clinical outcome in patients with locally advanced bladder carcinoma treated with conservative multimodality therapy. Urology. 2004;64(3):488–93. PubMed PMID: 15351577.
9. Gospodarowicz MK, Hawkins NV, Rawlings GA, Connolly JG, Jewett MA, Thomas GM, et al. Radical radiotherapy for muscle invasive transitional cell carcinoma of the bladder: failure analysis. J Urol. 1989;142(6):1448–53. discussion 53-4, PubMed PMID: 2585617.
10. Shipley WU, Rose MA, Perrone TL, Mannix CM, Heney NM, Prout Jr GR. Full-dose irradiation for patients with invasive bladder carcinoma: clinical and histological factors prognostic of improved survival. J Urol. 1985;134(4):679–83. PubMed PMID: 4032570.
11. Hart S, Skinner EC, Meyerowitz BE, Boyd S, Lieskovsky G, Skinner DG. Quality of life after radical cystectomy for bladder cancer in patients with an ileal conduit, cutaneous or urethral kock pouch. J Urol. 1999;162(1):77–81. PubMed PMID: 10379744.
12. Jenkins BJ, Caulfield MJ, Fowler CG, Badenoch DF, Tiptaft RC, Paris AM, et al. Reappraisal of the role of radical radiotherapy and salvage cystectomy in the treatment of invasive (T2/T3) bladder cancer. Br J Urol. 1988;62(4):343–6. PubMed PMID: 3191360.
13. Shearer RJ, Chilvers CF, Bloom HJ, Bliss JM, Horwich A, Babiker A. Adjuvant chemotherapy in T3 carcinoma of the bladder. A prospective trial: preliminary report. Br J Urol. 1988;62(6):558–64. PubMed PMID: 3064861.
14. De Neve W, Lybeert ML, Goor C, Crommelin MA, Ribot JG. Radiotherapy for T2 and T3 carcinoma of the bladder: the influence of overall treatment time. Radiother Oncol. 1995;36(3):183–8. PubMed PMID: 8532904.
15. Mameghan H, Fisher R, Mameghan J, Brook S. Analysis of failure following definitive radiotherapy for invasive transitional cell carcinoma of the bladder. Int J Radiat Oncol Biol Phys. 1995;31(2):247–54. PubMed PMID: 7836076.
16. Shipley WU, Zietman AL, Kaufman DS, Althausen AF, Heney NM. Invasive bladder cancer: treatment strategies using transurethral surgery, chemotherapy and radiation therapy with selection for bladder conservation. Int J Radiat Oncol Biol Phys. 1997;39(4):937–43. PubMed PMID: 9369144.
17. Miller LS. Bladder cancer: superiority of preoperative irradiation and cystectomy in clinical stages B2 and C. Cancer. 1977;39(2 Suppl):973–80. PubMed PMID: 402205.
18. Bloom HJ, Hendry WF, Wallace DM, Skeet RG. Treatment of T3 bladder cancer: controlled trial of pre-operative radiotherapy and radical cystectomy versus radical radiotherapy. Br J Urol. 1982;54(2):136–51. PubMed PMID: 7044462.
19. Sell A, Jakobsen A, Nerstrom B, Sorensen BL, Steven K, Barlebo H. Treatment of advanced bladder cancer category T2 T3 and T4a. A randomized multicenter

study of preoperative irradiation and cystectomy versus radical irradiation and early salvage cystectomy for residual tumor. DAVECA protocol 8201. Danish Vesical Cancer Group. Scand J Urol Nephrol Suppl. 1991;138:193–201. PubMed PMID: 1785004.

20. Svatek RS, Shariat SF, Novara G, Skinner EC, Fradet Y, Bastian PJ, et al. Discrepancy between clinical and pathological stage: external validation of the impact on prognosis in an international radical cystectomy cohort. BJU Int. 2011;107(6):898–904. PubMed PMID: 21244604.

21. Nepple KG, O'Donnell MA. The optimal management of T1 high-grade bladder cancer. Can Urol Assoc J. 2009;3(6 Suppl 4):S188–92. PubMed PMID: 20019983. Pubmed Central PMCID: 2792452.

22. Harland SJ, Kynaston H, Grigor K, Wallace DM, Beacock C, Kockelbergh R, et al. A randomized trial of radical radiotherapy for the management of pT1G3 NXM0 transitional cell carcinoma of the bladder. J Urol. 2007;178(3 Pt 1):807–13. discussion 13, PubMed PMID: 17631326.

23. Weiss C, Wolze C, Engehausen DG, Ott OJ, Krause FS, Schrott KM, et al. Radiochemotherapy after transurethral resection for high-risk T1 bladder cancer: an alternative to intravesical therapy or early cystectomy? J Clin Oncol. 2006;24(15):2318–24. PubMed PMID: 16710030.

24. Leissner J, Ghoneim MA, Abol-Enein H, Thuroff JW, Franzaring L, Fisch M, et al. Extended radical lymphadenectomy in patients with urothelial bladder cancer: results of a prospective multicenter study. J Urol. 2004;171(1):139–44. PubMed PMID: 14665862.

25. Poulsen AL, Horn T, Steven K. Radical cystectomy: extending the limits of pelvic lymph node dissection improves survival for patients with bladder cancer confined to the bladder wall. J Urol. 1998;160(6 Pt 1): 2015–9. Discussion 20, PubMed PMID: 9817313.

26. Harris SJ, Buchanan RB. An audit and evaluation of bladder movements during radical radiotherapy. Clin Oncol. 1998;10(4):262–4. PubMed PMID: 9764380.

27. McBain CA, Logue JP. Radiation therapy for muscle-invasive bladder cancer: treatment planning and delivery in the 21st century. Semin Radiat Oncol. 2005;15(1):42–8. PubMed PMID: 15662606.

28. Thariat J, Trimaud R, Angellier G, Caullery M, Amiel J, Bondiau PY, et al. Innovative image-guided CyberKnife stereotactic radiotherapy for bladder cancer. Br J Radiol. 2010;83(990):e118–21. PubMed PMID: 20505025, Pubmed Central PMCID: 3473597.

29. Eswara JR, Efstathiou JA, Heney NM, Paly J, Kaufman DS, McDougal WS, et al. Complications and long-term results of salvage cystectomy after failed bladder sparing therapy for muscle invasive bladder cancer. J Urol. 2012;187(2):463–8. PubMed PMID: 22177159.

30. Lynch TH, Waymont B, Dunn JA, Wallace DM. Urologists' attitudes to the management of bladder cancer. Br J Urol. 1992;70(5):522–5. PubMed PMID: 1467859.

31. Henningsohn L, Wijkstrom H, Dickman PW, Bergmark K, Steineck G. Distressful symptoms after radical radiotherapy for urinary bladder cancer. Radiother Oncol. 2002;62(2):215–25. PubMed PMID: 11937249.

32. Efstathiou JA, Bae K, Shipley WU, Kaufman DS, Hagan MP, Heney NM, et al. Late pelvic toxicity after bladder-sparing therapy in patients with invasive bladder cancer: RTOG 89-03, 95-06, 97-06, 99-06. J Clin Oncol. 2009;27(25):4055–61. PubMed PMID: 19636019, Pubmed Central PMCID: 2734419.

Gautam Jha, Guru Sonpavde, and Zeeshan Ahmad

30.1 Introduction

Urinary bladder cancer is the fifth most common solid tumor, and urothelial (transitional cell) carcinoma (UC) is the most common type of bladder cancer. Even after surgical resection for localized muscle invasive bladder cancer (MIBC), nearly

G. Jha, M.B.B.S., M.S. (✉)
Division of Hematology, Oncology and
Transplantation, Department of Medicine,
University of Minnesota, 516 Delaware Street SE,
14-150 PWB, MMC 8480, Minneapolis,
MN 55455, USA
c-mail: jhaxx014@umn.cdu

G. Sonpavde, M.D.
Department of Hematology/Oncology,
University of Birmingham Alabama,
1802 6th Avenue South, NP 2540B,
Birmingham, AL 35294, USA

Division of Hematology and Oncology,
University of Alabama, 1720 2nd Avenue South,
WTI5, Birmingham, AL 35294-3300, USA
e-mail: sonpavde@uab.edu

Z. Ahmad, M.D.
Division of Hematology, Oncology and
Transplantation, Department of Medicine,
University of Minnesota, 516 Delaware Street SE,
14-150 PWB, MMC 8480, Minneapolis,
MN 55455, USA

Department of Internal Medicine, Unity Hospital,
Fridley, MN, USA
e-mail: ahmadzeeshanmd@gmail.com

half eventually develop metastatic disease [1, 2]. UC is sensitive to chemotherapy, and high response rates (RR) up to 70 % have been noted to platinum-based chemotherapies when used prior to cystectomy [1]. Chemotherapy has been studied in the definitive setting concurrent with radiation, the neoadjuvant setting prior to surgical resection, the adjuvant setting post cystectomy and in patients with metastatic disease with palliative intent. The majority of studies have excluded histologic subtypes other than UC, and there is little objective information on the role of chemotherapy for nonurothelial cancer of the bladder.

30.2 Neoadjuvant Versus Adjuvant Chemotherapy

Neoadjuvant chemotherapy (NCT) offers the earliest opportunity to target the distant micrometastases that are responsible for most failures. Patients should be in the optimum state of health to tolerate chemotherapy in the presurgical setting [3]. Histopathologic evaluation of the cystectomy specimen offers in vivo chemotherapy sensitivity and can offer prognostic information—pathologic complete responses are markers of good prognosis [1, 4]. A good response to locoregionally advanced tumors can assist complete surgical resection.

However, with neoadjuvant therapy concerns remain of delaying definitive curative cystectomy

B.R. Konety and S.S. Chang (eds.), *Management of Bladder Cancer:*
A Comprehensive Text With Clinical Scenarios, DOI 10.1007/978-1-4939-1881-2_30,
© Springer Science+Business Media New York 2015

and the possibility of disease progression in a small subset of patients while on chemotherapy. A fraction of patients, e.g., pT2a (superficial muscle-invasive disease), is overtreated with NCT. Conversely, the adjuvant chemotherapy (ACT) strategy permits complete pathological assessment and risk stratification before offering chemotherapy to high-risk patients (with extravesical or node-positive disease).

30.3 Neoadjuvant Chemotherapy (NCT)

Initial clinical trials with the single agent cisplatin conducted in the 1980s failed to show any survival benefit and suggested combination with other agents [5–7]. Two large randomized phase III trials conducted in Europe studied cisplatin with doxorubicin or methotrexate. The Nordic Cystectomy Trial 1 randomized a total of 311 patients with cT1G3, T2-T4NxM0 invasive bladder cancer [8]. In the chemotherapy arm, 151 patients were treated with two cycles of cisplatin and doxorubicin, while 160 patients in the control arm received no chemotherapy. Patients in both arms received 20 Gy of radiation prior to cystectomy. Treatment with NCT did not attain statistically significant improvement in overall survival (OS), although subset analysis of patients with pT3-T4 disease did show 15 % improvement in survival in favor of the chemotherapy arm.

The Nordic Cystectomy Trial 2 randomized 317 patients with T2-T4aNxM0 UC to receive three cycles of cisplatin with methotrexate or no chemotherapy prior to cystectomy [9]. This trial again had a trend toward improved survival for the chemotherapy arm, but did not reach statistical significance. However, a combined analysis to the two Nordic trials did reveal improvement in 5-year survival from 56 % in the chemotherapy arms as compared to 48 % in the control arms without chemotherapy, $P=0.049$ [10].

In the largest NCT study to date, the International Collaborative Trialist study group randomized 976 patients with T2 grade 3, T3/4, N0, M0 UC to receive three cycles of cisplatin, methotrexate and vinblastine (CMV) or no therapy

prior to definitive local therapy [11]. Local therapy ranged from definitive radiation therapy (43 %) to radical cystectomy with (8 %) or without (53 %) low-dose radiation therapy. An update on the results of this trial revealed an improvement in 10-year OS in the chemotherapy group (36 % vs. 30 %, HR 0.84; $P=0.03$). Neoadjuvant CMV was similarly effective when followed by either radiotherapy or cystectomy as definitive local therapy, and the reductions in the risk of death were 20 and 26 % compared to the radiotherapy alone and cystectomy alone groups, respectively (radiotherapy alone: HR, 0.80; 95 % CI, 0.63–1.02; $P=0.070$; cystectomy alone: HR, 0.74; 95 % CI, 0.57–0.96; $P=0.022$).

Learning from studies in the metastatic setting, the Southwest Oncology group led a US intergroup trial to test MVAC (methotrexate, vinblastine, adriamycin, cisplatin) in the neoadjuvant setting and randomized 311 patients with cT2-T4,N0M0 UC to either three cycles of MVAC or no chemotherapy prior to radical cystectomy [12]. Unfortunately, this trial took over 11 years to accrue 317 patients from 126 institutions. Median OS did improve in the chemotherapy arm: 77 months as compared to 46 months in the control arm without chemotherapy, $P=0.06$. Treatment with MVAC resulted in significantly higher rates of pathologic complete remission (pCR) as compared to cystectomy alone (38 % vs. 15 %; $P<0.001$) in the control arm subjects. Both pCR and $<$pT2N0 disease following MVAC therapy were associated with improved median survival (13.6 and 12.5 years, respectively), while residual muscle-invasive disease or lymph node-positive disease led to poor survival—median survival 3.4 and 2.4 years, respectively [4]. Similar improvement in pathologic complete responses reported for other major trials correlated with improvement in survival, suggesting pCR as a surrogate prognostic marker for improved survival [4, 13–16].

In a large phase III trial for patients with locally advanced or metastatic UC, cisplatin with gemcitabine (GC) was much better tolerated and revealed efficacy similar to MVAC [17, 18]. Based on this study with improved tolerability, GC has emerged as the favored regimen in common practice. However, there have been no large studies to assess the efficacy of GC combination therapy in the neoadjuvant setting. In smaller phase II trials and retrospective studies, GC combination therapy has produced pathologic complete response rates similar to those of MVAC and is widely used [19–21].

The Advanced Bladder Cancer Meta-analysis Collaboration reported an individual patient data level meta-analysis of clinical trials conducted by the Medical Research Council Clinical Trials Unit [22]. This meta-analysis from 11 randomized trials, which included 3,005 patients, found a 5 % absolute survival benefit at 5 years (HR = 0.86, 95 % CI 0.77–0.95; $P = 0.003$) favoring NCT. Furthermore, while cisplatin-based chemotherapy was associated with benefits, no particular regimen or choice of definitive therapy (radical cystectomy versus radiation therapy versus the combination) was associated with a survival advantage. In a recent Cochrane review of neoadjuvant platinum-based combination chemotherapy trials, a similar 14 % relative risk reduction was noted in the combination chemotherapy regimen.

A significant proportion of patients are deemed cisplatin-ineligible owing to impaired renal function, advanced age and other comorbidities. Although carboplatin is often substituted for cisplatin for patients considered unfit for cisplatin, there are fairly limited data supporting the use of carboplatin-based regimens. In a 47-patient single-arm phase II trial, patients with T2-4N0M0 bladder cancer were treated with carboplatin, methotrexate and vinblastine [23]. Of the 47 patients, 38 underwent cystectomy post chemotherapy (7 progressed; 1 died; 1 was unfit for surgery). Twelve patients had pathologic CR (pCR 26.5 %; 95 % CI, 15–42 %) and six PR (pPR 13.5 %; 95 % CI, 5–27 %).

Aggressive multiple drug regimens with carboplatin have recently been studied. SWOG conducted a phase II trial of carboplatin, paclitaxel and gemcitabine to study cystoscopic surveillance versus immediate cystectomy post NCT. Although 34 patients (cT0 46 %; CI 34–58 %) had clinical T0 based on post-chemotherapy TURBT, ten of these opted for immediate cystectomy and six had gross residual

disease. Since a majority of patients did not undergo immediate cystectomy, the actual pT0 rates are unknown, and clearly cT0 does not provide a fair estimate of pT0. There was 75 % grade 3 or more hematologic toxicity and one death from infection with neutropenia. Another study with the same regimen enrolled 71 patients and had unacceptable toxicity with 7 treatment-related deaths [24]. In a similar phase II trial of neoadjuvant nab-paclitaxel, carboplatin and gemcitabine in patients with locally advanced bladder cancer, all of the 29 patients enrolled experienced grade 3–4 hematologic toxicities and 1 patient died of toxicity [25]. By intent-to-treat analysis, the pT0 rate was 27.6 %.

30.4 Neoadjuvant Chemotherapy and Controversies

While neoadjuvant therapy is recommended for locally advanced disease, there is a huge disparity between the clinical and pathologic staging. Nearly 66 % of patients with pT2 disease may be incorrectly staged, with 42 % upstaged after radical cystectomy [26]. Importantly, ≥T2 disease is found at RC in 40 % of patients clinically staged as having non-muscle invasive disease prior to RC. Despite a clear trend toward improved survival, most clinical trials studying NCT did not reach statistical significance, limited by inadequate sample size, poor accrual or non-standard and possibly less effective regimens.

Although GC is one of the most widely utilized regimens in the neoadjuvant setting, there are no phase III trials supporting its use, and none have compared it to either conventional or dose-dense MVAC regimens. Dose-dense MVAC with G-CSF support is being investigated to improve response rates, abbreviate the duration of NCT and improve tolerability.

A small fraction of patients eligible for NCT receive therapy, often limited by inappropriate staging, advanced age, poor renal function or comorbidity limiting cisplatin use [27]. Carboplatin substituted for patients deemed to be cisplatin ineligible lacks randomized trials supporting improved outcomes with its use.

Table 30.1 Phase III trials for NCT in UC

Trial	No. of patients	Neoadjuvant regimen	No. of cycles	Survival benefit	5-year OS	OS months	% Path CR	Significance for pT0
Nordic Cystectomy Trial 1 [8]	151	Cisplatin, doxorubicin	2	NO (15 % benefit for T3-4a; $P=0.03$)	59 %	NR	NR	Yes; combined Nordic I and II
	160	None	NA		51 %	NR	NR	
Nordic Cystectomy Trial 2 [9]	155	Cisplatin, methotrexate	3	No	53 %	NR	26.4	Yes
	154	None	NA		46 %	NR	11.5	
SWOG 8710 [12]	153	MVAC	3	Yes	57 %	77	38	Yes
	154	None	NA		43 %	46	15	
BA06 30894 [11]	491	CMV	3	Yes	49 %	44	32.5	NR
	485	None	NA		43 %	37	12.3	
JCOG 0209 [30]	64	MVAC	2	No	NR	102	34	Yes
	66	None	0		NR	81	9	

NA not applicable; *NR* not reported; *path CR* pathological complete response; *SWOG* Southwest Oncology Group; *JCOG* Japanese Clinical Oncology Group

The Genitourinary Malignancy Group at MD Anderson Cancer center conducted a phase III trial to assess the impact of timing on response to chemotherapy in patients with high-risk resectable UC [28]. In this study, 140 patients were randomized to receive two cycles of neoadjuvant MVAC and three cycles post cystectomy versus five cycles of adjuvant MVAC. NCT was better tolerated, and 97 % of patients completed at least two cycles of chemotherapy as compared to only 77 % in the adjuvant therapy arm, while seven patients in the ACT arm had positive margins as compared to one patient in the neoadjuvant group. However, there were six treatment-related deaths in each group and no difference in survival between the two treatment arms. Moreover, a retrospective study suggests that a third of patients are not candidates for ACT following radical cystectomy because of postoperative complications [29]. These limited data suggest that NCT is probably more feasible than ACT (Table 30.1).

30.5 Adjuvant Chemotherapy

Radical cystectomy with nerve-sparing techniques has a failure rate as high as 50 % [31–34]. While 10–20 % of patients will relapse in the pelvis after cystectomy, distant relapse is more common, suggesting a role for ACT [32, 35, 36]. ACT does not delay definitive therapy in patients with chemotherapy-resistant tumors and permits selection of high-risk patients for chemotherapy [32, 37]. Systemic treatment of micrometastasis is delayed, and the ability to assess chemosenstivity and thereby prognostic information from tumor downstaging is lost [38].

A retrospective study compared 71 patients treated with adjuvant cisplatin, adriamycin and cytoxan to stage-matched controls [39]. This nonrandomized study suggested improvement in disease-free survival and rates of 2-year survival (70 % vs. 37 %; $P=0.00012$) for high-risk patients, but no benefit for patients with low-risk disease [32, 39]. Another prospective study examined the same chemotherapy regimen in 91 patients with PT3-T4a or node-positive bladder cancer [3, 40]. There was significant improvement in median survival in the ACT arm (4.3 years) when compared with the observation arm (2.4 years; $P=0.0062$). Both of these studies were limited by low statistical power due to the small sample size.

A large retrospective study analyzed a cohort of 3,947 post-cystectomy patients, of whom 932 had received ACT. ACT was independently associated with improved survival (HR 0.83; $P=0.017$), and this benefit was most pronounced for higher risk groups [41]. A number of other trials failed to show a similar survival advantage for ACT. A retrospective review of 129 patients treated with GC or MVAC in the adjuvant setting within a group of 958 patients treated with radical cystectomy did not suggest any benefit of ACT [42].

Several large randomized clinical trials have closed prematurely owing to poor accrual. A prospective multicenter randomized phase III study by the Italian group closed after accruing only 194 of the planned 610 patients over a nearly 6-year period [43]. Ninety-two patients were randomized to the control arm of deferred chemotherapy at the time of relapse, and 102 were randomized to four cycles of GC-based chemotherapy. Only 62 % of patients completed planned chemotherapy, suggesting difficulty in administering chemotherapy in the post-surgical setting. At a median follow-up of 35 months, there was no difference in 5-year OS (53.7 % and 43.4 %, $P=0.24$, HR 1.29, 95 % CI 0.84–1.99) or 5-year disease-free survival (42.3 % and 37.2 %, $P=0.70$) in the control and ACT arms.

The Spanish Oncology Genitourinary Group (SOGUG) compared a triplet chemotherapy combination of cisplatin, gemcitabine and paclitaxel to observation in high-risk patients with pT3-4 and or pN+disease post cystectomy in a randomized phase III trial (99/01). The trial was closed prematurely because of poor accrual, and the results were presented in abstract form at the American Society of Clinical Oncology annual meeting. The study enrolled 142 of the planned 340 patients over 7 years (74 patients randomized to chemotherapy and 68 to observation). In the chemotherapy arm, 76 % of patients completed all four cycles of planned chemotherapy, and 41 % had grade III/IV neutropenia, 8 % had febrile neutropenia, and there was one death with sepsis. At a median follow-up of 30 months, median OS was not reached in the chemotherapy arm and was 26 months in the observation arm (HR: 0.44; $P<0.0009$). The 5-year OS was 60 % in the chemotherapy arm as compared to 31 % in the control group. In an intent-to-treat analysis, PFS (HR 0.38; $P<0.0001$), TTP (HR 0.36; $P<0.0001$) and disease-specific survival (HR

0.37; $P<0.0002$) all favored the chemotherapy treatment arm [44].

The EORTC conducted a randomized phase III trial (protocol 30994) comparing immediate versus deferred chemotherapy after radical cystectomy in patients with pT3-pT4 and/or N+M0 transitional cell carcinoma (TCC) of the bladder, which closed after accruing 284 of the planned 660 patients [45]. Chemotherapy either in the adjuvant setting or at the time of relapse could include one of three approved regimens of MVAC, high-dose MVAC and GC. CALGB also compared a sequential chemotherapy regimen of gemcitabine and doxorubicin followed by paclitaxel and cisplatin with cisplatin and gemcitabine, which similarly closed because of poor accrual [46].

There are very few randomized clinical trials to guide ACT in high-risk patients with bladder cancer. The ABC meta-analysis collaboration conducted a review and meta-analysis of all available randomized clinical trials until September 2004 and identified 6 RCTs randomizing 491 patients to cisplatin-based chemotherapy [47]. While there was a 25 % reduction in mortality in favor of chemotherapy (95 % CI 0.60–0.69, $P=0.019$) and absolute improvement in survival of 9 % (95 % CI 1–16 %) at 3 years, the study clearly had limited power, and the authors admitted insufficient evidence to recommend adjuvant chemotherapy routinely.

30.6 Adjuvant Chemotherapy and Controversies

Almost all published randomized controlled trials (RCTs) have compared ACT after cystectomy with cystectomy alone, have struggled with premature closures and lack the statistical power to make any definitive recommendations [48–56]. A benefit of chemotherapy in the setting of metastatic bladder cancer and in the neoadjuvant setting suggests a benefit for adjuvant therapy, contributing to difficulty in enrolling for randomized trials. Unlike NCT, ACT lacks level 1 evidence in the form of randomized clinical trials and yet it is more widely administered in routine practice [27].

The EORTC has completed a phase III trial (EORTC 30994) comparing ACT post cystectomy (one of three regimens: MVAC, dose-escalated MVAC, GC) versus intervention at disease recurrence in patients with pT3-4 and/or node-positive disease. Results are awaited for this and other recent randomized studies to provide guidance for the use of chemotherapy in this setting.

Patients who have > pT2 and or N1 disease at cystectomy despite receiving NCT have a very high risk of recurrent disease [4]. These patients should be enrolled in clinical trials whenever possible as there are no evidence-based recommendations. Non-cross-resistant chemotherapy should be considered when patients are eligible and are at high risk of recurrent disease.

30.7 Chemotherapy for Metastatic Disease

30.7.1 First-Line Chemotherapy

Locally advanced bladder cancer has a very high rate of failure locally and systemically within 2 years after curative cystectomy with or without perioperative chemotherapy [12, 22, 47]. In the absence of systemic treatment, this disease is progressive and universally fatal with only 30 % of patients living to 1 year beyond the first year despite local therapies including surgery and radiation therapy [57]. Systematic phase II studies in the late 1970s already established cisplatin, methotrexate, vinblastine and adriamycin as active agents. Furthermore, two-drug combinations appeared to be more active than single agents, suggesting a role for poly-chemotherapy regimens with all four of the known active agents.

As a logical next step, all of the four active agents were studied together (MVAC: methotrexate, vinblastine, adriamycin and cisplatin) at Memorial Sloan-Kettering Cancer Center (MSKCC), and preliminary findings were published in 1985 [58]. In this 25-patient study, significant clinical response was noted in 17 patients with 12 complete clinical remissions. A follow-up to this study with additional patients (133 patients with advanced bladder cancer) continued to show a similar impressive clinical response: 72 % clinical RR and 36 % complete responses [59]. While responses were noted at all of the metastatic sites, there was significant toxicity with four (3 %) treatment-related deaths.

A phase III intergroup study randomized 269 patients to either single-agent cisplatin or MVAC combination in patients with metastatic or locally advanced bladder cancer [7]. The MVAC combination was clearly demonstrated to be superior to single-agent cisplatin in terms of RR (39 % vs. 12 %), median progression-free survival (PFS) of 10.0 vs. 4.3 months and median OS of 12.5 vs. 8.2 months. With long-term follow-up, MVAC continued to demonstrate a similar benefit in survival ($P=0.00015$, log-rank test) [60]. The MVAC regimen was associated with significant mucositis, myelosuppression and a 3 % treatment-related mortality rate similar to the experience with MSKCC.

A number of subsequent studies compared MVAC to other chemotherapy combinations, attempted dose intensification to improve efficacy or used prophylactic G-CSF to improve safety. A phase I/II study evaluated G-CSF at five dose levels (1, 3, 10, 30 and 60 µg/kg/day) in 27 patients [61]. A dose-dependent increase in absolute neutrophil count (ANC) was noted at all dose levels and was associated with markedly diminished time with ANC less than 1,000 per microliter, diminished incidence of neutropenic fevers and mucositis, and permitted treatment completion. Use of G-CSF could permit dose escalation as it improved the myelosuppression associated with MVAC therapy, but other clinical trials had variable results [62–64].

A phase III trial randomized 263 patients with advanced bladder cancer to high-dose-intensity MVAC (HD-MVAC) administered over 2 weeks along with G-CSF to standard MVAC therapy [65]. HD-MVAC was associated with markedly improved complete RR (21 % vs. 9 %; $P=0.009$) and PFS ($P=0.037$; HR=0.75), but failed to show statistically significant improvement in survival or time to progression. A longer follow-up at 7 years suggested improved survival in the HD-MVAC arm (24.6 % are alive on the HD-MVAC arm vs. 13.2 % on the M-VAC arm) [66].

In a randomized phase III trial, MVAC was compared to cisplatin with cyclophosphamide and adriamycin (CISCA) [67]. Compared to CISCA, MVAC was associated with increased RR (65 % vs. 46 %; $P<0.05$) and median survival (48.3 vs. 36.1 weeks).

Phase I/II studies established activity for paclitaxel, docetaxel, gemcitabine and ifosfamide either as single agents or in combination with platinum in patients with advanced or metastatic. Urothelial cancer instead of transitional cell for uniformity with previous text carcinoma [68–72]. Based on promise in phase II studies for taxanes as above, docetaxel with cisplatin was compared to MVAC [73]. All of 220 patients in this study received prophylactic G-CSF. MVAC demonstrated higher efficacy including RR (54.2 % vs. 37.4 %; $P=0.017$), median time to progression (9.4 vs. 6.1 months; $P=0.003$) and median survival (14.2 vs. 9.3 months; $P=0.026$). Although MVAC was more myelosuppressive than cisplatin with taxotere, it was lower than expected with MVAC without G-CSF.

As a single agent, gemcitabine was very well tolerated and revealed RRs up to 23–28 % in various phase I and phase II trials with activity even in patients previously treated with MVAC [72, 74–76]. Forty-six patients were treated with GC in a phase II trial of patients with metastatic bladder cancer without previous chemotherapy exposure [77]. GC combination therapy was well tolerated and was very promising with a median OS of 14.3 months, 10 (22 %) CR, 9 (19 %) PR, 41 % ORR and stable disease observed in an additional 18 patients (39 %). Results from this and other promising phase II trials led to large phase III trials comparing GC with MVAC [77, 78]. Four hundred five patients with metastatic bladder cancer and no previous therapy were randomized to either GC or MVAC every 28 days for a maximum of six cycles [17]. Both the treatment combinations had a similar median OS (13.8 vs. 14.8 months, HR 1.04; $P=0.75$), as well as time to progressive disease (7.4 months in both groups, HR 1.05) and RR (GC, 49 %; MVAC, 46 %). GC had much less myelosuppression, resulting in fewer neutropenic fevers (2 % vs. 14 %), neutropenic sepsis (1 % vs. 12 %) and grade 3–4 mucositis (1 % vs. 22 %). GC had a favorable safety profile and similar efficacy at a long-term follow-up, establishing it as a preferred regimen for patients with newly diagnosed metastatic bladder cancer [18].

Subsequent studies have tried to improve on the GC combination with the addition of a third active agent. A large intergroup phase III study conducted by EORTC randomized 607 patients to GC with or without paclitaxel [79]. The addition of paclitaxel improved the ORR (55.5 % vs. 43.6 %), but failed to make a statistically significant improvement in survival (15.8 months vs. 12.7 months; HR=0.85, $P=0.075$) and had more febrile neutropenia (13.2 % vs. 4.3 %). Thus, this trial failed to make a case for the three-drug combination of cisplatin, gemcitabine and paclitaxel.

Cisplatin use is often challenging and substituted by carboplatin in patients with metastatic disease owing to inadequate renal function, poor performance status, marked neuropathy, ototoxicity and comorbidities. Indeed, the majority of patients with metastatic UC are not receiving cisplatin-based chemotherapy as suggested in a large retrospective analysis [80]. Several relatively small trials have assessed carboplatin-based regimens in cisplatin-ineligible patients. A carboplatin-based regimen was noted to be feasible in patients with inadequate renal function or other comorbidities, limiting cisplatin use with an overall RR of 45–63 % [81–86]. A phase II/III EORTC carboplatin-gemcitabine feasibility study in "unfit" patients with advanced bladder cancer determined that carboplatin AUC of 4.5 was better tolerated with less severe hematological toxicities, and the combination with gemcitabine had an overall response of 44 % and was similar in efficacy to the combination of carboplatin with methotrexate and vinblastine and appeared less toxic [81]. Based on the promising single activity of paclitaxel in bladder cancer and extensive experience in cancers of the lung and ovary for the combination of carboplatin with paclitaxel, this combination was studied in phase II clinical trials in patients deemed ineligible for cisplatin therapy [87, 88]. In phase I/II trials carboplatin with paclitaxel was well tolerated with primarily neuropathy as the non-hematologic toxicity and an overall RR of approximately 50 %.

Table 30.2 Single-agent phase II trials of second-line therapy for metastatic bladder cancer

Chemotherapy	Sample size	RR (%)	PFS (months)	OS (months)
Weekly paclitaxel [108]	31	10	2.2	7.2
Docetaxe l [70]	30	13	–	9.0
Nab-paclitaxel [104]	47	27.7	6.0	10.8
Pemetrexed [109]	47	27.7	2.9	9.6
Pemetrexed [110]	12	8	–	–
Vinflunine [95]	51	18	3.0	6.6
Vinflunine [98]	151	14.6	2.8	8.2
Irinotecan [93]	40	5	2.1	5.4
Ixabepilone [111]	42	11.9	2.7	8
Bortezomib [112]	25	0	1.4	5.7
Oxaliplatin [113]	18	6	1.5	7
Ifosfamide [69]	56	20	2.4	5.5

A phase II study randomized 57 patients to cisplatin or carboplatin with methotrexate, vinblastine and epirubicin treatment. While the carboplatin-based regimen was well tolerated with lower gastrointestinal, renal, neurologic and otologic toxicities, it appeared less effective with a clinical RR of 41 % compared to 71 % in the cisplatin arm [89]. Another phase II study compared cisplatin or carboplatin with gemcitabine and had similar toxicity for both agents, but median survival was 12.8 months for the cisplatin arm and 9.8 months for the carboplatin arm [90]. Standard MVAC was compared to carboplatin with paclitaxel in a phase III study, which failed to meet its accrual goal. For the 85 randomized patients, the RR and OS were similar for both arms, although numerically favoring the MVAC arm. The MVAC arm had predictably higher toxicity as compared to carboplatin with paclitaxel [91]. Phase II trials suggest that fractionated weekly GC may be feasible and more active than carboplatin-based regimens in patients with renal dysfunction [92].

30.7.2 Second-Line Chemotherapy

Multiple single agents such as taxanes [paclitaxel, docetaxel, nano-albumin-bound paclitaxel (nab-paclitaxel), gemcitabine, pemetrexed, oxaliplatin and irinotecan] have demonstrated limited activity in the second-line setting, with RRs of 0–28 %, median progression-free survival (PFS) of 2–4 months and a median OS of 6–9 months as listed in Table 30.2 [93–105]. Prognostic factors appear similar to those in the first-line setting and include performance status, liver metastasis, anemia and time from prior chemotherapy [106, 107] (Table 30.2).

Taxanes have been studied as maintenance after GC or at the time of progression as a single agent or a combination. Weekly paclitaxel and docetaxel every 3 weeks as a single agent had limited activity with RRs of 10 and 13 % in two separate phase II trials [70, 108]. An open-label phase II study of nab-paclitaxel in the second-line setting after progression on or after a cisplatin-based regimen within a year in patients with metastatic bladder cancer was conducted at five centers in Canada [104]. Nab-paclitaxel was well tolerated and led to 1 CR, 12 PRs and 10 stable diseases from 47 evaluable patients resulting in an ORR of 27.7 % (95 % CI 17.3–44.4) and disease control rate (CR plus PR plus SD of >4 months) of 49 % (95 % CI 36.1–63.9). Median PFS of 6 months and OS of 10.8 months were noted in this study. Fifteen of 47 patients had not received chemotherapy for metastatic disease and had progressed on perioperative chemotherapy within the preceding year, and patient selection bias in phase II trials might possibly contribute to this significant activity.

Pemetrexed, a multitargeted antifolate agent, appeared promising in the Hoosier Oncology Group study with a promising RR of 28 % and median OS of 9.6 months [109]. However, another phase II study did not confirm this activity and had poor activity, again likely due to patient selection bias with differing risk characteristics [110].

Based on promising results in phase II studies, vinflunine was studied in a randomized phase III trial that accrued 370 patients and compared vinflunine plus best supportive care (BSC) to BSC alone as second-line therapy [98, 100]. This trial permitted patients progressing after frontline platinum-containing chemotherapy for metastatic disease only. While an extension of survival, the primary endpoint, was not demonstrated with vinflunine compared to placebo by an intention-to-treat analysis (6.9 vs. 4.6 months, $P=0.287$), there was a statistical improvement in RR (8.6 vs. 0 %) and median PFS (3.0 vs. 1.5 months). Multivariate Cox analysis adjusting for front-line prognostic factors showed a statistically significant extension of OS with vinflunine ($P=0.036$), reducing the risk of death by 23 %. Moreover, in the eligible population ($n=357$), the median OS was significantly longer for vinflunine + BSC compared to BSC (6.9 vs. 4.3 months, $P=0.04$). Based on this study, vinflunine has been approved by the European Medicine Agency (EMEA). Nevertheless, the activity of vinflunine is modest and appears similar to the activity of other agents that have been evaluated in smaller phase II trials, e.g., taxanes and pemetrexed.

Tyrosine kinase inhibitors, sunitinib, sorafenib and gefitinib, had poor activity as single agents in phase II trials [96, 114, 115]. Pazopanib had a modest activity in a phase II study with 7 partial responses (17.1 %) of 41 patients [105].

Multiple chemotherapy combinations have been studied in phase II trials with RRs higher than single agents in the second-line setting. Gemcitabine with paclitaxel has been investigated in several phase II trials with RRs ranging from 44 to 60 % [97, 116, 117]. Every-3-week dosing appeared more effective as compared to biweekly dosing in a small, randomized phase II study [117].

Thirty patients with metastatic bladder cancer after progression on GC were treated with MVAC in a small phase II study to evaluate the safety and efficacy. Patients with adequate organ function and performance status were treated with the MVAC regimen after confirmation of disease relapse or progression on or after GC [118]. The median treatment-free interval before initiating MVAC was 2.5 months (range: 0.5–20.4), and patients received a median of three cycles of the M-VAC regimen (range: 1–12). In this relatively small Korean study, the authors reported that MVAC in the second-line setting was well tolerated and led to CR in two patients, PR in seven patients and stable disease in an additional six patients with an overall disease control rate of 50 %. Re-administration of the same first-line chemotherapy regimen is often utilized in the setting of durable response of typically more than a year, although there are limited data supporting this strategy [119].

30.8 Chemoradiation

Radiotherapy alone has poor outcomes for definitive treatment in patients with MIBC and appears inferior to surgery despite the lack of randomized clinical trials [120–122].

Subsequent strategies to improve the effectiveness of radiation therapy and permit bladder preservation have focused on multimodality therapies, which include maximal transurethral resection of the bladder tumor, chemotherapy administered concurrent to radiation and perioperatively as a neoadjuvant or adjuvant to chemoradiation.

From 1981 to 1986 the National Bladder Cancer Group enrolled 70 patients with MIBC, unfit for surgery, to a protocol of chemoradiation with cisplatin as a radiation sensitizer and found it safe and effective with a very promising 70 % complete RR [123]. From 1985 to 2001, the RTOG has enrolled 415 patients in 6 phase I/II chemoradiation trials with T2-4A MIBC and fit for cystectomy with a primary objective of maximizing cure rates and secondary objective of bladder preservation [124]. In the RTOG-0233 randomized phase 2 trial, 97 patients with T2-4a transitional cell carcinoma of the bladder were enrolled to receive paclitaxel plus cisplatin or

Table 30.3 Phase I/II chemoradiation trials conducted by the Radiation Therapy Oncology Group (RTOG)

RTOG protocol	Perioperative chemotherapy	Radiation sensitizer	No. of patients	5-year survival (%)	CR (%) post-chemoradiation
85-12 [126]	None	Cisplatin	42	NA	66
88-02 [127]	CMV (NCT)	Cisplatin	91	51	75
89-03 [128]	CMV (NCT) or none	Cisplatin	123	49	59
95-06 [129]	None	Cisplatin, 5-FU	34	NA	67
97-06 [130]	CMV (ACT)	Cisplatin	52	NA	74
99-06 [131]	CG (ACT)	Cisplatin, paclitaxel	80	56	81

CMV Cisplatin, methotrexate and vinblastine; *NCT* neoadjuvant chemotherapy; *ACT* adjuvant chemotherapy; *NA* not available

fluorouracil plus cisplatin with twice-daily radiation [125]. In this trial, cisplatin-based chemoradiotherapy, combined with either paclitaxel or fluorouracil, frequently induced complete responses with bladder-intact survival and OS, but both regimens were accompanied by adverse effects, and only about half of the patients were able to complete the entire regimen including ACT.

All of these trials incorporated maximal transurethral resection of the bladder tumor followed by chemoradiation therapy with a planned cystectomy in patients who failed to achieve complete response with cystoscopy after 40 Gy of radiation therapy. Those with complete response at cystoscopy receive additional consolidation chemoradiation therapy. These six trials have explored perioperative chemotherapy (none, cisplatin with methotrexate and vinblastine, GC), a radiation sensitizer regimen (cisplatin alone or combined with 5-FU, paclitaxel) and a radiation schedule (single vs. twice daily fractionation). Complete RR in these RTOG trials after initial therapy has ranged from 59 to 81 % and 5-year OS 49–56 %, as detailed in Table 30.3.

RTOG 89-03 is the only phase III study from the above six trials that evaluated two cycles of neoadjuvant CMV before concurrent cisplatin with radiation therapy. No improvement in 5-year survival was observed in this study, and the trial was prematurely closed because of excessive toxicities including neutropenia, sepsis and treatment-related deaths [128].

All of the above RTOG trials utilized cisplatin as the radiation sensitizer, which is often very difficult to administer, especially in patients with bladder cancer, because of inadequate renal function and poor performance status. A phase III clinical trial compared a noncisplatin-based synchronous chemotherapy regimen of fluorouracil and mitomycin C to radiation therapy alone based on previous phase I and II experiences [132, 133]. Radiotherapy was delivered at either 55 Gy in 20 fractions over a 4-week period or 64-Gy in 32 fractions over 6.5 weeks. Unlike the RTOG protocols, there was no break in radiation therapy for evaluation of response to determine continuation consolidation treatment versus cystectomy. Locoregional disease-free survival at 2 years was significantly better in the chemoradiotherapy group compared to the radiotherapy group (67 % vs. 54 %, HR 0.68, $P=0.03$). Survival at 5 years, although numerically improved with chemoradiation, was not statistically significant (48 % vs. 35 %, HR 0.82, $P=0.16$). This study offers an alternative chemotherapy regimen for patients with renal insufficiency or other contraindications to cisplatin use.

There has been no randomized clinical trial comparing bladder preservation strategies with cystectomy. Cystectomy remains the gold standard for now with concerns about the efficacy with bladder preservation protocols. The function of the preserved bladder is often poor after an aggressive multimodality bladder preservation strategy, although this is being refuted by a single-institution experience, which noted preserved bladder function as measured by urodynamic monitoring in 75 % of patients [134, 135]. In this analysis of patients treated on primarily RTOG and a few on local protocols, 29 % of patients needed cystectomy (17 % immediately after failure to achieve CR and 12 % salvage for recurrent disease noted during surveillance). Similarly, follow-up of patients from four of the RTOG trials revealed only 7 % late pelvic toxicity (5.7 % experiencing genitourinary symptoms of urinary urgency/frequency and 1.9 % with gastrointestinal toxicity) [136].

30.9 Chemoradiation and Controversies

Chemoradiation has never been compared to cystectomy, which remains the gold standard in the management of patients with MIBC. Chemoradiation is an alternative for patients who are unwilling to undergo cystectomy or are medically unfit. There is no chemotherapy regimen used synchronously with radiation that has been established to be superior, and cisplatin as a single agent remains the most widely studied.

Chemotherapy preceding (neoadjuvant) or following (adjuvant) radiation therapy has not been adequately studied. Neoadjuvant CMV is poorly tolerated and does not show a survival benefit. A benefit from NCT preceding cystectomy cannot be extrapolated for radiation therapy, and newer combinations need to be tested prospectively.

30.10 Conclusion

UC is a chemosensitive malignancy, and cisplatin-based combination chemotherapy has been established as a standard for metastatic disease and as neoadjuvant therapy. However, increments in advances are necessary and may be attainable by combinations of chemotherapy with biologic agents. GC has become the preferred platform for such combinations, as exemplified by an ongoing phase III Intergroup US trial comparing GC combined with either placebo or bevacizumab. Eribulin mesylate is undergoing evaluation in a randomized phase II trial in combination with GC. Despite the absence of definitive trials establishing the role of ACT, the body of data from different trials suggests that ACT is reasonable in those with muscle-invasive high-risk, extravesical or node-positive disease following radical cystectomy if the performance status and renal function allow it. In conjunction with the development of chemobiologic combinations, other chemotherapeutics are undergoing further development, e.g., nab-paclitaxel will be compared with docetaxel in the second-line setting. The development of predictive biomarkers for the efficacy of chemotherapy needs a special focus going forward.

References

1. Agarwal N, Hussain M. Management of bladder cancer: current and emerging strategies. Drugs. 2009;69(9):1173–87.
2. Stein JP. Improving outcomes with radical cystectomy for high-grade invasive bladder cancer. World J Urol. 2006;24(5):509–16.
3. Calabro F, Sternberg CN. Neoadjuvant and adjuvant chemotherapy in muscle-invasive bladder cancer. Eur Urol. 2009;55(2):348–58.
4. Sonpavde G, Goldman BH, Speights VO, Lerner SP, Wood DP, Vogelzang NJ, et al. Quality of pathologic response and surgery correlate with survival for patients with completely resected bladder cancer after neoadjuvant chemotherapy. Cancer. 2009;115(18): 4104–9.
5. Martinez-Pineiro JA, Gonzalez Martin M, Arocena F, Flores N, Roncero CR, Portillo JA, et al. Neoadjuvant cisplatin chemotherapy before radical cystectomy in invasive transitional cell carcinoma of the bladder: a prospective randomized phase III study. J Urol. 1995;153(3 Pt 2):964–73.
6. Wallace DM, Raghavan D, Kelly KA, Sandeman TF, Conn IG, Teriana N, et al. Neo-adjuvant (pre-emptive) cisplatin therapy in invasive transitional cell carcinoma of the bladder. Br J Urol. 1991;67(6): 608–15.
7. Loehrer Sr PJ, Einhorn LH, Elson PJ, Crawford ED, Kuebler P, Tannock I, et al. A randomized comparison of cisplatin alone or in combination with methotrexate, vinblastine, and doxorubicin in patients with metastatic urothelial carcinoma: a cooperative group study. J Clin Oncol. 1992;10(7):1066–73.
8. Malmstrom PU, Rintala E, Wahlqvist R, Hellstrom P, Hellsten S, Hannisdal E. Five-year followup of a prospective trial of radical cystectomy and neoadjuvant chemotherapy: Nordic Cystectomy Trial I. The Nordic Cooperative Bladder Cancer Study Group. J Urol. 1996;155(6):1903–6.
9. Sherif A, Rintala E, Mestad O, Nilsson J, Holmberg L, Nilsson S, et al. Neoadjuvant cisplatin-methotrexate chemotherapy for invasive bladder cancer—Nordic

cystectomy trial 2. Scand J Urol Nephrol. 2002; 36(6):419–25.

10. Sherif A, Holmberg L, Rintala E, Mestad O, Nilsson J, Nilsson S, et al. Neoadjuvant cisplatinum based combination chemotherapy in patients with invasive bladder cancer: a combined analysis of two Nordic studies. Eur Urol. 2004;45(3):297–303.

11. Griffiths G, Hall R, Sylvester R, Raghavan D, Parmar MK. International phase III trial assessing neoadjuvant cisplatin, methotrexate, and vinblastine chemotherapy for muscle-invasive bladder cancer: long-term results of the BA06 30894 trial. J Clin Oncol. 2011;29(16):2171–7.

12. Grossman HB, Natale RB, Tangen CM, Speights VO, Vogelzang NJ, Trump DL, et al. Neoadjuvant chemotherapy plus cystectomy compared with cystectomy alone for locally advanced bladder cancer. N Engl J Med. 2003;349(9):859–66.

13. Rosenblatt R, Sherif A, Rintala E, Wahlqvist R, Ullen A, Nilsson S, et al. Pathologic downstaging is a surrogate marker for efficacy and increased survival following neoadjuvant chemotherapy and radical cystectomy for muscle-invasive urothelial bladder cancer. Eur Urol. 2012;61(6):1229–38.

14. Winquist E, Kirchner TS, Segal R, Chin J, Lukka H, Genitourinary Cancer Disease Site Group CCOPiE-bCPGI. Neoadjuvant chemotherapy for transitional cell carcinoma of the bladder: a systematic review and meta-analysis. J Urol. 2004;171(2 Pt 1):561–9.

15. Schultz PK, Herr HW, Zhang ZF, Bajorin DF, Seidman A, Sarkis A, et al. Neoadjuvant chemotherapy for invasive bladder cancer: prognostic factors for survival of patients treated with M-VAC with 5-year follow-up. J Clin Oncol. 1994;12(7):1394–401.

16. Petrelli F, Coinu A, Cabiddu M, Ghilardi M, Vavassori I, Barni S. Correlation of pathologic complete response with survival after neoadjuvant chemotherapy in bladder cancer treated with cystectomy: a meta-analysis. Eur Urol. 2013;65(2):350–7.

17. von der Maase H, Hansen SW, Roberts JT, Dogliotti L, Oliver T, Moore MJ, et al. Gemcitabine and cisplatin versus methotrexate, vinblastine, doxorubicin, and cisplatin in advanced or metastatic bladder cancer: results of a large, randomized, multinational, multicenter, phase III study. J Clin Oncol. 2000; 18(17):3068–77.

18. von der Maase H, Sengelov L, Roberts JT, Ricci S, Dogliotti L, Oliver T, et al. Long-term survival results of a randomized trial comparing gemcitabine plus cisplatin, with methotrexate, vinblastine, doxorubicin, plus cisplatin in patients with bladder cancer. J Clin Oncol. 2005;23(21):4602–8.

19. Dash A, Pettus JA, Herr HW, Bochner BH, Dalbagni G, Donat SM, et al. A role for neoadjuvant gemcitabine plus cisplatin in muscle-invasive urothelial carcinoma of the bladder: a retrospective experience. Cancer. 2008;113(9):2471–7.

20. Herchenhorn D, Dienstmann R, Peixoto FA, de Campos FS, Santos VO, Moreira DM, et al. Phase II trial of neoadjuvant gemcitabine and cisplatin in patients with resectable bladder carcinoma. Int Braz J Urol. 2007;33(5):630–8. discussion 8.

21. Scosyrev E, Messing EM, van Wijngaarden E, Peterson DR, Sahasrabudhe D, Golijanin D, et al. Neoadjuvant gemcitabine and cisplatin chemotherapy for locally advanced urothelial cancer of the bladder. Cancer. 2012;118(1):72–81.

22. Advanced Bladder Cancer Meta-analysis Collaboration. Neoadjuvant chemotherapy in invasive bladder cancer: update of a systematic review and meta-analysis of individual patient data advanced bladder cancer (ABC) meta-analysis collaboration. Eur Urol. 2005;48(2):202–5. discussion 5–6.

23. Bellmunt J, Ribas A, Albanell J, Bermejo B, Vera R, De Torres JA, et al. M-CAVI, a neoadjuvant carboplatin-based regimen for the treatment of T2-4N0M0 carcinoma of the bladder. Am J Clin Oncol. 1996;19(4):344–8.

24. Smith DC, Mackler NJ, Dunn RL, Hussain M, Wood D, Lee CT, et al. Phase II trial of paclitaxel, carboplatin and gemcitabine in patients with locally advanced carcinoma of the bladder. J Urol. 2008; 180(6):2384–8. discussion 8.

25. Grivas PD, Hussain M, Hafez K, Daignault-Newton S, Wood D, Lee CT, et al. A phase II Trial of neoadjuvant nab-paclitaxel, carboplatin, and gemcitabine (ACaG) in patients with locally advanced carcinoma of the bladder. Urology. 2013;82(1):111–7.

26. Svatek RS, Shariat SF, Novara G, Skinner EC, Fradet Y, Bastian PJ, et al. Discrepancy between clinical and pathological stage: external validation of the impact on prognosis in an international radical cystectomy cohort. BJU Int. 2011;107(6):898–904.

27. David KA, Milowsky MI, Ritchey J, Carroll PR, Nanus DM. Low incidence of perioperative chemotherapy for stage III bladder cancer 1998 to 2003: a report from the National Cancer Data Base. J Urol. 2007;178(2):451–4.

28. Millikan R, Dinney C, Swanson D, Sweeney P, Ro JY, Smith TL, et al. Integrated therapy for locally advanced bladder cancer: final report of a randomized trial of cystectomy plus adjuvant M-VAC versus cystectomy with both preoperative and postoperative M-VAC. J Clin Oncol. 2001;19(20):4005–13.

29. Shabsigh A, Korets R, Vora KC, Brooks CM, Cronin AM, Savage C, et al. Defining early morbidity of radical cystectomy for patients with bladder cancer using a standardized reporting methodology. Eur Urol. 2009;55(1):164–74.

30. Hiroshi Kitamura TT, Masumori N, Shibata T, Kunieda F, Fujimoto H, Hirao Y, Kitamura Y, Tomita Y, Tobisu K, Niwakawa M, Naito S, Eto M, Kakehi Y. Randomized phase III trial of neoadjuvant chemotherapy (NAC) with methotrexate, doxorubicin, vinblastine, and cisplatin (MVAC) followed by radical cystectomy (RC) compared with RC alone for muscle-invasive bladder cancer (MIBC): Japan Clinical Oncology Group study, JCOG0209. J Clin Oncol. 2013;31(Suppl):abstr 4526.

31. Brendler CB, Steinberg GD, Marshall FF, Mostwin JL, Walsh PC. Local recurrence and survival following nerve-sparing radical cystoprostatectomy. J Urol. 1990;144(5):1137–40. discussion 40–1.

32. Dimopoulos MA, Moulopoulos LA. Role of adjuvant chemotherapy in the treatment of invasive carcinoma of the urinary bladder. J Clin Oncol. 1998;16(4):1601–12.

33. Skinner DG, Lieskovsky G, Boyd SD. Continuing experience with the continent ileal reservoir (Kock pouch) as an alternative to cutaneous urinary diversion: an update after 250 cases. J Urol. 1987;137(6):1140–5.

34. Hautmann RE, Miller K, Steiner U, Wenderoth U. The ileal neobladder: 6 years of experience with more than 200 patients. J Urol. 1993;150(1):40–5.

35. Prout Jr GR, Griffin PP, Shipley WU. Bladder carcinoma as a systemic disease. Cancer. 1979;43(6):2532–9.

36. Greven KM, Spera JA, Solin LJ, Morgan T, Hanks GE. Local recurrence after cystectomy alone for bladder carcinoma. Cancer. 1992;69(11):2767–70.

37. Rosenberg JE, Carroll PR, Small EJ. Update on chemotherapy for advanced bladder cancer. J Urol. 2005;174(1):14–20.

38. Marini L, Sternberg CN. Neoadjuvant and adjuvant chemotherapy in locally advanced bladder cancer. Urol Oncol. 1997;3(5–6):133–40.

39. Logothetis CJ, Johnson DE, Chong C, Dexeus FH, Sella A, Ogden S, et al. Adjuvant cyclophosphamide, doxorubicin, and cisplatin chemotherapy for bladder cancer: an update. J Clin Oncol. 1988;6(10):1590–6.

40. Skinner DG, Daniels JR, Russell CA, Lieskovsky G, Boyd SD, Nichols P, et al. The role of adjuvant chemotherapy following cystectomy for invasive bladder cancer: a prospective comparative trial. J Urol. 1991;145(3):459–64. discussion 64–7.

41. Svatek RS, Shariat SF, Lasky RE, Skinner EC, Novara G, Lerner SP, et al. The effectiveness of off-protocol adjuvant chemotherapy for patients with urothelial carcinoma of the urinary bladder. Clin Cancer Res. 2010;16(17):4461–7.

42. Walz J, Shariat SF, Suardi N, Perrotte P, Lotan Y, Palapattu GS, et al. Adjuvant chemotherapy for bladder cancer does not alter cancer-specific survival after cystectomy in a matched case-control study. BJU Int. 2008;101(11):1356–61.

43. Cognetti F, Ruggeri EM, Felici A, Gallucci M, Muto G, Pollera CF, et al. Adjuvant chemotherapy with cisplatin and gemcitabine versus chemotherapy at relapse in patients with muscle-invasive bladder cancer submitted to radical cystectomy: an Italian, multicenter, randomized phase III trial. Ann Oncol. 2012;23(3):695–700.

44. Paz-Ares LG, Solsona E, Esteban E, Saez A, Gonzalez-Larriba J, Anton A, et al. Randomized phase III trial comparing adjuvant paclitaxel/gemcitabine/cisplatin (PGC) to observation in patients with resected invasive bladder cancer: Results of the Spanish Oncology Genitourinary Group (SOGUG) 99/01 study. J Clin Oncol. 2010;28(18s).

45. Comparison of immediate and delayed adjuvant chemotherapy in treating patients who have undergone a radical cystectomy for stage III or stage IV transitional cell carcinoma of the bladder urothelium: EORTC 30994. [Internet]. Available from: http://clinicaltrials.gov/ct2/show/NCT00028756

46. Phase III study comparing sequential chemotherapy (AG-ITP) to cisplatin and gemcitabine as adjuvant treatment after cystectomy for transitional cell carcinoma of the bladder [Internet]. Available from: http://clinicaltrials.gov/ct2/show/NCT00014534

47. Advanced Bladder Cancer Meta-analysis Collaboration. Adjuvant chemotherapy for invasive bladder cancer (individual patient data). The Cochrane Database of systematic reviews. 2006(2):CD006018.

48. Advanced Bladder Cancer (ABC) Meta-analysis Collaboration. Adjuvant chemotherapy in invasive bladder cancer: a systematic review and meta-analysis of individual patient data. Advanced Bladder Cancer (ABC) Meta-analysis Collaboration. Eur Urol. 2005;48(2):189–99.

49. Richards B, Bastable JR, Freedman L, Glashan RW, Harris G, Newling DW, et al. Adjuvant chemotherapy with doxorubicin (adriamycin) and 5-fluorouracil in T3, NX, MO bladder cancer treated with radiotherapy. Br J Urol. 1983;55(4):386–91.

50. Einstein Jr AB, Shipley W, Coombs J, Cummings KB, Soloway MS, Hawkins I. Cisplatin as adjunctive treatment for invasive bladder carcinoma: tolerance and toxicities. Urology. 1984;23(4 Suppl):110–7.

51. Stockle M, Meyenburg W, Wellek S, Voges GE, Rossmann M, Gertenbach U, et al. Adjuvant polychemotherapy of nonorgan-confined bladder cancer after radical cystectomy revisited: long-term results of a controlled prospective study and further clinical experience. J Urol. 1995;153(1):47–52.

52. Studer UE, Bacchi M, Biedermann C, Jaeger P, Kraft R, Mazzucchelli L, et al. Adjuvant cisplatin chemotherapy following cystectomy for bladder cancer: results of a prospective randomized trial. J Urol. 1994;152(1):81–4.

53. Freiha F, Reese J, Torti FM. A randomized trial of radical cystectomy versus radical cystectomy plus cisplatin, vinblastine and methotrexate chemotherapy for muscle invasive bladder cancer. J Urol. 1996;155(2):495–9. discussion 9–500.

54. Skinner DG, Daniels JR, Russell CA, Lieskovsky G, Boyd SD, Krailo M, et al. Adjuvant chemotherapy following cystectomy benefits patients with deeply invasive bladder cancer. Semin Urol. 1990;8(4):279–84.

55. Shearer RJ, Chilvers CF, Bloom HJ, Bliss JM, Horwich A, Babiker A. Adjuvant chemotherapy in T3 carcinoma of the bladder. A prospective trial: preliminary report. Br J Urol. 1988;62(6):558–64.

56. Ruggeri EM, Giannarelli D, Bria E, Carlini P, Felici A, Nelli F, et al. Adjuvant chemotherapy in muscle-invasive bladder carcinoma: a pooled analysis from phase III studies. Cancer. 2006;106(4):783–8.

57. Yagoda A. Phase-II trials in patients with urothelial tract tumors. Memorial Sloan-Kettering Cancer Center. Cancer Chemother Pharmacol. 1983;11(Suppl): S9–12.

58. Sternberg CN, Yagoda A, Scher HI, Watson RC, Ahmed T, Weiselberg LR, et al. Preliminary results of M-VAC (methotrexate, vinblastine, doxorubicin and cisplatin) for transitional cell carcinoma of the urothelium. J Urol. 1985;133(3):403–7.

59. Sternberg CN, Yagoda A, Scher HI, Watson RC, Geller N, Herr HW, et al. Methotrexate, vinblastine, doxorubicin, and cisplatin for advanced transitional cell carcinoma of the urothelium. Efficacy and patterns of response and relapse. Cancer. 1989;64(12): 2448–58.

60. Saxman SB, Propert KJ, Einhorn LH, Crawford ED, Tannock I, Raghavan D, et al. Long-term follow-up of a phase III intergroup study of cisplatin alone or in combination with methotrexate, vinblastine, and doxorubicin in patients with metastatic urothelial carcinoma: a cooperative group study. J Clin Oncol. 1997;15(7):2564–9.

61. Gabrilove JL, Jakubowski A, Scher H, Sternberg C, Wong G, Grous J, et al. Effect of granulocyte colony-stimulating factor on neutropenia and associated morbidity due to chemotherapy for transitional-cell carcinoma of the urothelium. N Engl J Med. 1988; 318(22):1414–22.

62. Logothetis CJ, Finn LD, Smith T, Kilbourn RG, Ellerhorst JA, Zukiwski AA, et al. Escalated MVAC with or without recombinant human granulocyte-macrophage colony-stimulating factor for the initial treatment of advanced malignant urothelial tumors: results of a randomized trial. J Clin Oncol. 1995;13(9):2272–7.

63. Moore MJ, Iscoe N, Tannock IF. A phase II study of methotrexate, vinblastine, doxorubicin and cisplatin plus recombinant human granulocyte-macrophage colony stimulating factors in patients with advanced transitional cell carcinoma. J Urol. 1993;150(4): 1131–4.

64. Seidman AD, Scher HI, Gabrilove JL, Bajorin DF, Motzer RJ, O'Dell M, et al. Dose-intensification of MVAC with recombinant granulocyte colony-stimulating factor as initial therapy in advanced urothelial cancer. J Clin Oncol. 1993;11(3):408–14.

65. Sternberg CN, de Mulder PH, Schornagel JH, Theodore C, Fossa SD, van Oosterom AT, et al. Randomized phase III trial of high-dose-intensity methotrexate, vinblastine, doxorubicin, and cisplatin (MVAC) chemotherapy and recombinant human granulocyte colony-stimulating factor versus classic MVAC in advanced urothelial tract tumors: European Organization for Research and Treatment of Cancer Protocol no. 30924. J Clin Oncol. 2001;19(10): 2638–46.

66. Sternberg CN, de Mulder P, Schornagel JH, Theodore C, Fossa SD, van Oosterom AT, et al. Seven year update of an EORTC phase III trial of high-dose intensity M-VAC chemotherapy and G-CSF versus classic M-VAC in advanced urothelial tract tumours. Eur J Cancer. 2006;42(1):50–4.

67. Logothetis CJ, Dexeus FH, Finn L, Sella A, Amato RJ, Ayala AG, et al. A prospective randomized trial comparing MVAC and CISCA chemotherapy for patients with metastatic urothelial tumors. J Clin Oncol. 1990;8(6):1050–5.

68. Roth BJ, Dreicer R, Einhorn LH, Neuberg D, Johnson DH, Smith JL, et al. Significant activity of paclitaxel in advanced transitional-cell carcinoma of the urothelium: a phase II trial of the Eastern Cooperative Oncology Group. J Clin Oncol. 1994; 12(11):2264–70.

69. Witte RS, Elson P, Bono B, Knop R, Richardson RR, Dreicer R, et al. Eastern Cooperative Oncology Group phase II trial of ifosfamide in the treatment of previously treated advanced urothelial carcinoma. J Clin Oncol. 1997;15(2):589–93.

70. McCaffrey JA, Hilton S, Mazumdar M, Sadan S, Kelly WK, Scher HI, et al. Phase II trial of docetaxel in patients with advanced or metastatic transitional-cell carcinoma. J Clin Oncol. 1997;15(5):1853–7.

71. Dreicer R, Manola J, Roth BJ, Cohen MB, Hatfield AK, Wilding G. Phase II study of cisplatin and paclitaxel in advanced carcinoma of the urothelium: an Eastern Cooperative Oncology Group Study. J Clin Oncol. 2000;18(5):1058–61.

72. Stadler WM, Kuzel T, Roth B, Raghavan D, Dorr FA. Phase II study of single-agent gemcitabine in previously untreated patients with metastatic urothelial cancer. J Clin Oncol. 1997;15(11):3394–8.

73. Bamias A, Aravantinos G, Deliveliotis C, Bafaloukos D, Kalofonos C, Xiros N, et al. Docetaxel and cisplatin with granulocyte colony-stimulating factor (G-CSF) versus MVAC with G-CSF in advanced urothelial carcinoma: a multicenter, randomized, phase III study from the Hellenic Cooperative Oncology Group. J Clin Oncol. 2004;22(2):220–8.

74. Pollera CF, Ceribelli A, Crecco M, Calabresi F. Weekly gemcitabine in advanced bladder cancer: a preliminary report from a phase I study. Ann Oncol. 1994;5(2):182–4.

75. Lorusso V, Pollera CF, Antimi M, Luporini G, Gridelli C, Frassineti GL, et al. A phase II study of gemcitabine in patients with transitional cell carcinoma of the urinary tract previously treated with platinum. Italian Co-operative Group on Bladder Cancer. Eur J Cancer. 1998;34(8):1208–12.

76. Moore MJ, Tannock IF, Ernst DS, Huan S, Murray N. Gemcitabine: a promising new agent in the treatment of advanced urothelial cancer. J Clin Oncol. 1997;15(12):3441–5.

77. Kaufman D, Raghavan D, Carducci M, Levine EG, Murphy B, Aisner J, et al. Phase II trial of gemcitabine plus cisplatin in patients with metastatic urothelial cancer. J Clin Oncol. 2000;18(9):1921–7.

78. Moore MJ, Winquist EW, Murray N, Tannock IF, Huan S, Bennett K, et al. Gemcitabine plus cisplatin, an active regimen in advanced urothelial cancer: a phase II trial of the National Cancer Institute of

Canada Clinical Trials Group. J Clin Oncol. 1999; 17(9):2876–81.

79. Bellmunt J, von der Maase H, Mead GM, Skoneczna I, De Santis M, Daugaard G, et al. Randomized phase III study comparing paclitaxel/cisplatin/gemcitabine and gemcitabine/cisplatin in patients with locally advanced or metastatic urothelial cancer without prior systemic therapy: EORTC Intergroup Study 30987. J Clin Oncol. 2012;30(10):1107–13.

80. Sonpavde G, Watson D, Tourtellott M, Cowey CL, Hellerstedt B, Hutson TE, et al. Administration of cisplatin-based chemotherapy for advanced urothelial carcinoma in the community. Clin Genitourin Cancer. 2012;10(1):1–5.

81. Bellmunt J, de Wit R, Albanell J, Baselga J. A feasibility study of carboplatin with fixed dose of gemcitabine in "unfit" patients with advanced bladder cancer. Eur J Cancer. 2001;37(17):2212–5.

82. de Wit R, Tesselaar M, Kok TC, Seynaeve C, Rodenburg CJ, Verweij J, et al. Randomised phase II trial of carboplatin and iproplatin in advanced urothelial cancer. Eur J Cancer. 1991;27(11):1383–5.

83. Klocker J, Pont J, Schumer J, Pruger J, Kienzer H. Carboplatin, methotrexate and vinblastin (Carbo-MV) for advanced urothelial cancer. A phase II trial. Am J Clin Oncol. 1991;14(4):328–30.

84. Bellmunt J, Albanell J, Gallego OS, Ribas A, Vicente P, Carulla J, et al. Carboplatin, methotrexate, and vinblastine in patients with bladder cancer who were ineligible for cisplatin-based chemotherapy. Cancer. 1992;70(7):1974–9.

85. Waxman J, Barton C. Carboplatin-based chemotherapy for bladder cancer. Cancer Treat Rev. 1993; 19(Suppl):21–5.

86. Small EJ, Fippin LJ, Ernest ML, Carroll PR. A carboplatin-based regimen for the treatment of patients with advanced transitional cell carcinoma of the urothelium. Cancer. 1996;78(8):1775–80.

87. Vaughn DJ, Malkowicz SB, Zoltick B, Mick R, Ramchandani P, Holroyde C, et al. Paclitaxel plus carboplatin in advanced carcinoma of the urothelium: an active and tolerable outpatient regimen. J Clin Oncol. 1998;16(1):255–60.

88. Redman BG, Smith DC, Flaherty L, Du W, Hussain M. Phase II trial of paclitaxel and carboplatin in the treatment of advanced urothelial carcinoma. J Clin Oncol. 1998;16(5):1844–8.

89. Petrioli R, Frediani B, Manganelli A, Barbanti G, De Capua B, De Lauretis A, et al. Comparison between a cisplatin-containing regimen and a carboplatin-containing regimen for recurrent or metastatic bladder cancer patients. A randomized phase II study. Cancer. 1996;77(2):344–51.

90. Dogliotti L, Carteni G, Siena S, Bertetto O, Martoni A, Bono A, et al. Gemcitabine plus cisplatin versus gemcitabine plus carboplatin as first-line chemotherapy in advanced transitional cell carcinoma of the urothelium: results of a randomized phase 2 trial. Eur Urol. 2007;52(1):134–41.

91. Dreicer R, Manola J, Roth BJ, See WA, Kuross S, Edelman MJ, et al. Phase III trial of methotrexate, vinblastine, doxorubicin, and cisplatin versus carboplatin and paclitaxel in patients with advanced carcinoma of the urothelium. Cancer. 2004;100(8):1639–45.

92. Hussain SA, Stocken DD, Riley P, Palmer DH, Peake DR, Geh JI, et al. A phase I/II study of gemcitabine and fractionated cisplatin in an outpatient setting using a 21-day schedule in patients with advanced and metastatic bladder cancer. Br J Cancer. 2004;91(5):844–9.

93. Beer TM, Goldman B, Nichols CR, Petrylak DP, Agarwal M, Ryan CW, et al. Southwest Oncology Group phase II study of irinotecan in patients with advanced transitional cell carcinoma of the urothelium that progressed after platinum-based chemotherapy. Clin Genitourin Cancer. 2008;6(1):36–9.

94. Choueiri TK, Vaishampayan U, Rosenberg JE, Logan TF, Harzstark AL, Bukowski RM, et al. Phase II and biomarker study of the dual MET/VEGFR2 inhibitor foretinib in patients with papillary renal cell carcinoma. J Clin Oncol. 2013;31(2):181–6.

95. Culine S, Theodore C, De Santis M, Bui B, Demkow T, Lorenz J, et al. A phase II study of vinflunine in bladder cancer patients progressing after first-line platinum-containing regimen. Br J Cancer. 2006; 94(10):1395–401.

96. Petrylak DP, Tangen CM, Van Veldhuizen Jr PJ, Goodwin JW, Twardowski PW, Atkins JN, et al. Results of the Southwest Oncology Group phase II evaluation (study S0031) of ZD1839 for advanced transitional cell carcinoma of the urothelium. BJU Int. 2010;105(3):317–21.

97. Sternberg CN, Calabro F, Pizzocaro G, Marini L, Schnetzer S, Sella A. Chemotherapy with an every-2-week regimen of gemcitabine and paclitaxel in patients with transitional cell carcinoma who have received prior cisplatin-based therapy. Cancer. 2001;92(12):2993–8.

98. Vaughn DJ, Srinivas S, Stadler WM, Pili R, Petrylak D, Sternberg CN, et al. Vinflunine in platinum-pretreated patients with locally advanced or metastatic urothelial carcinoma: results of a large phase 2 study. Cancer. 2009;115(18):4110–7.

99. Wong Y, Litwin S, Vaughn DJ, Plimack ER, Song W, Lee JW, Dabrow MB, Brody M, Tuttle H, Hudes GR. Effect of EGFR inhibition with cetuximab (CET) on the efficacy of paclitaxel (TAX) in previously treated metastatic (MET) urothelial cancer. J Clin Oncol 2011;29 (suppl); abstr 4617.

100. Bellmunt J, Theodore C, Demkov T, Komyakov B, Sengelov L, Daugaard G, et al. Phase III trial of vinflunine plus best supportive care compared with best supportive care alone after a platinum-containing regimen in patients with advanced transitional cell carcinoma of the urothelial tract. J Clin Oncol. 2009;27(27):4454–61.

101. Albers P, Park SI, Niegisch G, Fechner G, Steiner U, Lehmann J, et al. Randomized phase III trial of 2nd

line gemcitabine and paclitaxel chemotherapy in patients with advanced bladder cancer: short-term versus prolonged treatment [German Association of Urological Oncology (AUO) trial AB 20/99]. Ann Oncol. 2011;22(2):288–94.

102. Pili R, Qin R, Flynn PJ, Picus J, Millward M, Ho WM, Pitot HC, Tan W, Erlichman C, Vaishampayan UN. MC0553: A phase II safety and efficacy study with the VEGF receptor tyrosine kinase inhibitor pazopanib in patients with metastatic urothelial cancer. J Clin Oncol 29; 2011 (suppl 7); abstr 259.

103. Sonpavde G, Sternberg CN, Rosenberg JE, Hahn NM, Galsky MD, Vogelzang NJ. Second-line systemic therapy and emerging drugs for metastatic transitional-cell carcinoma of the urothelium. Lancet Oncol. 2010;11(9):861–70.

104. Ko YJ, Canil CM, Mukherjee SD, Winquist E, Elser C, Eisen A, et al. Nanoparticle albumin-bound paclitaxel for second-line treatment of metastatic urothelial carcinoma: a single group, multicentre, phase 2 study. Lancet Oncol. 2013;14(8):769–76.

105. Necchi A, Mariani L, Zaffaroni N, Schwartz LH, Giannatempo P, Crippa F, et al. Pazopanib in advanced and platinum-resistant urothelial cancer: an open-label, single group, phase 2 trial. Lancet Oncol. 2012;13(8):810–6.

106. Bellmunt J, Choueiri TK, Fougeray R, Schutz FA, Salhi Y, Winquist E, et al. Prognostic factors in patients with advanced transitional cell carcinoma of the urothelial tract experiencing treatment failure with platinum-containing regimens. J Clin Oncol. 2010;28(11):1850–5.

107. Sonpavde G, Pond GR, Fougeray R, Choueiri TK, Qu AQ, Vaughn DJ, et al. Time from prior chemotherapy enhances prognostic risk grouping in the second-line setting of advanced urothelial carcinoma: a retrospective analysis of pooled, prospective phase 2 trials. Eur Urol. 2013;63(4):717–23.

108. Vaughn DJ, Broome CM, Hussain M, Gutheil JC, Markowitz AB. Phase II trial of weekly paclitaxel in patients with previously treated advanced urothelial cancer. J Clin Oncol. 2002;20(4):937–40.

109. Sweeney CJ, Roth BJ, Kabbinavar FF, Vaughn DJ, Arning M, Curiel RE, et al. Phase II study of pemetrexed for second-line treatment of transitional cell cancer of the urothelium. J Clin Oncol. 2006;24(21):3451–7.

110. Galsky MD, Mironov S, Iasonos A, Scattergood J, Boyle MG, Bajorin DF. Phase II trial of pemetrexed as second-line therapy in patients with metastatic urothelial carcinoma. Invest New Drugs. 2007;25(3):265–70.

111. Dreicer R, Li S, Manola J, Haas NB, Roth BJ, Wilding G, et al. Phase 2 trial of epothilone B analog BMS-247550 (ixabepilone) in advanced carcinoma of the urothelium (E3800): a trial of the Eastern Cooperative Oncology Group. Cancer. 2007;110(4):759–63.

112. Rosenberg JE, Halabi S, Sanford BL, Himelstein AL, Atkins JN, Hohl RJ, et al. Phase II study of bortezomib in patients with previously treated advanced urothelial tract transitional cell carcinoma: CALGB 90207. Ann Oncol. 2008;19(5):946–50.

113. Winquist E, Vokes E, Moore MJ, Schumm LP, Hoving K, Stadler WM. A Phase II study of oxaliplatin in urothelial cancer. Urol Oncol. 2005;23(3):150–4.

114. Dreicer R, Li H, Stein M, DiPaola R, Eleff M, Roth BJ, et al. Phase 2 trial of sorafenib in patients with advanced urothelial cancer: a trial of the Eastern Cooperative Oncology Group. Cancer. 2009;115(18):4090–5.

115. Gallagher DJ, Milowsky MI, Gerst SR, Lasonos A, Boyle MG, Trout A, et al. Final results of a phase II study of sunitinib in patients (pts) with relapsed or refractory urothelial carcinoma (UC). J Clin Oncol. 2008;26(15S):5082.

116. Meluch AA, Greco FA, Burris 3rd HA, O'Rourke T, Ortega G, Steis RG, et al. Paclitaxel and gemcitabine chemotherapy for advanced transitional-cell carcinoma of the urothelial tract: a phase II trial of the Minnie Pearl Cancer Research Network. J Clin Oncol. 2001;19(12):3018–24.

117. Fechner G, Siener R, Reimann M, Kobalz L, Albers P, German Association of Urologic Oncology Bladder Cancer Study G. Randomised phase II trial of gemcitabine and paclitaxel second-line chemotherapy in patients with transitional cell carcinoma (AUO Trial AB 20/99). Int J Clin Pract. 2006;60(1):27–31.

118. Han KS, Joung JY, Kim TS, Jeong IG, Seo HK, Chung J, et al. Methotrexate, vinblastine, doxorubicin and cisplatin combination regimen as salvage chemotherapy for patients with advanced or metastatic transitional cell carcinoma after failure of gemcitabine and cisplatin chemotherapy. Br J Cancer. 2008;98(1):86–90.

119. Kattan J, Culine S, Theodore C, Droz JP. Second-line M-VAC therapy in patients previously treated with the M-VAC regimen for metastatic urothelial cancer. Ann Oncol. 1993;4(9):793–4.

120. Goffinet DR, Schneider MJ, Glatstein EJ, Ludwig H, Ray GR, Dunnick NR, et al. Bladder cancer: results of radiation therapy in 384 patients. Radiology. 1975;117(1):149–53.

121. Mameghan H, Fisher R, Mameghan J, Brook S. Analysis of failure following definitive radiotherapy for invasive transitional cell carcinoma of the bladder. Int J Radiat Oncol Biol Phys. 1995;31(2):247–54.

122. Birkenhake S, Martus P, Kuhn R, Schrott KM, Sauer R. Radiotherapy alone or radiochemotherapy with platin derivatives following transurethral resection of the bladder. Organ preservation and survival after treatment of bladder cancer. Strahlenther Onkol. 1998;174(3):121–7.

123. Shipley WU, Prout Jr GR, Einstein AB, Coombs LJ, Wajsman Z, Soloway MS, et al. Treatment of invasive bladder cancer by cisplatin and radiation in patients unsuited for surgery. JAMA. 1987;258(7): 931–5.

124. Shipley WU, Kaufman DS, Tester WJ, Pilepich MV, Sandler HM. Overview of bladder cancer trials in the Radiation Therapy Oncology Group. Cancer. 2003;97(8 Suppl):2115–9.

125. Mitin T, Hunt D, Shipley WU, Kaufman DS, Uzzo R, Wu CL, et al. Transurethral surgery and twice-daily radiation plus paclitaxel-cisplatin or fluorouracil-cisplatin with selective bladder preservation and adjuvant chemotherapy for patients with muscle invasive bladder cancer (RTOG 0233): a randomised multicentre phase 2 trial. Lancet Oncol. 2013;14(9):863–72.

126. Tester W, Porter A, Asbell S, Coughlin C, Heaney J, Krall J, et al. Combined modality program with possible organ preservation for invasive bladder carcinoma: results of RTOG protocol 85-12. Int J Radiat Oncol Biol Phys. 1993;25(5):783–90.

127. Tester W, Caplan R, Heaney J, Venner P, Whittington R, Byhardt R, et al. Neoadjuvant combined modality program with selective organ preservation for invasive bladder cancer: results of Radiation Therapy Oncology Group phase II trial 8802. J Clin Oncol. 1996;14(1):119–26.

128. Shipley WU, Winter KA, Kaufman DS, Lee WR, Heney NM, Tester WR, et al. Phase III trial of neoadjuvant chemotherapy in patients with invasive bladder cancer treated with selective bladder preservation by combined radiation therapy and chemotherapy: initial results of Radiation Therapy Oncology Group 89-03. J Clin Oncol. 1998;16(11): 3576–83.

129. Kaufman DS, Winter KA, Shipley WU, Heney NM, Chetner MP, Souhami L, et al. The initial results in muscle-invading bladder cancer of RTOG 95-06: phase I/II trial of transurethral surgery plus radiation therapy with concurrent cisplatin and 5-fluorouracil followed by selective bladder preservation or cystec-tomy depending on the initial response. Oncologist. 2000;5(6):471–6.

130. Hagan MP, Winter KA, Kaufman DS, Wajsman Z, Zietman AL, Heney NM, et al. RTOG 97-06: initial report of a phase I-II trial of selective bladder conservation using TURBT, twice-daily accelerated irradiation sensitized with cisplatin, and adjuvant MCV combination chemotherapy. Int J Radiat Oncol Biol Phys. 2003;57(3):665–72.

131. Kaufman DS, Winter KA, Shipley WU, Heney NM, Wallace 3rd HJ, Toonkel LM, et al. Phase I-II RTOG study (99-06) of patients with muscle-invasive bladder cancer undergoing transurethral surgery, paclitaxel, cisplatin, and twice-daily radiotherapy followed by selective bladder preservation or radical cystectomy and adjuvant chemotherapy. Urology. 2009;73(4):833–7.

132. Hussain SA, Moffitt DD, Glaholm JG, Peake D, Wallace DM, James ND. A phase I-II study of synchronous chemoradiotherapy for poor prognosis locally advanced bladder cancer. Ann Oncol. 2001;12(7):929–35.

133. Hussain SA, Moffitt DD, Glaholm JG, Peake D, Wallace DMA, James ND. A phase II study of synchronous chemo-radiotherapy for locally advanced bladder cancer. Br J Cancer. 2001;85:16.

134. Zietman AL, Sacco D, Skowronski U, Gomery P, Kaufman DS, Clark JA, et al. Organ conservation in invasive bladder cancer by transurethral resection, chemotherapy and radiation: results of a urodynamic and quality of life study on long-term survivors. J Urol. 2003;170(5):1772–6.

135. Efstathiou JA, Spiegel DY, Shipley WU, Heney NM, Kaufman DS, Niemierko A, et al. Long-term outcomes of selective bladder preservation by combined-modality therapy for invasive bladder cancer: the MGH experience. Eur Urol. 2012;61(4):705–11.

136. Efstathiou JA, Bae K, Shipley WU, Kaufman DS, Hagan MP, Heney NM, et al. Late pelvic toxicity after bladder-sparing therapy in patients with invasive bladder cancer: RTOG 89-03, 95-06, 97-06, 99-06. J Clin Oncol. 2009;27(25):4055–61.

72-year-old man with a bulky, although mobile T2 urothelial carcinoma without evidence of metastasis

Chad R. Ritch and Michael S. Cookson

Abbreviations

AC	Adjuvant chemotherapy
CR	Complete response
ECOG	Eastern Cooperative Oncology Group
GC	Gemcitabine cisplatin
MIBC	Muscle-invasive bladder cancer
M-VAC	Methotrexate vinblastine, adriamycin, cisplatin
NAC	Neoadjuvant chemotherapy
PS	Performance status
RC	Radical cystectomy
TURBT	Transurethral resection of the bladder

31.1 Introduction

31.1.1 Clinical Scenario

A 72-year-old male presented with a history of intermittent painless gross hematuria. His past medical history was significant for benign pros-

C.R. Ritch, M.D., M.B.A. (✉)
University of Miami, Miller School of Medicine,
1120 NW 14th Ave, Miami, FL 33129, USA
e-mail: critch@miami.edu

M.S. Cookson, M.D., M.M.H.C.
University of Oklahoma Medical Center,
920 Stanton L Young Blvd, Oklahoma City,
OK 73104, USA
e-mail: michael-cookson@ouhsc.edu

tatic hypertrophy and his surgical history was unremarkable. He had a 19-year history of tobacco smoking and stopped 40 years ago. His Eastern Cooperative Oncology Group (ECOG) performance status was 0. Initial work-up involved a CT scan of the abdomen and pelvis that revealed an 8 cm intravesical mass extending along the lateral aspects of the bladder bilaterally as well as perivesical stranding concerning for extravesical tumor extension (Fig. 31.1). There was no evidence of hydronephrosis or lymphadenopathy. The patient's laboratory analysis was unremarkable and his renal function was stable with a serum Cr of 0.7 mg/dL. On bimanual exam, the bladder and prostate were mobile. A cystoscopy and transurethral resection of the bladder (TURBT) was performed which revealed a significant tumor burden involving up to 80 % of his bladder. The final pathology demonstrated high-grade papillary urothelial carcinoma invading muscularis propria (clinical stage T2).

31.1.2 Considerations for Neoadjuvant Chemotherapy

The decision to proceed directly to radical cystectomy (RC) versus neoadjuvant chemotherapy (NAC) followed by RC is based on multiple factors. The ICUD-EAU 2012 recommendations on bladder cancer support the use of NAC prior to

B.R. Konety and S.S. Chang (eds.), *Management of Bladder Cancer:
A Comprehensive Text With Clinical Scenarios*, DOI 10.1007/978-1-4939-1881-2_31,
© Springer Science+Business Media New York 2015

Fig. 31.1 CT scan demonstrating bulky T2 bladder cancer at the time of initial presentation

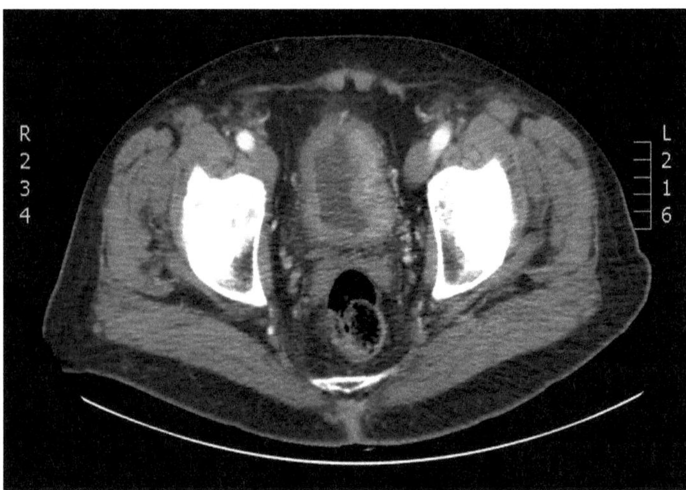

RC with approximately a 5 % overall survival advantage as compared to RC alone [1]. Furthermore, level I evidence from the Southwest Oncology Group 8710 trial (SWOG 8710) supports good pT0 response rates (38 % vs. 15 %, $P<0.001$) and a trend toward longer median survival (77 vs. 46 months, $P=0.06$) for patients undergoing neoadjuvant chemotherapy with M-VAC (methotrexate, vinblastine, adriamycin, and cisplatin) plus surgery compared to surgery alone (2). Despite the evidence in support of its usage, observational data demonstrate that it is still only administered to less than one-third of patients undergoing RC in the U.S. [2]. However, there are a variety of barriers that exist including surgeon bias, patient acceptance as well as a multitude of practical limitations and patient factors that may limit this recommendation despite the potential for survival advantage.

Patient factors are critical in the decision making for consideration of NAC. The patient's performance status (PS) should be considered as one of the main deciding factors whether or not to proceed with NAC. Those patients with "fair" to "poor" PS will most likely not tolerate NAC. The exception to this would be the patient whose poor performance status was directly related to their cancer symptoms. Reported adverse events with cisplatin-based chemotherapy include: hematologic (neutropenia, anemia, thrombocytopenia), gastrointestinal (nausea, vomiting, diarrhea), nephrotoxicity, neuropathy, and fatigue [3].

Though the majority of these are typically moderate (grade 3) adverse events, patients with poor PS who experience such toxicity are unlikely to complete treatment and may potentially experience undesired surgical delay or ultimately progress to the point that they are no longer surgical candidates. In our experience, based on the current clinical scenario, this patient's excellent PS makes him a good candidate for consideration of NAC.

Gemcitabine and Cisplatinum (GC) is a chemotherapeutic regimen that is commonly used at our institution in the neoadjuvant setting. While there are no randomized controlled trials comparing GC to M-VAC in the neoadjuvant setting, there is evidence to support less toxicity and non-inferiority with GC as compared to M-VAC [4]. Results from a large randomized phase III study of GC versus M-VAC in metastatic bladder cancer demonstrated lower rates of neutropenic fever, neutropenic sepsis, and toxic deaths with GC [4]. While the majority of data in support of GC non-inferiority is derived from retrospective series, these studies show pT0 rates of 35 % that is comparable to MVAC in the neoadjuvant setting [5].

Renal impairment is also a relative contraindication to full dose cisplatin-based chemotherapy. In the setting of impaired renal function, dose reduction of the cisplatin or alternative regimens such as those containing carboplatin have been considered in these situations [6]. However, caution should be exercised in extrapolating the results of cisplatin-based trials to the clinical use of carboplatin as there are currently no randomized trials demonstrating benefit in the neoadjuvant setting. A phase II trial of neoadjuvant paclitaxel, carboplatin, and gemcitabine demonstrated a 32 % complete response rate in patients undergoing RC [7]. However, other phase II studies comparing cisplatin to carboplatin containing regimens have demonstrated lower response rates and overall survival leading to concerns of inferior efficacy [8].

Prior to offering alternative chemotherapy regimens in patients with renal impairment who are being considered for NAC, attempts should be made to optimize renal function with either percutaneous nephrostomy or ureteral stenting if obstruction is the source of failure. Then, it is recommended that the patient be offered NAC utilizing a cisplatin-based regimen once renal function improves. Otherwise, in a patient with muscle-invasive bladder cancer (MIBC) and good PS and non-obstructive renal impairment, proceeding directly to RC may be appropriate.

Nutritional status should also play a role in deciding in whom to offer NAC. It has been demonstrated that nutritional deficiency is a strong predictor of 90-day mortality in patients undergoing RC [9]. In our experience, patients with nutritional deficiency defined as such as these with increased risk of mortality from surgery alone are unlikely to achieve benefit from NAC. Their inability to tolerate chemotherapy as well as the probability of chemotherapy-induced toxicity often precludes them from being considered candidates for NAC. In this clinical situation, we recommend they should be nutritionally optimized first and then proceed directly to surgery.

In considering NAC, there are certain clinical factors that predict more advanced pathology and subsequent adverse outcomes. These factors include a delay in presentation or treatment beyond 3 months, clinically locally advanced tumors (T3b-T4), presence of hydronephrosis and/or suspicion of lymphadenopathy on cross-sectional imaging. These features suggest more aggressive tumors and are therefore best managed by multimodal therapy with chemotherapy up-front followed by RC. In addition, the presence of lymphovascular invasion on the TURBT specimen is suggestive of more aggressive disease and influences our decision to proceed with NAC.

As a part of our NAC protocol, we recommend obtain repeat imaging with a CT scan of the abdomen and pelvis following completion of the first 2 cycles. Any evidence of tumor progression on imaging is a poor prognostic indicator as these patients unlikely to achieve any additional response, and in most settings we will abort chemotherapy and proceed directly to surgery. Patients who experience a complete response (CR–cT0) on TURBT after chemotherapy should still be treated with RC. The rationale for surgery is that despite evidence of response, there can still be significant discordance between clinical and pathological stage. Studies have shown that despite 57 % of patients achieving a clinical CR following neoadjuvant MVAC, only 30 % actually had a pathological CR [10].

Given these considerations and caveats, the patient in this clinical scenario has an ECOG PS of 0, no renal functional impairment and with good nutritional status is an optimal candidate for cisplatin-based NAC. He therefore underwent three cycles of NAC with GC. He tolerated the systemic therapy well with only mild fatigue and cold sensitivity. His post-chemotherapy CT scan demonstrated marked improvement with respect to his primary tumor. There was some residual thickening of the bladder wall but no perivesical stranding, hydronephrosis or evidence to suggest extravesical extension (Fig. 31.2). He underwent RC 4 weeks following his chemotherapy. Final pathology was pT2a, N0, Mx with 19 lymph nodes available for analysis. He was discharged on postoperative day 7 without complications. His 30- and 90-day follow-up visits were unremarkable overall he has been doing well.

31.1.3 When Would We Consider Adjuvant Chemotherapy?

We typically reserve adjuvant chemotherapy (AC) for those patients who have significant symptoms related to the primary tumor that necessitate urgent cystectomy but who are then found to harbor adverse features on final pathology.

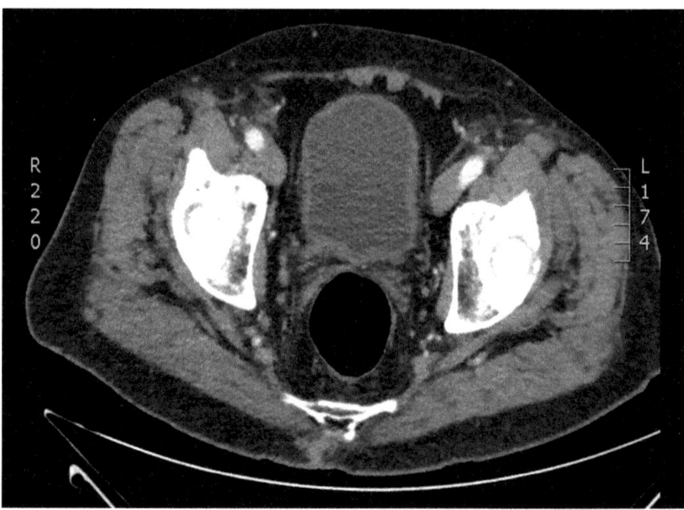

Fig. 31.2 CT scan demonstrating clinical response following 3 cycles of Gemcitabine/Cisplatin (GC) for T2 bladder cancer in the same patient (see Fig. 31.1)

For example, if a patient presents with gross hematuria or severe lower urinary tract symptoms they will often not tolerate NAC and can potentially be harmed by treatment-related anemia, infection and possibly sepsis. We would therefore proceed directly to RC in order to relieve their symptoms and treat their disease. Following RC, if the pathology demonstrates advanced stage (pT3b or T4) or multiple involved lymph nodes we will consider offering AC with the hope of eradicating residual micrometastatic disease. Again, as is the case with NAC, we would consider factors such as performance status, nutritional status and clinical comorbidities such as renal and cardiac function before offering AC. It is important to recognize the fact that despite being considered for AC based on pathological features, many RC patients do not go on to receive therapy based on a planned schedule due to the recovery period and postoperative morbidity [11, 12].

Patients who are not considered good candidates for AC are those who have poor PS and are nutritionally depleted with multiple comorbidities and no visible residual disease as they are unlikely to gain a significant overall survival benefit from chemotherapy and can potentially be harmed by treatment-related toxicity. We typically recommend surveillance with bi-annual CT imaging and offer chemotherapy for any visible evidence of systemic disease recurrence in these patients. In contrast, relatively healthy patients with adverse findings on final pathology despite no visible residual disease may derive a survival benefit from adjuvant chemotherapy. A meta-analysis of six randomized trials of AC by the Advanced Bladder Cancer collaboration suggested a survival benefit for patients in the treatment arms [13]. There was an absolute improvement of 9 % in overall survival and of 12 % in disease-free survival at 3 years in the AC group [13]. However, a notable limitation to interpreting these data is the fact that the majority of these trials were individually underpowered and precluded any definitive recommendation in support of AC by the authors based on these studies. Poor trial accrual reflects the limited practicality of AC in the clinical setting due to the high morbidity of RC and urinary diversion. With complication rates of up to 64 % reported by high-volume centers and 90-day readmission rates of 27 % reported by our institution, implementing adjuvant therapy in this patient population is challenging [14, 15].

31.1.4 Surveillance

We routinely perform a 6-month CT scan or MRI of the abdomen and pelvis with contrast along with a chest X-ray in follow-up for patients who undergo NAC and RC. We will continue cross-sectional imaging every 6 months for 2 years then annually thereafter in patients who are pT2, N0.

Due to a high risk of recurrence for patients who have persistent lymph node involvement following NAC and RC, we recommend close surveillance with repeat cross-sectional imaging every 3–6 months and referral to medical oncology for enrollment in a clinical trial. These patients often have a poor outcome with low 5-year overall survival rates.

31.2 Conclusion

Level 1 evidence supports the use of NAC with modest survival advantage over RC alone for patients with clinically organ-confined muscle-invasive urothelial cell carcinoma of the bladder. In this patient who presented with bulky non-metastatic cT2 bladder cancer, minimal symptoms and good PS, based on available evidence we recommend the use of NAC with three cycles of GC followed by RC. We reserve adjuvant chemotherapy for those patients who are markedly symptomatic at presentation thereby necessitating urgent local control with RC, as well as those with adverse pathological features (N+, positive margins, advanced pT stage) in whom NAC was not administered.

References

1. Sternberg CN, Bellmunt J, Sonpavde G, Siefker-Radtke AO, Stadler WM, Bajorin DF, et al. ICUD-EAU International Consultation on Bladder Cancer 2012: chemotherapy for urothelial carcinoma-neoadjuvant and adjuvant settings. Eur Urol. 2013;63(1):58–66. Epub 2012/08/25.
2. Porter MP, Kerrigan MC, Donato BM, Ramsey SD. Patterns of use of systemic chemotherapy for Medicare beneficiaries with urothelial bladder cancer. Urol Oncol. 2011;29(3):252–8. Epub 2009/05/20.
3. Grossman HB, Natale RB, Tangen CM, Speights VO, Vogelzang NJ, Trump DL, et al. Neoadjuvant chemotherapy plus cystectomy compared with cystectomy alone for locally advanced bladder cancer. N Engl J Med. 2003;349(9):859–66. Epub 2003/08/29.
4. von der Maase H, Hansen SW, Roberts JT, Dogliotti L, Oliver T, Moore MJ, et al. Gemcitabine and cisplatin versus methotrexate, vinblastine, doxorubicin, and cisplatin in advanced or metastatic bladder cancer: results of a large, randomized, multinational, multicenter, phase III study. J Clin Oncol. 2000;18(17):3068–77. Epub 2000/09/23.
5. Dash A, Pettus JA, Herr HW, Bochner BH, Dalbagni G, Donat SM, et al. A role for neoadjuvant gemcitabine plus cisplatin in muscle-invasive urothelial carcinoma of the bladder: a retrospective experience. Cancer. 2008;113(9):2471–7. Epub 2008/10/01.
6. Raghavan D, Burgess E, Gaston KE, Haake MR, Riggs SB. Neoadjuvant and adjuvant chemotherapy approaches for invasive bladder cancer. Semin Oncol. 2012;39(5):588–97. Epub 2012/10/09.
7. Smith DC, Mackler NJ, Dunn RL, Hussain M, Wood D, Lee CT, et al. Phase II trial of paclitaxel, carboplatin and gemcitabine in patients with locally advanced carcinoma of the bladder. J Urol. 2008;180(6):2384–8. discussion 8. Epub 2008/10/22.
8. Dogliotti L, Carteni G, Siena S, Bertetto O, Martoni A, Bono A, et al. Gemcitabine plus cisplatin versus gemcitabine plus carboplatin as first-line chemotherapy in advanced transitional cell carcinoma of the urothelium: results of a randomized phase 2 trial. Eur Urol. 2007;52(1):134–41. Epub 2007/01/09.
9. Gregg JR, Cookson MS, Phillips S, Salem S, Chang SS, Clark PE, et al. Effect of preoperative nutritional deficiency on mortality after radical cystectomy for bladder cancer. J Urol. 2011;185(1):90–6. Epub 2010/11/16.
10. Scher HI, Yagoda A, Herr HW, Sternberg CN, Bosl G, Morse MJ, et al. Neoadjuvant M-VAC (methotrexate, vinblastine, doxorubicin and cisplatin) effect on the primary bladder lesion. J Urol. 1988;139(3):470–4. Epub 1988/03/01.
11. Apolo AB, Grossman HB, Bajorin D, Steinberg G, Kamat AM. Practical use of perioperative chemotherapy for muscle-invasive bladder cancer: summary of session at the Society of Urologic Oncology annual meeting. Urol Oncol. 2012;30(6):772–80. Epub 2012/12/12.
12. Eldefrawy A, Soloway MS, Katkoori D, Singal R, Pan D, Manoharan M. Neoadjuvant and adjuvant chemotherapy for muscle-invasive bladder cancer: The likelihood of initiation and completion. Indian J Urol. 2012;28(4):424–6. Epub 2013/03/02.
13. Advanced Bladder Cancer Meta-analysis C. Adjuvant chemotherapy in invasive bladder cancer: a systematic review and meta-analysis of individual patient data Advanced Bladder Cancer (ABC) Meta-analysis Collaboration. Eur Urol. 2005;48(2):189–99; discussion 99–201. Epub 2005/06/09.
14. Shabsigh A, Korets R, Vora KC, Brooks CM, Cronin AM, Savage C, et al. Defining early morbidity of radical cystectomy for patients with bladder cancer using a standardized reporting methodology. Eur Urol. 2009;55(1):164–74. Epub 2008/08/05.
15. Stimson CJ, Chang SS, Barocas DA, Humphrey JE, Patel SG, Clark PE, et al. Early and late perioperative outcomes following radical cystectomy: 90-day readmissions, morbidity and mortality in a contemporary series. J Urol. 2010;184(4):1296–300. Epub 2010/08/21.

Samuel D. Kaffenberger, Todd M. Morgan, and Anne K. Schuckman

32.1 Introduction

For patients with muscle-invasive bladder cancer, the critical diagnostic and therapeutic role of lymph node dissection (LND) has been demonstrated repeatedly [1]. Studies have shown that lymph node count is correlated with patient survival in both lymph node-positive patients and node-negative patients [2–5]. Lymph node status is a major driver of patient outcome, and plays a key role in defining adjuvant therapy. Despite the widespread acceptance of the importance of LND, the extent of lymph node dissection is a subject of great controversy [6]. Additionally, the relevance of lymph node count as a metric of the completeness of dissection, the definition of a quality lymph node dissection, and even the

S.D. Kaffenberger, M.D.
Department of Urologic Surgery, Vanderbilt University, A-1302 Medical Center North, Nashville, TN 37232, USA
e-mail: samuel.d.kaffenberger@vanderbilt.edu

T.M. Morgan, M.D. (✉)
Department of Urology, University of Michigan, 1500 E. Medical Center Dr., CCC 7308, Ann Arbor, MI 48109, USA
e-mail: tomorgan@med.umich.edu

A.K. Schuckman, M.D.
USC Institute of Urology, Keck Medical Center of the University of Southern California, 1441 Eastlake Ave, Ste., 7416, Los Angeles, CA 90089, USA
e-mail: schuckma@usc.edu

proper interpretation of the significance of positive nodes are all areas of controversy [7–9]. The goal of this chapter is to summarize the key current concepts surrounding the performance of lymphadenectomy at the time of radical cystectomy (RC) for bladder cancer.

32.2 Lymph Node Anatomy and Distribution of Nodal Metastases

To date, there are not yet any available data on prospective randomized trials directly comparing extended LND to standard LND. Additionally, standardized anatomic boundaries for classifying lymph node location are lacking. In lieu of prospective evidence, investigators have sought to determine appropriate dissection templates based on a number of mapping techniques—both experimental and descriptive. Given the low but real risk of LND-associated complications, these efforts have sought to maximize efficiency and minimize morbidity of LND [10, 11]. Therefore, the aim of these investigations has been to allow maximum sensitivity of LND for identifying and removing positive nodes, while minimizing the potential for morbidity.

In an effort to define the appropriate extent of LND in muscle-invasive bladder cancer, several groups have performed surgical lymph node mapping [7, 12–15]. By splitting the en bloc dissection into specific "packets" at the time of

B.R. Konety and S.S. Chang (eds.), *Management of Bladder Cancer: A Comprehensive Text With Clinical Scenarios*, DOI 10.1007/978-1-4939-1881-2_32,
© Springer Science+Business Media New York 2015

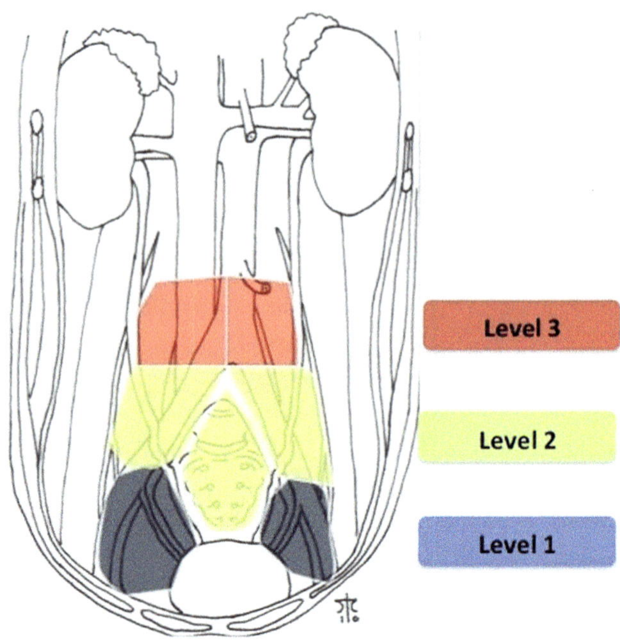

Fig. 32.1 Three levels of pelvic lymphadenectomy are described for bladder cancer. Standard lymphadenectomy typically includes level I lymph nodes and may extend over the common iliac arteries to the ureteroiliac junction. Extended dissection templates include levels I and II and may include level III nodes. Courtesy of Sia Daneshmand, M.D

LND, the precise frequency of node-positive disease in various zones has been described. Leissner et al. [12] prospectively evaluated 290 patients undergoing RC with extended LND for muscle-invasive bladder cancer. They defined the inferior mesenteric artery (IMA) as the upper limit of dissection, the genitofemoral nerve as the lateral border, and the pelvic floor as the caudal extent. A total of 81 patients (27 %) had positive nodes, and the distribution of positive sites ranged from 15.4 % in the obturator region to 4.0 % in the paracaval region.

The Leissner study was the first to classify nodal location according to the following levels that are now frequently utilized for reporting: level I (to common iliac bifurcation), level II (to aortic bifurcation), and level III (to IMA, including paracaval/para-aortic nodes) (Fig. 32.1). Importantly, only 20 patients (6.9 %) had positive nodes at level II alone and no patients had nodal metastases only at level III. Thus, while there were some patients who had "skip lesions" to level II, there were no patients with skip lesions directly to level III lymph nodes. However, if only a level I dissection was completed in this population, 6.8 % of node-positive patients and 74.1 % of all positive lymph nodes would have

been missed. Additionally, even in patients with unilateral tumors, a significant number of patients had positive nodes on the contralateral side. The resultant maps support the concept that a bilateral LND incorporating level I and level II lymph nodes is necessary for a quality dissection.

Vazina and colleagues [14] also performed mapping studies on 171 patients with either high-risk non-muscle-invasive or muscle-invasive bladder cancer. There were 13 patients (7.6 %) who received neoadjuvant chemotherapy. Consistent with other series, lymph node metastases were found in 43 patients (24 %) at the time of RC. Dissection limits were defined as in the Leissner study, and positive nodes were identified in the true pelvis in 22.7 % (level I), common iliacs in 8 % (level II), presacral in 5.1 % and at or above the aortic bifurcation in 4 % (level III). Tumor stage correlated closely with the proximal extent of nodal involvement.

Finally, in the largest series to date, Dorin et al. [7] retrospectively mapped nodal spread of bladder cancer in 674 patients undergoing RC and extended LND at either the University of Southern California (USC) or Oregon Health Sciences University (OHSU). They identified similar rates of lymph node metastases (23 %),

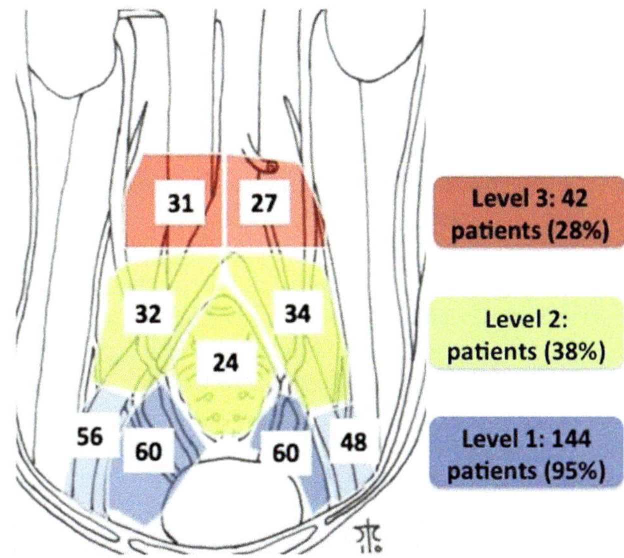

Fig. 32.2 Distribution of patients with positive lymph nodes in each location among 151 lymph node-positive patients reported by Dorin et al. (adapted with permission from authors) [7]. The number of patients with positive lymph nodes at each level is shown beside the number of patients with positive lymph nodes in each nodal packet. Courtesy of Sia Daneshmand, M.D

and again tumor and nodal stages were strongly correlated (Fig. 32.2). Using the same mapping scheme as Leissner and colleagues, they found that 41 % of node-positive patients had affected nodes above the common iliac bifurcation (level II or III), and that 18 % of the total positive nodes were above the aortic bifurcation in level III. Importantly, 7/151 node-positive patients (4.6 %) had positive nodes in level II and/or level III but not level I. Furthermore, in contrast to other series in which no level III skip lesions were seen, one patient was identified with nodal metastases only in level III. These authors concluded that an extended LND is supported in light of the rate of lymph node metastases outside of the anatomic boundaries of a standard LND.

While mapping studies are able to define the likelihood of finding positive nodes in large groups of patients, they do not help surgeons personalize treatment for a given patient. The primary tumor pathologic stage is not available at the time of RC, and therefore the probability of an individual patient harboring nodal metastases is very difficult to predict in the setting of clinically negative nodes. Additionally, the exact basin of nodes most likely to be affected in any single individual is unknown. As a result, many researchers have investigated whether sentinel lymph node dissections in bladder cancer can identify the key lymph node or nodal region that serves as the initial drainage site for the primary tumor [16]. This concept of identifying a sentinel lymph node has been widely applied in melanoma, penile, and breast cancer; however, it has had only an experimental role in bladder cancer to date. Identifying a sentinel node is attractive as a way to help individualize the extent of LND as well as to identify occult micrometastases in sentinel nodes, thus offering additional prognostic information.

The first sentinel lymph node studies used peri-tumoral blue dye as well as radioactive tracer injection in the peri-tumoral region [16, 17]. In these studies, lymphoscintigraphy was performed preoperatively. Sentinel nodes were identified intraoperatively by blue dye and intra- and postoperatively with a gamma probe. In both studies, 85 % of patients were found to have an identifiable sentinel node. However, there were several technical problems with this process that have prevented broader uptake of this concept. Preoperative lymphoscintigraphy was complicated by interference from the bladder injection sites, and no "blue" sentinel node was seen in many patients. Yet, in both studies, the false-negative rate was fairly low (0 and 19 %).

Newer techniques have sought to overcome some of the early technical problems with sentinel node identification. In a small study of six patients, single-photon emission computed tomography (SPECT-CT) combined with transurethral peritumoral injection was more accurate at identifying both positive and negative sentinel nodes than planar scintigraphy, blue dye, or intraoperative gamma detection. Remarkably, using SPECT-CT, all metastatic sentinel nodes were detected (0 % false-negative rate). One of the key findings from this study was the presence of multiple sentinel nodes, including bilateral sentinel nodes, in several of these patients. Thus, this study again implies that the drainage pattern of the bladder is highly variable, and bilateral dissection is required to accurately stage and treat patients undergoing RC.

Another important report combined the SPECT-CT technique with intraoperative gamma probe to "map" the lymphatic drainage of the bladder [18]. Rather than looking for the specific drainage of a given tumor, the authors sought to define if different areas of the bladder consistently drain via a predictable path. In this study, 60 patients underwent injection of technetium Tc 99 m nanocolloid into six predefined non-tumor-bearing areas of the bladder. Subsequent extended LND was performed, and a mean number of 24 lymph nodes draining the bladder were found per patient. The authors found a mean of four radioactive lymph nodes per injection site, and nodes from every one of the six evaluated regions of the bladder were seen draining to each area of the LND template. These authors found that 92 % of the radioactive nodes were located distal to the uretero-iliac junction, in the field of a standard LND. Interestingly, 4 % of nodes were found in the fossa of Marcille (dorsolateral to external iliac vessels), and 26 % were found in the internal iliac distribution. Based on this mapping study, the authors recommended a thorough LND to include all regions up to at least the uretero-iliac junction.

32.3 Nodal Staging for Bladder Cancer

Pathologic staging of bladder cancer is done based on evaluation of the cystectomy specimen and the regional lymph nodes, and the primary staging system is the joint International Union

Table 32.1 TNM staging system for bladder cancer

Primary tumor (T)	
TX	Primary tumor not assessed
T0	No evidence of primary tumor
Ta	Superficial, non-invasive papillary tumor
Tis	Carcinoma in situ
T1	Tumor invading into lamina propria
T2	Tumor invading into muscularis propria
pT2a	Tumor invading superficial muscularis propria
pT2b	Tumor invading deep muscularis propria
T3	Tumor invading perivesical fat
pT3a	Microscopic exravesical disease
pT3b	Gross extravesical disease
T4	Invasion into: prostatic stroma, seminal vesicle, uterus, vagina, pelvic sidewall, or abdominal wall
T4a	Prostatic stromal invasion (men) or uterus/vaginal invasion (women)
T4b	Invasion into pelvic sidewall or abdominal wall
Regional lymph nodes (N)	
NX	Lymph nodes not assessed
N0	No lymph node disease
N1	Single positive lymph node in one of the following locations: hypogastric, obturator, external iliac or presacral regions
N2	Multiple positive lymph nodes in the hypogastric, obturator, external iliac or presacral regions
N3	Common iliac lymph node metastasis
Distant metastasis (M)	
M0	No distant metastasis
M1	Distant metastasis

Adapted from Compton C, Byrd D, Garcia-Aguilar J, et al.: Urinary Bladder, in Compton CC, Byrd DR, Garcia-Aguilar J, Kurtzman SH, Olawaiye A and Washington MK: AJCC Cancer Staging Atlas, Springer New York, 2012, pp 575–582

Against Cancer (UICC) and the American Joint Committee on Cancer (AJCC) system. The 2010 UICC-AJCC staging system (7th edition) is given in Table 32.1, and has been modified from the prior 2002 staging system [19]. In particular, the classification of regional lymph node disease in the 2010 system has been altered from the previous version and no longer relies on size of lymph node involvement. Patients with N1 disease are those with a single positive node in the primary drainage regions of the bladder—the hypogastric, obturator, internal iliac, external iliac, perivesical, sacral, and presacral lymph nodes. Patients with multiple positive nodes in the primary drainage regions are classified as having N2 disease.

The common iliac lymph nodes are considered secondary drainage regions in the current staging system, and tumors involving these lymph nodes are classified as N3. Laterality is not a factor in lymph node staging. Patients with disease beyond the regional lymph nodes, such as lung, bone, or retroperitoneal lymph nodes, are classified as stage M1. Patients are considered Nx or Mx if the status of their lymph nodes or distant sites has not been determined.

32.4 Measures of Lymph Node Dissection Quality

In light of the controversy regarding the extent of LND, there is a need for reproducible metrics that can be utilized to evaluate and compare dissection adequacy. Lymph node count during pathologic examination is far and away the mostly commonly utilized measure, and numerous studies have shown an association between higher node counts and improved survival after RC [3, 20–25]. This association has remained even after controlling for pathologic lymph node stage. Building upon this, various lymph node count cutoffs ranging from 10 to 16 have been proposed as minimum standards for lymph node dissection adequacy [3, 20–23]. While minimum node count standards are convenient and easy to interpret, it has been demonstrated that there may be a linear relationship between node count and survival, suggesting that a binary standard may not be appropriate or even feasible [26]. Moreover, there may be significant limitations in the interpretation of many of these studies due to retrospective analysis and confounding by indication. Specifically, LND extent may be impacted by patient and/or provider factors that are difficult to account for even with advanced statistical modeling, and these may create a selection bias that implies an association between node count and survival whether or not one truly exists [27].

Further complicating the utilization of node count as a measure of lymphadenectomy quality is the significant variability that exists in the pathologic quantification of lymph nodes in a specimen. The number of nodes counted in a specimen has been shown to differ based upon pathologic processing measures, the number of separate packets each specimen is divided into, inter- and intra-pathologist variability in the determination of what constitutes a lymph node, and biological and anatomical differences between patients [28–30]. This discrepancy has been demonstrated in a recent study by Dorin and colleagues comparing lymph node counts for identical dissection templates between USC and OHSU, both high-volume institutions for RC [7]. Marked differences in median node counts between the two institutions were found (72 versus 40 nodes) despite equivalent rates of node-positive disease and survival. Furthermore, substantial inter-individual variability exists in the number of nodes present in the extended LND template. In a human cadaveric study with all nodes counted by a single pathologist and utilizing the same extended template of dissection, Davies et al. reported total node counts ranging from 10 to 53 nodes [30].

Due in part to these concerns, other measures of LND adequacy have been evaluated. While subjective and less practical as an externally reviewable quality measure, dissection template may be a more natural determination of LND extent. This is further illustrated in the Dorin et al. study in which identical lymph node dissection templates utilized at two different institutions resulted in similar outcomes despite markedly different node counts [7]. By resecting all nodal tissue from within an anatomically defined dissection template, the inherent variability that exists between individuals, surgeons, pathologists, and institutions becomes immaterial.

Lymph node density, the ratio of positive lymph nodes to total resected lymph nodes, has been studied as a potentially important outcome measure after pelvic lymphadenectomy [31–34]. While node density may account for some of the pathologic variability in node counting between institutions, it may also provide additional prognostic significance when compared to TNM nodal staging alone. In a number of large retrospective experiences, patients with a node density of 20 % or more have been found to have decreased survival compared to those with less than 20 % positive node density [34–36]. Others, however, have not found lymph node density to be more informative than TNM nodal staging alone and thus the utility of node density as a variable of independent prognostic significance remains in question [37, 38].

32.5 Analysis of Data Comparing Dissection Extent and Outcomes

Despite a substantial burden of evidence linking extent of lymphadenectomy with survival, there remains a great deal of controversy surrounding this assertion. Some of the complexity in interpreting the available literature can be attributed to varying definitions of the anatomical boundaries of a standard versus an extended lymphadenectomy. A standard lymphadenectomy for bladder cancer is generally considered to include all level I nodes up to the common iliac bifurcation or to the crossing of the retracted ureter over the iliac artery proximally. While generally including all level I and II lymph nodes, the proximal extent of an "extended" lymphadenectomy has ranged from the aortic bifurcation to the inferior mesenteric artery. The inclusion of level III lymph nodes has sometimes been termed a "super-extended" lymphadenectomy. This lack of standardization of templates has made the comparison of studies on LND extent difficult.

In the absence of prospective randomized controlled trials, a number of studies have attempted to retrospectively compare outcomes between standard and extended pelvic lymphadenectomy templates [39, 40]. In a single-institution study of two high-volume surgeons, extended LND at the time of RC was associated with significantly improved disease-free survival in patients with node-positive disease compared to standard LND [40]. The non-randomized selection to perform extended pelvic lymphadenectomy was an intra-operative decision based upon "liver status," according to the published report. Few conclusions regarding the benefit of extended LND can be drawn, however, given the lack of randomization, inclusion of patients with non-urothelial carcinoma, and presence of built-in study biases.

Another study evaluated two high-volume centers—one of which routinely performed a standard pelvic lymphadenectomy (level I), and the other of which performed an extended pelvic lymphadenectomy (levels I–II) [39]. While findings were again impacted by differences in patient populations, lack of randomization, and methodological limitations, the authors concluded that extended LND resulted in improved survival, better local disease control, and more accurate nodal staging compared to standard lymphadenectomy. However, in a separate study evaluating survival and recurrence rates between a super-extended (levels I–III) lymphadenectomy template at one institution and an extended lymphadenectomy template (cephalad extent just proximal to the common iliac bifurcation) at another institution, no major differences were found [8].

In contrast to these studies comparing LND templates, the majority of studies evaluating LND extent and outcomes have utilized node count as a surrogate measure of dissection extent, as discussed earlier [3, 20–25]. Taken with the few retrospective studies comparing lymph node dissection templates, the burden of evidence does appear to favor a more extensive pelvic lymphadenectomy at the time of RC. Still, important considerations must be taken in the interpretation of these data. Beyond the difficulty in extrapolating causality from retrospective case series with significant selection bias, the question remains as to whether or not an extended template lymphadenectomy simply improves staging instead of survival [41].

There is little doubt that an extended LND template offers improved pathologic nodal staging compared to the standard lymph node dissection template [1]. When comparing outcomes of node-negative or node-positive patients between series, however, stage migration may account for survival differences seen without changing the overall course of the disease. That is, if patients with small volume nodal disease are correctly staged as pN+ after undergoing extended lymphadenectomy, the apparent outcomes of the cohort of pN0 patients in the same series will likely be improved relative to a cohort of pN0 patients undergoing standard LND. This is due to the misclassification of some small volume pN+ patients as pN0 in the standard lymphadenectomy cohort. Similarly, the pN+ patients in the standard lymphadenectomy group would appear to have worse survival compared to the pN+ patients in the extended lymphadenectomy cohort even in the absence of an actual change in the natural history of the disease. This is a result of the inclusion of patients with very small volume nodal disease in the extended LND pN+ group. This stage migration is often referred to as the "Will Rogers" phenomenon and may play a role in the survival differences observed between LND series.

Whether or not extended lymphadenectomy and increased nodal yield directly impacts recurrence and survival, perhaps through increased cancer cytoreduction, remains an open question. Evidence supporting a causal effect on the natural history of the disease includes the apparent improved local disease control in patients who undergo extended LND as well as the frequent finding of molecular indications of micrometastatic disease in patients with histologically negative lymph nodes [39, 42, 43]. While the relative contributions of improved staging and therapeutic benefit to the improved survival reported in the literature with extended LND are thus far unclear, the results of two ongoing prospective randomized trials (discussed below) should shed substantial light on the role of an extended LND in preventing recurrence and bladder cancer-specific mortality.

32.6   Additional Areas of Controversy

Given the increased operative time and potential increase in surgical and postoperative morbidity of an extended lymphadenectomy, some groups have sought a risk-stratified approach to LND extent. For example, given the low rate of skip lesions, some have advocated the utilization of frozen section pathologic analysis of level I nodes to guide the decision to proceed to level II and/or level III nodes [40, 44, 45]. The ability of frozen section pathologic analysis to detect lymph node-positive disease in bladder cancer has been shown to be robust. Ugurlu and colleagues assessed the performance of frozen section analysis in several nodal regions and found an overall sensitivity of 81 % and specificity of 100 % [45]. Baltaci et al. reported similar findings on frozen section analysis of obturator lymph nodes and, importantly, in patients with clinically stage ≤T2 disease, there were no false-negative frozen section analyses [44]. Thus, the utilization of frozen section analysis of level I lymph nodes to guide LND extent, possibly with the addition of clinical staging information, may be one avenue toward a selective approach to LND.

An alternative or perhaps complement to frozen section analysis could be the implementation of sentinel lymph node mapping to help determine LND extent. While further refinement of this technique would be required to improve its diagnostic accuracy, coupling this technique with frozen section analysis could allow for a more individualized approach to extended LND. If the potential survival benefit of extended LND were known to be limited to those with pathologic node-positive disease, a risk-stratified, targeted approach to extended LND would be an attractive option.

Another key area of controversy surrounds the utility of lymphadenectomy in the setting of gross lymphadenopathy. Despite the poor prognosis of patients who present with clinically positive regional lymph node disease, long-term survival is possible in a minority of patients. A multimodal approach using cisplatin-based combination chemotherapy with subsequent consolidative surgery in those who respond appears to offer the best chance of long-term survival in these individuals [46, 47]. This is evidenced by the fact that in patients who undergo chemotherapy alone and who have a complete clinical response, recurrence often occurs at the original site of nodal disease [48]. Furthermore, in a retrospective series, Herr et al. reported on 12 patients with advanced or regional node-positive disease who underwent chemotherapy and had a complete or partial response but refused consolidative surgery [46]. Only one (8 %) survived 5 years, whereas 10 of 31 patients (32 %) with regional nodal disease who had a complete or partial response to cisplatin-based combination chemotherapy and underwent consolidative surgery survived 5 years.

Long-term survival also appears to be possible in patients who present with non-regional nodal metastases in the absence of visceral involvement by tumor. Chemotherapy followed by consolidative RC, extended pelvic LND, and retroperitoneal lymphadenectomy demonstrated a 36 % 4-year disease-specific survival in a small series of 11 patients with retroperitoneal nodal disease and bladder cancer [49]. Herr et al. reported an 18 % 5-year disease-specific survival in 11 patients with distant nodal disease who underwent combination chemotherapy and consolidative surgery [46]. More recently, Nieuwenhuijzen and colleagues demonstrated a 42 % 5-year survival rate in patients with biopsy-proven node-positive bladder cancer with complete response to combination chemotherapy who underwent consolidative surgery [47]. Of the 15 patients with a complete clinical response, 4 had microscopic residual nodal disease at the time of RC with LND, all of which died within 2 years. Of those with a partial response to chemotherapy, 5-year survival was 19 %. In patients whose nodal disease does not respond to chemotherapy, prognosis is uniformly poor and surgery appears unlikely to offer a survival benefit.

Finally, the feasibility and reproducibility of an adequate LND using a robotic approach continues to be an area of debate, as robotic assistance is increasingly being utilized in the performance of RC [50]. While prospective randomized trial data for robotic-assisted radical cystectomy are limited and have not yet supported any improved outcomes of the minimally invasive approach, existing data do appear to show no difference in short-term oncologic outcomes [51–55]. Concerns over the extent of LND during robotic-assisted radical cystectomy appear to be abating, as a number of studies have now shown no differences in node counts, complications, or anatomic extent of LND [56]. Additionally, in a small series of patients, Davis et al. performed an extended bilateral robotic lymphadenectomy

followed by an open "second look" lymphadenectomy [53]. With a median operative time of 117 min during the robotic-assisted extended pelvic LND, a median count of 43 nodes was achieved with only four median additional nodes retrieved during second look open lymphadenectomy. Additional data from two multicenter prospective randomized controlled trials of robotic vs. open RC are pending, although whether these results can be generalized outside of high-volume centers remains to be seen.

32.7 Coming Soon: Phase III Trial Data

Currently, there is no level I evidence defining the proper extent of LND. However, there are two ongoing trials investigating the relationship between extent of LND and impact on disease progression and patient survival. The German AUO (Association of Urologic Oncology) study randomized patients with clinically localized (T2-4) bladder cancer to standard (level I) or extended (level I/II/III) LND. No neoadjuvant chemotherapy was allowed. The study completed accrual in 2010, and is powered for 90 % detection of a 15 % difference in progression-free survival [57]. The Southwest Oncology Group (SWOG) Trial S1011 is currently accruing patients. This study is powered to detect a 10–12 % improvement in disease-free survival (DFS) in patients undergoing extended LND. Patients with clinically localized (T2, T3, or T4a) urothelial carcinoma undergoing RC are randomized to either a standard (level I) or extended (level I/II/III) lymph node dissection. In contrast to the German AUO study, neoadjuvant chemotherapy is allowed. The study aims to accrue 620 patients, and has 85 % power to detect a 28 % reduction in the rate of progression or death in the extended group compared to the standard group. This corresponds to an improvement in 3-year DFS from 55 to 65 % [57].

The S1011 trial is being completed by experienced urologic oncologic surgeons with high-volume cystectomy practices. Laparoscopic and robotic approaches are not allowed. Credentialing is strictly monitored with surgeons submitting operative reports and photographic correlation of LND extent and completeness for several cystectomies prior to enrolling patients as well as for all patients on trial. The results of both of these phase III trials are eagerly awaited. Hopefully, these efforts will help provide level I evidence to guide the optimal extent of LND for patients undergoing RC.

32.8 Conclusions

Despite intense investigation, there remains tremendous debate regarding the appropriate extent of LND at the time of RC for bladder cancer. Observational studies have supplied a wealth of information; however, data from these studies have intrinsic limitations making it challenging to separate causality from association in many instances. A better understanding of the relationship between LND extent and oncologic outcomes will come through the two ongoing phase III trials. In the meantime, the current data clearly support a meticulous dissection that, at minimum, entirely covers the level I anatomic boundaries. Exactly where the proximal boundary of the dissection should be remains to be determined. Furthermore, additional research will hopefully enable LND extent to be tailored based on individual clinical and pathologic parameters, facilitating a more personalized approach to this vital oncologic procedure.

References

1. Stein J, Lieskovsky G, Cote R, Groshen S, Feng A, Boyd S, et al. Radical cystectomy in the treatment of invasive bladder cancer: long-term results in 1,054 patients. J Clin Oncol. 2001;19:666–75.
2. Herr HW. Extent of surgery and pathology evaluation has an impact on bladder cancer outcomes after radical cystectomy. Urology. 2003;61:105–8.
3. Leissner J, Hohenfellner R, Thüroff JW, Wolf HK. Lymphadenectomy in patients with transitional cell carcinoma of the urinary bladder; significance for staging and prognosis. BJU Int. 2000;85:817–23.
4. Herr HW, Bochner BH, Dalbagni G, Donat SM, Reuter VE, Bajorin DF. Impact of the number of lymph nodes retrieved on outcome in patients with muscle invasive bladder cancer. J Urol. 2002;167: 1295–8.
5. Karl A, Carroll PR, Gschwend JE, Knüchel R, Montorsi F, Stief CG, et al. The impact of lymphadenectomy and lymph node metastasis on the outcomes of radical cystectomy for bladder cancer. Eur Urol. 2009;55:826–35.
6. Stein JP. Lymphadenectomy in bladder cancer: how high is "high enough"? Urol Oncol. 2006;24:349–55.
7. Dorin RP, Daneshmand S, Eisenberg MS, Chandrasoma S, Cai J, Miranda G, et al. Lymph node dissection technique is more important than lymph node count in identifying nodal metastases in radical cystectomy patients: a comparative mapping study. Eur Urol. 2011;60:946–52.
8. Zehnder P, Studer UE, Skinner EC, Dorin RP, Cai J, Roth B, et al. Super extended versus extended pelvic lymph node dissection in patients undergoing radical cystectomy for bladder cancer: a comparative study. J Urol. 2011;186:1261–8.
9. Bochner BH, Cho D, Herr HW, Donat M, Kattan MW, Dalbagni G. Prospectively packaged lymph node dissections with radical cystectomy: evaluation of node count variability and node mapping. J Urol. 2004;172:1286–90.
10. Shabsigh A, Korets R, Vora KC, Brooks CM, Cronin AM, Savage C, et al. Defining early morbidity of radical cystectomy for patients with bladder cancer using a standardized reporting methodology. Eur Urol. 2009;55:164–74.
11. Lowrance WT, Rumohr JA, Chang SS, Clark PE, Smith JA, Cookson MS. Contemporary open radical cystectomy: analysis of perioperative outcomes. J Urol. 2008;179:1313–8.
12. Leissner J, Ghoneim MA, Abol-Enein H, Thüroff JW, Franzaring L, Fisch M, et al. Extended radical lymphadenectomy in patients with urothelial bladder cancer: results of a prospective multicenter study. J Urol. 2004;171:139–44.
13. Miocinovic R, Gong MC, Ghoneim IA, Fergany AF, Hansel DE, Stephenson AJ. Presacral and retroperitoneal lymph node involvement in urothelial bladder cancer: results of a prospective mapping study. J Urol. 2011;186(4):1269–73.
14. Vazina A, Dugi D, Shariat SF, Evans J, Link R, Lerner SP. Stage specific lymph node metastasis mapping in radical cystectomy specimens. J Urol. 2004;171:1830–4.
15. Jensen JB, Ulhøi BP, Jensen KM-E. Lymph node mapping in patients with bladder cancer undergoing radical cystectomy and lymph node dissection to the level of the inferior mesenteric artery. BJU Int. 2010;106:199–205.
16. Liedberg F, Chebil G, Davidsson T, Gudjonsson S, Månsson W. Intraoperative sentinel node detection improves nodal staging in invasive bladder cancer. J Urol. 2006;175:84–8.
17. Sherif A, Garske U, de La Torre M, Thörn M. Hybrid SPECT-CT: an additional technique for sentinel node detection of patients with invasive bladder cancer. Eur Urol. 2006;50:83–91.

18. Roth B, Wissmeyer MP, Zehnder P, Birkhäuser FD, Thalmann GN, Krause TM, et al. A new multimodality technique accurately maps the primary lymphatic landing sites of the bladder. Eur Urol. 2010;57:205–11.

19. Edge SB, Byrd DR, Compton CC, Fritz AG, Greene FL, Trotti A. AJCC cancer staging handbook. 7th ed. New York, NY: Springer; 2010.

20. Konety BR, Joslyn SA, O'Donnell MA. Extent of pelvic lymphadenectomy and its impact on outcome in patients diagnosed with bladder cancer: analysis of data from the Surveillance, Epidemiology and End Results Program data base. J Urol. 2003;169:946–50.

21. May M, Herrmann E, Bolenz C, Brookman-May S, Tiemann A, Moritz R, et al. Association between the number of dissected lymph nodes during pelvic lymphadenectomy and cancer-specific survival in patients with lymph node-negative urothelial carcinoma of the bladder undergoing radical cystectomy. Ann Surg Oncol. 2011;18:2018–25.

22. Wright JL, Lin DW, Porter MP. The association between extent of lymphadenectomy and survival among patients with lymph node metastases undergoing radical cystectomy. Cancer. 2008;112:2401–8.

23. Herr HW, Faulkner JR, Grossman HB, Natale RB, DeVere White R, Sarosdy MF, et al. Surgical factors influence bladder cancer outcomes: a cooperative group report. J Clin Oncol. 2004;22:2781–9.

24. Brunocilla E, Pernetti R, Schiavina R, Borghesi M, Vagnoni V, Rocca GC, et al. The number of nodes removed as well as the template of the dissection is independently correlated to cancer-specific survival after radical cystectomy for muscle-invasive bladder cancer. Int Urol Nephrol. 2013;45:711–9.

25. Morgan TM, Barocas DA, Penson DF, Chang SS, Ni S, Clark PE, et al. Lymph node yield at radical cystectomy predicts mortality in node-negative and not node-positive patients. Urology. 2012;80:632–40.

26. Koppie TM, Vickers AJ, Vora K, Dalbagni G, Bochner BH. Standardization of pelvic lymphadenectomy performed at radical cystectomy: can we establish a minimum number of lymph nodes that should be removed? Cancer. 2006;107:2368–74.

27. Gilbert SM. Separating surgical quality from causality–gaining perspective in the debate on lymph node count and extent of lymphadenectomy. Cancer. 2008;112:2331–3.

28. Bochner BH, Herr HW, Reuter VE. Impact of separate versus en bloc pelvic lymph node dissection on the number of lymph nodes retrieved in cystectomy specimens. J Urol. 2001;166:2295–6.

29. Parkash V, Bifulco C, Feinn R, Concato J, Jain D. To count and how to count, that is the question: interobserver and intraobserver variability among pathologists in lymph node counting. Am J Clin Pathol. 2010;134:42–9.

30. Davies JD, Simons CM, Ruhotina N, Barocas DA, Clark PE, Morgan TM. Anatomic basis for lymph node counts as measure of lymph node dissection extent: a cadaveric study. Urology. 2013;81:358–63.

31. Kassouf W, Agarwal PK, Herr HW, Munsell MF, Spiess PE, Brown GA, et al. Lymph node density is superior to TNM nodal status in predicting disease-specific survival after radical cystectomy for bladder cancer: analysis of pooled data from MDACC and MSKCC. J Clin Oncol. 2008;26:121–6.

32. Bruins HM, Huang GJ, Cai J, Skinner DG, Stein JP, Penson DF. Clinical outcomes and recurrence predictors of lymph node positive urothelial cancer after cystectomy. J Urol. 2009;182:2182–7.

33. Stein JP, Cai J, Groshen S, Skinner DG. Risk factors for patients with pelvic lymph node metastases following radical cystectomy with en bloc pelvic lymphadenectomy: concept of lymph node density. J Urol. 2003;170:35–41.

34. Herr HW. Superiority of ratio based lymph node staging for bladder cancer. J Urol. 2003;169:943–5.

35. Herr H. The concept of lymph node density—is it ready for clinical practice? J Urol. 2007;177:1273–6.

36. Wiesner C, Salzer A, Thomas C, Gellermann-Schultes C, Gillitzer R, Hampel C, et al. Cancer-specific survival after radical cystectomy and standardized extended lymphadenectomy for node-positive bladder cancer: prediction by lymph node positivity and density. BJU Int. 2009;104:331–5.

37. Tarin TV, Power NE, Ehdaie B, Sfakianos JP, Silberstein JL, Savage CJ, et al. Lymph node-positive bladder cancer treated with radical cystectomy and lymphadenectomy: effect of the level of node positivity. Eur Urol. 2012;61:1025–30.

38. Jensen JB, Ulhøi BP, Jensen KM-E. Evaluation of different lymph node (LN) variables as prognostic markers in patients undergoing radical cystectomy and extended LN dissection to the level of the inferior mesenteric artery. BJU Int. 2012;109:388–93.

39. Dhar NB, Klein EA, Reuther AM, Thalmann GN, Madersbacher S, Studer UE. Outcome after radical cystectomy with limited or extended pelvic lymph node dissection. J Urol. 2008;179:873–8.

40. Abol-Enein H, Tilki D, Mosbah A, El-Baz M, Shokeir A, Nabeeh A, et al. Does the extent of lymphadenectomy in radical cystectomy for bladder cancer influence disease-free survival? A prospective single-center study. Eur Urol. 2011;60:572–7.

41. Morgan TM, Kaffenberger SD, Cookson MS. Surgical and chemotherapeutic management of regional lymph nodes in bladder cancer. J Urol. 2012;188:1081–8.

42. Marín-Aguilera M, Mengual L, Burset M, Oliver A, Ars E, Ribal MJ, et al. Molecular lymph node staging in bladder urothelial carcinoma: impact on survival. Eur Urol. 2008;54:1363–72.

43. Kurahashi T. Detection of micrometastases in pelvic lymph nodes in patients undergoing radical cystectomy for focally invasive bladder cancer by real-time reverse transcriptase-pcr for cytokeratin 19 and uroplakin II. Clin Cancer Res. 2005;11:3773–7.

44. Baltaci S, Adsan O, Ugurlu O, Aslan G, Can C, Gunaydin G, et al. Reliability of frozen section examination of obturator lymph nodes and impact on

lymph node dissection borders during radical cystectomy: results of a prospective multicentre study by the Turkish Society of Urooncology. BJU Int. 2011;107: 547–53.

45. Ugurlu O, Adsan O, Tul M, Kosan M, Inal G, Cetinkaya M. Value of frozen sections of lymph nodes in pelvic lymphadenectomy in patients with invasive bladder tumor. Int J Urol. 2006;13:699–702.

46. Herr HW, Donat SM, Bajorin DF. Post-chemotherapy surgery in patients with unresectable or regionally metastatic bladder cancer. J Urol. 2001;165:811–4.

47. Nieuwenhuijzen JA, Bex A, Meinhardt W, Kerst JM, Schornagel JH, van Tinteren H, et al. Neoadjuvant methotrexate, vinblastine, doxorubicin and cisplatin for histologically proven lymph node positive bladder cancer. J Urol. 2005;174:80–5.

48. Dimopoulos MA, Finn L, Logothetis CJ. Pattern of failure and survival of patients with metastatic urothelial tumors relapsing after cis-platinum-based chemotherapy. J Urol. 1994;151:598–600.

49. Sweeney P, Millikan R, Donat M, Wood CG, Radtke AS, Pettaway CA, et al. Is there a therapeutic role for post-chemotherapy retroperitoneal lymph node dissection in metastatic transitional cell carcinoma of the bladder? J Urol. 2003;169:2113–7.

50. Li K, Lin T, Fan X, Xu K, Bi L, Duan Y, et al. Systematic review and meta-analysis of comparative studies reporting early outcomes after robot-assisted radical cystectomy versus open radical cystectomy. Cancer Treat Rev. 2013;39:551–60.

51. Hellenthal NJ, Hussain A, Andrews PE, Carpentier P, Castle E, Dasgupta P, et al. Lymphadenectomy at the time of robot-assisted radical cystectomy: results from the International Robotic Cystectomy Consortium. BJU Int. 2011;107:642–6.

52. Nix J, Smith A, Kurpad R, Nielsen ME, Wallen EM, Pruthi RS. Prospective randomized controlled trial of robotic versus open radical cystectomy for bladder cancer: perioperative and pathologic results. Eur Urol. 2010;57:196–201.

53. Davis JW, Gaston K, Anderson R, Dinney CPN, Grossman HB, Munsell MF, et al. Robot assisted extended pelvic lymphadenectomy at radical cystectomy: lymph node yield compared with second look open dissection. J Urol. 2011;185:79–83.

54. Parekh DJ, Messer J, Fitzgerald J, Ercole B, Svatek R. Perioperative outcomes and oncologic efficacy from a pilot prospective randomized clinical trial of open versus robotic assisted radical cystectomy. J Urol. 2013;189:474–9.

55. Davis JW, Kamat AM. Lymphadenectomy with robotic cystectomy. Curr Urol Rep. 2013;14:59–63.

56. Lavery HJ, Martinez-Suarez HJ, Abaza R. Robotic extended pelvic lymphadenectomy for bladder cancer with increased nodal yield. BJU Int. 2011;107: 1802–5.

57. Tilki D, Brausi M, Colombo R, Evans CP, Fradet Y, Fritsche H-M, et al. Lymphadenectomy for bladder cancer at the time of radical cystectomy. Eur Urol. 2013;64:266–76.

63-year-old man at radical cystectomy
for T2 tumor has unexpected grossly
positive lymph nodes

Christian Thomas and Joachim W. Thüroff

33.1 Clinical Scenario

A 63-year-old patient with clinical T2 bladder cancer is planned for radical cystectomy. Lymph node dissection during surgery reveals unexpected grossly positive lymph nodes. At this point the urologic surgeon must make decisions about continuation of cystectomy as well as the extent of lymphadenectomy. The following chapter discusses important issues that arise in this difficult intraoperative situation.

33.2 How Frequent Are Positive Lymph Nodes at Radical Cystectomy?

In general, positive lymph nodes at radical cystecomy are found in 20–30 % [1–3]. Thereby, nodal involvement significantly correlates with tumor stage. While patients with a pT2a and pT2b disease have positive lymph nodes in approximately 14 and 24 % of cases, this rate increases up to 42 % in patients with pT3/4 disease [3]. One-third of these patients show lymph node involvement in ≥ 5 nodes. While 5-year probability of recurrence-free survival is 78 % in the absence of nodal involvement, this number decreases to 35 % in case of positive lymph nodes. Table 33.1 shows the probability of positive lymph nodes depending on pT-stage [1]. Within the last 10 years, a uniform nomenclature has emerged dividing pelvic/paraaortic lymph node anatomy into three levels. Level I consists of lymph nodes up to the common iliac bifurcation including the internal iliac nodes. Level II consists of all lymph nodes above the common iliac bifurcation up to the aortic bifurcation. Level III consists of all lymph nodes between the aortic bifurcation up to the inferior mesenteric artery and in some descriptions, above this level as well. If a patient has nodal metastases at level I, 57 % of the patients also have positive nodes at level II and 31 % at level III [4]. In up to 22 % of patients with positive lymph nodes the primary landing side is level II–III [5]. Isolated level III metastases are found in up to 6 % [6]. A lymph node template consisting of levels I–III is shown in Fig. 33.1.

C. Thomas, M.D. (✉) • J.W. Thüroff, M.D.
Department of Urology, University Medical Center,
Johannes Gutenberg University,
Langenbeckstrasse 1, Mainz 55131, Germany
e-mail: christian.thomas@unimedizin-mainz.de;
joachim.thueroff@unimedizin-mainz.de

B.R. Konety and S.S. Chang (eds.), *Management of Bladder Cancer:
A Comprehensive Text With Clinical Scenarios*, DOI 10.1007/978-1-4939-1881-2_33,
© Springer Science+Business Media New York 2015

Table 33.1 Probability of positive lymph nodes depending on pT-stage [1]

pT-stage	Positive lymph nodes (%)
pTa, Cis	2.4
pT1	6.7
pT2	18.2
pT3a	26.3
pT3b	45.6
pT4a	42.3

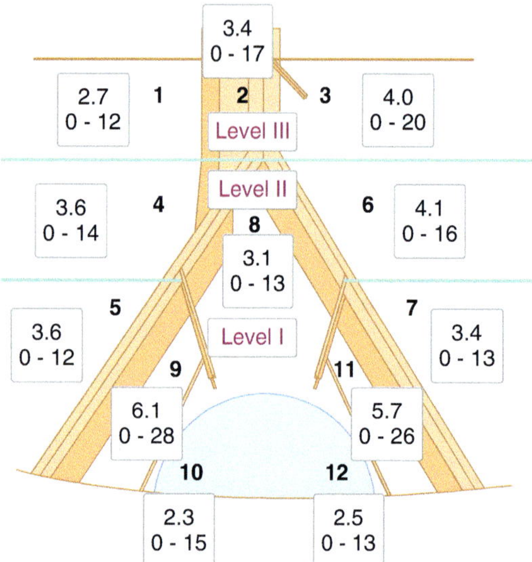

Fig. 33.1 Example of a lymph node template (level I–III) for lymph node dissection in bladder cancer [4]. Total number of lymph nodes removed from each anatomical region in 290 patients with extended lymphadenectomy. Values are means and minimum to maximum of regional lymph node counts

33.3 How Reliable Is Preoperative Imaging?

In patients planned for radical cystectomy for bladder cancer, multi-detector row computerized tomography (MDCT) is performed routinely to assess local tumor stage and lymph node status. However, its value for predicting local tumor stage and lymph node status has been questioned due to an overall accuracy of only approximately 50–60 % in routine clinical practice [7]. MR techniques seem to provide a higher accuracy for lymph node staging in the pelvis. Using T2-weighted imaging, DW imaging or the combination of both, the accuracy for pelvic lymph node staging and prediction of local tumor stage is approximately 80 % [8]. A further improvement seems to be the combination of DW imaging with superparamagnetic nanoparticles of iron oxide, revealing a diagnostic accuracy of 90 % in detecting lymph node metastases [9].

However, as long as clinical staging of lymph node status still relies on computerized tomography in the majority of cases and availability of novel imaging techniques is scarce, approximately 25 % of patients will have lymph node metastases that are missed on current preoperative staging [10, 11]. Notably, the majority of preoperatively undetected lymph node metastases with CT imaging are micrometastaes without gross enlargement of the involved lymph node(s). Therefore, our presented clinical scenario of unexpected grossly involved lymph nodes at radical cystectomy is rather rare.

33.4 What Is the Extent of Lymphadenectomy That Should Be Performed in Case of Unexpected Grossly Lymph Nodes?

The association between the extent of lymphadenectomy and survival remains conflicting in the literature. In general, positive lymph nodes at radical cystectomy are associated with a poor prognosis [1, 3, 5]. However, if <3 lymph nodes are positive durable long-term cancer-free survival is up to 35 % [1]. Several studies have shown that a larger number of removed nodes are associated with better long-term recurrence-free and survival rates, independent of presence or absence of lymph node metastases [12–15]. Therefore, a minimum number of 15 lymph nodes should be removed [12, 16]. However, just focusing on the number of lymph nodes removed seems to be problematic due to differences in pathological processing, individual anatomical variations and sampling errors. Using a standardized lymph node dissection technique based on lymph node anatomy levels I–III [4] and sending in the material for processing in separate packets yields higher count of lymph nodes than en-block resection of the same template [17]. Despite significantly different lymph node counts, two high-volume centers using the same anatomical template demonstrated no differences in positive lymph nodes or oncologic outcomes [18]. While standard lymphadenectomy should at least consist of level I and II, level III should be included in case of positive lymph nodes. The reason therefore is that lymph node density is an independent prognosticator in those patients [3, 16, 19]. Depending on the study, less than five positive lymph nodes are associated with an improved survival [1, 3, 16]. Concerning our clinical scenario presented above, when lymph node metastases are grossly positive as confirmed by frozen section, we recommend performing a so-called "super-extended" lymph node dissection including level III. Even when lymph node metastases are per se associated with a worse oncologic outcome, a lymph node density less than 25 % or even 12 % might have a positive impact on survival [3, 19]. If less than five lymph nodes are positive at extended lymphadenectomy (stage I–II), a curative prognosis is likely in up to one-third of the patients [1].

33.5 Should Cystectomy Be Continued in This Situation?

Radical cystectomy is typically performed in a curative intent for muscle-invasive bladder cancer. In the presence of positive lymph nodes, the chance to cure the patient with radical surgery markedly decreases. However, in up to one-third of cases a multimodal approach of cystectomy, extended lymphadenectomy and adjuvant chemotherapy is curative [1]. Therefore, cystectomy should be performed even in the presence of grossly positive lymph nodes. Another indication for cystectomy in a metastatic state is local tumor control. Even if the patient cannot be cured and

further treatment will be in a palliative setting, the risks of recurrent gross hematuria, bladder pain, and/or ureteral obstruction with a need of palliative upper tract diversion can be obviated. Unfortunately, literature regarding these aspects does not exist and recommendations are based on expert opinion. While cystectomy in the presence of grossly positive lymph nodes is feasible and reasonable from the oncologic point of view, the question might arise if an incontinent rather than continent urinary diversion should be favored to reduce postoperative complications and accelerate rehabilitation. It is known to be important to start adjuvant systemic treatment as quickly as possible. However, as shown in the literature available on urinary diversion, rates of postoperative complications including strictures, urinary leaks and rate of reoperations do not significantly differ between both types of diversion [20]. Therefore, if the type of urinary diversion would not compromise the extent of pelvic exenteration (e.g. orthotopic pouch/neobladder), the urinary diversion may be performed as preoperatively planned. However, a planned nerve-sparing approach for preservation of potency should be abandoned in the presence of grossly positive lymph nodes since it would interfere with the completeness of lymph node dissection. In this setting, the oncologic outcome has priority over other aspects and a complete lymph node dissection has to be performed including the presacral, deep internal iliac and deep obturator areas, which bears a high risk of insufficient preservation of erectile function.

33.6 Conclusion

Approximately one out of five patients undergoing radical cystectomy for bladder cancer will present unexpected positive lymph nodes intraoperatively. One-third of these patients will have tumor involvement in >5 nodes. In case of grossly positive lymph nodes, a super-extended lymph node dissection up to the paraaortal/paracaval regions is recommended (stage I–III) to possibly improve oncologic outcome. In all other cases, lymph node dissection should be performed at least up to the common iliac vessels, preferably up to the aortic bifurcation. Cystectomy should be performed independently of lymph node condition in patients with invasive bladder cancer to reduce local tumor complications. The type of urinary diversion should not be altered by lymph node positivity unless the diversion would otherwise negatively influence radicality of the procedure (e.g. orthotopic pouch/neobladder). Current advances in imaging might help to reduce the rate of unexpected grossly positive lymph node positivity in the future.

References

1. Stein JP, Lieskovsky G, Cote R, Groshen S, Feng AC, Boyd S, Skinner E, Bochner B, Thangathurai D, Mikhail M, Raghavan D, Skinner DG. Radical cystectomy in the treatment of invasive bladder cancer: long-term results in 1,054 patients. J Clin Oncol. 2001;19(3):666–75.
2. Morgan TM, Kaffenberger SD, Cookson MS. Surgical and chemotherapeutic management of regional lymph nodes in bladder cancer. J Urol. 2012;188:1081–8.
3. Steven K, Poulson AL. Radical cystectomy and extended pelvic lymphadenectomy: survival of patients with lymph node metastasis above the bifurcation of the common iliac vessels treated with surgery only. J Urol. 2007;178:1218–23.
4. Leissner J, Ghoneim MA, Abol-Enein H, Thüroff JW, Franzaring L, Fisch M, Schulze H, Managadze G, Allhoff EP, El-Baz MA, Kastendieck H, Buhtz P, Kropf S, Hohenfellern R, Wolf HK. Extended radical lymphadenectomy in patients with urothelial bladder cancer: results of a prospective multicenter study. J Urol. 2004;171:139–44.
5. Wiesner C, Salzer A, Thomas C, Gellermann-Schultes C, Gillitzer R, Hampel C, Thüroff JW. Cancer-specific survival after radical cystectomy and standardized extended lymphadenectomy for node-positive bladder cancer: prediction by lymph node positivity and density. BJU Int. 2009;104:331–5.
6. Miocinovic R, Gong MC, Ghoneim IA, Fergany AF, Hansel DE, Stephenson AJ. Presacral and retroperitoneal lymph node involvement in urothelial bladder cancer: results of a prospective mapping study. J Urol. 2011;186:1269–73.
7. Tritschler S, Mosler C, Straub J, Buchner A, Karl A, Graser A, Stief C, Tilki D. Staging of muscle-invasive bladder cancer: can computerized tomography help us to decide on local treatment? World J Urol. 2012;30:827–31.
8. Thoeny HC, Forstner R, De Keyzer F. Genitourinary applications of diffusion-weighted MR imaging in the pelvis. Radiology. 2013;263:326–42.
9. Thoeny HC, Triantafyllou M, Birkhaeuser FD, Froehlich JM, Tshering DW, Binser T, Fleischmann A, Vermathen P, Studer UE. Combined ultrasmall superparamagnetic particles of iron oxide-enhanced and diffusion-weighted magnetic resonance imaging reliably detect pelvic lymph node metastases in normal-sized nodes of bladder and prostate cancer patients. Eur Urol. 2009;55:761–9.
10. Shariat SF, Palapattu GS, Karakiewicz PI, Rogers CG, Vazina A, Bastian PJ, Schoenberg MP, Lerner SP, Sagalowsky AI, Lotan Y. Discrepancy between clinical and pathologic stage: impact on prognosis after radical cystectomy. Eur Urol. 2007;51:137–49.
11. Svatek RS, Shariat SF, Novara G, Skinner EC, Fradet Y, Bastian PJ, Kamat AM, Kassouf W, Karakiewicz PI, Fritsche HM, Izawa JI, Tilki D, Ficarra V, Volkmer BG, Isbarn H, Dinney CP. Discrepancy between clinical and pathological stage: external validation of the impact on prognosis in an international radical cystectomy cohort. BJU Int. 2011;107:898–904.
12. Leissner J, Hohenfellner R, Thüroff JW, Wolf HK. Lymphadenectomy in patients with transitional cell carcinoma of the urinary bladder: significance for staging and prognosis. BJU Int. 2000;85:817–23.
13. Konety BR, Joslyn SA, O'Donnell MA. Extent of pelvic lymphadenectomy and its impact on outcome in patients diagnosed with bladder cancer: analysis of data from the Surveillance, Epidemiology and End Results Program data base. J Urol. 2003;169:946–50.
14. May M, Herrmann E, Bolenz C, Brookman-May S, Tiemann A, Moritz R, Fritsche HM, Burger M, Trojan L, Michel MS, Wülfing C, Müller SC, Ellinger J, Buchner A, Stief CG, Tilki D, Wieland WF, Gilfrich C, Höfner T, Hohenfellner M, Haferkamp A, Roigas J, Zacharias M, Bastian PJ. Association between the number of dissected lymph nodes during pelvic lymphadenectomy and cancer-specific survival in patients with lymph node negative urothelial carcinoma of the bladder undergoing radical cystectomy. Ann Surg Oncol. 2011;18:2018–25.
15. Wright JL, Lin DW, Porter MP. The association between extent of lymphadenectomy and survival among patients with lymph node metastases undergoing radical cystectomy. Cancer. 2008;112:2401–8.
16. Fleischmann A, Thalmann GN, Narkwalder R, Studer UE. Extracapsular extension of pelvic lymph node metastases from urothelial carcinoma of the bladder is an independent prognostic factor. J Clin Oncol. 2005;23:2358–65.
17. Stein JP, Cai J, Groshen S, Skinner DG. Risk factors for patients with pelvic lymph node metastases following radical cystectomy with en bloc pelvic lymphadenectomy: concept of lymph node density. J Urol. 2003;170:35–41.

18. Dorin RP, Daneshmand S, Eisenberg MS, Chandrasoma S, Cai J, Miranda G, Nichols PW, Skinner DG, Skinner EC. Lymph node dissection technique is more important than lymph node count in identifying nodal metastases in radical cystectomy patients: a comparative mapping study. Eur Urol. 2011;60:946–52.

19. Osawa T, Abe T, Shinohara N, Harabayashi T, Sazawa A, Kubota K, Matsuno Y, Shibata T, Shinno Y, Kamota S, Minami K, Sakashita S, Kumagai A, Mori T, Nonomura K. Role of lymph node density in predicting survival of patients with lymph node metastases after radical cystectomy: a multi-institutional study. Int J Urol. 2009;16:274–8.

20. Urh A, Soliman PT, Schmeler KM, Estin S, Frumovitz M, Nick AM, Fellman B, Urbauer DL, Ramirez PT. Postoperative outcomes after continent versus incontinent urinary diversion at the time of pelvic exenteration for gynecologic malignancies. Gynecol Oncol. 2013;129:580–5.

Daniel J. Canter, Joseph Zabell, Stephen A. Boorjian, and Christopher J. Weight

Abbreviations

RC	Radical cystectomy
GFR	Glomerular filtration rate
BCS	Bladder cancer-specific survival
PFS	Progression-free survival
NCCN	National Comprehensive Cancer Network
ICUD	International Consultation on Urologic Diseases
EAU	European Association of Urology
UUT	Upper urinary tract

34.1 Introduction

While the majority of patients with newly diag nosed bladder cancer present with non-muscle invasive tumors, approximately 20–40 % continue to present with or to progress to muscle invasion.

D.J. Canter
Urologic Institute of Southeastern Pennsylvania,
Einstein Healthcare Network, 5501 Old York Road,
Philadelphia, PA, 19141, USA
e-mail: canterda@einstein.edu

J. Zabell • C.J. Weight (✉)
Department of Urology, University of Minnesota,
420 Delaware Sr. SE MMC 394, Minneapolis,
MN 55455, USA
e-mail: zabe0034@umn.edu; cjweight@umn.edu

S.A. Boorjian
Mayo Clinic, 200 First Street SW, Rochester,
MN 55905, USA
e-mail: boorjian.stephen@mayo.edu

Radical cystectomy (RC) with pelvic lymph node dissection and urinary diversion remains the gold standard treatment for patients with muscle-invasive disease, as well as for patients with high-risk non-muscle-invasive tumors. However, despite definitive surgery, disease recurrence has been documented in up to half of these patients [1]. Various regimens have been outlined for surveillance of patients following RC, often with disparate recommendations regarding the intensity of follow-up and choice of imaging. Nevertheless, postoperative cancer surveillance for the early detection of recurrent disease is only useful in as much as it may improve patient outcomes.

However, continued debate exists as to whether routine oncologic follow-up does in fact impact patient survival, and as such the value of oncologic surveillance has been questioned, particularly given the high noted costs associated with bladder cancer care [2]. At the same time, considering the reconstructive nature of radical cystectomy with urinary diversion, surveillance after radical cystectomy should also be considered to evaluate the metabolic abnormalities associated with urinary diversion, and to facilitate the identification of renal obstruction that may result from ureteroenteric anastomotic stricture. Herein, we review data regarding surveillance following radical cystectomy, both with regard to oncologic monitoring and for the metabolic consequences of urinary diversion and detail existing (and often contrasting) established guidelines.

B.R. Konety and S.S. Chang (eds.), *Management of Bladder Cancer:*
A Comprehensive Text With Clinical Scenarios, DOI 10.1007/978-1-4939-1881-2_34,
© Springer Science+Business Media New York 2015

34.2   Metastatic Surveillance Following Radical Cystectomy

Recurrence following RC may be broadly categorized in a site-specific fashion as urothelial (upper tract + urethra), which will be covered in separate sections below, and non-urothelial. Non-urothelial recurrences include both local pelvic relapse of tumor and distant (soft tissue, lymph node, viscera, other) disease. Notably, the rates of metastases following RC in published series to date have been variable, as from both single institutional and multi-institutional studies, recurrent disease has been described in 21–50 % of patients [1, 3–6]. Understanding the factors associated with disease recurrence is important for patient counseling, clinical trial development, and the establishment of guidelines for postoperative surveillance.

Not surprisingly, patients' risk of recurrence has been found to be highly correlated with pathologic stage at RC [1, 4, 7, 8]. For example, Shariat et al. reported the experience of three high-volume RC centers, comprising 888 patients, and found that the 5-year progression-free (PFS) and bladder cancer-specific (B-CS) survival was 88.8, 75.3, 80.8, 71.6, 44.2, and 28.4 %, respectively, and 93.9, 87.2, 85.9, 78.9, 47.7, and 31.0 %, respectively, for pTa, pTis, pT1, pT2, pT3, and pT4 tumors [4]. Meanwhile, patients with lymph node positive disease at the time of RC had a 3-year PFS and B-CS survival of 29.1 and 37.5 %, respectively [4]. Likewise, Madersbacher et al. noted a 5-year recurrence-free survival after RC of 73 % among patients with ≤pT2 disease, versus 56 % with >pT2 tumors [7]. Similarly, Hautmann and colleagues reported a stage-specific 5-year recurrence-free survival of 89.8 % for pTa/pTis/pT1 tumors, 71.6 % for pT2 disease, 43 % for pT3, and 27.9 % with pT4 disease [8].

In addition to incorporating risk factors for disease recurrence, the optimal surveillance strategy after RC should also incorporate an understanding of the site predilection and documented timing of recurrences. As noted, metastases may be characterized as either local (disease recurring in the surgical bed or regional pelvic lymph nodes) or distant. The most common distant sites of recurrence include the lungs, bone, and abdomen (including visceral and soft tissue) [3, 9, 10]. Meanwhile, the rate of isolated pelvic recurrence has been suggested to be relatively infrequent, at 5–10 % [11]. The risk of pelvic relapse has been associated with locally advanced tumor stage at RC and the presence of lymph node-positive disease [11]. With regard to the timing of tumor recurrence after RC, the median time to recurrence is approximately 12 months, with most recurrences occurring within 2–3 years.

Indeed, in a series from Vanderbilt University examining patterns of recurrence after RC, only 3.9 % of recurrences were diagnosed more than 3 years after surgery [3]. Similarly, data from the Canadian Bladder Cancer Network demonstrated that 90 % of patients experiencing a recurrence were diagnosed within the first two years after RC [9]. Meanwhile, in a recent multi-institutional series of 2,724 patients from various European and North American centers, 80.9 and 90.6 % of recurrences occurred within 2 and 3 years after RC, respectively [12]. Furthermore, the study also documented a correlation between disease-free survival at 2 and 3 years and 5-year overall survival, suggesting that recurrence status at 2–3 years after RC could serve as a surrogate measure for 5-year overall survival [12].

Notably, inconsistent recommendations for surveillance following RC have been published to date (Table 34.1). For example, the National Comprehensive Cancer Network (NCCN) guidelines for follow-up of patients after RC suggest "imaging of the chest, abdomen, and pelvis every 3 to 12 months for 2 years based on risk of recurrence and then as clinically indicated" [13]. These guidelines do not, however, detail a preferred model for risk stratification, nor recommend a specific imaging modality. Similarly the International Consultation on Urologic Diseases (ICUD) guidelines contain only the statement that "Surveillance regimens for local, distant, and secondary urothelial recurrences after RC should be based on risk-adapted strategies" [6], without providing further detail regarding risk stratification for metastatic surveillance.

Table 34.1 Guideline recommendations for chest, abdomen, and pelvis imaging for metastatic surveillance following radical cystectomy

Source	Recommendation
NCCN [13]	Q 3–12 months for 2 years based on risk of recurrence, and then as clinically indicated[a]
EAU [14]	< pT1: Yearly cross-sectional imaging×5 years
	pT2: Q6 months cross-sectional imaging for 2 years, then yearly until year 5 after surgery
	> pT3 or N+: Cross-sectional imaging at 3 and 6 months, then Q6 months until year 3, then yearly until year 5 after surgery
Bochner et al [11]	CT or MRI of the abdomen/pelvis at 3, 6, 12, 18, and 24 months after surgery, yearly until year 5, then every other year[b]
	Chest x-ray or chest CT at 3 and 12 months after surgery, yearly until year 5, then every other year

[a]Guidelines do not recommend risk model or specific imaging modality

[b]For patients with ≤pT2N0M0 disease, imaging of the abdomen/pelvis may be omitted at 6 and 12 months, and stopped altogether at 24 months after surgery

The European Association of Urology (EAU) guidelines propose risk-stratified follow-up for metastatic surveillance after RC, although the authors acknowledge that these recommendations are based on level 4 evidence [14]. Specifically, yearly cross-sectional imaging of the chest, abdomen, and pelvis for 5 years after RC is recommended for patients with non-muscle-invasive disease at RC, starting 12 months after surgery [14]. In contrast, for patients with pT2 tumors, imaging is recommended to be initiated 6 months postoperatively, and to continue at 6-month intervals for 2 years, and then annually for 5 years [14]. Meanwhile, for patients with pT3 or N+disease, surveillance imaging is recommended to begin at 3 months after surgery, and to be performed then at 6 months postoperatively and at 6-month intervals for 3 years, and then annually until year 5 after surgery [14]. Despite these recommendations, the authors note that "any advice related to follow-up is entirely based on expert consensus and level-4 evidence data" [14]. Likewise, Bochner et al. described a similar stage-specific metastatic surveillance schedule. With this regimen, imaging begins at 3 months after RC and is repeated at 6 months [11]. After that, the surveillance schedule extends to every 6 months until 2 years, after which the schedule becomes yearly [11]. After 5 years, radiographic follow-up can be reduced to every other year [11]. Interestingly, Umbreit et al. describe a model stratifying site-specific recurrence risk based on patient preoperative factors as well as pathologic data [15]. In this model, scores were assigned to variables found to be significant predictors for recurrence on multivariable analysis [15]. For example, according to this model, a patient with a unifocal pT3 bladder tumor at cystectomy with negative surgical margins and with eight negative lymph nodes removed would have a 67.9 % 3-year recurrence-free survival in the abdomen/pelvis, and a 87.1 % 3-year thoracic recurrence-free survival [15]. Of note, a patient with the same pathology but with 15 negative lymph nodes removed at surgery would have a 3-year recurrence-free survival of 78.1 and 92.4 % for the abdomen/pelvis and thoracic region, respectively [15]. Meanwhile, a patient with multifocal CIS at cystectomy with 20 negative lymph nodes removed and with a positive ureteral margin would have a 3-year recurrence-free survival of 86.4 % in the upper tract, 95.2 % in the thoracic region, and 94.4 % in bone [15]. Such tools aim to provide an evidence based framework to guide surveillance following RC, and warrant prospective evaluation.

Consistent with the lack of uniformity in published guidelines for surveillance following RC (and perhaps a contributing factor to these discrepancies) are the findings that: (1) the majority of recurrences after RC are diagnosed in the setting of symptoms [7] and (2) conflicting data have been reported as to the survival benefit of early (i.e. asymptomatic) detection of recurrent disease after RC. Indeed, responses of metastatic urothelial carcinoma to chemotherapy are usually transient, with a median survival in such patients of 12–14 months [16]. Not surprisingly, then, Volkmer et al., in a single-institution study that included 1,270 patients who underwent RC with 20 years of follow-up, determined that overall survival was not significantly different among patients who experienced disease recurrence when stratified by presentation of recurrent disease as asymptomatic versus symptomatic [17].

On the other hand, a separate study by Boorjian and colleagues [7] demonstrated that detection of asymptomatic recurrence following RC was in fact associated with improved overall survival. Specifically, 5 and 10-year overall survival for patients with asymptomatic versus symptomatic recurrence were 46 and 26 %, respectively, versus 22 and 10 % ($p<0.0001$) [10]. The potential mechanisms responsible for the noted association between detection of asymptomatic disease and improved survival include improved efficacy of systemic therapy in patients without symptoms, as well as the delivery of therapy with lower disease burden [7]. Such patients with minimal tumor burden may indeed be considered for a multimodal approach to therapy, including systemic therapy and surgical resection [18, 19].

In summary, the best predictors for disease relapse after RC remain pathologic tumor stage and lymph node status. The majority of recurrences have been documented within the first 2–3 years after surgery. While conflicting evidence has been reported regarding a benefit to the detection of asymptomatic recurrence, we suggest that surveillance imaging following surgery may be considered with a risk-stratified regimen tailored in intensity over time.

34.3 Surveillance of the Upper Urinary Tract Following Radical Cystectomy

Urothelial carcinoma has been considered a "field-change" disease, such that the entire urothelium remains at risk in patients with bladder cancer. Thus, upper urinary tract (UUT) surveillance represents a relevant component of consideration for follow-up after RC, with UUT recurrences noted in 2–9 % of patients after RC [6, 20–24]. Interestingly, patients have been found to remain at prolonged risk for metachronous tumors in the UUT, with a median time to diagnosis after RC noted between 24 and 41 months [6, 20–24]. Moreover, one series has demonstrated that the risk of UUT recurrence did not decrease over time after RC [25], such that the UUT represents the most common site of late recurrence following RC [26]. Risk factors identified for UUT recurrence include a history of carcinoma in situ, recurrent bladder cancer, non-muscle-invasive bladder cancer, and distal ureteral involvement with tumor at RC [26].

Surveillance of the UUT after RC involves both imaging and urine cytology [11, 26]. In the setting of a known or suspected UUT lesion, ureterorenoscopy with biopsy is then recommended to establish histological diagnosis [6]. Classically, upper tract imaging has been in the form of intravenous pyelography. More recently, however, CT urography has become the standard surveillance modality, which allows for monitoring of abdominopelvic adenopathy and visceral metastatic disease as well as UUT tumor recurrence and the development of ureteroenteric anastomotic stricturing [11]. MR urography offers an alternative for monitoring after RC in patients who cannot receive intravenous contrast. Importantly, retrograde pyelography (loopogram) remains an option for UUT surveillance in patients who cannot receive contrast and are ineligible for an MRI.

Meanwhile, urine cytology represents a noninvasive (and, relative to imaging, lower-cost) assay which has been associated with a high specificity albeit relatively low sensitivity for urothelial carcinoma. Although the interpretation of urine cytology may be obscured following urinary diversion by concurrent intestinal mucosal cells as well as mucous [27], nevertheless cytology remains the preferred urine test to date for bladder cancer surveillance to detect UUT recurrence [11]. Indeed, one series study found that, among patients with positive cytology after radical cystectomy, 9 % had documented urothelial recurrence at the time of positive cytology, and 57 % ultimately developed radiologic evidence of urothelial recurrence, at a median of 2.1 years after the positive cytology [28]. As such, the use of cytology may facilitate the identification of patients most likely to benefit from additional interrogation of the UUT with radiologic or ureteroscopic evaluation.

Table 34.2 Guideline recommendations for upper tract surveillance following radical cystectomy

Source	Recommendation
NCCN [13]	No specific UUT imaging regimen recommended. See Table 34.1 recommendations for abdomen/pelvis surveillance
	Urine cytology every 3–6 months for 2 years, and then "as clinically indicated"
ICUD [6]	"Surveillance regimens should be based on a risk-adapted strategy[a]," such that "The number of risk factors for upper tract tumors…predicts the risk of recurrence"
	However, "…the optimal interval for follow-up imaging remains unclear"
EAU [14]	Imaging follows metastatic surveillance guidelines (Table 34.1)
	Urine cytology at 3, 6, and 12 months, then annually (not specified beyond year 5)

[a]Noted risk factors for upper tract recurrence in these guidelines = "(1) positive ureteral margin, (2) carcinoma in situ of the bladder and ureter, (3) tumor multifocality, (4) urethral tumor, and (5) male gender"

Importantly, the question again exists as to whether early detection of UTT recurrence translates into improved patient survival, and again conflicting evidence has been reported. The routine use of imaging or cytology after RC has been found in one series to improve detection of UUT recurrences [29], while recurrences identified via surveillance have also been associated with slightly higher survival rates compared to recurrences identified secondary to symptoms (i.e. gross hematuria, flank pain) [30]. On the other hand, up to 80 % of UUT recurrences have been found to present symptomatically, and separate series have demonstrated no improvement in clinicopathologic outcomes or patient survival among patients diagnosed with a secondary UUT tumor during routine surveillance versus patients who presented symptomatically [10, 15, 20, 21].

Reflecting this controversy regarding the benefit to routine UUT follow-up, similar to the guidelines for metastatic surveillance above, with regard to UUT follow-up after RC, guideline recommendations (Table 34.2) are often conflicting, and are notably largely based on expert opinion and level-4 evidence [26]. Notably, the NCCN guidelines do not specify a UUT imaging follow-up protocol separate from the recommended abdomen/pelvis surveillance (Table 34.1) [13]. In addition, urine cytology is advised "every 3–6 months for 2 years and then as clinically indicated" [13]. Likewise, Bochner and colleagues suggest a protocol for periodic cross-sectional imaging with CT urography, and recommend urine cytology testing at 3, 6, 12, 18, 24 months, and then annually through year 5, and then every 2 years following RC [11]. Interestingly, the EAU guidelines provide a Grade B recommendation that "specific upper urinary tract imaging is only indicated in case of clinical symptoms," but outline a regimen for imaging which mirrors the metastatic surveillance schedule, and only suggest interval urine cytology as well [14].

Meanwhile, the ICUD guidelines suggest "risk-adapted" follow-up, with risk factors identified for UUT recurrence including a positive ureteral margin at RC, carcinoma in situ of the bladder and ureter, tumor multifocality, the presence of a urethral tumor, and male gender [6]. While these guidelines suggest that "cytology should be considered for monitoring of the upper tract after urinary diversion," the ICUD further asserts that "routine upper tract imaging is indicated only in patients who are at high risk or have clinical symptoms suspicious for a metachronous upper tract recurrence" [6]. Our practice has been to obtain annual urine cytology after cystectomy, and to evaluate the upper tract with cross-sectional imaging as scheduled for metastatic surveillance outlined in the section above.

34.4 Surveillance of the Urethra Following Radical Cystectomy

Urethrectomy at the time of RC is typically performed in female patients unless orthotopic diversion is planned, thus removing in the majority of women the urethra as a potential site for subsequent disease recurrence. While urethrectomy at the time of RC had historically been advised for men [31], the added operative morbidity of this procedure, together with the potential impact on patients' subsequent sexual function [32–34], and the increased use of orthotopic reconstruction, have resulted in urethrectomy currently being relatively infrequently performed in men undergoing RC [35].

The incidence of subsequent urethral recurrence in patients undergoing RC has been reported between 0 and 18 % [31, 36–41], with a recent large series demonstrating a recurrence rate of 5.6 % [42]. The biology of metachronous urothelial cancer in the remnant urethra has not been definitively established as representing recurrence of disease versus a second primary cancer [35]. Nevertheless, because urethrectomy is not routinely performed at the time of RC in men, understanding the factors associated with urethral recurrence is important to help guide postoperative surveillance.

Not surprisingly, the presence of tumor at the urethral margin of the surgical specimen has been found to be highly predictive for urethral recurrence [41], and as such obtaining a negative frozen section urethral margin has been recommended for patients in whom an orthotopic reconstruction is planned [39]. The most consistent risk factor for urethral recurrence following RC has been prostatic urethral involvement with cancer, with evidence suggesting a correlation between the depth of tumor invasion into the prostate and the risk of subsequent recurrence [34, 39, 40, 42, 43]. Interestingly, conflicting data have been reported regarding a potential independent association between the type of urinary diversion and the risk of urethral recurrence [37, 40, 42–44]. That is, several series have reported a decreased rate of urethral recurrence among patients receiving an orthotopic reconstruction versus a cutaneous diversion [37, 40, 42, 44]. Some authors have postulated that the exposure of the remaining urothelium to urine confers an anticancer effect [37]; however, others have argued that this finding can be explained by careful patient selection, with those undergoing neobladder reconstruction having more favorable pathologic features [43].

Urethral wash cytology was proposed for monitoring of the urethra following RC by Wolinska, and has since represented the mainstay of surveillance for the remnant urethra [45].

Table 34.3 Guideline recommendations for obtaining urethral cytology following radical cystectomy

Source	Recommendation
NCCN [13]	Q 6–12 months "particularly if Tis was found within the bladder or prostatic urethra"
ICUD [6]	"Routine surveillance…in asymptomatic patients has not shown a survival benefit… it seems reasonable to tailor surveillance according to the patients' risk profile[a]"
EAU [14]	"Urethral washes and cytology are not recommended as standard follow-up"
Bochner et al [11]	Biannually × 3 years and then annually if moderate–high risk[b]
	Annually in low risk patients × 5 years
	Biannually × 5 years and then annually after neobladder

[a]Noted risk factors for urethral recurrence in these guidelines = "prostatic tumor involvement (either superficial or invasive) in male patients and bladder-neck involvement in female patients"
[b]High risk as specified here = prostatic tumor involvement; moderate risk = multiple bladder tumors or evidence of carcinoma in situ of the bladder, bladder neck, or trigone; low risk = solitary tumor away from the bladder neck or trigone

Cytology can be obtained by voiding in patients with an orthotopic reconstruction (although UUT recurrence must also be considered in such cases). For patients without orthotopic diversion, urethral washing may be obtained by advancing a 14 or 16 French catheter to the proximal (blind) end of the urethra, washing with 10–15 ml of normal saline, and collecting the efflux for analysis [46]. Patients with a positive urethral cytology, as well as those presenting with urethral bleeding/discharge, pain, or a palpable mass after RC, should be evaluated further with urethroscopy.

Unfortunately, little consistency again exists among the guideline recommendations for surveillance of the urethra following RC (Table 34.3). That is, Bochner and colleagues recommended a surveillance schedule for patients with a cutaneous diversion of "urethral washes biannually for the first 3 years and annually thereafter in moderate-to-high risk patients and annually in low-risk patients for a period of 5 years" [11]. For patients with an orthotopic diversion, the same authors recommend "a voided urine cytology…should be performed biannually for the first 5 years and then annually". Meanwhile, the most recent NCCN guidelines recommend "Urethral wash cytology, every 6 to 12 months; particularly if Tis was found within the bladder or prostatic urethra" [13]. Likewise, the ICUD guidelines state that "it seems reasonable to tailor surveillance according to the patient's risk profile" [6]. These recommendations are likely based on the findings as noted above from multiple retrospective analyses which have demonstrated a significant association between prostatic urethral involvement of tumor at cystectomy and patients' subsequent risk of urethral recurrence [11, 40–43]. Indeed, the ICUD guidelines assign a Grade B recommendation, with level 3 evidence, to the assertion that "Risk factors for urethral recurrence are prostatic tumor involvement (either superficial or invasive) in male patients and bladder-neck involvement in female patients" [6].

Notably, however the ICUD guidelines do include the statement that "From an oncologic perspective, the use of routine surveillance urinary cytology, urethral washings, and diagnostic urethroscopy in asymptomatic patients has not shown a survival benefit" [6], although this recommendation is also Grade B, based on level 3 evidence. Similarly, then, the EAU guidelines for follow-up of patients with muscle-invasive bladder cancer after radical cystectomy include a Grade Λ recommendation that "urethral washes and cytology are not recommended as standard follow-up" [14].

These disparate recommendations largely result from the fact that conflicting evidence exists regarding the clinical benefit to routine urethral washing/cytology following RC [42, 43, 46–48]. Indeed, Lin et al. compared the outcomes of 17 patients who underwent urethrectomy after RC for an asymptomatic positive urethral wash cytology versus 7 patients not followed by urethral wash who presented with bleeding/urethral discharge [46]. These investigators noted no significant difference in survival between the two cohorts, and in fact the mode of presentation (asymptomatic versus symptomatic) was not found to be independently associated with patients' risk of death on multivariate analysis [46]. Meanwhile, Boorjian et al., in a series of 85 patients with urethral recurrence following cystectomy, demonstrated that the detection of asymptomatic urethral recurrence was associated with significantly lower stage disease and improved patient survival, suggesting the importance of continued, if potentially risk-stratified, postoperative surveillance of the remnant urethra [42].

34.5 Surveillance Following Bladder Preservation in the Setting of Muscle-Invasive Bladder Cancer

A number of strategies have been described for bladder preservation in patients with muscle-invasive disease, including partial cystectomy [49], chemoradiation [50], transurethral resection alone [51], and chemotherapy alone [52]. Surveillance in such patients should be guided by tumor stage, and should include evaluation of the UTT, with imaging of the chest/abdomen/pelvis as after RC [13]. In addition, these patients required continued monitoring of the bladder for disease recurrence, which has been reported for example in approximately one-third of patients undergoing transurethral resection alone or partial cystectomy [49, 51]. As such, NCCN guidelines advise "cystoscopy and urine cytology ± selected mapping biopsies every 3–6 months for 2 years, then increasing intervals as appropriate" [13].

34.6 Surveillance of Renal Function and Metabolic Complications of Urinary Diversion

Following cystectomy, a variety of intestinal segments can be used for reconstruction of the urinary tract, including stomach, jejunum, ileum, and colon. While a wide variety of urinary reconstruction methods are available, the most commonly used segment used is ileum, either in the form of an ileal conduit or orthotopic neobladder. Colon is often the next bowel segment used if ileum is unavailable for various anatomic or medical reasons. With the use of these bowel segments in the urinary tract, absorptive anomalies can develop, leading to a variety electrolyte derangements from altered solute absorption across the intestinal segment. In addition, urinary diversion carries the risk of long-term renal failure. Thus, following cystectomy with urinary diversion, electrolyte and renal function surveillance is an important component of long-term postoperative care.

The type of electrolyte abnormality for which patients are at risk after diversion depends on the type and length of intestinal segment used [26]. For example, the use of stomach has been associated with the development of hypochloremic metabolic alkalosis, while the use of jejunum confers a risk of hyponatremia, hyperkalemic metabolic acidosis. Importantly, both ileum and colon are associated with the development of hyperchloremic, hypokalemic metabolic acidosis that often presents with abdominal pain, fatigue, anorexia, lethargy, and weakness. Acidosis results from the absorption of urinary components through the bowel mucosa [53], specifically, the absorption of ammonium chloride and secretion of sodium bicarbonate [11]. Indeed, electrolyte abnormalities are relatively common following urinary diversion, with a recent study identifying an incidence of approximately 23 % after ileal conduit and 28 % after neobladder [54]. Studer et al. in fact noted that approximately 4.4 % of patients required hospitalization for metabolic acidosis after orthotopic neobladder [55]. As chronic metabolic acidosis can lead to bone demineralization [26], patients should be followed after urinary diversion to facilitate early detection and correction.

In addition to these metabolic complications, patients are also at risk for progressive renal deterioration after urinary diversion. The etiology for chronic kidney disease in this setting is likely multifactorial, and includes preexisting renal disease in such a patient population [56], the frequent presence of comorbid conditions such as diabetes and hypertension, the impact of aforementioned metabolic derangements, and the sequelae of reflux, obstruction, and infection that may occur after ureteroenteric anastomosis [53,

57]. As such, Madersbacher et al. reported morphologic/functional deterioration in approximately 27 % of patients after ileal conduit [58], while Studer et al. identified increased serum creatinine levels in 3.8 % of patients at 5 years after orthotopic urinary diversion [55]. In addition, Samuel and colleagues found that 29 % of patients undergoing ileal conduit experienced a worsening of glomerular filtration rate (GFR) > 5 % at a mean of 8.2 years after surgery [59]. Most recently, Jin et al., in a study of patients who survived ≥10 years after surgery, noted a decline in GFR >10 in 36 % of patients after ileal conduit and 21 % after orthotopic ileal neobladder [57]. In accordance with these findings, NCCN guidelines recommend monitoring of serum creatinine and electrolytes following cystectomy with urinary diversion every 3–6 months for the first two years after surgery, and then as clinically indicated [13]. EAU guidelines likewise advise blood chemistry, including serum creatinine, and blood gas analysis at 3, 6, and 12 months postoperatively, and then yearly [14]. Moreover, given the noted risk for long-term renal function decline after urinary diversion [57], the EAU guidelines suggest that "follow-up oncologic surveillance can be stopped after 5 years, but continuation with functional surveillance… is recommended" [14]. Likewise, Bochner and colleagues advised monitoring of electrolytes at 3, 6, 12, 18, and 24 months after surgery, then annually through year 5, and then at 2-year intervals [11]. Our practice has been to obtain a serum electrolyte panel with creatinine at 3, 6, 12, 18, and 24 months after surgery, and then annually thereafter.

The use of the terminal ileum for urinary diversion has implications for vitamin B12 metabolism, as the terminal ileum represents a critical site for absorption of this vitamin. The consequences of vitamin B12 deficiency include megaloblastic anemia and impaired myelin production, which may in turn lead to irreversible neurologic symptoms [11]. Resection of >60 cm of terminal ileum has in particular been associated with an increased risk of B12 malabsorption, and it has been estimated that, given the body's stores of this vitamin, complete depletion of normal B12 levels would take 3–4 years [11]. In a review of urinary diversions [54], Nieuwenhuijzen identified low vitamin B12 in 23 % of patients after ileal conduit and 15 % after orthotopic diversion. Meanwhile, Studer et al. identified a 12 % rate of subnormal vitamin B12 at some time during follow-up, with 5 % receiving B12 substitution [55]. Although clinically significant risk of B12 deficiency is rare following urinary diversion, surveillance and subsequent treatment with B12 replacement are relatively inexpensive and non-invasive. Accordingly, NCCN guidelines recommend annual serum B12 surveillance for patients with a continent diversion [13]. Meanwhile, Bochner and colleagues recommend checking vitamin B12 at annually from years 2 to 5 following urinary diversion, and subsequently every other year [11].

34.7 Conclusions

Though high levels of evidence are lacking, guideline recommendations continue to recommend monitoring patients after RC for cancer recurrence and metabolic disturbances associated with urinary diversion. The optimal surveillance strategy and the extent to which oncologic follow-up may improve patient outcomes have yet to be defined, and remain areas of important future research.

References

1. Stein JP et al. Radical cystectomy in the treatment of invasive bladder cancer: long-term results in 1,054 patients. J Clin Oncol. 2001;19(3):666–75.
2. Riley GF et al. Medicare payments from diagnosis to death for elderly cancer patients by stage at diagnosis. Med Care. 1995;33(8):828–41.
3. Hassan JM et al. Patterns of initial transitional cell recurrence in patients after cystectomy. J Urol. 2006;175(6):2054–7.
4. Shariat SF et al. Outcomes of radical cystectomy for transitional cell carcinoma of the bladder: a contemporary series from the Bladder Cancer Research Consortium. J Urol. 2006;176(6 Pt 1):2414–22. discussion 2422.
5. Rink M et al. Stage-specific impact of tumor location on oncologic outcomes in patients with upper and lower tract urothelial carcinoma following radical surgery. Eur Urol. 2012;62(4):677–84.
6. Gakis G et al. ICUD-EAU International Consultation on Bladder Cancer 2012: radical cystectomy and bladder preservation for muscle-invasive urothelial carcinoma of the bladder. Eur Urol. 2013;63(1): 45–57.
7. Madersbacher S et al. Radical cystectomy for bladder cancer today–a homogeneous series without neoadjuvant therapy. J Clin Oncol. 2003;21(4):690–6.
8. Hautmann RE et al. Cystectomy for transitional cell carcinoma of the bladder: results of a surgery only series in the neobladder era. J Urol. 2006;176(2):486–92. discussion 491-2.
9. Yafi FA et al. Surveillance guidelines based on recurrence patterns after radical cystectomy for bladder cancer: the Canadian Bladder Cancer Network experience. BJU Int. 2012;110(9):1317–23.
10. Boorjian SA et al. Detection of asymptomatic recurrence during routine oncological followup after radical cystectomy is associated with improved patient survival. J Urol. 2011;186(5):1796–802.
11. Bochner BH, Montie JE, Lee CT. Follow-up strategies and management of recurrence in urologic oncology bladder cancer: invasive bladder cancer. Urol Clin North Am. 2003;30(4):777–89.
12. Sonpavde G et al. Disease-free survival at 2 or 3 years correlates with 5-year overall survival of patients undergoing radical cystectomy for muscle invasive bladder cancer. J Urol. 2011;185(2):456–61.
13. Clark PE et al. Bladder cancer. J Natl Compr Canc Netw. 2013;11(4):446–75.
14. Stenzl A et al. The updated EAU guidelines on muscle-invasive and metastatic bladder cancer. Eur Urol. 2009;55(4):815–25.
15. Umbreit EC et al. Multifactorial, site-specific recurrence model after radical cystectomy for urothelial carcinoma. Cancer. 2010;116(14):3399–407.
16. Sternberg CN et al. Randomized phase III trial of high-dose-intensity methotrexate, vinblastine, doxorubicin, and cisplatin (MVAC) chemotherapy and recombinant human granulocyte colony-stimulating factor versus classic MVAC in advanced urothelial tract tumors: European Organization for Research and Treatment of Cancer Protocol no. 30924. J Clin Oncol. 2001;19(10):2638–46.
17. Volkmer BG et al. Oncological followup after radical cystectomy for bladder cancer-is there any benefit? J Urol. 2009;181(4):1587–93. discussion 1593.
18. Siefker-Radtke AO et al. Is there a role for surgery in the management of metastatic urothelial cancer? The M.D. Anderson experience. J Urol. 2004;171(1):145–8.
19. Lehmann J et al. Surgery for metastatic urothelial carcinoma with curative intent: the German experience (AUO AB 30/05). Eur Urol. 2009;55(6):1293–9.
20. Sanderson KM et al. Upper tract urothelial recurrence following radical cystectomy for transitional cell carcinoma of the bladder: an analysis of 1,069 patients with 10-year followup. J Urol. 2007;177(6):2088–94.
21. Meissner C et al. The efficiency of excretory urography to detect upper urinary tract tumors after cystectomy for urothelial cancer. J Urol. 2007;178(6): 2287–90.

22. Tollefson MK et al. Significance of distal ureteral margin at radical cystectomy for urothelial carcinoma. J Urol. 2010;183(1):81–6.
23. Schoenberg MP, Carter HB, Epstein JI. Ureteral frozen section analysis during cystectomy: a reassessment. J Urol. 1996;155(4):1218–20.
24. Gakis G et al. Sequential resection of malignant ureteral margins at radical cystectomy: a critical assessment of the value of frozen section analysis. World J Urol. 2011;29(4):451–6.
25. Tran W et al. Longitudinal risk of upper tract recurrence following radical cystectomy for urothelial cancer and the potential implications for long-term surveillance. J Urol. 2008;179(1):96–100.
26. Soukup V et al. Follow-up after surgical treatment of bladder cancer: a critical analysis of the literature. Eur Urol. 2012;62(2):290–302.
27. Yoshimine S et al. The clinical significance of urine cytology after a radical cystectomy for urothelial cancer. Int J Urol. 2010;17(6):527–32.
28. Raj GV et al. Natural history of positive urinary cytology after radical cystectomy. J Urol. 2006;176(5):2000–5. discussion 2005.
29. Slaton JW et al. A stage specific approach to tumor surveillance after radical cystectomy for transitional cell carcinoma of the bladder. J Urol. 1999;162(3 Pt 1):710–4.
30. Giannarini G et al. Do patients benefit from routine follow-up to detect recurrences after radical cystectomy and ileal orthotopic bladder substitution? Eur Urol. 2010;58(4):486–94.
31. Schellhammer PF, Whitmore Jr WF. Transitional cell carcinoma of the urethra in men having cystectomy for bladder cancer. J Urol. 1976;115(1):56–60.
32. Kitamura T et al. Urethrectomy is harmful for preserving potency after radical cystectomy. Urol Int. 1987;42(5):375–9.
33. Tomic R, Sjodin JG. Sexual function in men after radical cystectomy with or without urethrectomy. Scand J Urol Nephrol. 1992;26(2):127–9.
34. Ingimarsson JP, Seigne JD. The conundrum of prostatic urethral involvement. Urol Clin North Am. 2013;40(2):249–59.
35. Nelles JL et al. Urethrectomy following cystectomy for bladder cancer in men: practice patterns and impact on survival. J Urol. 2008;180(5):1933–6. discussion 1936-7.
36. Hardeman SW, Soloway MS. Urethral recurrence following radical cystectomy. J Urol. 1990;144(3):666–9.
37. Freeman JA et al. Urethral recurrence in patients with orthotopic ileal neobladders. J Urol. 1996;156(5):1615–9.
38. Stenzl A, Bartsch G, Rogatsch H. The remnant urothelium after reconstructive bladder surgery. Eur Urol. 2002;41(2):124–31.
39. Clark PE, Hall MC. Contemporary management of the urethra in patients after radical cystectomy for bladder cancer. Urol Clin North Am. 2005;32(2):199–206.
40. Stein JP et al. Urethral tumor recurrence following cystectomy and urinary diversion: clinical and pathological characteristics in 768 male patients. J Urol. 2005;173(4):1163–8.
41. Cho KS et al. The risk factor for urethral recurrence after radical cystectomy in patients with transitional cell carcinoma of the bladder. Urol Int. 2009;82(3):306–11.
42. Boorjian SA et al. Risk factors and outcomes of urethral recurrence following radical cystectomy. Eur Urol. 2011;60(6):1266–72.
43. Huguet J et al. Diagnosis, risk factors, and outcome of urethral recurrences following radical cystectomy for bladder cancer in 729 male patients. Eur Urol. 2008;53(4):785–92. discussion 792-3.
44. Nieder AM et al. Urethral recurrence after cystoprostatectomy: implications for urinary diversion and monitoring. Urology. 2004;64(5):950–4.
45. Wolinska WH et al. Urethral cytology following cystectomy for bladder carcinoma. Am J Surg Pathol. 1977;1(3):225–34.
46. Lin DW, Herr HW, Dalbagni G. Value of urethral wash cytology in the retained male urethra after radical cystoprostatectomy. J Urol. 2003;169(3):961–3.
47. Knapik JA, Murphy WM. Urethral wash cytopathology for monitoring patients after cystoprostatectomy with urinary diversion. Cancer. 2003;99(6):352–6.
48. Clark PE et al. The management of urethral transitional cell carcinoma after radical cystectomy for invasive bladder cancer. J Urol. 2004;172(4 Pt 1):1342–7.
49. Knoedler JJ et al. Does partial cystectomy compromise oncologic outcomes for patients with bladder cancer compared to radical cystectomy? A matched case-control analysis. J Urol. 2012;188(4):1115–9.
50. James ND et al. Radiotherapy with or without chemotherapy in muscle-invasive bladder cancer. N Engl J Med. 2012;366(16):1477–88.
51. Herr HW. Transurethral resection of muscle-invasive bladder cancer: 10-year outcome. J Clin Oncol. 2001;19(1):89–93.
52. Herr HW. Outcome of patients who refuse cystectomy after receiving neoadjuvant chemotherapy for muscle-invasive bladder cancer. Eur Urol. 2008;54(1):126–32.
53. Hautmann RE et al. ICUD-EAU International Consultation on Bladder Cancer 2012: urinary diversion. Eur Urol. 2013;63(1):67–80.
54. Nieuwenhuijzen JA et al. Urinary diversions after cystectomy: the association of clinical factors, complications and functional results of four different diversions. Eur Urol. 2008;53(4):834–42. discussion 842-4.
55. Studer UE et al. Twenty years experience with an ileal orthotopic low pressure bladder substitute-lessons to be learned. J Urol. 2006;176(1):161–6.
56. Canter D et al. Baseline renal function status limits patient eligibility to receive perioperative chemotherapy for invasive bladder cancer and is minimally affected by radical cystectomy. Urology. 2011;77(1):160–5.

57. Jin XD et al. Long-term renal function after urinary diversion by ileal conduit or orthotopic ileal bladder substitution. Eur Urol. 2012;61(3): 491–7.
58. Madersbacher S et al. Long-term outcome of ileal conduit diversion. J Urol. 2003;169(3):985–90.
59. Samuel JD et al. The natural history of postoperative renal function in patients undergoing ileal conduit diversion for cancer measured using serial isotopic glomerular filtration rate and 99 m technetium-mercaptoacetyltriglycine renography. J Urol. 2006; 176(6 Pt 1):2518–22. discussion 2522.

A 61-year-old man received neoadjuvant
chemotherapy and radical cystectomy, with
final pathology showing pT3aN0M0 disease

Eila C. Skinner

Abbreviations

CMV   Cisplatin, methotrexate, vinblastine
GC   Gemcitabine, cisplatin
MVAC Methotrexate, vinblastine, adriamycin
      (doxorubicin), cisplatin

35.1   Introduction

Neoadjuvant chemotherapy followed by cystectomy is considered by many to be the standard of care for muscle-invasive bladder cancer. This is based on prospective randomized trial evidence that the neoadjuvant chemotherapy confers an approximate 5 % absolute benefit in survival compared to cystectomy alone [1]. There have now been more than ten such trials completed in the US and Europe. Trial designs have varied somewhat in enrollment criteria and specific chemotherapy agents tested, and some have allowed definitive radiation instead of cystectomy [2]. The majority have reported a benefit of neoadjuvant chemotherapy in terms of recurrence-free and overall survival. There are flaws in the trial designs of most of these trials, including the fact that surgical technique such as extent of pelvic node dissection was not standardized in these trials and may have confounded the results [3]. In addition, most of the trials excluded patients with poor renal function or performance status, which accounts for many of our typical cystectomy candidates. In spite of these drawbacks, several meta-analyses have concluded that the benefit is real [4, 5].

Urologists have only recently begun to embrace this approach, even in academic centers, and still only a minority of patients with muscle-invasive disease today receive neoadjuvant chemotherapy prior to cystectomy, though that number appears to be increasing [6]. For the patients who do receive these treatments, however, there are still a number of questions remaining.

35.2   What Are the Predictors of Prognosis for Patients Treated with Chemotherapy Followed by Cystectomy?

The most powerful predictor of prognosis appears to be the pathologic stage from the cystectomy specimen. Studies of patients treated with neoadjuvant platinum-based chemotherapy have reported pT0 rates of up to 46 % at cystectomy

E.C. Skinner, M.D. (✉)
Department of Urology, Thomas A. Stamey Research
Chair of Urology, 300 Pasteur Drive, Suite S-287,
Stanford, CA 94305, USA
e-mail: skinnere@stanford.edu

B.R. Konety and S.S. Chang (eds.), *Management of Bladder Cancer:*
A Comprehensive Text With Clinical Scenarios, DOI 10.1007/978-1-4939-1881-2_35,
© Springer Science+Business Media New York 2015

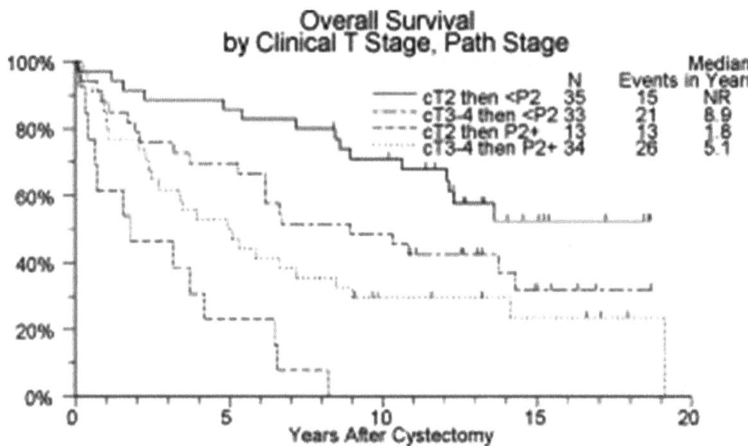

Fig. 35.1 Post-cystectomy survival by baseline clinical stage and pathologic (Path) stage (<p2 vs. p2+) after therapy with MVAC. Adapted from Sonpavde G, Goldman BH, Speights VO, et al. Quality of pathologic response and surgery correlate with survival for patients with completely resected bladder cancer after neoadjuvant chemotherapy. Cancer 2009; 115:4104–09

(mean 28 %) [7]. Two phase III prospective randomized trials, SWOG 8710 and the Nordic trial, had pT0 rates of 38 and 23 % respectively [1, 8]. Downstaging to pT0 is more common in patients with initial smaller and lower stage tumors [8]. Nearly all studies reported have shown a very significant survival advantage for patients who achieved downstaging to <pT2 status compared to those who did not [9] (Fig. 35.1). Patients with non-muscle-invasive residual disease, or even organ-confined invasive disease also appear to have an advantage compared to those who have extravesical or node-positive disease following chemotherapy [8]. Although patients at all clinical stages appear to benefit from neoadjuvant chemotherapy, the greatest benefit is seen in patients who had clinical T3 disease preoperatively.

In addition to pathologic stage, demographic features such as age and gender and other pathologic features such as the presence of lymphovascular invasion even in node-negative patients have been shown to impact recurrence and survival in patients treated with cystectomy with or without chemotherapy. Nomograms have been developed based on large databases that physicians and patients can use to estimate recurrence risk in an individual patient. Two that are available publicly include the Memorial Sloan Kettering prediction tool (available at http://www.mskcc.org/cancer-care/adult/bladder/prediction-tools) and the Cancer Prognostics and Health Outcomes Unit of the University of Montreal nomogram (available at www.nomogram.org). Many others have been developed to include other variables such as molecular markers that are still not widely available [10].

Other researchers have evaluated molecular markers as predictors for response to neoadjuvant chemotherapy [11]. These have included evaluation of specific markers such as the p53 family or ERCC1, as well as genome-wide approaches using panels of genes found to be differentially expressed in responders vs. nonresponders [12]. It would be extremely useful to identify robust markers based on TURBT specimens that are not just prognostic of tumor behavior but that can specifically predict patient response to neoadjuvant chemotherapy. This would allow avoidance of the toxicity from chemotherapy and the resultant delay in surgery for patients in whom the treatment is unlikely to achieve a benefit. Alternative neoadjuvant approaches could also be tested in patients who have high-risk invasive disease but are predicted to not respond to standard therapy. Many researchers are working on this problem using panels of tissue and blood markers, or other novel techniques such as COXEN [13, 14]. Although some of these are commercially available, none are widely accepted yet for standard use outside of a research setting.

35.3 If He Had Not Received Neoadjuvant Chemotherapy, Should He Receive Postoperative Chemotherapy with this Pathology?

The benefit of adjuvant chemotherapy is less well established in the literature than neoadjuvant therapy. Multiple adjuvant chemotherapy trials have been closed prematurely due to poor accrual or were underpowered to show a significant difference in survival. The Advanced Bladder Cancer (ABC) Meta-analysis Collaboration in 2005 evaluated six trials that included only 491 total patients. Five of the trials showed a benefit, and they estimated a 25 % reduction in risk of recurrence (approximately a 5 % absolute advantage) [15] (Fig. 35.2). Four additional prospective randomized studies since then all closed prematurely due to poor accrual (Spanish SOGUG 99/01, CALGB 90104, Italian Multicenter and EORTC 30994) [16]. For the patients who were randomized in all of these studies, many either did not receive chemotherapy at all or did not complete all of the prescribed therapy, attesting to the difficulty of delivering chemotherapy in the post-cystectomy setting. Thus these studies may actually underestimate the potential benefit of adjuvant chemotherapy in a patient such as this one.

The patient in our scenario has the best prognosis of patients with extravesical disease, but still has an estimated recurrence-free survival at 5 years of less than 70 % using the MSKCC nomogram. He is young, and if he recovers smoothly after cystectomy with good renal function he should be advised to receive adjuvant chemotherapy.

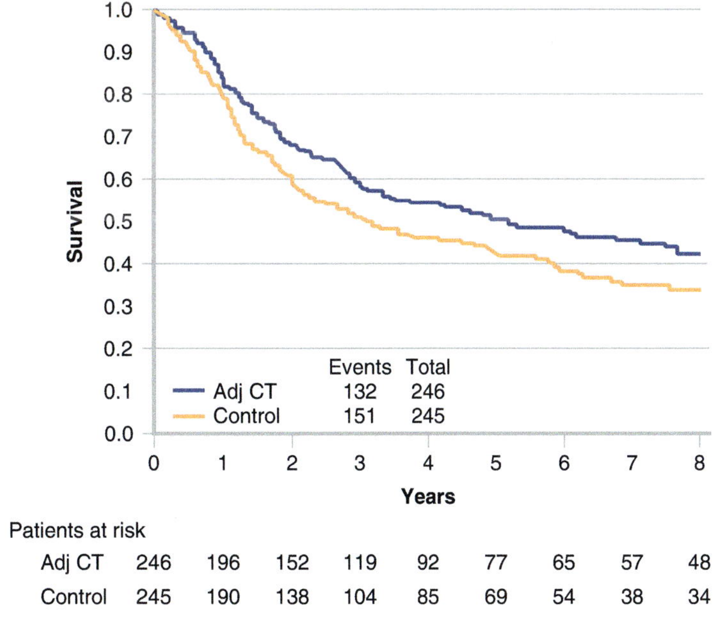

Fig. 35.2 Kaplan–Meier curve for survival from individual patient meta-analysis of six trials of adjuvant chemotherapy after radical cystectomy. Adapted from Vale, Claire L and the Advanced Bladder Cancer (ABC) Meta-Analysis Collaboration. Adjuvant chemotherapy in invasive bladder cancer: a systematic review and meta-analysis of individual patient data. Eur Urol 2005; 48:189–201

35.4 Since He Did Receive Neoadjuvant Chemotherapy and Still Has Significant Residual Disease, Should He Receive Additional Adjuvant Chemotherapy?

The ideal drug combination or number of cycles of perioperative chemotherapy for cystectomy patients has not yet been elucidated. Prospective and retrospective studies have used a variety of platinum-containing regimens, including MVAC, CMV, and a number of others, with varying numbers of cycles delivered. There are no completed randomized trials comparing one regimen to another in the perioperative setting, though a few such trials are planned or underway. In the US, gemcitabine and cisplatin (GC) have been used by most oncologists as a substitute for the more toxic standard MVAC combination based on similar outcomes in the metastatic setting. Retrospective non-randomized studies suggest these agents may have similar results as MVAC [17]. Recently many academic centers have begun using dose-dense MVAC as a better tolerated neoadjuvant combination that may have better efficacy. A large prospective intergroup study comparing neoadjuvant ddMVAC to GC is being planned.

An even less studied question is whether there is any role for additional chemotherapy after surgery in patients who already received neoadjuvant treatment, for example switching from GC to MVAC or to another second-line regimen such as the one containing a taxane. The good prognosis for patients who achieved a pT0 response after 3 or 4 cycles of preoperative chemotherapy suggests that there might not be much additional benefit of further treatment after surgery for them. On the other hand, patients with persistent extravesical disease after neoadjuvant cisplatin chemotherapy have a high risk of recurrence and a poor prognosis, but are also likely to have chemo-resistant disease. Thus additional platinum-based chemotherapy may only add toxicity without impacting the ultimate cure rate. The role of adjuvant radiation therapy or alternative chemotherapy agents is similarly unknown in this setting.

Today there is no established postoperative treatment that is known to impact the high recurrence rate in patients with persistent extravesical disease after neoadjuvant chemotherapy and cystectomy. This patient population is ideal for clinical trials of new agents. Although these patients do not have measurable disease, the high recurrence rate suggests that the vast majority of these patients harbor micrometastatic disease. It is particularly attractive to consider such treatments as immunotherapy or biologic response modifiers which may have less toxicity for these debilitated patients and have a better chance of working in low-volume disease settings. A few such trials are underway including a trial with an autologous cellular immunotherapy against Her2 for tumors expressing Her2 (NCT01353222). The challenge in this setting is the surgical recovery and postoperative complications that may delay any adjuvant treatment or make patients ineligible for participation in clinical trials.

35.5 What Is the Ideal Follow-Up Schedule for These Patients

There is no consensus about the ideal follow-up program for patients after cystectomy, regardless of the stage, grade, or prior chemotherapy. Regimens vary considerably by institution and country in terms of both intensity of follow-up and imaging used. There is some suggestion that the degree and intensity of follow-up is essentially irrelevant because the vast majority of patients who recur will die of their disease and there is little evidence that early detection of the recurrence changes that outcome [18]. Nevertheless, at most institutions some standard follow-up regimen is customary, including periodic imaging, lab tests and physical exam.

A number of consensus guidelines are available to guide the surgeon in developing a follow-up schedule (Table 35.1). The NCCN guidelines (available at http://www.nccn.org/professionals/physician_gls/pdf/bladder.pdf) suggest routine follow-up only out to 2 years and then as clinically indicated thereafter. This is somewhat surprising considering that the median time to recurrence is

Table 35.1 Published guidelines for follow-up after radical cystectomy

NCCN guidelines

(*Available at*: http://www.nccn.org/professionals/physician_gls/pdf/bladder.pdf)

- Urine cytology, creatinine, and electrolytes every 3–6 months for 2 years then as clinically indicated
- Imaging of the chest, abdomen, and pelvis every 3–12 months for 2 years based on risk of recurrence, then as clinically indicated
- Urethral wash cytology every 6–12 months, particularly if Tis was found within the bladder or prostatic urethra
- If a continent diversion was created, monitor for vitamin B12 deficiency annually

EAU guidelines

(Available at: http://www.uroweb.org/gls/pdf/07_%20Bladder%20Cancer.pdf)

Based on pathologic stage:

<p T2

- Labs, cytology at 3, 6, 12 months then annually
- Ultrasound at 3 months
- CT C/A/P (or MRI) annually to 5 years

pT2

- Labs, cytology at 3, 6, 12 months then annually
- Ultrasound at 3 months
- CT C/A/P (or MRI) every 6 months to 2 years, then annually to 5 years

pT3-4 or N+

- Labs, cytology at 3 and 6 months, then every 6 months to 3 years, then annually to 5 years
- Ultrasound at 3 months
- CT C/A/P (or MRI) at 3 and 6 months, then every 6 months to 3 years, then annually to 5 years.

12–18 months and the risk of recurrence persists at least out to 5 years, especially in patients with lower pathologic stage [19]. The EAU guidelines are based on the pathologic stage and the risk of recurrence, with more frequent scans for patients with higher stage disease (available at http://www.uroweb.org/gls/pdf/07_%20Bladder%20Cancer.pdf). Both sets of guidelines are based on expert opinion rather than strong evidence comparing outcomes with different programs.

The goal of follow-up is to identify correctable or treatable problems early to attempt to decrease morbidity. Although very rapid recurrences are occasionally seen, the initial evaluation at 3 or 4 months is primarily looking at surgical recovery and evaluating whether the ureteral anastomoses have healed without stricture, evaluating renal function and acid–base balance, and checking whether the patient with a neobladder is emptying adequately. This can be accomplished with renal and bladder ultrasound or abdominal/pelvic CT, labs, and a physical exam. In patients at low risk of recurrence one might check labs including a urinary cytology and a chest X-ray every 6 months during the first 3 years and then yearly, with a CT abdomen and pelvis with intravenous contrast (or MRI) once yearly out to 5 years. Vitamin B12 level should also be checked yearly if a continent diversion is performed. Urethral wash cytology should be performed annually if the patient had CIS, especially in the prostatic urethra. Even beyond the period of risk for cancer recurrence renal ultrasound and labs should be performed every 1–2 years for life because of the risk of late ureteral obstruction, stones, and renal deterioration. The advisability of long-term routine upper tract imaging with a contrast CT scan is unknown. Ureteral recurrences often happen later, but even with surveillance are often symptomatic by the time they are picked up [20].

In higher risk patients (such as this one) the most common sites of recurrence are in the retroperitoneum, lungs, liver, and bones. More frequent scans and labs are reasonable, although the ideal frequency is unknown. Changing the frequency from every 3 months (as recommended in the EAU guidelines) to every 4 months, for example, eliminates one scan per year, with significant cost saving and decreased radiation exposure. It is unlikely that any measurable difference in outcome would be seen with this approach. It may also be reasonable to substitute the chest CT scan with a CXR in many if not most cases. A suggested follow-up schedule for this patient would include CT Chest/Abdomen/Pelvis with IV contrast, chemistry labs and urine cytology every 4 months the first year, then every 6 months to 3 years, and annually thereafter, with CXR replacing the chest CT after 3 years. After 5 years a renal ultrasound and chemistry panel can be done every 1–2 years, with other studies as clinically indicated.

35.6   Conclusions

There is quite convincing evidence that neoadjuvant chemotherapy should be considered for the majority of patients with muscle-invasive bladder cancer unless they have compromised renal function. Cisplatin-based combinations have been most widely tested and so far have shown the best results, although the exact best regimen is not known. Patients who have favorable pathology after this combination treatment (pT0 or <pT2 disease) have an excellent prognosis of long-term cure and do not require additional chemotherapy after surgery. Follow-up should be adapted to the risk of recurrence and is generally continued for at least 3–5 years. Questions that remain unanswered include how to accurately predict pretreatment who is likely to respond to the chemotherapy, and what to do for those who have adverse pathologic features at cystectomy following neoadjuvant chemotherapy.

References

1. Grossman HB, Natale RB, Tangen CM, Speights VO, Vogelzang NJ, Trump DL, deVere White RW, Sarosdy MF, Wood DP, Raghavan D, Crawford ED. Neoadjuvant chemotherapy plus cystectomy compared with cystectomy alone for locally advanced bladder cancer. N Engl J Med. 2003;349:859–66.
2. International Collaboration of Trialists, Medical Research Council Advanced Bladder Cancer Working Party, European Organisation for Research and Treatment of Cancer Genito-Urinary Tract Cancer Group. International phase III trial assessing neoadjuvant cisplatin, methotrexate, and vinblastine chemotherapy for muscle-invasive bladder cancer: long-term results of the BA06 30894 trial. J Clin Oncol. 2011;29:2171–7.
3. Herr HW, Faulkner JR, Grossman HB, et al. Surgical factors influence bladder cancer outcomes: a cooperative group report. J Clini Oncol. 2004;22:2781–9.
4. Vale CL, Advanced Bladder Cancer (ABC) Meta-analysis Collaboration. Neoadjuvant chemotherapy in invasive bladder cancer: update of a systematic review and meta-analysis of individual patient data. Eur Urol. 2005;48:202–6.
5. Wynquist E, Kirchner TS, Segal R, Chin J, Lukka H. Neoadjuvant chemotherapy for transitional cell carcinoma of the bladder: a systematic review and meta-analysis. J Urol. 2004;171:561–9.
6. Porter MP, Kerrigan C, Donato BM, Ramsey SD. Patterns of use of systemic chemotherapy for Medicare beneficiaries with urothelial bladder cancer. Urol Oncol. 2011;29:252–8.
7. Petrelli F, Coinu A, Cabiddu M, Ghilardi M, Vavassori I, Barni S. Correlation of pathologic complete response with survival after neoadjuvant chemotherapy in bladder cancer treated with cystectomy: a meta-analysis. Eur Urol. 2013;65:350–7.
8. Rosenblatt R, Sherif A, Rintala E, Wahlqvist R, Ullen A, Nilsson S, Malstrom P-U, The Nordic Urothelial Cancer Group. Pathologic downstaging is a surrogate marker for efficacy and increased survival following neoadjuvant chemotherapy and radical cystectomy for muscle-invasive urothelial bladder cancer. Eur Urol. 2012;61:1229–38.
9. Sonpavde G, Goldman BH, Speights VO, Lerner SP, David P. Wood MD, Vogelzang NJ, Trump DL, Natale RB, Grossman HB, Crawford ED. Quality of pathologic response and surgery correlate with survival for patients with completely resected bladder cancer after neoadjuvant chemotherapy. Cancer. 2009;115:4104–9.
10. Shariat SF, Chromecki TF, Cha EK, Karakiewicz PI, Sun M, Fradet Y, Isbarn H, Scherr DS, Bastian PJ, Plummer K, Fajkovic H, Sagalowsky AI, Ashfaq R, Doblinger M, Cote RJ, Lotan Y. Risk stratification of organ confined bladder cancer after radical cystectomy using cell cycle related biomarkers. J Urol. 2012;187:457–62.
11. Raghavan D, Burgess E, Gaston KE, Haake MR, Riggs B. Neoadjuvant and adjuvant chemotherapy approaches for invasive bladder cancer. Sem Oncol. 2012;39:588–97.
12. Takata R, Katagiri T, Kanehir M, Tsunoda T, Suin T, Miki T, Namiki M, Kohri K, Atsushita Y, Fujioka T, Nakamura Y. Predicting response to methotrexate, vinblastine, doxorubicin and cisplatin neoadjuvant chemotherapy for bladder cancers through genome-wide gene expression profiling. Clin Cancer Res. 2005;11:2625.

13. Bellmut J, Pons F, Orsola A. Molecular determinants of response to cisplatin-based neoadjuvant chemotherapy. Curr Opin Urol. 2013;23(5):466–71.
14. Smith SC, Baras AS, Lee JK, Theodorescu D. The COXEN principle: translating signatures of in vivo chemosensitivity into tools for clinical outcome prediction and drug discovery in cancer. Cancer Res. 2010;70:1753–8.
15. Vale CL, Advanced Bladder Cancer (ABC) Meta-analysis Collaboration. Adjuvant chemotherapy in invasive bladder cancer: a systematic review and meta-analysis of individual patient data. Eur Urol. 2005;48:189–201.
16. Sternberg CN, Bellmunt J, Sonpavde G, Siefer-Radtke AO, Stadler WM, Bajorin DF, Dreicer R, George DJ, Milowsky MI, Thodorescu D, Vaughn DJ, Galsky MD, Soloway MS, Quinn DA. ICUD-EAU International Consultation on Bladder Cancer 2012: Chemotherapy for urothelial carcinoma—neoadjuvant and adjuvant settings. Eur Urol. 2013;63:58–66.
17. Fairey AS, Daneshmand S, Quinn D, Dorff T, Dorin R, Lieskovsky G, Schuckman A, Cai J, Miranda G, Skinner EC. Neoadjuvant chemotherapy with gemcitabine/cisplatin vs methotrexate/vinblastine/doxorubicin/cisplatin for muscle-invasive urothelial carcinoma of the bladder: a retrospective analysis from the University of Southern California. Urol Oncol. 2012;31:1737–43.
18. Volkmer BG, Kuefer R, Bartsch Jr GC, Gust K, Hautmann RE. Oncological followup after radical cystectomy for bladder cancer: Is there any benefit? J Urol. 2009;181:1587–93.
19. Stein JP, Lieskovsky G, Cote R, et al. Radical cystectomy in the treatment of invasive bladder cancer: long-term results in 1,054 patients. J Clin Oncol. 2001;19:666.
20. Sanderson KM, Stein JP, Cai J, et al. Upper tract recurrence following radical cystectomy for transitional cell carcinoma. An analysis of 1069 patients with 10-year follow-up. J Urol. 2007;177:2008–94.

Clinical Scenario: Clinical Pelvic Nodal Metastases After Complete Response to Chemotherapy

52-Year-old man with T2 N1 M0 urothelial carcinoma who undergoes platinum-based chemotherapy with complete response

Adam C. Reese and Mark Schoenberg

36.1 Introduction

Approximately 25 % of patients with muscle invasive bladder cancer will either present with metastatic disease or subsequently develop metastases later in their disease course. The prognosis of these patients is poor; however, the literature suggests that patients with regional lymph node involvement fair better than those with visceral metastases [1]. Systemic chemotherapy is the standard first-line treatment in patients presenting with lymph node metastases [2].

A.C. Reese, M.D. (✉)
Assistant Professor, Department of Urology,
Temple University School of Medicine,
3401 North Broad St., Suite 340, Philadelphia,
PA 19140, USA
e-mail: adam.reese@gmail.com

M. Schoenberg, M.D.
The Department of Urology, Albert Einstein College
of Medicine & The Montefiore Medical Center,
Medical Arts Pavilion, 5th Floor, 111 East 210th
Street, Bronx, NY 10467, USA
e-mail: mschoenb@montefiore.org;
mark.schoenberg@einstein.yu.edu

Traditionally, a chemotherapy regimen of methotrexate, vinblastine, doxorubicin, and cisplatin (MVAC) has been used in these patients. More recently, however, studies have shown a cisplatin-based combination to have comparable efficacy but with less toxicity, and thus this has become the preferred regimen in medically fit patients [3].

Response to chemotherapy in individual patients is variable and difficult to predict. Studies of patients with locally advanced or lymph-node positive bladder cancer at presentation suggest that approximately 30 % of patients will have a complete clinical response to chemotherapy, 50–60 % will have a partial response, and roughly 15 % will have no response or will progress through chemotherapy [4, 5]. However, these clinical response rates are based on changes in size of metastatic deposits on imaging studies [6], and are notoriously inaccurate when correlated with pathological response rates after radical cystectomy. For example, in a study of 152 patients with locally advanced or lymph node-positive bladder cancer, 37.5 % of patients with a complete clinical response to chemotherapy were ultimately found to have residual disease after radical cystectomy [4].

B.R. Konety and S.S. Chang (eds.), *Management of Bladder Cancer:*
A Comprehensive Text With Clinical Scenarios, DOI 10.1007/978-1-4939-1881-2_36,
© Springer Science+Business Media New York 2015

36.2 Assessing Response to Chemotherapy

This failure to identify persistent disease after the completion of systemic chemotherapy underscores the limitations of contemporary imaging modalities. Response to chemotherapy, as defined by the RECIST criteria [6], is determined by a decrease in size of suspicious lymph nodes to <10 mm in the short axis on computed tomography (CT) or magnetic resonance imaging (MRI) (Fig. 36.1). However, this definition fails to identify lymph nodes that decrease in size but harbor persistent micrometastatic disease after the completion of chemotherapy, resulting in a substantial false-negative rate. In fact, studies have suggested that approximately 20 % of lymph node metastases are not visible on conventional CT scans [7]. Furthermore, enlarged lymph nodes on CT or MRI are often reactive, and do not harbor viable tumor when removed surgically [8]. Thus, there is a significant risk of false-positive, as well as false-negative, findings when using conventional imaging modalities to identify lymph node metastases.

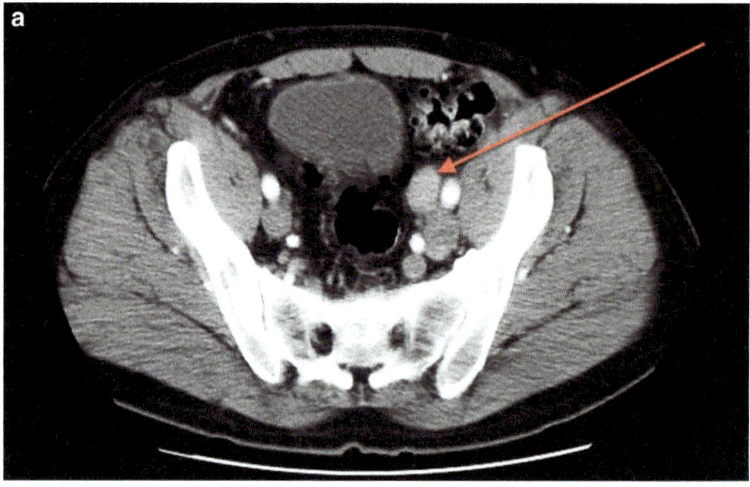

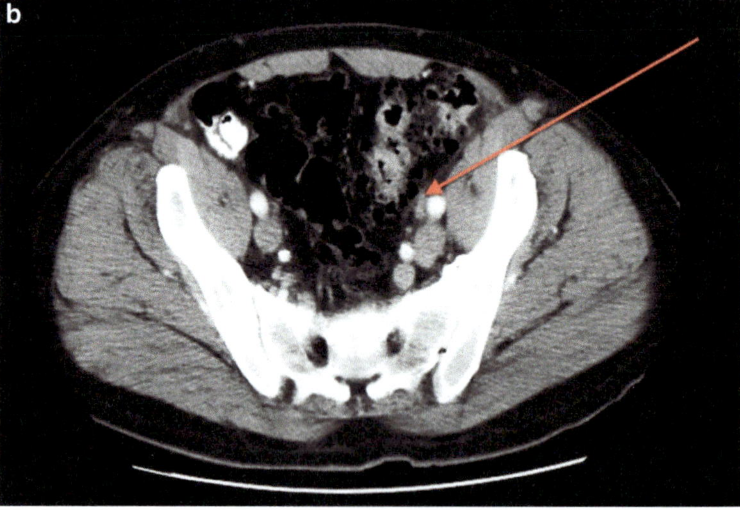

Fig. 36.1 A 64-year-old man with urothelial carcinoma of the bladder. (**a**) Computed tomography of the abdomen and pelvis at the time of diagnosis (on *left*) shows a 2.7×1.7 cm enhancing left external iliac lymph node (*red arrow*). (**b**) Cross-sectional imaging performed after chemotherapy (on *right*) shows resolution of this lymph node

Because of the poor performance of CT and MRI in identifying nodal metastases, investigators have attempted to identify new imaging modalities to better discriminate positive from negative lymph nodes. One such imaging modality is fast dynamic contrast-enhanced MRI, which is capable of measuring tumor neovascularization due to increased uptake of contrast agent in tumors. This technique has shown promise in assessing response to chemotherapy. A prospective study of 40 patients with N1–N2 TCC of the bladder treated with chemotherapy followed by consolidative cystectomy compared fast dynamic contrast-enhanced MRI to conventional MRI in predicting response to chemotherapy [9]. After the second cycle of chemotherapy, fast dynamic contrast-enhanced MRI correctly identified 20/21 patients with a pathological response to chemo, and 13/15 with no response. In comparison, conventional MRI only identified 18/25 responders and 7/11 non-responders.

Positron emission tomography (PET) is another technique that hypothetically should offer additional discriminative ability beyond that of CT or MRI. Traditional PET uses FDG, an analog of glucose, which is preferentially taken up by metabolically active tissues such as tumor metastases. PET, when combined with CT, may allow for detection of micrometastatic disease in lymph nodes that do not reach traditional size criteria for metastases. However, most studies of FDG PET/CT in detecting bladder cancer lymph node metastases have been disappointing. Two studies performed PET/CT prior to radical cystectomy and determined the accuracy of this imaging modality in detecting lymph node metastases, using final pathology as the gold standard. These studies concluded that PET/CT offered no greater discriminative ability than conventional CT or MRI alone [10, 11]. Other studies have shown a marginal increase in accuracy with PET/CT relative to CT alone [12]. Even studies that reported PET/CT to be more accurate that CT alone have reported that up to 30 % of lymph node metastases were not detected by preoperative PET/CT [13].

36.3 Likelihood of Residual Disease Following Chemotherapy

A complete radiographic response in a patient receiving chemotherapy for regional lymph node involvement is a favorable sign, however it does not definitively rule out the possibility of persistent micrometastatic disease in regional lymph nodes. What is the likelihood of persistent malignancy in the setting of a complete radiographic response? This question is difficult to answer given a paucity of literature on patients with regional lymph node involvement treated with chemotherapy followed by cystectomy. One can potentially extrapolate from the neoadjuvant chemotherapy studies of node negative patients, for which there is higher quality data, in an attempt to answer this question. These situations are not completely analogous, however, as the chemotherapeutic response of disease in the bladder is potentially different than that of regional lymph nodes.

The Southwest Oncology Group (SWOG) trial 8710 was the first study to show a survival benefit for neoadjuvant chemotherapy followed by radical cystectomy [14]. This trial randomized 317 patients with clinical T2N0M0 to T4aN0M0 bladder cancer to neoadjuvant chemotherapy followed by radical cystectomy vs. cystectomy alone. Of the 154 patients randomized to the neoadjuvant chemotherapy arm, 46 (30 %) had pathological T0 disease after radical cystectomy, 22 (14 %) had <T2 disease (Ta, T1, TIS), and the remaining 86 (56 %) had persistent or progressive tumors [15]. Not surprisingly, patients with stable or progressive disease despite chemotherapy had markedly inferior survival compared to pT0 patients, while patients with persistent <T2 disease had intermediate outcomes.

Which patients are likely to benefit from consolidative cystectomy after neoadjuvant chemotherapy? Most would argue that cystectomy for patients rendered pT0 after neoadjuvant chemotherapy likely represents overtreatment, and bladder preservation protocols may be appropriate in these patients. However, studies have reported 5- and 10-year survival rates for pT0 patients of only 92 and 86 %, respectively, arguing that not all pT0 patients are truly free of disease [16]. Patients with persistent, but not progressive, disease after neoadjuvant chemotherapy are those who are most likely to benefit from consolidative surgery. Unfortunately, it is difficult to accurately stage patients prior to radical cystectomy [17], and thus identifying these patients prior to surgery is often not possible. Finally, patients with progressive disease despite chemotherapy are thought to have chemotherapy-resistant tumors and have markedly inferior survival despite radical cystectomy [18]. Whether the marginal benefit offered by surgery for these aggressive tumors justifies the morbidity of radical cystectomy remains in question.

36.4 Response to Chemotherapy in Patients with Nodal Metastases

Interestingly, data from Memorial Sloan Kettering Cancer Center suggest that the response to chemotherapy of pelvic lymph node metastases may differ from the response of the primary bladder tumor. Kaag et al. studied patients found to be pT0 at the time of radical cystectomy, and compared two patient groups based on their clinical presentation: (1) patients with localized, resectable disease receiving neoadjuvant chemotherapy (clinical stage <T4aN0); and (2) patients with locally extensive unresectable disease or pelvic lymph node metastases (clinical stage T4bN0, or N+) [19]. The authors found that no patients rendered pT0 after receiving neoadjuvant chemotherapy for clinically localized tumors had pathological lymph node involvement. In contrast, 35 % of patients with locally extensive disease or pelvic lymph node metastases at presentation had pathological lymph node involvement despite the absence of disease in the bladder (pT0). These data suggest that pelvic lymph node metastases may be less responsive to chemotherapy, and that rates of persistent disease after

chemotherapy may be higher for patients presenting with N+ disease than patients receiving neoadjuvant chemotherapy for localized tumors.

The published data investigating the optimal treatment for patients with pelvic nodal metastases are scarce, and the clinical response to chemotherapy for patients with N+ disease is less well characterized. Furthermore, the optimal management strategy following chemotherapy remains controversial. Chemotherapy alone typically elicits a favorable response in up to two-thirds of patients, however most of these patients will relapse at a median of 12 months, and median survival following relapse is only 9 months [1]. In recent years there has been a movement towards combined modality therapy using concurrent cisplatin-based chemotherapy and radiotherapy for muscle invasive bladder cancer, however the majority of these trials excluded patients with nodal metastases and thus the efficacy of this regimen in N+ patients remains unknown [20, 21]. Thus, consolidative surgery remains the best studied and most commonly employed treatment strategy following chemotherapy in patients with regional lymph node involvement. Advocates for post-chemotherapy surgery cite data showing that patients with an initial response to cisplatin-based chemotherapy alone tend to relapse at the site of original disease [1], and resecting these sites could prevent disease recurrence.

Herr et al. studied 207 patients with unresectable primary tumors or pelvic/regional nodal metastases treated with systemic chemotherapy [22]. Of these patients, 127 did not undergo surgery after chemotherapy due to disease progression, comorbidity or poor performance status, or refusal to undergo surgery. The remaining 80 patients who underwent radical cystectomy after chemotherapy were selected based on a favorable response to chemotherapy; 24 (30 %) had a complete clinical response to chemotherapy, 44 (55 %) a partial response, and 12 (15 %) had no response. After radical cystectomy, 24 (30 %) of these patients were found that have pathological T0 disease, whereas 49 (61 %) had residual cancer, and 7 (9 %) were unresectable. In patients treated with MVAC, 5-year survival for patients

Table 36.1 Studies investigating outcomes of patients with nodal metastases treated with chemotherapy +/− radical cystectomy (RC)

Author	Study population	Clinical response to chemotherapy	Pathological response after radical cystectomy	Survival
Herr et al. [22]	– 207 Patients with cT4bNxMo or cT3-T4, N2-N3 disease – 80 Underwent cystectomy after chemotherapy	– Complete response—30 % – Partial response—55 % – Stable or progressive disease—15 %	– pT0—30 % – Persistent disease—61 % – Unresectable tumor—9 %	– pT0 after RC—29 % 5-year survival – Persistent disease after RC—29 % 5-year survival – Unresectable—0 % 5-year survival
Nieuwenhuijzen et al. [5]	– 52 Patients with cN1–N3, M0 disease	– Complete response—29 % – Partial response—57 % – Stable or progressive disease—14 %	Persistent positive lymph nodes in 42 %	– Complete clinical response to chemotherapy—42 % 5-year survival – Partial clinical response to chemotherapy—19 % 5-year survival – Progressive disease—0 % 5-year survival
Meijer et al. [4]	– 152 Patients with c ≥T3 and/or ≥N1 disease	– Complete response—32 % – Partial response—52 % – Stable disease—8 % – Progressive disease—9 %	– pT0—26 % – Partial response—29 % – Stable disease—24 % – Progressive disease—11 % – Not evaluable—10 %	– pT0 after RC—74 month median survival – Partial response after RC—22-month median survival – Stable disease after RC—15-month median survival – Progressive disease after RC—10-month median survival

with pT0 disease was 41 %, compared to 29 % for patients with residual disease at the time of cystectomy. Interestingly, of the 12 patients with a major response to chemotherapy who refused surgery, only 1 (8 %) survived beyond 3 years. These findings argue that consolidative cystectomy provided a survival benefit beyond that offered by chemotherapy alone, even in the setting of a favorable response to chemotherapy (Table 36.1).

A group from the Netherlands Cancer Institute has published the most extensive experience of patients with pelvic nodal metastases treated with chemotherapy followed by radical cystectomy [4, 5]. They first published a series of 52 patients with lymph node metastases confirmed histologically, either by lymph node dissection or aspiration cytology, prior to the initiation of chemotherapy. Following chemotherapy, a complete clinical response with resolution of all visible disease was seen in 29 % of patients, a partial response in 57 %, and 14 % had progressive disease. At the time of cystectomy 19 patients underwent pelvic lymph node dissection, of whom 8 had persistent node positive disease. Patients with resolution of visible nodal metastases after chemotherapy had significantly improved survival compared to those with persistent nodal disease. All patients with persistent node positivity despite chemotherapy died within 2 years of treatment.

More recently, the same group reported on a larger series of 152 patients with locally advanced and/or lymph node positive bladder cancer treated with induction chemotherapy. Following chemotherapy, 125 patients (82 %) underwent cystectomy, 12 (8 %) received radiotherapy, and 15 (10 %) did not undergo additional treatment. Presumably due to the small number of patients who did not undergo cystectomy, the authors did not compare outcomes between these three groups. Similar to prior studies, they found that response to chemotherapy was significantly associated with survival. Patients with a complete clinical response had superior survival to those with a partial response; patients with stable or progressive disease had the worst overall survival. Likewise, patients with persistent evidence of nodal involvement following chemotherapy had markedly inferior survival compared to patients with radiographic resolution of lymph node involvement.

36.5 Conclusions

Although there are numerous unanswered questions regarding the optimal management of patients with clinically node-positive disease, several conclusions can be drawn from the literature. First, survival is poor for patients with progressive disease despite chemotherapy, and surgery does not appear improve survival compared to chemotherapy alone in this group of patients [4, 22]. Second, the response to chemotherapy is highly variable among individuals, and current imaging modalities are unable to differentiate patients with persistent micrometastatic disease from those with a complete pathological response [4]. Thus, pathological evaluation of the bladder and regional lymph nodes after radical cystectomy is the only way to accurately evaluate response to chemotherapy. In this manner, surgery is the most effective manner of staging these patients, and pathology after radical cystectomy is strongly correlated with patient prognosis.

As such, in the current scenario of a 52-year-old man with T2 No M1 urothelial carcinoma exhibiting a complete response to chemotherapy, we would recommend proceeding with radical cystectomy in the patient who is otherwise fit for surgery. We feel that either an open or robotic approach is acceptable, assuming the surgeon has sufficient technical proficiency to perform an appropriate pelvic lymphadenectomy. We would favor a non-orthotopic urinary diversion in this setting, as this patient is likely at increased risk of pelvic disease recurrence, which could interfere with neobladder function.

In this scenario, it is important to remember that the independent contribution of surgery, above and beyond that of chemotherapy, in improving survival remains unclear. Additional study is needed to clarify those patients who will benefit from radical cystectomy versus chemotherapy alone. Furthermore, the role of radiation therapy in this setting remains poorly characterized. Further research is needed to determine the optimal treatment modalities, and the correct sequencing of these modalities, in managing patients with regional lymph node metastases.

References

1. Dimopoulos MA, Finn L, Logothetis CJ. Pattern of failure and survival of patients with metastatic urothelial tumors relapsing after cis-platinum-based chemotherapy. J Urol. 1994;151:598.
2. Sternberg CN, Yagoda A, Scher HI, et al. Methotrexate, vinblastine, doxorubicin, and cisplatin for advanced transitional cell carcinoma of the urothelium. Efficacy and patterns of response and relapse. Cancer. 1989; 64:2448.
3. von der Maase H, Hansen SW, Roberts JT, et al. Gemcitabine and cisplatin versus methotrexate, vinblastine, doxorubicin, and cisplatin in advanced or metastatic bladder cancer: results of a large, randomized, multinational, multicenter, phase III study. J Clin Oncol. 2000;18:3068.
4. Meijer RP, Nieuwenhuijzen JA, Meinhardt W, et al. Response to induction chemotherapy and surgery in non-organ confined bladder cancer: a single institution experience. Eur J Surg Oncol. 2013;39:365.
5. Nieuwenhuijzen JA, Bex A, Meinhardt W, et al. Neoadjuvant methotrexate, vinblastine, doxorubicin and cisplatin for histologically proven lymph node positive bladder cancer. J Urol. 2005;174:80.
6. Eisenhauer EA, Therasse P, Bogaerts J, et al. New response evaluation criteria in solid tumours: revised RECIST guideline (version 1.1). Eur J Cancer. 2009; 45:228.
7. Paik ML, Scolieri MJ, Brown SL, et al. Limitations of computerized tomography in staging invasive bladder cancer before radical cystectomy. J Urol. 2000;163: 1693.

8. Herr HW. Routine CT scan in cystectomy patients: does it change management? Urology. 1996;47:324.

9. Schrier BP, Peters M, Barentsz JO, et al. Evaluation of chemotherapy with magnetic resonance imaging in patients with regionally metastatic or unresectable bladder cancer. Eur Urol. 2006;49:698.

10. Jensen TK, Holt P, Gerke O, et al. Preoperative lymph-node staging of invasive urothelial bladder cancer with 18F-fluorodeoxyglucose positron emission tomography/computed axial tomography and magnetic resonance imaging: correlation with histopathology. Scand J Urol Nephrol. 2011;45:122.

11. Swinnen G, Maes A, Pottel H, et al. FDG-PET/CT for the preoperative lymph node staging of invasive bladder cancer. Eur Urol. 2010;57:641.

12. Drieskens O, Oyen R, Van Poppel H, et al. FDG-PET for preoperative staging of bladder cancer. Eur J Nucl Med Mol Imaging. 2005;32:1412.

13. Kibel AS, Dehdashti F, Katz MD, et al. Prospective study of [18F]fluorodeoxyglucose positron emission tomography/computed tomography for staging of muscle-invasive bladder carcinoma. J Clin Oncol. 2009;27:4314.

14. Grossman HB, Natale RB, Tangen CM, et al. Neoadjuvant chemotherapy plus cystectomy compared with cystectomy alone for locally advanced bladder cancer. N Engl J Med. 2003;349:859.

15. Sonpavde G, Goldman BH, Speights VO, et al. Quality of pathologic response and surgery correlate with survival for patients with completely resected bladder cancer after neoadjuvant chemotherapy. Cancer. 2009;115:4104.

16. Stein JP, Lieskovsky G, Cote R, et al. Radical cystectomy in the treatment of invasive bladder cancer: long-term results in 1,054 patients. J Clin Oncol. 2001;19:666.

17. Ploeg M, Kiemeney LA, Smits GA, et al. Discrepancy between clinical staging through bimanual palpation and pathological staging after cystectomy. Urol Oncol. 2012;30:247.

18. Weight CJ, Garcia JA, Hansel DE, et al. Lack of pathologic down-staging with neoadjuvant chemotherapy for muscle-invasive urothelial carcinoma of the bladder: a contemporary series. Cancer. 2009;115:792.

19. Kaag MG, Milowsky MI, Dalbagni G, et al. Regional lymph node status in patients with bladder cancer found to be pathological stage T0 at radical cystectomy following systemic chemotherapy. BJU Int. 2011;108:E272.

20. Efstathiou JA, Spiegel DY, Shipley WU, et al. Long-term outcomes of selective bladder preservation by combined-modality therapy for invasive bladder cancer: the MGH experience. Eur Urol. 2012;61:705.

21. Rodel C, Weiss C, Sauer R. Trimodality treatment and selective organ preservation for bladder cancer. J Clin Oncol. 2006;24:5536.

22. Herr HW, Donat SM, Bajorin DF. Post-chemotherapy surgery in patients with unresectable or regionally metastatic bladder cancer. J Urol. 2001;165:811.

Amanda N. Calhoun and Kamal S. Pohar

37.1 Introduction

Muscle-invasive bladder cancer is a serious and complex disease that requires knowledgeable and expert management to achieve the best treatment outcomes. Treatment strategies for muscle-invasive bladder cancer include radical or partial cystectomy, chemotherapy, and radiotherapy, either alone or in combination.

Consensus guidelines are useful as they serve as a summary of the best available evidence that allows the clinician to more easily put evidence into practice. Consensus guidelines for muscle-invasive bladder cancer have been generated by authorities in the field and published by the National Comprehensive Cancer Network (NCCN), International Consultation of Urologic Disease (ICUD), and European Association of Urology (EAU). However, guidelines may vary from organization or location and guidelines may have a different interpretation of the same evidence causing conflicting recommendations. In this chapter, we have reviewed and compared the clinical practice guidelines for the management of muscle-invasive bladder cancer of the NCCN, ICUD, and EAU [1–4].

37.2 Radical Cystectomy and Lymphadenectomy

Radical cystectomy is widely accepted as the gold standard treatment for muscle-invasive bladder cancer. Radical cystectomy involves removal of the bladder, prostate, seminal vesicles and distal ureters in males, as well as the entire urethra, adjacent vagina, and uterus in females [5]. In addition, a meticulous pelvic lymphadenectomy is important to accurately stage for nodal disease, improve locoregional disease control and cure a subset of patients with lymph node metastases [6].

A standard pelvic lymphadenectomy includes removal of the external iliac, obturator, and internal iliac lymph nodes. An extended lymphadenectomy also includes the removal of the common iliac and presacral lymph nodes. Accumulating evidence suggests an extended lymphadenectomy is associated with an improvement in progression-free and disease-free survival when compared to lesser templates of lymphadenectomy [7, 8]. Thus the NCCN, ICUD, and EAU recommend performing an extended lymphadenectomy at the time of radical cystectomy.

A.N. Calhoun, M.S.
Department of Urology, Ohio State University
Wexner Medical Center, 410 West 10th Avenue,
N924 Doan Hall, Columbus, OH 43210, USA
e-mail: Amanda.Calhoun@osumc.edu

K.S. Pohar, M.D., F.R.C.S.C. (✉)
Department of Urology, Ohio State University
Wexner Medical Center, 915 Olentangy River Road,
Suite 2000, Columbus, OH 43212, USA
e-mail: Kamal.Pohar@osumc.edu

B.R. Konety and S.S. Chang (eds.), *Management of Bladder Cancer:
A Comprehensive Text With Clinical Scenarios*, DOI 10.1007/978-1-4939-1881-2_37,
© Springer Science+Business Media New York 2015

It should be mentioned that the value of a well-performed lymph node dissection by an experienced surgeon is considered significant.

37.3 Timing of Cystectomy

Patients who are candidates for cystectomy should not have a delay in surgery beyond 12 weeks from the date of initial diagnosis of muscle-invasive bladder cancer. A delay in planned cystectomy can have a potential negative outcome on both the stage of disease and survival. A retrospective study of 441 patients with stage II bladder cancer from the Surveillance, Epidemiology and End Results (SEER)-Medicare database found that a delay in cystectomy greater than 12 weeks from diagnosis had a significant decrease in both disease-specific and overall survival. Specifically, patients who underwent a cystectomy 12–24 weeks after initial diagnosis were twice as likely to die of their disease when compared to patients who underwent a cystectomy 4–8 weeks after diagnosis. Those delayed 8–12 weeks had no significant change in mortality risk when compared to patients who had surgery within 4–8 weeks [9]. Importantly, it was recently demonstrated that timely delivery of cystectomy (i.e. within 12 weeks) after completing neoadjuvant chemotherapy is possible in a multidisciplinary setting with good communication among health care providers [10].

Both the EAU and the ICUD recommend definitive treatment of muscle-invasive bladder cancer within 3 months of diagnosis. The NCCN guidelines do not comment on the timing of cystectomy.

37.4 Neoadjuvant Chemotherapy

The benefit of treating micrometastatic disease early with the use of neoadjuvant chemotherapy has been investigated by several randomized trials. Meta-analyses of the benefit of neoadjuvant cisplatin-based chemotherapy has shown a 9 % improvement in disease-free and 5 % improvement in overall survival at 5 years [11]. Four of the reported trials also found that a favorable pathologic response to neoadjuvant chemotherapy (i.e. downstaging) was associated with improved overall survival [12]. MVAC (methotrexate, vinblastine, doxorubicin, and cisplatin) is considered the standard neoadjuvant chemotherapy regimen for muscle-invasive bladder cancer. There has been interest in substituting other regimens for MVAC to obtain better tolerability of therapy but none have been validated with prospective comparison trials. A retrospective study from Memorial Sloan-Kettering Cancer Center (MSKCC) demonstrated that gemcitabine and cisplatin (GC) given neoadjuvantly produced similar rates of down-staging and disease-free survival when compared to a similar cohort of patients treated with MVAC [13]. However, a report from the Cleveland clinic identified that only 2 of 20 patients treated with neoadjuvant GC achieved a pathologic complete response [14]. Importantly, there are no data that support substituting carboplatin for cisplatin in the neoadjuvant setting.

Neoadjuvant cisplatin-based combination chemotherapy for cT2-T4a bladder cancer is recommended by the NCCN, ICUD, and EAU based on level 1 evidence. The ICUD recommends M-VAC as the only neoadjuvant regimen that has proven efficacy. The ICUD also has a level 2 [15] recommendation that those with high-risk disease, such as cT3b cancers or lymph node metastasis, likely receive a more substantial benefit from neoadjuvant chemotherapy. Similarly, the NCCN recommends MVAC as the preferred neoadjuvant regimen but suggests a schedule of dose-dense (DD) administration based on category 1 evidence in unresectable or metastatic patients that demonstrated DD-MVAC to be both more effective and better tolerated than traditional MVAC [16]. However, the NCCN also recommends GC as an acceptable alternative to DD-MVAC based on comparison trials in the locally advanced and metastatic setting [17]. The EAU recommends cisplatin-containing combination chemotherapy without specifying a particular regimen. Neoadjuvant chemotherapy is not recommended by any of the guidelines if cisplatin cannot be safely administered.

37.5 Adjuvant Chemotherapy

Currently, there is not enough evidence to support the routine use of adjuvant chemotherapy. The adjuvant chemotherapy trials for muscle-invasive bladder cancer have suffered from poor accrual and/or early closure [18]. Also there are practical benefits to neoadjuvant as opposed to adjuvant chemotherapy. The benefits include an ability to objectively assess response of the primary tumor and better tolerance of chemotherapy given the relatively high rate of post-cystectomy complications that often delay starting adjuvant chemotherapy in a timely fashion [19]. Despite this neoadjuvant chemotherapy is underutilized prior to radical cystectomy and clinicians are often faced with a patient at high risk of disease relapse following radical cystectomy [20]. A recent retrospective analysis suggested that patients with $\geq$pT3 disease or nodal involvement benefited most from adjuvant chemotherapy [21]. Studies are currently underway to determine if patients who did not receive neoadjuvant chemotherapy may benefit from immediate adjuvant chemotherapy versus observation.

The EAU does not recommend adjuvant therapy outside of the setting of a clinical trial. The NCCN and the ICUD recommend considering adjuvant chemotherapy only if neoadjuvant chemotherapy was not given in patients with $\geq$pT3 or node-positive disease. All guidelines recommend against using non-cisplatin-based adjuvant chemotherapy.

37.6 Histologic Variants

Urothelial carcinoma is the most common type of bladder cancer, however many other histologic types of carcinoma can occur in the bladder alone or in combination with urothelial cancer. Histologic variants of carcinoma include squamous cell carcinoma, adenocarcinoma, micropapillary, nested variant, plasmacytoid, sarcomatoid, small cell carcinoma, among others. A retrospective analysis of the Southwest Oncology Group (SWOG) 8710 neoadjuvant chemotherapy trial reported that mixed histologic tumors of the bladder with an urothelial component also benefited from neoadjuvant chemotherapy, as both pathologic downstaging of the primary tumor and improved survival were identified [22].

The NCCN recommends that mixed histologies with an urothelial component should be treated similar to pure urothelial tumors with the qualification that these cancers have the potential to be more aggressive. The ICUD has a grade C [15] recommendation that muscle-invasive urothelial carcinoma with squamous or adenocarcinomatous elements should be treated with neoadjuvant cisplatin-based combination chemotherapy prior to cystectomy. No specific comment is made about other histologic variants. The EAU states the assessment of mixed or non-urothelial histology can be helpful for treatment and prognosis but does not have any histology-specific treatment recommendations.

Treatment recommendations for pure histologic variants of urothelial cancer are often different given the more aggressive nature of the disease or lack of response to certain treatments. The NCCN recommends that pure squamous cell cancer be treated with immediate cystectomy. For unresectable tumors radiation combined with chemotherapy traditionally used for squamous cancers of other sites may be considered. Similarly, pure adenocarcinoma is best treated by radical cystectomy. The ICUD has a grade B recommendation [15] to consider immediate radical cystectomy for nested variant and micropapillary histology due to the poor prognosis associated with the histology. Each of the guidelines agree that pure small cell carcinoma of the bladder should be treated as a systemic disease with upfront neoadjuvant chemotherapy with agents specific for this histology followed by radical cystectomy or radiotherapy for definitive local treatment [23].

37.7 Bladder Preservation

While bladder preservation is not often the treatment of choice for the majority of patients with muscle-invasive bladder cancer, it can provide suitable outcomes compared to radical cystectomy in a highly selected subset of patients.

Bladder preservation can consist of partial cystectomy, radical transurethral resection (TUR), external beam radiation, chemotherapy, or a multimodality approach. Those with favorable tumor characteristics including a single organ-confined primary tumor, small tumor size and no evidence of hydronephrosis could be considered for bladder preservation. Patients who refuse cystectomy can also be considered for bladder preservation. Patients who are medically unfit because of comorbidities or poor performance status and at high risk of major complications or death following radical cystectomy should also be considered for bladder preservation treatment.

37.7.1　Partial Cystectomy

Partial cystectomy is usually only considered in a highly select group of patients with a solitary tumor in a location that allows for segmental resection with a wide margin without diffuse CIS of the bladder. A single institution report of 58 patients confirmed that most patients with invasive bladder cancer selected for a partial cystectomy were alive with an intact bladder after a mean follow-up of 33 months. Seven patients recurred with superficial bladder cancer and all were treated successfully and retained their bladder [24]. Neoadjuvant chemotherapy and a thorough pelvic lymphadenectomy are considered necessary in the overall treatment plan.

The NCCN recommends partial cystectomy in highly selected patients with tumor in a suitable location. They also recommend considering neoadjuvant cisplatin-based chemotherapy. The ICUD has a level 3 [15] recommendation that very highly selected patients with focal invasive cancers and/or cT0 or minimal residual disease after neoadjuvant chemotherapy may be candidates for bladder preservation with partial cystectomy.

37.7.2　Radical TUR Alone

TUR alone can be considered for patients with cT2N0 disease whose tumors are likely to be completely resected by TUR. However, the limited amount of data that support maximal TUR as the sole treatment for muscle-invasive bladder cancer are observational, non-randomized, and uncontrolled [2]. A non-randomized prospective study of 151 patients with muscle-invasive bladder cancer who were downstaged to $\leq$pT1 on repeat TUR were treated by either TUR alone (surveillance) or radical cystectomy. In this study, the 99 patients treated with TUR alone had a comparable 10-year disease-specific survival when compared with the 52 patients treated with immediate cystectomy. At last follow-up 57 % of patients treated with TUR alone were alive with an intact bladder [25]. Further analysis determined that patients with organ-confined, unifocal and smaller tumors ($<$5 cm) and without evidence of hydronephrosis were less likely to recur after radical TUR alone. Repeat resection of the primary tumor to document pT0 stage is important for prognosis [26].

The NCCN recommends TURBT alone be considered for those with extensive comorbidities or poor performance status. The EAU does not recommend radical TURBT alone as a treatment option for most patients. The ICUD has a level 3 [15] recommendation that very highly selected patients with focal invasive cancers and cT0 or minimal residual disease after neoadjuvant chemotherapy may be candidates for bladder preservation with TUR.

37.7.3　Maximal TUR Followed by Chemoradiation

Multimodality bladder preservation therapy for selected patients would optimally include maximal TUR followed by concurrent chemoradiation. Combined chemoradiation has been shown to be superior to radiation alone in two randomized trials [27, 28]. Radiosensitizing chemotherapy has traditionally utilized the combination of cisplatin and 5-fluorouracil. However, even patients with poor renal function benefit from concurrent chemoradiation, as the combination of mitomycin C and 5-fluorouracil improves locoregional control when compared to radiation [28]. Follow-up after bladder preservation should include routine cystoscopy and immediate cystectomy for non-responders or evidence of high-risk recurrent disease [2].

The NCCN has a category 2B recommendation [15] for multimodality therapy with maximal TUR followed by concurrent chemoradiation if one is considering bladder preservation. The EAU recommends that the decision regarding radical cystectomy versus a bladder sparing approach be made based on the tumor stage and patient comorbidity that is best measured by a validated score, such as the Charlson Comorbidity Index [29]. The ICUD feels that bladder-preserving therapy is a valid alternative to radical cystectomy in selected patients [2].

37.8 Long-Term Follow-Up

It is not uncommon following treatment for muscle-invasive bladder cancer that patients relapse with disseminated metastases or recur locally in the true pelvis. Higher tumor stage (i.e. $\geq$pT3) and the presence of lymph node metastasis predict for a high risk of recurrent disease as does a positive soft tissue surgical margin [30].

Following cystectomy or bladder preservation for muscle-invasive bladder cancer, the NCCN recommends urine cytology, liver function tests, creatinine, and electrolytes every 3–6 months for 2 years and then as clinically indicated. Imaging of the chest, abdomen, and pelvis is recommended every 3–6 months for 2 years based on the risk of recurrence and then as clinically indicated. The ICUD and EAU recommend that surveillance for disease recurrence should be based on patient risk (i.e. pT and pN stage), and how long it has been since treatment was completed.

Some patients are also more likely to develop a new primary urothelial upper tract or urethral recurrence. A retrospective study of 1,420 patients who underwent radical cystectomy found that upper tract recurrence occurred in 0.8 % of patients with zero risk factors, versus 13.5 % in those with three to four risk factors [31]. Risk factors included a history of carcinoma in situ, tumor multifocality, cystectomy for non-muscle-invasive bladder cancer and a positive ureteral or urethral margin in the cystectomy specimen. The risk of urethral recurrence is low in men and women, however some recommend routine surveillance with urethral washings of the non-functional urethra and urine cytology in the setting of an orthotopic neobladder.

The NCCN recommends imaging of the upper tracts every 3–6 months for 2 years based on the risk of recurrence and then as clinically indicated. Annual urine cytology is also recommended. In addition, the NCCN recommends urethral wash cytology every 6–12 months, particularly if stromal invasion of the prostate or CIS was identified in the bladder or prostatic urethra. The ICUD recommends upper tract surveillance with imaging only in patients who are at high risk for upper tract tumors or those with symptoms. The ICUD does not recommend routine urethral washings or urine cytology in asymptomatic patients as there is no known survival benefit. The EAU recommendation is similar to that of the ICUD, however it is suggested that males at high risk of urethral recurrence (i.e. prostate involvement) should be monitored by urethral wash cytology as a survival advantage may be present if the tumor is diagnosed before it becomes symptomatic.

37.9 Conclusion

Muscle-invasive bladder cancer is a complex disease that requires dedicated and often multidisciplinary management. It is imperative that clinicians are well-informed of the most recent practice guidelines in the care of muscle-invasive bladder cancer to ensure optimum delivery of care. Guidelines should be updated continuously to reflect the most current advances in practice. As such, clinicians should familiarize themselves with the content of the guidelines and be aware of practice updates.

References

1. National Comprehensive Cancer Network Clinical Practice Guidelines in Oncology. Bladder Cancer (Version 1.2013) [cited September 25, 2013]. Available from: http://www.nccn.org/professionals/physician_gls/pdf/bladder.pdf

2. Gakis G, Efstathiou J, Lerner SP, Cookson MS, Keegan KA, Khurshid AG, et al. ICUD-EAU International Consultation on Bladder Cancer 2012: radical cystectomy and bladder preservation for muscle-invasive urothelial carcinoma of the bladder. Eur Urol. 2013;63:45–57.

3. Sternberg CN, Bellmunt J, Sonpavde G, Siefker-Radtke AO, Stadler WM, Bajorin DF, et al. ICUD-EAU International Consultation on Bladder Cancer 2012: chemotherapy for urothelial carcinoma—neoadjuvant and adjuvant settings. Eur Urol. 2013;63:58–66.

4. Witjies JA, Compérat E, Cowan NC, De Santis M, Gakis G, Lebret T, et al. European Association of Urology Guidelines on Muscle-invasive and Metastatic Bladder Cancer [cited September 25, 2013]. Available from: http://www.uroweb.org/gls/pdf/07_Bladder%20Cancer_LRV2.pdf

5. Stenzl A, Nagele U, Kuczyk M, Sievert KD, Anastasiadis A, Seibold J, et al. Cystectomy—technical considerations in male and female patients. Eur Urol Suppl. 2005;3:138–46.

6. Herr HW, Faulkner JR, Grossman HB, Natale RB, deVere White R, Sarosdy MF, et al. Surgical factors influence bladder cancer outcomes: a cooperative group report. J Clin Oncol. 2004;22:2781–9.

7. Dhar NB, Klein EA, Reuther AM, Thalmann GN, Madersbacher S, Studer UE. Outcome after radical cystectomy with limited or extended pelvic lymph node dissection. J Urol. 2008;179:873–8.

8. Abol-Enein H, Tilki D, Mosbah A, El-Baz M, Shokeir A, Nabeeh A, et al. Does the extent of lymphadenectomy in radical cystectomy for bladder cancer influence disease-free survival? A prospective single-center study. Eur Urol. 2011;60:572–7.

9. Gore JL, Lia J, Setodji CM, Litwin MS, Saigal CS. Mortality increases when radical cystectomy is delayed more than 12 weeks: results from a Surveillance, Epidemiology, and End Results-Medicare Analysis. Cancer. 2009;115(5):988–96.

10. Alva AS, Tallman CT, He C, Hussain MH, Hafez K, Montie JE, et al. Efficient delivery of radical cystectomy after neoadjuvant chemotherapy for muscle-invasive bladder cancer. Cancer. 2012;118:44–53.

11. Advanced Bladder Cancer (ABC) Meta-analysis Collaboration. Neoadjuvant chemotherapy in invasive bladder cancer: update of a systematic review and meta-analysis of individual patient data. Eur Urol. 2005;48:202–6. discussion 205–6.

12. Winquist E, Kirchner TS, Segal R, Chin J, Lukka H. Neoadjuvant chemotherapy for transitional cell carcinoma of the bladder: a systematic review and meta-analysis. J Urol. 2004;171:561–9.

13. Dash A, Pettus JA, Herr HW, Bochner BH, Dalbagni G, Donat SM, et al. A role for neoadjuvant gemcitabine plus cisplatin in muscle-invasive urothelial carcinoma of the bladder: a retrospective experience. Cancer. 2008;113:2471–7.

14. Weight CJ, Garcia JA, Hansel DE, Fergany AF, Campbell SC, Gong MC, et al. Lack of pathologic down-staging with neoadjuvant chemotherapy for muscle-invasive urothelial carcinoma of the bladder: a contemporary series. Cancer. 2009;115:792–9.

15. Oxford Centre for Evidence-based Medicine Levels of Evidence (May 2009). Produced by Bob Phillips, Chris Ball, Dave Sackett, Doug Badenoch, Sharon Straus, Brian Haynes, Martin Dawes since November 1998. Updated by Jeremy Howick March 2009. http://www.cebm.net/index.aspx?o=1025. Accessed Jan 2014)

16. Sternberg CN, de Mulder P, Schornagel JH, Theodore C, Fossa SD, van Oosterom AT, et al. Seven year update of an EORTC phase III trial of high-dose intensity M-VAC chemotherapy and G-CSF versus classic M-VAC in advanced urothelial tract tumors. Eur J Cancer. 2006;42:50–4.

17. Von der Maase H, Sengelov L, Roberts JT, Ricci S, Dogliotti L, Oliver T, et al. Long-term survival results of a randomized trial comparing gemcitabine plus cisplatin, with methotrexate, vinblastine, doxorubicin, plus cisplatin in patients with bladder cancer. J Clin Oncol. 2005;23:4602–8.

18. Advanced Bladder Cancer Meta-analysis Collaboration. Adjuvant chemotherapy for invasive bladder cancer (individual patient data). Cochrane Database Sys Rev 2006:CD006018.

19. Donat SM, Shabsigh A, Savage C, Cronin AM, Bochner BH, Dalbagni G, et al. Potential impact of postoperative early complications on the timing of adjuvant chemotherapy in patients undergoing radical cystectomy: a high-volume tertiary cancer center experience. Eur Urol. 2009;55:177–86.

20. Meeks JJ, Joaquim B, Bochner BH, Clarke NW, Daneshmand S, Galsky MD, et al. A systematic review of neoadjuvant and adjuvant chemotherapy for muscle-invasive bladder cancer. Eur Urol. 2012;62:523–33.

21. Svatek RS, Shariat SF, Lasky RE, Skinner EC, Novara G, Lerner SP, et al. The effectiveness of off-protocol adjuvant chemotherapy for patients with urothelial carcinoma of the bladder. Clin Cancer Res. 2010;16:4461–7.

22. Scosyrev E, Ely BW, Messing EM, Speights VO, Grossman HB, Wood DP, et al. Do mixed histological features affect survival benefit from neoadjuvant platinum-based combination therapy in patients with locally advanced bladder cancer? A secondary analysis of Southwest Oncology Group-Directed Intergroup Study (S8710). BJU Int. 2011;108(5):693–9.

23. Lynch SP, Shen Y, Kamat A, Grossman HB, Shah JB, Millikan RE, et al. Neoadjuvant chemotherapy in small cell urothelial cancer improves pathologic downstaging and long-term outcomes: results from a retrospective study at the MD Anderson Cancer Center. Eur Urol. 2013;64(2):307–13.

24. Holzbeierlein JM, Lopez-Corona E, Bochner BH, Herr HW, Donat SM, Russo P, et al. Partial cystectomy: a contemporary review of the Memorial Sloan-Kettering Cancer Center experience and recommendations for patient selection. J Urol. 2004;172:878–81.

25. Herr HW. Transurethral resection of muscle-invasive bladder cancer: 10-year outcome. J Clin Oncol. 2001;19:89–93.

26. Solsona E, Iborra I, Ricos JV, Monros JL, Casanova J, Calabuig C. Feasibility of transurethral resection for muscle invasive infiltrating carcinoma of the bladder: long term follow up of a prospective study. J Urol. 1998;159:95–8.

27. Coppin CM, Gospodarowicz MK, James K, Tannock IF, Zee B, Carson J, et al. Improved local control of invasive bladder cancer by concurrent cisplatin and preoperative or definitive radiation. The National Cancer Institute of Canada Clinical Trials Group. J Clin Oncol. 1996;14:2901–7.

28. James JD, Hussain SA, Hall E, Jenkins P, Tremlett J, Rawlings C, et al. Radiotherapy with or without chemotherapy in muscle-invasive bladder cancer. N Engl J Med. 2012;366:1477–88.

29. Charlson ME, Pompei P, Ales KL, MacKenzie CR. A new method of classifying prognostic comorbidity in longitudinal studies: development and validation. J Chronic Dis. 1987;40(5):373–83.

30. Ghoneim MA, Abdel-Latif M, El-Mekresh M, Abol-Enein H, Mosbah A, Ashamallah A, et al. Radical cystectomy for carcinoma of the bladder: 2,720 consecutive cases 5 years later. J Urol. 2008;180(1): 121–7.

31. Volkmer BG, Schnoeller T, Kuefer R, Gust K, Finter F, Hautmann RE. Upper urinary tract recurrence after radical cystectomy for bladder cancer—who is at risk? J Urol. 2009;182:2632–7.

Index

B.R. Konety and S.S. Chang (eds.), *Management of Bladder Cancer:*   465
A Comprehensive Text With Clinical Scenarios, DOI 10.1007/978-1-4939-1881-2,
© Springer Science+Business Media New York 2015

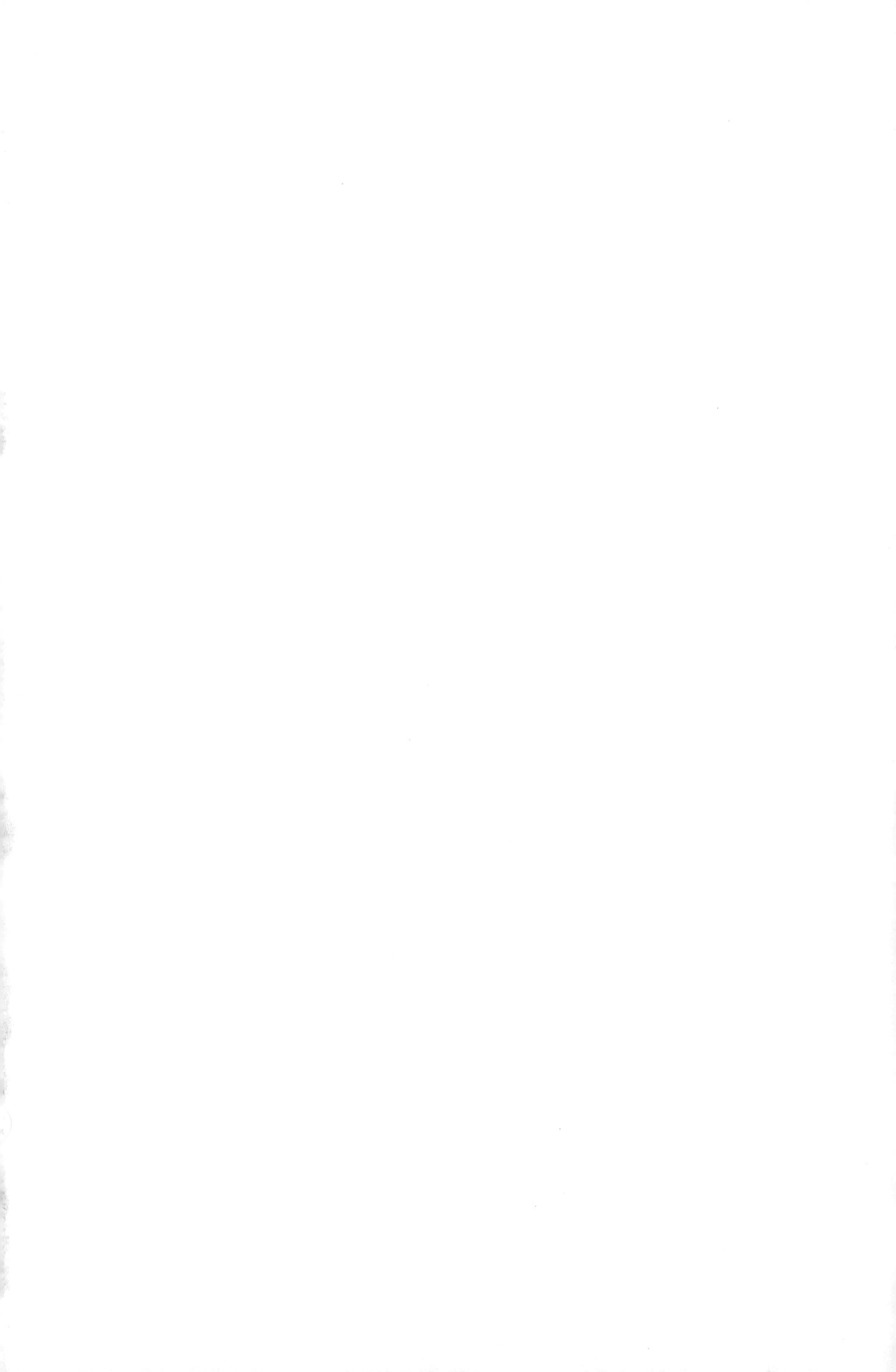